HUMAN PHYSIOLOGY

Dr Shipra Chandra

ALLIED
HEALTH
PRESS

Human Physiology

Author: **Dr Shipra Chandra**

Allied Health Press
4164 Lakeshore Road
Burlington ON L7L 1A4
Canada
www.alliedhealthpress.com
Email: orders@arclereducation.com

ISBN: 978-1-77956-213-5

ABOUT THE AUTHOR

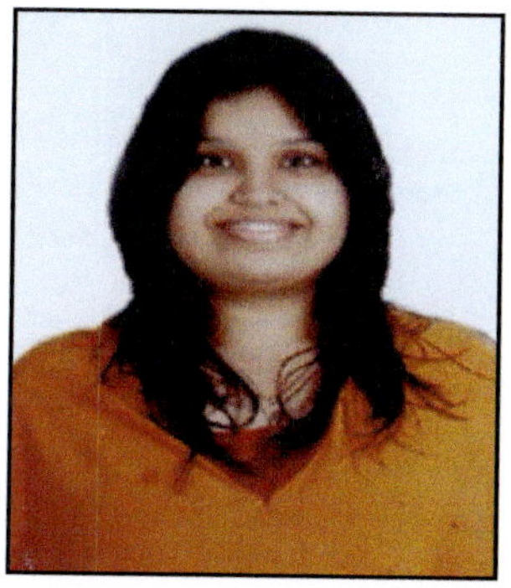

Dr. Shipra Chandra born in Delhi in 1983, completed school from a government school in Delhi in 2001 with First division. Being a science student , took admission in Chemistry Honors at Kirori Mal College, Delhi University. But the wonders of Human Body always fascinated me and I continued preparing for Pre Medical Test (PMT) despite being in a reputed college and course.

By the Grace of God and blessings of my family I secured 5th rank in CPMT 2002 along-with being waitlisted at DPMT and securing rank in AIEEE exam. Joined MBBS on 14/11/2002 at the most prestigious King George Medical College, Lucknow, U.P. Completed MBBS in First division in 2008 and joined AIIMS, New Delhi Department of Emergency Medicine for work experience in 2009 but continued the preparation for Post Graduation Entrance Test and cracked the UP-PGME in 2010 and was allotted MD Physiology from King George Medical University. After completing the MD in 2013, I again cleared AIIMS, New Delhi entrance test for Senior Residency. Learned a lot during my 3 year tenure from 2013 to 2016 at AIIMS. Following which I joined Fortis Hospital Shalimar Bagh and continued search for a Government Job. Gave the interview at U.P. Public Service Commission in 2017, cracked it and joined as Assistant Professor at Sarojini Naidu Medical College, Agra in 2017. I have 7 research publications , one book chapter and guided 3 MD students during my tenure . Promoted to the post of Associate Professor in 2022 and currently working in the same capacity.

Word Roots, Prefixes, and Suffixes by Chapter

Chapter 1 Introduction to Physiology: The Cell and General Physiology

a-, an atypical, anoxia

ab- abduction

ad- adduction

ante- antepartum

anti- antipsychotic

Chapter 2 Body Tissues

Adipo-: Fat

Chondr-: Cartilage

-cyt: Cell

Epi-: Upon, after, in addition

-glia: Glue

Chapter 3 The Integumentary System

Aden/o Gland

Adip/o Fat

Albin/o White

Aut/o Self

Bi/o Life

Chapter 4 Nervous System

Algesi/o Excessive sensitivity to pain

Cephal/o Head

Cerebell/o Cerebellum

Cerebr/o Brain, cerebrum

Crani/o Cranium (skull)

Dur/o Dura mater

Chapter 5 Cardiovascular System

myocarditis muscle layer of heart inflamed

pericarditis outer layer of heart inflamed

endocarditis inner layer of heart inflamed

cardiologist a physician specializing in the heart

cardiomyopathy damage to heart muscle layer

Chapter 6 Human Skeletal System

Lamin/o Lamina (part of the vertebral arch)

Lord/oCurve or swayback (lordosis: anterior curvature in lumbar spine)

Lumb/o Lower back, lumbar region

Myel/o Bone marrow

Chapter 7 Immune System Physiology

splen(o)- spleen Splenomegaly = enlargement of the spleen

thym(o)- thymus Thymectomy = surgical removal of the thymus

tox(o)- poison

Chapter 8 Human Reproductive System

Bartholin/o: Bartholin gland

Cervic/o: Cervix

Chori/o: Chorion

Colp/o: Vagina

Culd/o: Cul-de-sac

Chapter 9 Human Musculature System

myo Muscles

scapula Shoulder

brachi or brachio Arm

carp or carpo Wrist

cost or costo Rib

Chapter 10 Renal System

cyst/o urinary bladder cystitis

nephr/o kidney nephrectomy

pyel/o renal pelvis pyeloplasty

ren/o kidney renal

Table of Contents

2 Body Tissues 53

3 The Integumentary System 89

4 Nervous System 117

5 Cardiovascular System 145

6 Human Skeletal System 179

7 Immune System Physiology 203

8 Human Reproductive System 239

9 Human Musculature System 291

10 Renal System 321

LIST OF FIGURES

LIST OF TABLES

PREFACE

Human physiology is a cornerstone of medical knowledge, contributing to our understanding of health, disease, and the complexities of human biology. This field encompasses the study of various systems within the body, including the circulatory, respiratory, nervous, and digestive systems, among others. It investigates how these systems interact to maintain homeostasis, enabling the body to respond to internal and external changes.

Recent research and innovations in human physiology have led to groundbreaking discoveries that not only enhance our understanding of the human body but also pave the way for novel treatments and technologies. Researchers have begun to elucidate the profound impact of microorganisms in our bodies on health and disease. Studies have shown that the gut microbiome, in particular, plays a crucial role in digestion, immune function, and even mental health. This has led to the development of new probiotic treatments and dietary recommendations aimed at promoting a healthy microbiome balance. The field of neurophysiology, where advances in brain imaging techniques, such as functional MRI (fMRI) and electroencephalography (EEG), have revolutionized our understanding of brain function. These technologies allow scientists to observe brain activity in real-time, providing insights into how different areas of the brain interact during various tasks and under different conditions. Furthermore, the field of cardiovascular physiology has seen remarkable innovations, particularly in the development of wearable technology that monitors heart rate, blood pressure, and other vital signs. These devices provide continuous, real-time data that can be used for personalized health monitoring and early detection of cardiovascular diseases. Additionally, advancements in regenerative medicine, including stem cell therapy and tissue engineering, hold the promise of repairing or replacing damaged tissues and organs, offering new hope for patients with previously untreatable conditions.

"Human Physiology" is written with the aim of providing an in-depth and comprehensive exploration of the mechanisms and functions of the human body. Its primary goal is to facilitate a deep understanding of how various physiological systems interact and maintain homeostasis, enabling the body to function optimally in a wide range of environments. Tailored for students and professionals in the fields of medicine, biology, and health sciences, this textbook serves as a foundational resource, offering clear explanations, detailed diagrams, and up-to-date research findings. By bridging the gap between basic biological concepts and their clinical applications, the book empowers learners with the knowledge and critical thinking skills necessary to navigate the complexities of human biology and to contribute effectively to advancements in healthcare and medical research. Through this comprehensive guide, readers are encouraged to engage with the material actively, nurturing a lifelong curiosity and appreciation for the study of human physiology.

Chapter 1

INTRODUCTION TO PHYSIOLOGY: THE CELL AND GENERAL PHYSIOLOGY

Contents

Unit Introduction

Trillions of cells constitute the human body, and they all collaborate to sustain the organism as a whole. Despite each cell having a distinct function, they all possess very similar metabolic requirements. The welfare of individual cells as well as the well-being of the entire body relies on maintaining a constant internal milieu that encompasses everything the cells require to survive (oxygen, glucose, mineral ions, waste removal, etc.). The term "homeostasis" pertains to the various mechanisms that the body employs to regulate its internal environment.

The study of physiology encompasses biological processes necessary for living things to function. The fundamental idea is homeostasis, which preserves a steady internal environment despite external changes. Maintaining homeostasis ensures critical variables like pH, body temperature, and nutrient levels remain within specific ranges supporting cellular activity. Cells, the basic building blocks of life, have diverse structures and functions. From specialized neurons transmitting electrical signals to muscle cells generating mechanical force, understanding organ systems and the body requires knowledge of cellular physiology. Membrane transport, energy metabolism, signal transduction, and gene expression are important concepts. Physiologists study how cells respond to environmental changes and maintain homeostasis to learn about health, illness, and potential therapies. This overview sets the foundation for exploring the intricate details of physiology and bridging the gap between molecular mechanisms and organism function.

Orientation and Directional Terms

Term	Definition	Illustration
Homeostasis	Homeostasis is a self-regulating process that allows living organisms to maintain internal stability while adjusting to external conditions.	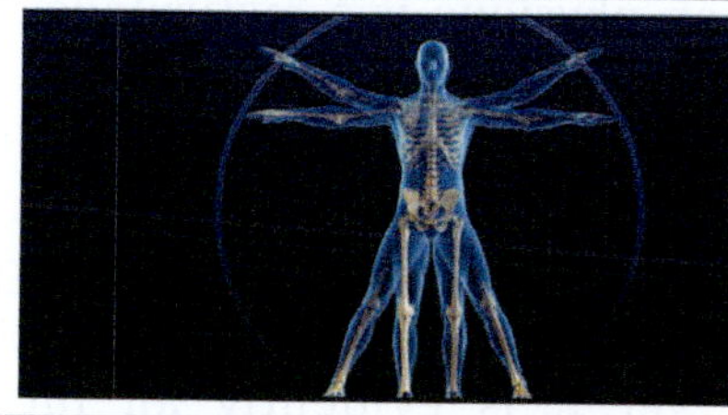
Meninges	Meninges are three membrane layers that cover and protect your brain and spinal cord.	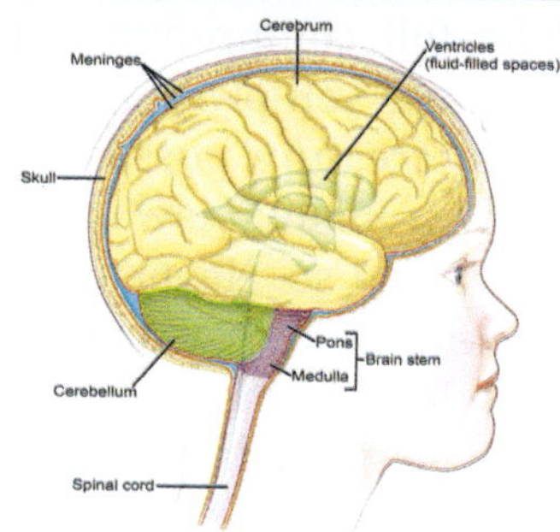
Organ system	An organ system is a group of organs that work together to perform a function in the body.	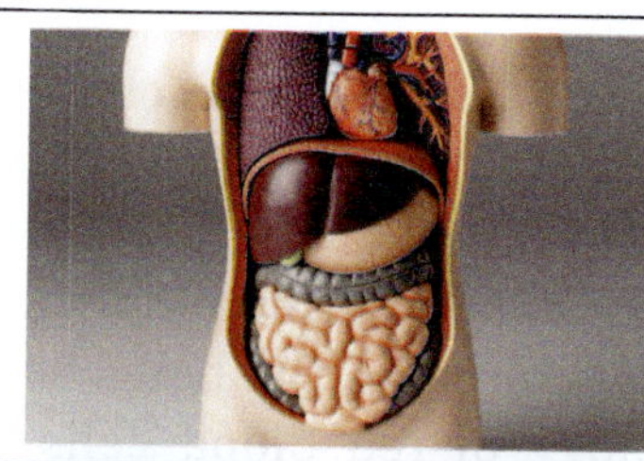
Pathophysiology	Pathophysiology is a medical science that studies the changes in regulatory mechanisms related to the development, onset, and outcome of diseases.	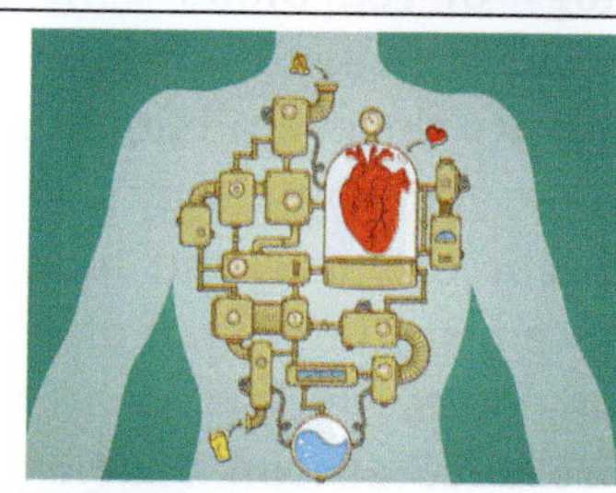
Mesentery	A mesentery is a double layer of peritoneum that attaches the vasculature and nerves to the intraperitoneal organs.	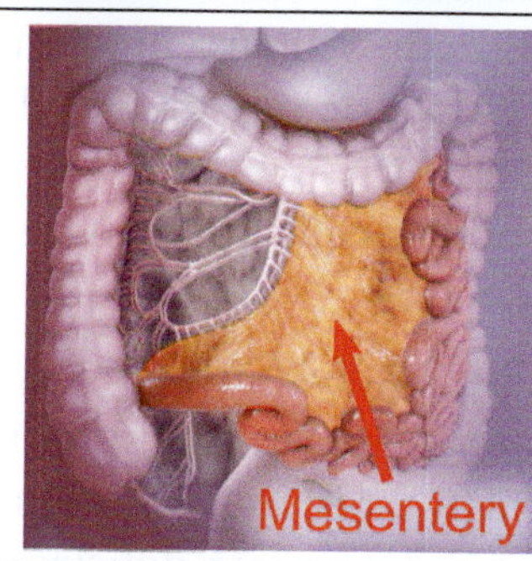

1.1. Organization and General Plan of the Body

The human physique is a meticulously crafted reactor for chemical processes. The body is comprised of trillions of cells arranged in precise manners and thousands of chemical reactions that occur in a highly organized manner. This succinctly encapsulates our essence, yet it is evidently an incomplete narrative. The full comprehension of human consciousness and self-awareness still eludes us. As no other creature possesses the ability to introspect, we remain unaware of the factors that enable us to do so. Nevertheless, we have amassed a wealth of knowledge regarding our composition and internal mechanisms. A portion of this knowledge is encompassed within the fundamental human anatomy and physiology course you are about to undertake.

The study of anatomy centers on the composition, dimensions, configuration, and conceivably even the hue of the body. The study of physiology, on the other hand, delves into the functioning of the body. For instance, the physiology of red blood cells elucidates their purpose, modus operandi, and their interrelation with the overall functioning of the body. Anatomy and physiology are intimately intertwined. For example, red blood cells are anatomically constituted by molecules of the protein hemoglobin, which contains the mineral iron. The presence of iron enables red blood cells to fulfill their primary function of oxygen transport. The physiology of red blood cells is indispensable to the overall physiology of the body, as all bodily cells necessitate oxygen for proper functioning.

The study of dysfunctions is known as pathophysiology, and understanding normal physiology facilitates understanding of these disorders. For instance, iron deficiency anemia is a type of anemia that you are probably familiar with. The symptoms of iron-deficiency disorder arise from low iron levels in the diet because low iron levels in hemoglobin, which is carried by red blood cells, reduce the amount of oxygen carried throughout the body. An illustration of the connection between anatomy, physiology, and pathophysiology is provided here.

With a focus on normal structure and function, the aim of this text is to help you understand anatomy and physiology. However, a large number of pathophysiology examples have been included to show how disease relates to normal physiology and to explain some of the techniques involved in disease diagnosis. Many of the examples are clinical applications designed to help you start putting what you've learned into practice and show how your anatomy and physiology knowledge will serve as the foundation for your future studies in the health professions.

1.1.1. Levels of Organization

The structural and functional layers of the human body are arranged in increasing complexity. As you'll see, every subsequent level builds upon the structures and features of the one before it. Starting at the most basic level – the chem level – we'll move on to discuss cells, tissues, organs, and organ systems. Figure 1.1. shows each level of organization in detail.

1.1.1.1. Chemicals

The two main types of chemicals that comprise the human body are inorganic and organic. With a few notable exceptions, inorganic chemicals are primarily simple molecules composed of one or two elements other than carbon. Water (H_2O), oxygen (O_2), carbon dioxide (CO_2), with one exception, and minerals like iron (Fe), calcium (Ca), and sodium (Na) are examples of inorganic chemicals. The elements carbon and hydrogen are always present in organic compounds, which are frequently extremely complex. Nucleic acids, proteins, fats, and carbohydrates fall under this group of organic compounds.

1.1.1.2. Cells

Cells are the smallest structurally and functionally units of living organisms. Human cells exhibit a wide range of forms, yet they possess common characteristics. Comprised of various chemicals, each type of cell carries out distinct chemical reactions.

1.1.1.3. Tissues

A tissue is a group of cells that share a common structure and function. Tissues are categorized into four groups:

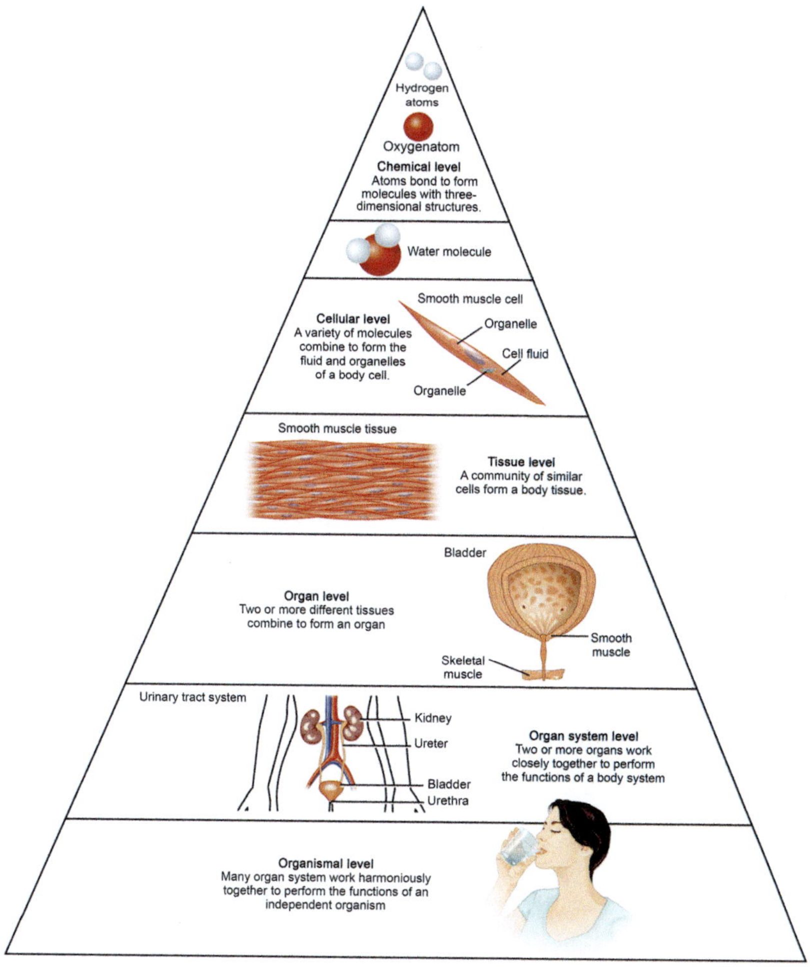

Figure 1.1. Levels of structural organization of the human body, depicted from the simplest (chemical) to the most complex (organism). The organ system shown here is the urinary system.

Source: https://courses.lumenlearning.com/suny-ap1/chapter/structural-organization-of-the-human-body/.

1. **Epithelial Tissues:** These tissues cover or line body surfaces and some have the ability to produce secretions with specific functions. Examples of epithelial tissues include the outer layer of the skin and sweat glands. Internal epithelial tissues consist of the walls of capillaries (squamous epithelium) and kidney tubules (cuboidal epithelium), as depicted in Figure 1.1.
2. **Connective Tissues:** Connect and support parts of the body, while some transport or store materials. Examples of this group include blood, bone, cartilage, and adipose tissue.
3. **Muscle Tissues:** This are specialized for contraction, which brings about movement. Examples of muscle tissue include our skeletal muscles and the heart. In Figure 1.1, you can see smooth muscle tissue, which is found in organs such as the urinary bladder and stomach.
4. **Nerve Tissue:** It is specialized to generate and transmit electrochemical impulses that regulate body functions. Examples of nerve tissue include the brain and optic nerves.

1.1.1.4. Organs

An organ is a collection of tissues that have been carefully positioned to carry out specific tasks. Examples of organs include the kidneys, individual bones, liver, lungs, and stomach. The kidneys utilize various epithelial tissues to perform their absorption function. The stomach's epithelial tissue secretes gastric juice to aid in digestion. Smooth muscle tissue in the stomach wall contracts to mix food with gastric juice and move it into the small intestine. Nerve tissue carries impulses that regulate the contraction of the stomach.

1.1.1.5. Organ Systems

An organ system is a collection of organs that collaborate to support a specific purpose. Examples include the digestive, respiratory, and urinary systems. The urinary system consists of the kidneys, ureters, bladder, and urethra. Each of these organs contributes to the production and elimination of urine.

Table 1.1 provides an overview of the organ systems and their general functions in the human body, along with a list of some representative organs. Figure 1.2 shows every organ system. Certain organs belong to more than one organ system; the diaphragm is a component of both the respiratory and muscular systems, and the pancreas is both an endocrine and a digestive organ. A person is made up of all the organ systems.

Table 1.1. *The Organ Systems*

System	Subsystem	Body Parts	Organs	Organ Parts
Musculoskeletal	Musculoskeletal	Human skeleton	Human Skeleton	List of bones of the human skeleton
		Joints	Joints	–
		Ligaments	Ligaments	–
		Muscular system	Muscles	List of skeletal muscles of the human body (sub: Muscles of breathing).
		Tendons	Tendons	Tendon#List of Tendons
Digestive	Digestive	Mouth	Teeth	–
			Tongue	–
			Lips	–
		Salivary glands	Parotid glands	–
			Submandibular glands	–
			Sublingual glands	–
		Pharynx	Pharynx	–
		Esophagus	Esophagus	–
		Stomach	Stomach	–
		Small intestine	Duodenum	–
			Jejunum	–
			Ileum	–
		Large intestine	Cecum	–
			Ascending colon	–
			Transverse colon	–
			Descending colon	–
			Sigmoid colon	–
		Rectum	Rectum	–
		Liver	Liver	–
		Gallbladder	Gallbladder	–
		Mesentery	Mesentery	–
		Pancreas	Pancreas	–
		Anal canal	Anal canal	–

Respiratory	Respiratory	Nasal cavity	Nasal cavity	–
		Pharynx	Pharynx	–
		Larynx	Larynx	–
		Trachea	Trachea	–
		Bronchi	Bronchi	–
		Bronchioles and smaller air passages	Bronchioles and smaller air passages	–
		Lungs	Lungs	–
		Muscles of breathing	Muscles of breathing	–
Urinary	Urinary	Kidneys	Kidneys	–
		Ureter	Ureter	–
		Bladder	Bladder	–
		Urethra	Urethra	–
Reproductive	Female	Ovaries	Ovaries	–
		Fallopian tubes	Fallopian tubes	–
		Uterus	Uterus	–
		Cervix	Cervix	–
		Placenta	Placenta	–
		Vulva	Vulva	–
		Clitoris	Clitoris	–
		Vagina	Vagina	–
Reproductive	Male	Testes	Testes	–
		Epididymis	Epididymis	–
		Vas deferens	Vas deferens	–
		Seminal vesicles	Seminal vesicles	–
		Prostate	Prostate	–
		Bulborethral glands	Bulborethral glands	–
		Penis	Penis	–
		Scrotum	Scrotum	–

Endocrine	Endocrine	Pituitary gland	Pituitary gland	–
		Pineal gland	Pineal gland	–
		Thyroid gland	Thyroid gland	–
		Parathyroid glands	Parathyroid glands	–
		Adrenal glands	Adrenal glands	–
		Pancreas	Pancreas	–
Circulatory	Circulatory	Heart	Heart	–
		Arteries	Arteries	–
		Veins	Veins	–
		Capillaries	Capillaries	–
	Lymphatic	Lymphatic vessel	Lymphatic vessel	–
		Lymph node	Lymph node	–
		Bone marrow	Bone marrow	–
		Thymus	Thymus	–
		Spleen	Spleen	–
		Gut-associated lymphoid tissue	Tonsils	–
		Interstitium	Interstitium	–
Nervous	(Brain +)	Brain	Cerebral hemispheres	–
			Thalamus	–
			Hypothalamus	–
			Midbrain	–
			Cerebellum	–
			Pons	–
			Medulla oblongata	–
		The spinal cord	The spinal cord	List of nerves of the human body
		Choroid plexus	Choroid plexus	–

	Peripheral nervous	Nerves	Cranial nerves	List of nerves of the human body
			Spinal nerves	List of nerves of the human body
			Ganglia	–
			Enteric nervous system	–
	Sensory organs	Eye	Cornea	–
			Iris	–
			Ciliary body	–
			Lens	–
			Retina	–
		Ear	Outer ear (Earlobe)	–
			Eardrum	–
			Middle ear (Ossicles)	–
			Cochlea	–
			Vestibule of the ear	–
			Semicircular canals	–
		Olfactory epithelium	Olfactory epithelium	–
		Tongue	Taste buds	–
Integumentary	Integumentary	Mammary glands	Mammary glands	–
		Skin	Skin	–
		Subcutaneous tissue	Subcutaneous tissue	–

Source: https://en.wikipedia.org/wiki/List_of_organs_of_the_human_body.

1.2. Metabolism and Homeostasis

All of the chemical reactions and physical processes that occur inside the body are collectively referred to as metabolism. All of the biological processes—growing, repairing, reacting, and reproducing—are included in metabolism. Among the thousands of processes involved in metabolism are the heart's pumping action, the stomach's food digestion, the diffusion of gases in the lungs and tissues, and the body's cellular energy production.

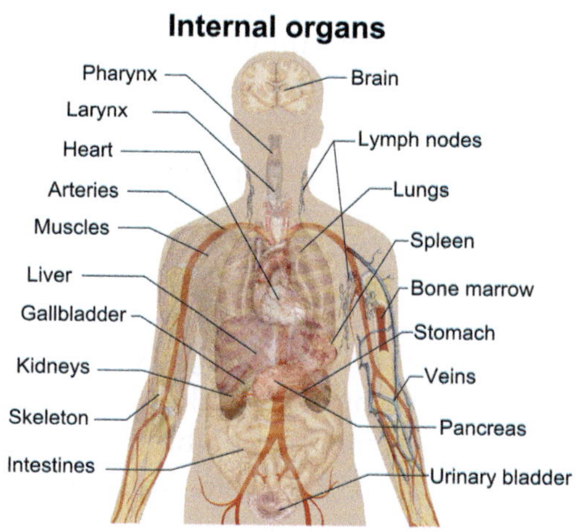

Figure 1.2. *Organ systems: Compare the depiction of each system to its description in Table 1.1.*

Source: Häggström, M., (2014). "Medical gallery of Mikael Häggström 2014." WikiJournal of Medicine, 1(2). doi: 10.15347/wjm/2014.008. ISSN 2002-4436. Public Domain.orBy Mikael Häggström, used with permission. All used images are in public domain., Public Domain, https://commons.wikimedia.org/w/index.php?curid=10709118.

The word "metabolism" is Greek for "change," and the body is constantly changing in three different ways: visibly (e.g., walking down the street), microscopic (e.g., cells dividing in the skin to produce new epidermis), and submicroscopic (e.g., RNA an d enzymes synthesizing new proteins). A related idea called metabolic rate is most commonly used to describe how quickly the body generates heat and energy, or alternatively, how much energy is produced in a given amount of time, like a day. Thus, one component of metabolism is metabolic rate. One could say that someone in good health is in a state of homeostasis. The body's capacity to sustain a steady metabolism and carry out regular functions in the face of ongoing changes is reflected in homeostasis. The body must react appropriately to any changes that occur as part of normal metabolism, whether they are internal or external.

Consuming breakfast causes a change within the body. As food enters the stomach, the body begins digesting it into simpler chemicals that can be utilized. For instance, the protein in a hard-boiled egg is broken down into amino acids, which are the essential building blocks needed by cells to create specialized proteins.

An increase in the outside temperature is an illustration of an external change. The body's temperature would also tend to rise on a hot day. To support normal functioning, however, body temperature needs to be maintained within its typical range of roughly 97° to 99°F (36° to 38°C). What happens? The body reacts to a rise in outside temperature by increasing sweating, which allows extra body heat to be released through the evaporation of sweat on the skin's surface. Dehydration, on the other hand, is an unwanted internal change that could result from this reaction. What happens is that we experience thirst and drink fluids to replace the water lost through perspiration as our body's water content decreases. Observe how certain bodily reactions always go back to the original situation that caused them. In the example above, a rising body temperature causes more sweating, which in turn causes a lower body temperature, which in turn causes a decrease in sweating. Sweating that is not necessary and would waste water is avoided. This exemplifies a negative feedback mechanism, whereby the body's reaction counteracts the stimulus (essentially shutting it off for a while) and maintains a portion of the body's metabolism within normal bounds.

Examine Figure 1.3 for a different negative feedback mechanism in which the body's metabolic rate is regulated by the hormone thyroxine. The pituitary gland and hypothalamus, two regions of the brain, detect a decrease in metabolic rate and release hormones to stimulate the thyroid gland, located just below the larynx on the front of the neck, to secrete thyroxine. Thyroxine stimulates the cellular enzyme systems responsible for converting food into energy, thereby increasing the metabolic rate. The brain and pituitary gland sense an increase in heat and energy production, subsequently reducing the release of their hormones. This prevents the release of thyroxine until the metabolic rate decreases once again. The metabolic rate fluctuates but remains within typical limits.

You may be wondering if positive feedback mechanisms actually exist. They do, but they differ significantly from negative feedback mechanisms in the body and are relatively uncommon. Positive feedback mechanisms maintain the progression of events by responding to stimuli rather than reversing or halting them. A prime example is childbirth, where the sequence of events is as follows: The posterior pituitary gland secretes oxytocin in response to stretching of the uterine cervix. Oxytocin causes the uterine muscle to contract, leading to further stretching, which triggers more oxytocin and more contractions. This cycle continues until the baby and placenta are delivered, at which point the mechanism comes to an end. This serves as the "brake," causing a pause in the process. Any positive feedback system requires an external "brake" to prevent it from becoming overactive. One example of such a mechanism is blood clotting, which can turn into a harmful cycle of excessive clotting without external controls. This can cause more harm than good. Similarly, after an injury, inflammation is initially beneficial and necessary for the healing process to begin. However, if left unchecked, it can become a destructive cycle of further damage. Another instance of positive feedback can occur with the onset of fever. For instance, bacteria can impact the hypothalamic thermostat in the body, leading to a fever. As the metabolic rate increases, body temperature rises, which further intensifies the fever, creating a self-perpetuating cycle. In this case, the inhibition or "brake" is provided by white blood cells that eliminate the bacteria causing the fever. An external disruption to the cycle is necessary. Positive feedback mechanisms are relatively rare in the body due to their potential for harm and self-perpetuation.

On the other hand, negative feedback mechanisms have built-in brakes because the body possesses numerous inhibitory pathways that are integral to the cycle. Most hormone secretion is regulated by negative feedback systems. Multiple negative feedback mechanisms are involved in the control of blood pressure and heart rate.

When all of these processes come together, the body's functioning, including metabolism, is maintained within normal bounds, creating a steady state or equilibrium. This is known as equilibrium.

You will find many more examples of homeostasis in the upcoming chapters. It is important to remember that homeostasis is facilitated by the healthy operation of every organ and system in the human body as you continue your studies. Additionally, it is important to note that the values of metabolism that we refer to as normal are frequently ranges rather than single figures. For example, the typical range for body temperature is between 97° and 99°F (36° and 38°C). Another example is the normal respiratory rate, which ranges from 12 to 20 breaths per minute, and the normal pulse rate, which ranges from 60 to 80 beats per minute. It is also important to understand that normal metabolism includes deviations from the normal range.

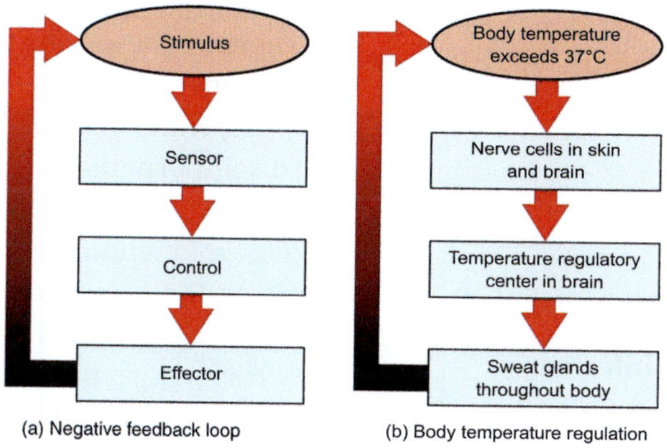

Figure 1.3. *Feedback mechanisms. (A) The negative feedback mechanism of regulation of metabolic rate. (B) The positive feedback mechanism triggered by a fever.*

Source: https://bio.libretexts.org/Bookshelves/Human_Biology/Human_Biology_%28Wakim_and_Grewal%29/10%3A_Introduction_to_the_Human_Body/10.7%3A_Homeostasis_and_Feedback

1.3. Terminology and General Plan of the Body

Throughout your anatomy and physiology course, you will encounter a plethora of unfamiliar vocabulary. At times, you may even feel as though you are delving into a second language, which is indeed the case. Each term possesses a distinct meaning that is well-known to other language learners. To effectively communicate with colleagues and potential patients, it is imperative that you attain proficiency in the language employed within your field. Despite the initial abundance of new terms, you will swiftly discover that utilizing them becomes second nature to you.

The organ systems will be discussed throughout the text, employing the terminology introduced in this chapter. This approach will serve to reinforce the definitions of these terms and transform these novel words into knowledge.

1.3.1. Body Parts and Areas

Every part is indicated in figure 1.2 and listed in Table 1.2. Figure 1.4 designates a particular bodily part or region. For instance, when we talk about the thigh, we always say "femoral." The quadriceps femoris is a sizable muscle group located in the thigh, and the femoral artery is a blood vessel that flows through it.

As in the case of pulmonary artery, pulmonary edema, and pulmonary embolism, pulmonary is another word that always refers to the lungs. Even though you might not be familiar with all of these terms right now, you are aware that they are all related to the lungs.

1.3.2. Terms of Location and Position

The body is always assumed to be in anatomic position when describing relative locations: upright, facing forward, arms at the sides, palms facing forward, feet slightly apart. Table 1.3 lists the terms of location along with definitions and examples for each. Locate the body parts that the figures provide examples for as you read each term. Observe further that each pair of terms in this list consists of a set of opposites. This will assist you in remembering the terms and their definitions.

Table 1.2. *Descriptive Terms for Body Parts and Areas*

The cranial region encompasses the upper part of the head, while the facial region encompasses the lower half of the head, starting below the ears.
The forehead is known as the frontal region.
The eyes are referred to as the orbital or ocular region.
The cheeks are referred to as the buccal region.
The ears are referred to as the auricle or otic region.
The nose is referred to as the nasal region.
The mouth is referred to as the oral region.
The chin is referred to as the mental region.
The neck is referred to as the cervical region.
The trunk of the body contains, from superior to inferior.
The thoracic region encompassing the chest
The mammary region encompasses each breast.
The sternal region encompasses the sternum.
The abdominal region encompasses the stomach area.
The umbilical region is located around the navel.
The coxal region (hip region) encompasses the lateral (side) of the hips.
The pubic region encompasses the area above the genitals.
The pelvis and legs contain, from superior to inferior.
The inguinal or groin region between the thigh and the abdomen.
The pubic region surrounding the genitals.
The femoral region encompassing the thighs.
The patellar region encompassing the front of the knee.
The crural region encompassing the lower leg, between the knee and ankle.
The fibular region encompassing the outside of the lower leg.
The tarsal region encompassing the ankle.

The pedal region encompassing the foot.

The digital/phalangeal region encompasses the toes.

The great toe is referred to as the hallux.

The regions of the upper limbs, from superior to inferior, are the axillary region encompassing the armpit.

The brachial region encompassing the upper arm.

The antecubital region encompassing the front of the elbow.

The antebrachial region encompassing the forearm.

The carpal region encompassing the wrist.

The palmar region encompassing the palm, and the digital/phalangeal region encompassing the fingers.

The thumb is referred to as the pollex.

The posterior view contains, from superior to inferior, the cervical region encompassing the neck.

The scapular region encompassing the scapulae and the area around.

The dorsal region encompassing the upper back.

The lumbar region encompassing the lower back and the sacral region occurring at the end of the spine, directly above the buttocks.

The regions of the back of the arms, from superior to inferior, include the acromial region encompassing the shoulder.

The olecranal region encompassing the back of the elbow.

The antebrachial region encompasses the forearm, front and back and the manual or manus region encompassing the back of the hand.

The posterior regions of the legs, from superior to inferior, include the gluteal region encompassing the buttocks.

The femoral region encompassing the thigh.

The popliteal region encompassing the back of the knee.

The sural region encompassing the back of the lower leg.

The calcaneal region encompassing the heel, and the plantar region encompassing the sole of the foot.

Source: https://en.wikipedia.org/wiki/List_of_human_anatomical_regions

1.3.3. Body Cavities and Their Membranes

The dorsal cavity (posterior) and the ventral cavity (anterior) are the two main cavities in the body. There are additional subdivisions within each of these cavities, as depicted in Figure 1.5.

1.3.4. Dorsal Cavity

The cranial cavity and the vertebral or spinal cavity constitute the dorsal cavity, which houses the central nervous system. The dorsal cavity is continuous, with no partitions or boundaries separating its subdivisions. The skull forms the cranial cavity, where the brain is located. The spinal cavity, composed of the spine, contains the spinal cord. The meninges are the membranes that cover the brain and spinal cord and surround these cavities.

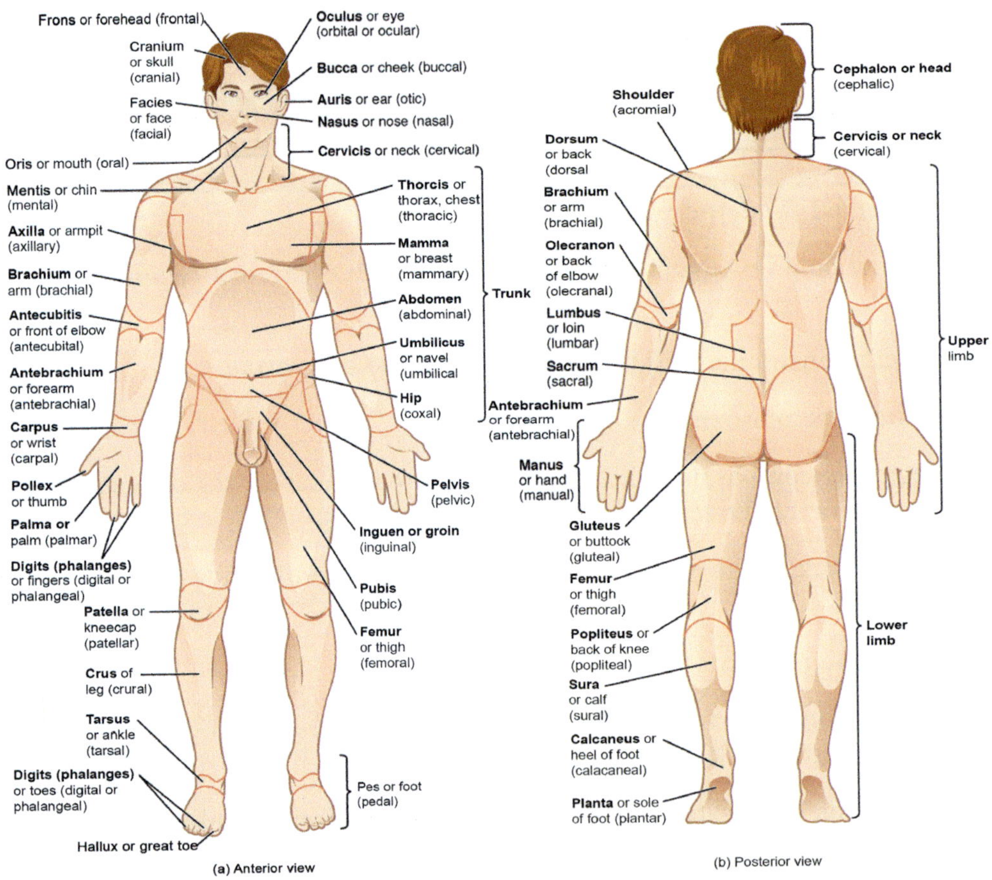

Figure 1.4. *Body parts and areas. The body is shown in anatomic position. (A) Anterior view; and (B) posterior view.*

Source: https://courses.lumenlearning.com/suny-ap1/chapter/anatomical-terminology/.

1.3.5. Ventral Cavity

The ventral cavity is divided into two compartments: the thoracic cavity and the abdominal cavity. These compartments are separated by the diaphragm, a large dome-shaped respiratory muscle.

The diaphragm contains openings for the esophagus and large blood vessels, acting as a barrier between the thoracic and abdominal cavities. The pelvic cavity can be considered a subdivision of the abdominal cavity or a separate cavity, as there is no physical wall between them.

The heart and lungs are among the organs located in the thoracic cavity. Pleural membranes are a type of serous membrane that line the thoracic cavity. The lungs are covered by the visceral pleura, while the parietal pleura lines the chest wall. The pericardial membranes are a unique set of serous membranes found in the heart. The heart muscle is covered by the visceral pericardium, while the parietal pericardium lines the fibrous pericardial sac.

he stomach, intestines, and liver are among the organs located within the abdominal cavity. The peritoneum and mesentery are two additional serous membranes that are found in the abdominal cavity. The membrane that covers the outside surfaces of the abdominal organs is called the mesentery, and it continues the peritoneum, which lines the entire abdominal wall.

The abdominal cavity is superior to the pelvic cavity. The peritoneum covers the free surfaces of several pelvic organs, but it does not actually line the pelvic cavity. The female uterus and the male prostate gland are reproductive organs that are located in the pelvic cavity, along with the bladder.

Table 1.3. *Terms of Location and Position*

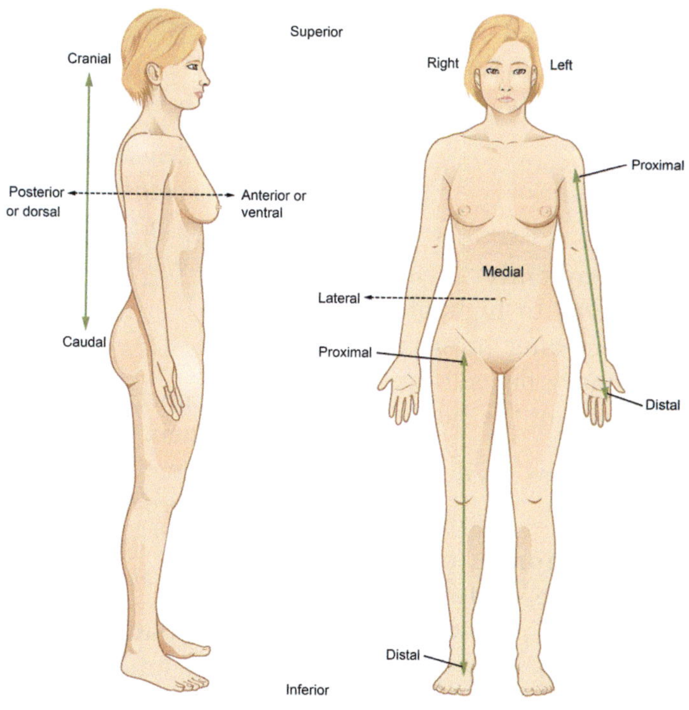

Source: https://courses.lumenlearning.com/suny-ap1/chapter/anatomical-terminology/.

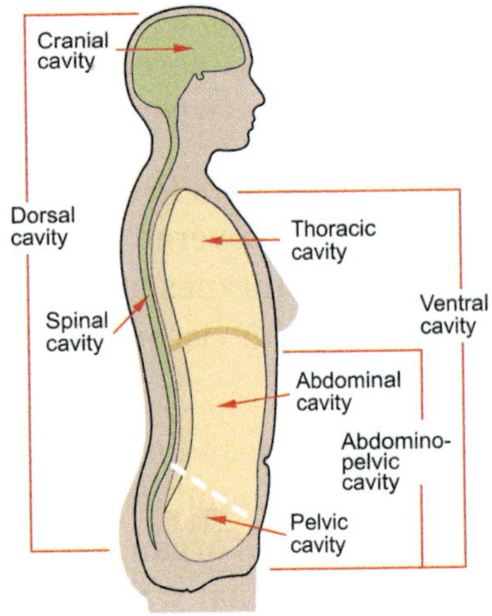

Figure 1.5. *Body cavities (lateral view from the left side).*

Source: By Vectorization: Mysid in Inkscape, based on http://training.seer.cancer.gov/module_anatomy/unit1_3_terminology3_cavities.html. Image renamed from File:Body cavities.svg (SVG), Public Domain, https://commons.wikimedia.org/w/index.php?curid=5678872.

1.3.6. Planes and Sections

The body or an organ is frequently sliced or sectioned in a particular way to highlight specific structures when describing internal anatomy. A plane is an imaginary flat surface that divides two organs or parts of the body.

These planes and sections are shown in Figure 1.6.

1. **Frontal (Coronal) Section:** A plane from side to side that separates the body into front and back portions.
2. **Sagittal Section:** A plane from front to back that separates the body into right and left portions. A midsagittal section creates equal right and left halves.
3. **Transverse Section:** A horizontal plane that separates the body into upper and lower portions.
4. **Cross-Section:** A plane perpendicular to the long axis of an organ. A cross-section of the small intestine (which is a tube) would look like a circle with the cavity of the intestine in the center.
5. **Longitudinal Section:** A plane along the long axis of an organ.

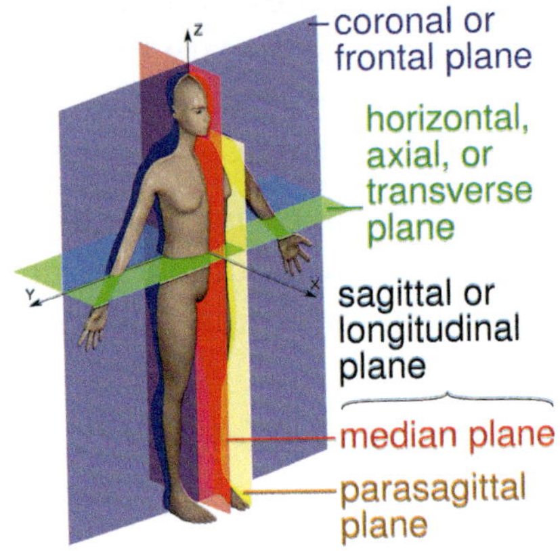

Figure 1.6. *Planes and sections of the body.*

Source: By David Richfield and Mikael Häggström, M.D. and cmglee – Human anatomy planes, labeled.jpg, CC BY-SA 4.0, https://commons.wikimedia.org/w/index.php?curid=91212408.

1.3.7. Areas of the Abdomen

A sizable portion of the body's lower trunk is the abdomen. If a patient complains of pain in the abdomen, the doctor or nurse would want to know more specific details about the location of the pain. The abdomen can be broken down into smaller sections.

1. **Quadrants:** A transverse plane and a midsagittal plane that cross at the umbilicus divide the abdomen into four quadrants. Clinically, this is probably the division used more frequently. The pain of gallstones might then be described as in the right upper quadrant.

2. **Nine Areas:** Two transverse planes and two sagittal planes divide the abdomen into nine areas:
3. **Upper Areas:** Above the level of the rib cartilages are the left hypochondriac, epigastric, and right hypochondriac.
4. **Middle Areas:** The left lumbar, umbilical, and right lumbar.
5. **Lower Areas:** Below the level of the top of the pelvic bone are the left iliac, hypogastric, and right iliac.

Anatomical studies frequently use these divisions to describe organ locations. For instance, the liver is located in the epigastric and right hypochondriac regions (Figure 1.7).

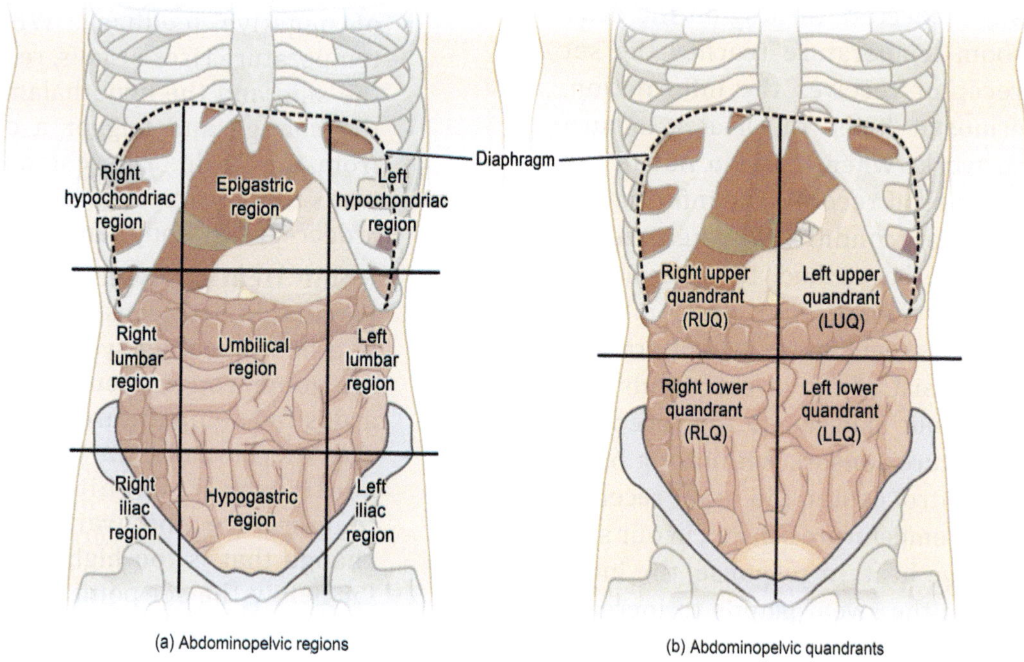

Figure 1.7. *Areas of the abdomen. (A) Four quadrants; and (B) nine regions.*

Source: By OpenStax. Download for free at http://cnx.org/contents/17e4eea8-a005-45af-b835-f756a014cd48@3., CC BY 3.0, https://commons.wikimedia.org/w/index.php?curid=29624324.

1.4. Homeostasis

In general, the terms stability, balance, and equilibrium are associated with homeostasis. It takes continuous observation and adaptation when circumstances change to maintain a stable internal environment. Homeostatic regulation is the term used to describe how the body adjusts its physiological systems. Three components or mechanisms are involved in homeostatic regulation: the receptor, the control center, and the effector. Information about a change in the environment is sent to the receptor. Information from the receptor is received and processed by the control center, also known as the integration center. Finally, the effector enhances or opposes the stimulus in response to the control center's commands. We can better comprehend this process by using the functioning of a thermostat as a metaphor. The thermostat regulates and keeps track of the room's temperature. The set point is the temperature at which the thermostat is set to be ideal. The thermostat's job is to maintain the room's temperature within a few degrees of its predetermined level. The thermometer (the receptor) notifies the thermostat that the room is too cold if the temperature drops below the set point. The room will then be warmed by the thermostat's effectors turning on the heat. When the room temperature reaches the set point, the receptor receives the information, and the thermostat "tells" the heater to turn off. This also works when it is too hot in the room. The thermostat receives the information and turns on the air conditioner. When the set point temperature is reached, the thermostat turns off the air conditioner. In a similar manner, our bodies regulate body temperature. The effectors consist of the sweat glands and blood vessels in our skin, while the receptors are the temperature sensors within our body. Acting as the control center, the brain receives signals from the temperature sensors in our skin when we perceive heat. In response, the brain sends a signal to the sweat glands to increase sweating and blood flow to the skin. Conversely, when we feel cold, the brain signals the sweat glands to stop sweating, reduce blood flow, and initiate shivering. The ultimate objective of this continuous process is to maintain and restore homeostasis. One way to conceptualize homeostasis is as a dynamic equilibrium, as it necessitates ongoing adjustments to remain at or close to the set point due to the ever-changing internal and external conditions of the body.

1.4.1. Positive and Negative Feedback

When a change of variable occurs, there are two main types of feedback to which the system reacts: Negative feedback and positive feedback.

1. **Negative Feedback:** A reaction in which the system responds in such a way as to reverse the direction of change. This mechanism helps maintain homeostasis by keeping things constant. For example, when the concentration of carbon dioxide in the human body increases, the lungs are signaled to increase their activity and expel more carbon dioxide. Thermoregulation is another example of negative feedback. When body temperature rises or falls, receptors in the skin and the hypothalamus sense the change and trigger a command from the brain. This command then leads to the correct response, such as a decrease in body temperature.
2. **Home Heating System vs. Negative Feedback:** Let's consider the example of a home heating system. When you are home, you set your thermostat to a desired temperature, let's say 70°. The thermometer in the thermostat continuously monitors the air temperature and waits to sense a change that is too high above or too far below the set point. When such a change occurs, the thermometer sends a message to the "Control Center" or thermostat. The thermostat then sends a message to the furnace to either shut off if the temperature is too high or kick back on if the temperature is too low. In this example, the air temperature serves as the "NEGATIVE FEEDBACK." When the Control Center receives negative feedback, it triggers a chain reaction to maintain the room temperature.
3. **Positive Feedback:** A mechanism that amplifies the change in a variable, leading to a destabilizing effect and preventing homeostasis. While less common than negative feedback in

naturally occurring systems, positive feedback has its applications. For instance, in nerves, a threshold electric potential triggers the generation of a much larger action potential. Blood clotting and events in childbirth are other examples of positive feedback.

4. **Harmful Positive Feedback:** However, positive feedback can also be harmful within homeostasis. In cases of high fever, for example, it can cause a metabolic change that further elevates the fever. In rare occurrences, when the body temperature reaches 113°, cellular proteins cease to function and metabolism stops, resulting in death.

Sustainable systems require a combination of both positive and negative feedback. Positive feedback is typically activated when divergence from the homeostatic condition is recognized, while negative feedback is used for fine-tuning responses as the homeostatic condition is approached. This creates a state of "metastability," where homeostatic conditions are maintained within fixed limits. However, if these limits are exceeded, the system can shift dramatically to a new and potentially less desirable state of homeostasis.

1.4.1.1. Homeostatic Systems Possess Several Properties

- They exhibit ultra-stability, allowing the system to determine how variables should be adjusted.
- The entire organization, including internal, structural, and functional aspects, contributes to maintaining balance.
- Physiology is primarily the study of processes related to homeostasis. While some of the functions discussed in this book may not be directly related to homeostasis (such as muscle contraction), a suitable internal environment is essential for all bodily processes to function properly. Therefore, homeostasis provides a suitable framework for the introductory study of physiology.

1.4.1.2. Where Did the Term "Homeostasis" Come From?

The term "Homeostasis" originated from the studies of the French scientist Claude Bernard (1813-1878) on the maintenance of stability in the "milieu interior." He stated, "All the vital mechanisms, despite their variations, have one common objective: to maintain constant the conditions of life in the internal environment" (from Leçons sur les Phénonèmes de la Vie Commune aux Animaux et aux Végétaux, 1879). The term itself was coined by the American physiologist Walter Cannon, author of The Wisdom of the Body (1932). It is derived from the Greek words *homoios* (meaning same, like, resembling) and *stasis* (meaning to stand, posture).

1.4.2. Pathways That Alter Homeostasis

Numerous homeostatic processes maintain the internal environment within acceptable limits. Either the body experiences various ailments or diseases, or homeostasis is preserved through multiple regulatory systems. The homeostatic balance is disrupted when the body's cells start to malfunction, eventually leading to illness or cellular dysfunction. There are two primary causes of disease and cellular malfunction: deficiency (cells not receiving sufficient nutrients) and toxicity (cells being harmed by unnecessary substances). Disruptions in homeostasis within your cells can either exacerbate or ameliorate the issue. In addition to internal regulatory mechanisms, the preservation of cellular health in our body is also influenced by external factors, primarily derived from lifestyle choices and environmental exposures.

1. **Nutrition:** Insufficient intake of specific vitamins or minerals in your diet can impair cellular function, potentially resulting in disease conditions. For instance, a menstruating woman with inadequate dietary iron intake may develop anemia. The lack of hemoglobin, a molecule that requires iron, leads to reduced oxygen-carrying capacity. In mild cases, symptoms may be nonspecific (e.g., fatigue), but severe anemia can prompt compensatory mechanisms such as increased cardiac output, leading to palpitations, diaphoresis, and potentially heart failure.
2. **Toxins:** Any substance that interferes with cellular function can cause cellular malfunction. This can occur through various means, including exposure to chemicals, plants, insecticides, or bites. A commonly observed example is drug overdoses. When an individual consumes an excessive amount of a drug, their vital signs begin to fluctuate, potentially causing complications such as coma, brain damage, and even death.
3. **Psychological:** Your physical health and mental health are inseparable. Our thoughts and emotions cause chemical changes to take place, either for the better, as with meditation, or for the worse, as with stress.
4. **Physical:** Maintaining our physical health is essential for our cells and bodies. Adequate rest, sunlight, and exercise are examples of physical mechanisms that influence homeostasis. Lack of sleep is related to a number of ailments, such as irregular cardiac rhythms, fatigue, anxiety, and headaches.
5. **Genetic/Reproductive:** Inheriting strengths and weaknesses can be part of our genetic makeup. Genes are sometimes turned off or on due to external factors, over which we may have some control, but at other times, little can be done to correct or improve genetic diseases. Beginning at the cellular level, a variety of diseases originate from mutated genes. For example, cancer can be genetically inherited or caused by a mutation from an external source, such as radiation or genes altered in a fetus when the mother uses drugs.
6. **Medical:** Due to genetic differences, some bodies need help in gaining or maintaining homeostasis. Through modern medicine, our bodies can be given different aids, from antibodies to help fight infections to chemotherapy to kill harmful cancer cells. Traditional and alternative medical practices have many benefits, but the potential for harmful effects is also present. Whether through nosocomial infections or the wrong dosage of medication, homeostasis can be altered by that which is trying to fix it. Trial and error with medications can cause potential harmful reactions and possibly death if not caught soon enough.

All of the aforementioned factors, whether adverse or favorable, have an influence on cells. There will almost invariably be a deleterious deviation in homeostasis as a consequence of inadequate beneficial pathways. Moreover, excessive toxicity results in homeostatic imbalance, which deteriorates cells. Your body is better equipped to self-regulate and self-repair, maintaining homeostasis, when negative health influences are eliminated and adequate positive health influences are provided.

1.5. Homeostasis Throughout the Body

Every bodily system supports the overall organism's homeostasis as well as that of the other systems. Every bodily system interacts with every other system to maintain overall health, and no system functions alone. Typically, a disturbance in one bodily system affects multiple other systems. Here are a few succinct explanations of how different body systems support homeostasis maintenance:

1.5.1. Nervous System

The nervous and endocrine systems are the main control centers of the body, operating below the level of consciousness. For instance, the hypothalamus in the brain serves as the body's "thermostat" and stimulates the pituitary gland to release various hormones that regulate the body's development and metabolism. The sympathetic and parasympathetic branches of the nervous system alternately stimulate and inhibit physiological responses such as heart rate and breathing rate to maintain appropriate levels. The nervous system also regulates skeletal muscle contractions, which contribute to body movement, bone maintenance, and thickening, thereby impacting bone composition. It also controls arrector pili muscles involved in thermoregulation. Additionally, the nervous system governs the respiratory system, which regulates breathing depth and pace, the cardiovascular system, which governs heart rate and blood pressure, the endocrine organs, which secrete oxytocin and ADH, the digestive system, which governs the movement and secretion of the digestive tract, and the urinary system, which controls bladder voiding and helps regulate renal blood pressure. The nervous system is also involved in our sexual behaviors and functions.

1.5.2. Endocrine System

The hormones secreted into the bloodstream by glands make up the endocrine system. Every hormone affects a target tissue or multiple target tissues. The majority of body systems and cells' growth and metabolism are thus regulated by the endocrine system. More precisely, the endocrine system contains sex hormones that can stimulate melanocytes on our skin, activate sebaceous glands, change dermal blood flow, and release lipids from adipocytes. Numerous hormones control the growth of our bones, and the endocrine system aids in the mobilization of calcium and calcitonin. Hormones regulate muscle growth, energy production, and metabolism in the muscular system. Hormones have an impact on neuronal metabolism, fluid and electrolyte balance, and reproductive hormones that impact CNS development and behavior in the nervous system. We require hormones in the cardiovascular system to control red blood cell production and to raise and lower blood pressure. Hormones also stimulate the lymphatic system and have anti-inflammatory effects. In conclusion, nearly every other bodily system is regulated by the endocrine system.

1.5.3. Integumentary System

The integumentary system is involved in controlling blood ion balances, regulating body temperature through sweating and vasodilation, or shivering and piloerection (goose bumps), and protecting the body from invasive microbes (primarily by forming a thick impenetrable layer). Additionally, changes in capillary permeability and blood flow are produced by mast cell stimulation, which may have an impact on the body's regulation of blood flow. Additionally, it aids in the synthesis of vitamin D, which interacts with the absorption of calcium and phosphorus to support bone growth and maintenance, such as in the event that a bone breaks and needs to be repaired. Skin hair protects the nasal cavity and other orifices, keeping pathogens from entering our bodies further. Because it excretes water and other solutes (i.e., minerals), our skin also aids in maintaining equilibrium. The skin's keratinized epidermis prevents fluid loss. In other words, it offers mechanical defense against environmental threats. As our first line of defense, our skin is integumentary, and maintaining its balance requires effort.

1.5.4. Skeletal System

One significant mineral reserve is the skeletal system. For instance, minerals are extracted from the bones when blood contains low levels of calcium or magnesium and the diet lacks these minerals. However, the skeletal system provides the necessary calcium for every muscle contraction. The bone marrow produces and stores lymphocytes and other immune response-related cells. The skeletal system also plays a protective role for essential organs such as the nervous system, endocrine organs, chest, and pelvic regions.

1.5.5. Muscular System

The muscular system, in turn, plays a major role in regulating body temperature by generating heat. It helps maintain blood glucose balance by storing energy as glycogen. Additionally, it indirectly contributes to overall health by enabling mobility, allowing individuals to find food, seek shelter from severe weather, and more. Muscles also enable facial expressions while protecting the skin. They assist the nervous system in monitoring body position and safeguard the digestive system and endocrine glands. Furthermore, muscles control contractions related to sexual sensations and enable the retention of urine when necessary. They also protect deep blood vessels, facilitate lymph flow through the lymphatic system, and assist in blood circulation through veins.

1.5.6. Cardiovascular System

The cardiovascular system, in addition to needing to maintain itself within certain levels, plays a role in the maintenance of other body systems by transporting hormones (the heart secretes ANP and BNP) and nutrients (such as oxygen and EPO to bones), removing waste products, and providing all living body cells with a fresh supply of oxygen while removing carbon dioxide. Homeostasis is disturbed if the cardiovascular or lymphatic systems are not functioning correctly. Our skin, bones, muscles, nervous system, endocrine system, lymphatic system, lungs, digestive tract, urinary system, and reproductive system all rely on the cardiovascular system as a "road" or "highway" for the distribution of substances within our body. There are many risk factors for an unhealthy cardiovascular system. Some diseases associated with it are typically labeled as "uncontrollable" or "controllable." The main uncontrollable risk factors include age, gender, and a family history of heart disease, especially at an early age.

1.5.7. Lymphatic System

There are three main functions of the lymphatic system. Firstly, it is responsible for maintaining the volume of tissue and blood. Without this function, excess fluid that escapes the capillaries would accumulate and result in edema. Secondly, the lymphatic system absorbs fatty acids and triglycerides from the digestion of fat, preventing them from directly entering the bloodstream. Lastly, the lymphatic system plays a crucial role in supporting the immune system and defending against invasive microbes. It also aids in the maintenance and healing of injured muscles and bones.

Additionally, maintaining an acidic pH in urine helps prevent urinary tract infections, serving as an additional line of defense. The tonsils in our body protect us from toxins and infections that enter through the digestive system, as well as guard against infections reaching our lungs.

1.5.8. Respiratory System

Moving on to the respiratory system, it collaborates with the cardiovascular system to supply oxygen to the cells in every bodily system for cellular metabolism. The respiratory system also eliminates carbon dioxide from the body. Furthermore, it contributes to maintaining appropriate blood pH levels, which is crucial for homeostasis. Carbon dioxide is primarily transported in the plasma as bicarbonate ions, which function as a chemical buffer. Hyperventilation lowers the blood's concentration of CO_2, resulting in a rise in the pH of bodily fluids. When acid levels exceed 7.45, respiratory alkalosis occurs. Conversely, excessive CO_2 lowers the pH below 7.35, leading to respiratory acidosis. The respiratory system also plays a protective role by trapping pathogens and aiding the lymphatic system. It is important to note that the contraction of respiratory muscles can generate abdominal pressure, which can assist in the passage of air. Let us not forget that our lungs serve as the gateway for the breath of life.

1.5.9. Digestive System

All body systems would quickly deteriorate in the absence of a consistent supply of nutrients and energy from the digestive system. The body requires water, ions, vitamins, and organic materials, all of which are absorbed by the digestive system. Lipids are transported by the digestive tract to the subcutaneous layer of the skin for storage. It is important to note that the body undergoes three distinct processes with food: digestion, absorption, and elimination. If any of these processes are not functioning properly, noticeable problems will arise. Chemical digestion, movements, ingestion, absorption, and elimination are all examples of digestive mechanics. To maintain proper functioning, it is essential to understand the different parts of the digestive system. Disruption of these parts can compromise the health of the digestive system.

1.5.10. Urinary System

The urinary system, specifically the kidneys, plays a vital role in eliminating toxic nitrogenous wastes that accumulate as proteins and nucleic acids are broken down and utilized for other purposes. Additionally, the urinary system directly contributes to maintaining appropriate blood pressure, blood volume, and blood ion concentration. The kidneys also produce the hormone erythropoietin, which stimulates the production of red blood cells. Furthermore, the kidneys are crucial in preserving the body's water balance and the proper salt composition of the extracellular fluid. When external factors lead to excessive fluid loss, feedback systems are activated to prevent further fluid loss and maintain the body's fluid balance.

1.5.11. Reproductive System

The reproductive system plays a distinct role by primarily focusing on the preservation of the species rather than the individual organism's homeostasis. However, the sex hormones produced by this system can impact other bodily functions, and an imbalance can result in disorders such as osteoporosis in individuals, like women who have their ovaries removed at an early age.

1.6. The Cell and Its Functions

A human being is made up of 100 trillion cells, each of which is a living structure that can endure for months or even years if the fluids around it provide the right nutrients. It is crucial that we comprehend the fundamental structure of the cell and the roles of its constituent parts before we can comprehend the operation of the organs and other bodily structures.

1.6.1. Organization of the Cell

Figure 1.8 displays a standard cell through a light microscope, highlighting the nucleus and cytoplasm as its main components. The nucleus is enclosed by the nuclear membrane, while the cytoplasm is surrounded by a cell membrane, also known as the plasma membrane, separating it from the surrounding fluids.

Protoplasm refers to the various materials that comprise a cell as a whole. The five fundamental components of protoplasm are water, electrolytes, proteins, lipids, and carbohydrates.

1. **Water:** Water is the principal fluid medium of the cell, present in most cells, except for fat cells, in a concentration of 70% to 85%. Many cellular chemicals are dissolved in the water, while others are suspended in the water as solid particulates. Chemical reactions take place among the dissolved chemicals or at the surfaces of the suspended particles or membranes.
2. **Ions:** Important ions in the cell include potassium, magnesium, phosphate, sulfate, bicarbonate, and smaller quantities of sodium, chloride, and calcium. These ions provide inorganic chemicals for cellular reactions and are necessary for the operation of some of the cellular control mechanisms. For instance, ions acting at the cell membrane are required for the transmission of electrochemical impulses in nerve and muscle fibers.
3. **Proteins:** After water, the most abundant substances in most cells are proteins, which normally constitute 10% to 20% of the cell mass. These proteins can be divided into two types: structural proteins and functional proteins.

   The primary form of structural proteins in a cell is as long filaments, which are polymers of numerous individual protein molecules. Intracellular filaments are widely utilized in the formation of microtubules, which serve as the "cytoskeletons" of various cellular organelles, including cilia, nerve axons, mitotic spindles, and a complex network of slender filamentous tubules that connect the cytoplasm and nucleoplasm in their respective compartments. Fibrillar proteins are found extracellularly in various tissues such as blood vessel walls, tendons, ligaments, and the collagen and elastin fibers of connective tissue.

   The functional proteins are a completely different class of protein, typically consisting of tubular-globular combinations of a few molecules. Unlike fibrillar proteins, which are often immobile in the cell fluid, these proteins are primarily the enzymes of the cell. Furthermore, a large number of them adhere to the cell's membrane structures. The enzymes catalyze particular intracellular chemical reactions when they come into direct contact with other substances in the cell fluid. For example, a variety of protein enzymes catalyze the chemical reactions that divide glucose into its constituent components and then combine these with oxygen to form carbon dioxide and water, all the while providing energy for cellular function.
4. **Lipids:** The fact that lipids are soluble in fat solvents unites a variety of substances under one umbrella category. Phospholipids and cholesterol are particularly significant lipids, constituting a mere 2% of the total mass of the cell. Due to their primary insolubility in water, phospholipids and cholesterol play a crucial role in

forming the cell membrane and intracellular membrane barriers that separate the different cell compartments.

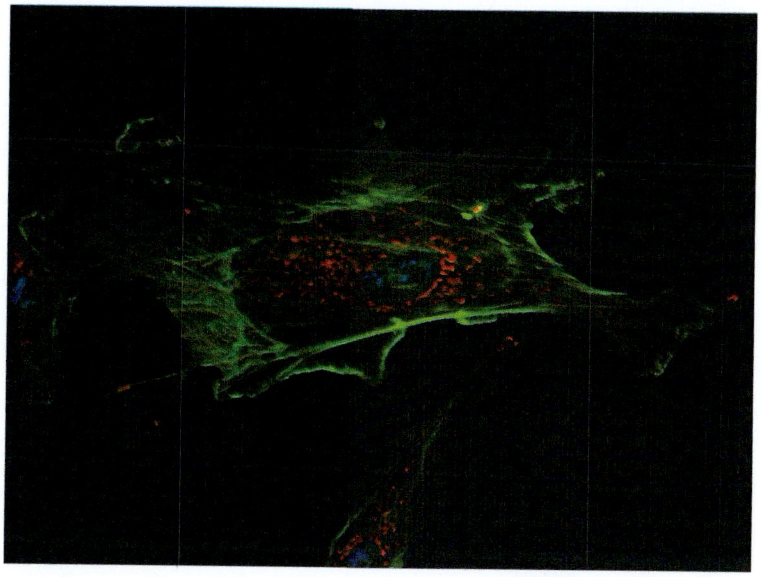

Figure 1.8. *Structure of the cell as seen with the fluorescent microscope.*

Source: By IP69.226.103.13 – Own work, CC BY-SA 3.0, https://commons.wikimedia.org/w/index.php?curid=8093704.

In addition to cholesterol and phospholipids, certain cells also contain high levels of triglycerides or neutral fat. Triglycerides often account for up to 95% of the mass of fat cells. The body predominantly stores its energy-producing nutrients in the form of fat, which can be dissolved and utilized to provide energy to any part of the body.

5. **Carbohydrates:** Despite having minimal structural value in the cell other than as components of glycoprotein molecules, are essential for cellular nutrition. Carbohydrate reserves are not stored in large quantities by the majority of human cells; they typically make up around 1% of the total mass. However, in muscle cells, they can occasionally reach 3%, and in liver cells, they can reach 6%. Nevertheless, extracellular fluid surrounding us always contains dissolved glucose, a form of carbohydrate that cells can easily access. Additionally, cells keep a small amount of carbohydrates in reserve as glycogen, an insoluble glucose polymer that can be rapidly depolymerized to meet the cells' energy needs.

1.6.2. Physical Structure of the Cell

The cell is more than just a collection of chemicals, fluid, and enzymes; intracellular organelles are highly ordered physical structures found within the cell. For a cell to function, each organelle's physical characteristics are just as crucial as its chemical components. For example, the cell would instantly stop releasing more than 95% of its energy from nutrients if it were missing one of the organelles, the mitochondria. Figure 1.9 depicts the key organelles as well as additional cell structures.

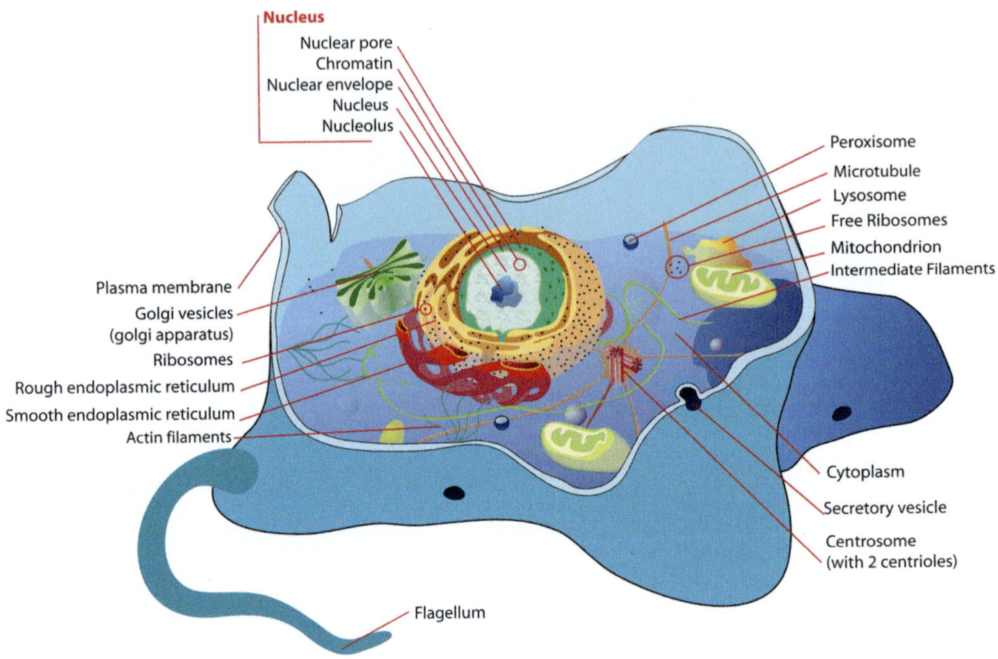

Figure 1.9. *Reconstruction of a typical cell, showing the internal organelles in the cytoplasm and in the nucleus.*

Source: By LadyofHats (Mariana Ruiz) - Own work using Adobe Illustrator. Image renamed from Image:Animal cell structure.svg, Public Domain, https://commons.wikimedia.org/w/index.php?curid=4266142.

1.6.3. Membranous Structures of the Cell

Membranes made mostly of lipids and proteins envelop the majority of the cell's organelles. These membranes consist of the Golgi apparatus, lysosomes, mitochondria, nuclear membrane, endoplasmic reticulum membrane, and cell membrane.

Since water is not soluble in lipids, the lipids in the membranes act as a barrier to prevent the flow of water and substances soluble in water from one cell compartment to another. However, the membrane's protein molecules frequently do permeate all the way through, offering specialized passageways—often arranged into actual pores—for the passage of particular substances through the membrane. Furthermore, a large number of other membrane proteins function as enzymes, catalyzing a wide range of diverse chemical reactions.

1.6.4. Cell Membrane

Enclosing the cell, the cell membrane (also known as the plasma membrane) is a thin, elastic, pliable structure that ranges in thickness from 7.5 to 10 nanometers. It is primarily composed of lipids and proteins. Proteins constitute approximately 55% of the composition, followed by phospholipids (25%), cholesterol (13%), other lipids (4%), and carbohydrates (3%).

1.6.4.1. Lipid Barrier of the Cell Membrane Impedes Water Penetration

The cell membrane's structure is depicted in Figure 1.10. Its fundamental structure is a lipid bilayer, which is a continuous, thin film of lipids that is double-layered and only one molecule thick on the cell surface. Giant globular protein molecules are dispersed throughout this lipid layer.

The fundamental lipid bilayer is composed of phospholipid molecules. Each phospholipid molecule has a hydrophilic end that is soluble in water, and a hydrophobic end that is only soluble in fats. The phospholipid consists of a hydrophilic phosphate end and a hydrophobic fatty acid portion.

As illustrated in Figure 1.10, the hydrophobic portions of the phospholipid molecules have a natural tendency to associate with each other in the middle of the membrane. This is because they are repelled by water but mutually attracted to one another. The two surfaces of the entire cell membrane are thus composed of the hydrophilic phosphate sections, which are in contact with extracellular water on the outside and intracellular water on the inside.

Water-soluble substances such as urea, glucose, and ions cannot pass through the lipid layer located in the middle of the membrane. Conversely, substances that are soluble in fat, such as alcohol, carbon dioxide, and oxygen, can easily traverse this part of the membrane.

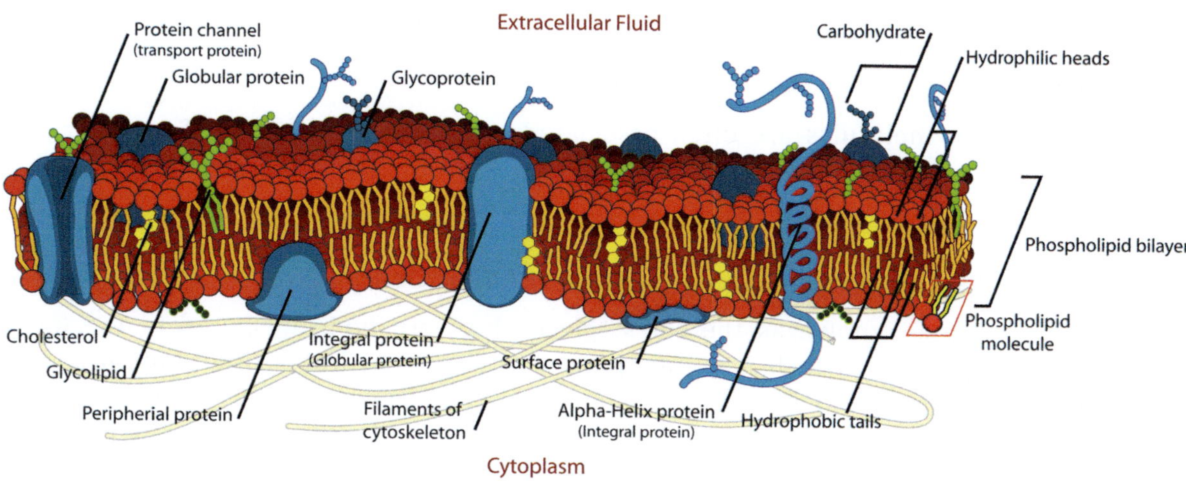

Figure 1.10. *The structure of the cell membrane shows that it is composed mainly of a lipid bilayer of phospholipid molecules, with large numbers of protein molecules protruding through the layer. Additionally, carbohydrate moieties are attached to the protein molecules on the outside of the membrane and to additional protein molecules on the inside.*

Source: By LadyofHats Mariana Ruiz – Own work. Image renamed from File:Cell membrane detailed diagram.svg, Public Domain, https://commons.wikimedia.org/w/index.php?curid=6027169.

Because the steroid nucleus of the cholesterol molecules in the membrane is highly fat soluble, the molecules themselves are lipids. These molecules are, in a sense, dissolved in the membrane's bilayer. They primarily contribute to determining the bilayer's degree of permeability (or impermeability) to components of bodily fluids that are soluble in water. Additionally, cholesterol regulates a significant portion of the membrane's fluidity. Figure 1.10 illustrates integral and peripheral cell membrane proteins. The image showcases dispersed globular masses within the lipid bilayer, known as glycoproteins. Integral proteins extend completely through the membrane, while peripheral proteins are attached to only one surface and do not penetrate entirely through.

The structural channels (or pores) that many integral proteins provide allow water molecules and water-soluble substances, particularly ions, to diffuse between the extracellular and intracellular fluids. Additionally, the selective characteristics of these protein channels enable the preferential diffusion of some substances over others.

Other crucial proteins act as carriers of materials that would not otherwise be able to cross the lipid bilayer. Occasionally, these proteins can even transport materials in the opposite direction of their electrochemical gradients for diffusion; this is known as "active transport." Others function as enzymes.

Water-soluble substances that are difficult to pass through cell membranes, such as peptide hormones, can also be recognized by integral membrane proteins. Conformational changes in the receptor protein are induced by the interaction of specific ligands with cell membrane receptors. The signal is then transmitted from the extracellular region of the receptor to the intracellular region of the cell through an enzymatic process that either activates the intracellular portion of the protein or facilitates interactions between the receptor and cytoplasmic proteins acting as second messengers. Therefore, integral proteins spanning the cell membrane provide a means for the cell's interior to receive environmental information.

Peripheral protein molecules are often associated with integral proteins. These peripheral proteins primarily function as enzymes or regulators of substance transport through the cell membrane "pores."

1.6.4.2. Membrane Carbohydrates – The Cell "Glycocalyx"

Membrane carbohydrates, known as the cell's "glycocalyx," are typically found in the form of glycoproteins or glycolipids, which are combinations of carbohydrates and proteins. In fact, glycolipids constitute approximately 10% of membrane lipid molecules and the majority of integral proteins. Generally, the "glyco" portions of these molecules extend outward from the cell surface and protrude outside the cell. Additionally, numerous carbohydrate compounds called proteoglycans are loosely attached to the cell's outer surface. These compounds consist mainly of carbohydrate substances bound to small protein cores. Consequently, a loose layer of carbohydrates, known as the glycocalyx, often covers the entire external surface of the cell.

The carbohydrate moieties affixed to the cell's outer surface serve multiple significant functions: (i) A large number of them possess a negative electrical charge, endowing most cells with an overall negative surface charge that deters other negatively charged objects. (ii) Cells are connected to one another by the glycocalyx of some cells adhering to that of other cells. (iii) A large number of carbohydrates function as receptors for hormones like insulin. When these substances are bound together, attached internal proteins are activated, which in turn triggers a series of intracellular enzymes. (iv) Certain carbohydrate moieties trigger immune responses.

1.6.5. Cytoplasm and Its Organelles

Organelles and small and large dispersed particles abound in the cytoplasm. The term "cytosol" refers to the transparent, fluid part of the cytoplasm where the particles are distributed; it primarily consists of dissolved glucose, proteins, and electrolytes.

Neutral fat globules, glycogen granules, ribosomes, secretory vesicles, and five particularly significant organelles—the endoplasmic reticulum, the Golgi apparatus, mitochondria, lysosomes, and peroxisomes—are scattered throughout the cytoplasm.

1.6.5.1. Endoplasmic Reticulum

The endoplasmic reticulum is a network of flat and tubular vesicular structures found in the cytoplasm, as seen in Figure 1.9. Vesicles and tubules are interconnected. Moreover, similar to cell membranes, their walls consist of lipid bilayer membranes that are abundant in proteins. In specific cells, such as liver cells, the total surface area of this structure can be up to 30–40 times larger than the area of the cell membrane.

Figure 1.11 illustrates the intricate structure of a small section of the endoplasmic reticulum. The endoplasmic matrix, a distinct watery substance from the fluid in the cytosol outside the endoplasmic reticulum, fills the space inside the tubules and vesicles. The space between the nuclear membrane's two surfaces and the endoplasmic reticulum are connected, as demonstrated by electron micrographs.

Upon entering the endoplasmic reticulum, substances produced in specific regions of the cell are transported to other areas of the cell. Additionally, a significant portion of the cell's metabolic processes are supported by the machinery present on the extensive surface area of this reticulum and the numerous enzyme systems connected to its membranes.

1.6.5.2. Ribosomes and the Granular Endoplasmic Reticulum

Numerous tiny granular particles, known as ribosomes, are attached to the exterior surfaces of various regions of the endoplasmic reticulum. In the presence of these ribosomes, the reticulum is referred to as the granular endoplasmic reticulum. The ribosomes function as the cell's factory for synthesizing new protein molecules. They are composed of a combination of RNA and proteins.

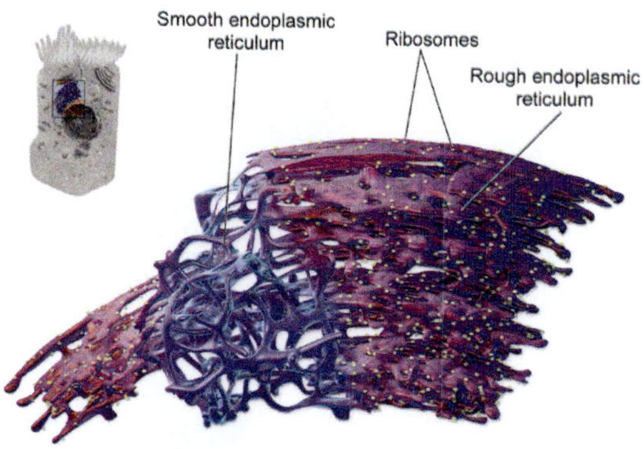

Figure 1.11. *Structure of the endoplasmic reticulum.*

Source: By BruceBlaus. When using this image in external sources, it can be cited as: Blausen.com staff (2014). "Medical gallery of Blausen Medical 2014" WikiJournal of Medicine, 1(2). doi: 10.15347/wjm/2014.010.ISSN 2002-4436. – Own work, CC BY 3.0, https://commons.wikimedia.org/w/index.php?curid=28223972 By Mariana Ruiz LadyofHats – I made it myself on Adobe Illustrator based on the information found on these websites: [1], [2], [3], [4], and [5]. Public Domain, https://commons.wikimedia.org/w/index.php?curid=8152684.

1.6.5.3. Agranular Endoplasmic Reticulum

The endoplasmic reticulum does not have ribosomes attached to it. The agranular, or smooth, endoplasmic reticulum is the name given to this section. The synthesis of lipids and other cellular functions supported by intrareticular enzymes are carried out by the agranular reticulum.

1.6.5.4. Golgi Apparatus

The Golgi apparatus is closely related to the endoplasmic reticulum. Figure 1.12 illustrates this relationship. Its membranes are comparable to those of the endoplasmic reticulum granule. Usually found close to one side of the nucleus, it is made up of four or more stacked layers of thin, flat, enclosed vesicles. This device, which is situated on the side of the cell where the secretory substances are extruded, is noticeable in secretory cells.

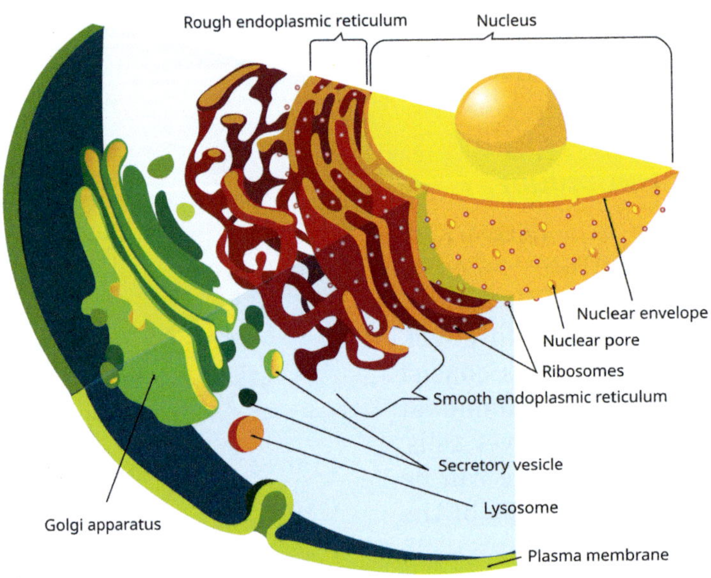

Figure 1.12. *A typical golgi apparatus and its relationship to the endoplasmic reticulum (ER) and the nucleus.*

Source: By Mariana Ruiz LadyofHats – I made it myself on Adobe Illustrator based on the information found on these websites: [1], [2], [3], [4], and [5]. Public Domain, https://commons.wikimedia.org/w/index.php?curid=8152684.

The endoplasmic reticulum and the Golgi apparatus collaborate to carry out numerous functions. Small "transport vesicles," also referred to as endoplasmic reticulum vesicles or ER vesicles, continuously bud off from the endoplasmic reticulum and rapidly merge with the Golgi apparatus, as depicted in Figure 1.12. Substances enclosed within endoplasmic reticulum vesicles are thus transferred from the ER to the Golgi apparatus. The transported materials are subsequently broken down into lysosomes, secretory vesicles, and other cytoplasmic components within the Golgi apparatus.

1.6.5.5. Lysosomes

Lysosomes, vesicular organelles illustrated in Figure 1.9, originate when they separate from the Golgi apparatus and disperse throughout the cytoplasm. The lysosomes function as an intracellular digestive system, enabling the cell to break down three types of material: (i) food particles that have entered the cell; (ii) damaged cellular structures; and (iii) undesired substances such as bacteria. The lysosome typically has a diameter of 250–750 nanometers, although it can vary significantly depending on the cell type. It is surrounded by a typical lipid bilayer membrane and contains a large number of tiny, 5–8 nanometer-diameter granules that are protein aggregates consisting of up to 40 distinct hydrolase (digestive) enzymes. By combining the hydrogen from a water molecule with one part of the compound and the hydroxyl portion of the water molecule with the other part of the compound, a hydrolytic enzyme can split an organic compound into two or more parts. For example, hydrolysis of protein yields amino acids, hydrolysis of glycogen yields glucose, and hydrolysis of lipids yields fatty acids and glycerol.

Normally, the lysosome's membrane keeps the confined hydrolytic enzymes from interacting with other materials inside the cell, which prevents the enzymes from breaking down food. However, under certain cell conditions, the membranes of some lysosomes are broken, releasing the digestive enzymes. The organic materials that these enzymes come into contact with are subsequently broken down into tiny, highly diffusible substances such as glucose and amino acids.

1.6.5.6. Peroxisomes

Physically, peroxisomes and lysosomes are similar, but there are two key distinctions between them. First, rather than emerging from the Golgi apparatus, they are thought to be formed by self-replication (or possibly by budding off from the smooth endoplasmic reticulum). Secondly, instead of hydrolases, they have oxidases. A number of the oxidases can produce hydrogen peroxide (H_2O_2) by combining oxygen with hydrogen ions obtained from various intracellular substances. When combined with catalase, another oxidase enzyme found in large amounts in peroxisomes, hydrogen peroxide, a highly oxidizing substance, can oxidize a variety of substances that would otherwise be harmful to cells. For example, the peroxisomes in liver cells detoxify approximately half of the alcohol an individual consumes in this manner.

1.6.5.7. Secretory Vesicles

The secretion of unique chemical substances is a crucial function for numerous cells. The Golgi apparatus releases almost all of these secretory substances into the cytoplasm in the form of storage vesicles known as secretory vesicles or secretory granules. These substances are formed by the endoplasmic reticulum-Golgi apparatus system. Pancreatic acinar cells contain normal secretory vesicles, which are used to store protein proenzymes (enzymes that have not yet been activated), as seen in Figure 1.13. After being secreted via the outer cell membrane, the proenzymes enter the pancreatic duct and the duodenum, where they activate and begin to break down food in the digestive tract.

1.6.5.8. Mitochondria

It is said that the mitochondria are the "powerhouses" of the cell; these can be seen in Figures 1.9 and 1.14. Without them, practically every cellular activity would come to an end since cells couldn't draw enough energy from the nutrients.

Every part of the cytoplasm of every cell contains mitochondria, but the total number of mitochondria in a cell can range from fewer than 100 to several 1,000, depending on the cell's energy requirements. Moreover, the regions of the cell that harbor the majority of its mitochondria are responsible for the majority of the cell's energy metabolism. The size and shape of mitochondria are also irregular, with some being globular with a diameter of only a few 100 nanometers, while others are elongated with a diameter of up to one micrometer and a length of seven micrometers. There are also filamentous and branching mitochondria.

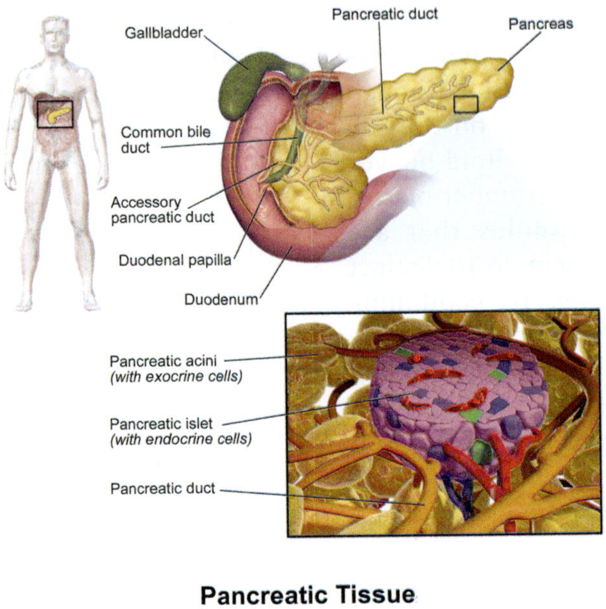

Figure 1.13. *Secretory granules (secretory vesicles) in acinar cells of the pancreas.*

Source: By BruceBlaus. When using this image in external sources it can be cited as: Blausen.com staff (2014). "Medical gallery of Blausen Medical 2014." WikiJournal of Medicine, 1(2). doi: 10.15347/wjm/2014.010. ISSN 2002-4436. - Own work, CC BY 3.0, https://commons.wikimedia.org/w/index.php?curid=28909220.

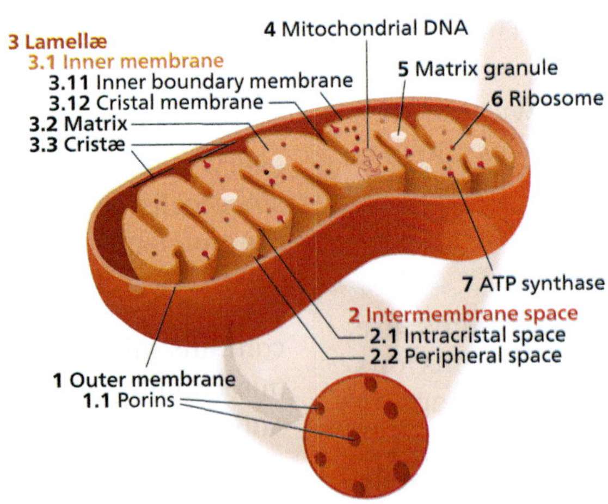

Figure 1.14. *Structure of a mitochondrion.*

Source: By Kelvin song - Own work, CC0, https://commons.wikimedia.org/w/index.php?curid=27715320.

The mitochondrion's basic structure consists of two lipid bilayer–protein membranes, namely the inner and outer membranes, as depicted in Figure 1.14. The inner membrane contains numerous infoldings that create folds to which oxidative enzymes are attached. Additionally, the inner cavity of the mitochondrion is filled with a matrix containing a significant amount of dissolved enzymes, which are crucial for extracting energy from nutrients. These enzymes work in conjunction with the oxidative enzymes present in the infoldings to initiate nutrient oxidation, resulting in the release of energy, carbon dioxide, and water. Adenosine triphosphate (ATP), a high-energy compound, is synthesized using the liberated energy. Once released from the mitochondrion, ATP diffuses throughout the cell, releasing its energy wherever it is needed to facilitate cellular processes.

Due to their capacity for self-replication, mitochondria have the ability to generate additional mitochondria whenever a cell requires an increased supply of ATP. This phenomenon is commonly referred to as self-replication. Interestingly, the DNA found within mitochondria is identical to that found within the cell nucleus. The nucleus contains a pivotal component known as DNA, which governs cell replication. Similarly, the DNA within mitochondria regulates the replication of mitochondria themselves.

1.6.5.9. Cell Cytoskeleton – Filament and Tubular Structures

The cell cytoskeleton consists of filamentous and tubular structures. Typically, the cell's fibrillar proteins are organized into tubules or filaments. These structures originate from precursor protein molecules synthesized by cytoplasmic ribosomes. Following polymerization, these precursor molecules give rise to filaments. For example, the outer region of the cytoplasm, known as the ectoplasm, contains a substantial number of actin filaments that function as an elastic support for the cell membrane. In muscle cells, actin and myosin filaments are arranged to form a distinctive contractile apparatus that serves as the basis for muscle contraction.

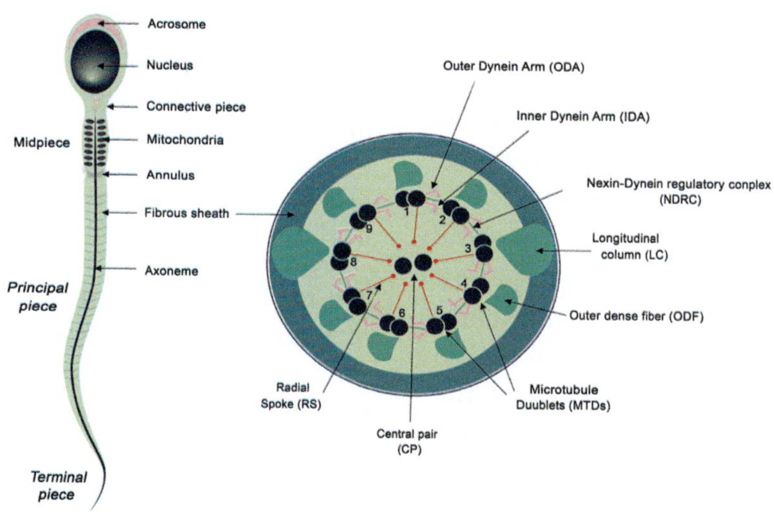

Figure 1.15. *Microtubules in the flagellum of a sperm.*

Source: Touré, A., (2019). Importance of SLC26 transmembrane anion exchangers in sperm post-testicular maturation and fertilization potential. Front. Cell Dev. Biol., 7, 230. doi: 10.3389/fcell.2019.00230.

All cells employ a specific type of rigid filament called microtubules, which are composed of polymerized tubulin molecules. Figure 1.15 illustrates typical microtubules found in the flagellum of a sperm.

The tubular skeleton that runs from the cytoplasm of each cell to the tip of each cilium is another illustration of microtubules. It is located in the center of each cilium. Moreover, stiff microtubules make up the mitotic spindle and centrioles of the dividing cell.

As a result, one of the main roles of microtubules is to serve as a cytoskeleton, providing stiff external structures for some cell components.

1.6.6. Nucleus

The nucleus functions as the central nervous system of the cell. In essence, it houses the genes, which are large amounts of DNA. The genes determine the characteristics of the cell's proteins, including structural proteins and intracellular enzymes that regulate nuclear and cytoplasmic activity.

The genes play a crucial role in the cell's reproduction. Through a unique process called mitosis, the cell divides into two daughter cells, with each receiving one set of DNA genes. Initially, the genes replicate to produce two identical sets.

Unfortunately, the microscopic appearance of the nucleus does not provide many clues about its regulatory functions. Figure 1.16 illustrates the light microscopic view of the interphase nucleus (during the interphase between mitoses), where the nucleoplasm contains darkly staining chromatin material. During mitosis, this chromatin material organizes into highly structured chromosomes, which are easily identifiable under a light microscope.

1.6.6.1. Nuclear Membrane

The nuclear membrane, known as the nuclear envelope, consists of two separate bilayer membranes that are nested within each other. The outer membrane is connected to the endoplasmic reticulum in the cell cytoplasm, and the gap between the two nuclear membranes is connected to the interior of the endoplasmic reticulum, as depicted in Figure 1.16.

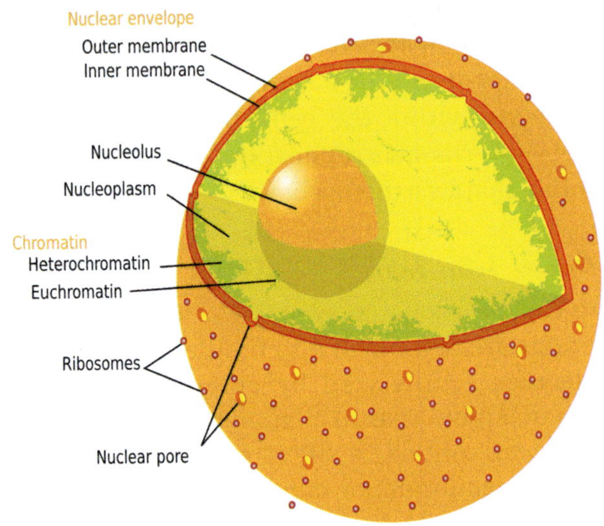

Figure 1.16. *Structure of the nucleus.*

Source: By Mariana Ruiz LadyofHats – I did it myself with adobe ilustrator using the information found here [1], [2],[3], [4] and [5], Public Domain, https://commons.wikimedia.org/w/index.php?curid=736389.

Several 1,000 nuclear pores penetrate the nuclear membrane, with large complexes of protein molecules attached at the edges. This results in the central area of each pore being approximately 9 nanometers in diameter, allowing molecules with a molecular weight of up to 44,000 to pass through easily.

1.6.7. Nucleoli and Formation of Ribosomes

Most cell nuclei include one or more nucleoli, which are highly staining structures. Unlike the majority of the other organelles covered here, the nucleolus lacks a limiting membrane. Rather, it is just a massive build-up of RNA and proteins similar to those in ribosomes. When the cell is actively making proteins, the nucleolus enlarges significantly.

The process of nucleoli formation, along with the assembly of ribosomes in the cytoplasm outside the nucleus, initiates within the nucleus. Initially, certain DNA genes within the chromosomes trigger the synthesis of RNA. While some of this RNA remains in the nucleoli, the majority is transported out through the nuclear pores into the cytoplasm. Once in the cytoplasm, the RNA combines with specific proteins to create functional ribosomes that are integral in the production of cytoplasmic proteins.

1.7. Functional Systems of the Cell

The remaining sections cover a number of illustrative cell functional systems that give rise to life.

1.7.1. Ingestion by the Cell – Endocytosis

For a cell to survive, thrive, and multiply, it needs to acquire nutrients and other substances from the surrounding fluids. The cell membrane facilitates this process through diffusion and active transport, allowing essential substances to enter the cell.

Substances move through cell membrane pores or, in the case of lipid-soluble substances, through the lipid matrix of the membrane due to diffusion, which is essentially simple movement through the membrane caused by the random motion of the substance's molecules.

Active transport is the process of physically moving a substance through the membrane using protein structures that extend through the entire membrane. These mechanisms are crucial for maintaining proper cell function and are essential for cell survival.

Endocytosis is a specialized function of the cell membrane that allows very large particles to enter the cell. Pinocytosis and phagocytosis are the two main types of endocytosis. Pinocytosis is the process by which small particles that are particulate constituents inside the cell cytoplasm and extracellular fluid vesicles are ingested. Ingestion of large particles, such as bacteria, entire cells, or sections of deteriorating tissue, is referred to as phagocytosis.

1.7.1.1. Pinocytosis

While pinocytosis is a continuous process in most cell membranes, in certain cells it occurs rapidly. For instance, in macrophages, it occurs at such a high rate that approximately 3% of the entire membrane is engulfed in the form of vesicles every minute. However, the majority of pinocytotic vesicles can only be observed under an electron microscope due to their extremely small size, typically ranging from 100 to 200 nanometers in diameter.

Most protein molecules and other large macromolecules can only enter cells through pinocytosis. The process of pinocytotic vesicle formation is typically enhanced when these macromolecules bind to the cell membrane.

The process of pinocytosis is depicted in Figure 1.17, where three protein molecules are observed adhering to the membrane. These molecules usually bind to specialized protein receptors on the membrane that are specific to the type of protein being absorbed.

The majority of the receptors are found in coated pits, which are tiny depressions on the exterior of the cell membrane. Below these pits in the cell membrane, there is a lattice of fibrillar proteins known as clathrin, along with other proteins such as contractile filaments of myosin and actin. The fibrillar proteins surrounding the invaginating pit cause the borders to close over the attached proteins and a small amount of extracellular fluid, resulting in the inward invagination of the entire pit once the protein molecules have bound to the receptors. Shortly after, the invaginated section of the membrane separates from the cell surface, forming a pinocytotic vesicle within the cell's cytoplasm.

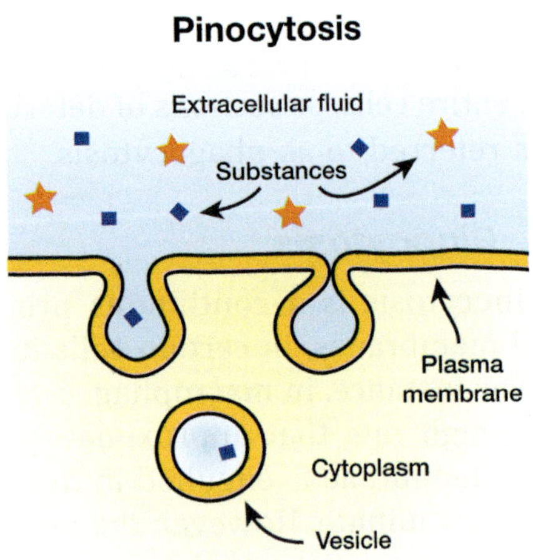

Figure 1.17. *Mechanism of pinocytosis.*

Source: By Jacek, F. H. – modified Image: Endocytosis types.svg, author Mariana Ruiz Villarreal LadyofHats, Public Domain, https://commons.wikimedia.org/w/index.php?curid=2738559.

The exact factors that trigger the necessary changes in the cell membrane to create pinocytotic vesicles are not yet fully understood. This mechanism relies on energy generated within the cell, provided by ATP, a high-energy molecule discussed further in the chapter. Additionally, the presence of calcium ions in the extracellular fluid is essential for this process, as they likely interact with contractile protein filaments located beneath the coated pits to facilitate the separation of vesicles from the cell membrane.

1.7.1.2. Phagocytosis

Pinocytosis and phagocytosis function similarly, but phagocytosis deals with larger particles rather than molecules. Phagocytosis is primarily carried out by specific cells, such as tissue macrophages and certain white blood cells.

During phagocytosis, when a particle such as a bacterium, dead cell, or tissue fragment attaches to receptors on the surface of the phagocyte, the process of phagocytosis is initiated. In the case of bacteria, each bacterium is typically already bound to a specific antibody, which binds to the phagocyte receptors and facilitates the engulfment of the bacterium. This antibody-mediated process is known as opsonization.

Phagocytosis occurs in the following steps:

1. The cell membrane receptors attach to the surface ligands of the particle.
2. The membrane edges surrounding the points of attachment rapidly extend outward to enclose the entire particle. More and more membrane receptors attach to the particle ligands in a sequential manner, forming a closed phagocytic vesicle.
3. Actin and other contractile fibrils in the cytoplasm surround the phagocytic vesicle and contract around its outer edge, propelling the vesicle towards the interior of the cell.
4. The contractile proteins then constrict the stem of the vesicle, causing it to separate from the cell membrane. This leaves the vesicle within the cell interior, similar to the formation of pinocytotic vesicles.

1.7.2. Digestion of Pinocytotic and Phagocytic Foreign Substances Inside the Cell – Function of the Lysosomes

As demonstrated in Figure 1.18, one or more lysosomes attach to a pinocytotic or phagocytic vesicle inside a cell almost immediately and release their acid hydrolases inside the vesicle. Consequently, a digestive vesicle is formed within the cytoplasm of the cell, wherein proteins, carbohydrates, lipids, and other materials are hydrolyzed by vesicular hydrolases. The byproducts of digestion, such as small molecules of amino acids, glucose, phosphates, and other compounds, can permeate through vesicle membranes and enter the cytoplasm. The residual body, composed of indigestible materials, remains after the breakdown of the digestive vesicle. In the majority of cases, exocytosis, which is essentially the opposite of endocytosis, is the process that ultimately excretes the residual body through the cell membrane.

Therefore, the pinocytotic and phagocytic vesicles containing lysosomes can be referred to as the cell's digestive organs.

1.7.2.1. Regression of Tissues and Autolysis of Cells

The body's tissues frequently undergo shrinkage. This phenomenon occurs, for instance, in the muscles during extended periods of inactivity, in the uterus following pregnancy, and in the mammary glands at the end of lactation. Lysosomes play a significant role in this contraction process. However, it remains unclear how lysosomes become more active when a tissue is not actively functioning.

The unique function of lysosomes also includes the removal of damaged cells or damaged cell parts from tissues. Lysosomes rupture when a cell sustains damage from heat, cold, trauma, chemicals, or any other source. The released hydrolases immediately begin to break down nearby organic materials. If the damage is minimal, only a portion of the cell is removed and the rest is repaired. In cases of severe damage, autolysis occurs, which is a process where the entire cell is broken down. As a result, the cell is completely eliminated and is typically replaced by a new cell of the same type that is generated through mitosis of an adjacent cell.

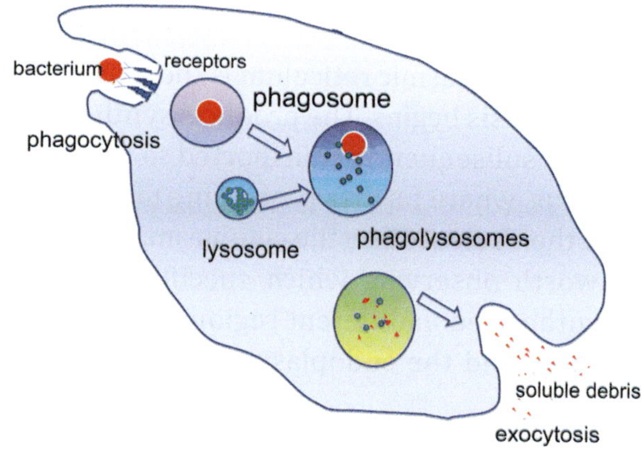

Figure 1.18. *Digestion of substances in pinocytotic or phagocytic vesicles by enzymes derived from lysosomes.*

Source: By GrahamColm at English Wikipedia, CC BY-SA 3.0, https://commons.wikimedia.org/w/index.php?curid=6811745.

Additionally, phagocytized bacteria can be killed by bactericidal agents found in lysosomes before they can harm cells. These agents include: (i) lysozyme, which breaks down the bacterial cell membrane; (ii) lysoferrin, which binds iron and other materials to prevent them from growing bacteria; and (iii) acid, which has a pH of roughly 5.0 and breaks down the bacterial metabolic systems and activates the hydrolases.

1.7.3. Synthesis and Formation of Cellular Structures by Endoplasmic Reticulum and Golgi Apparatus

1.7.3.1. Specific Functions of the Endoplasmic Reticulum

It has been previously noted that the Golgi apparatus and endoplasmic reticulum are extensive in secretory cells. These structures primarily consist of lipid bilayer membranes, resembling cell membranes. The walls of these structures are densely packed with protein enzymes that catalyze the synthesis of various compounds essential for the cell.

The endoplasmic reticulum is the site where most synthesis begins. The products synthesized there are subsequently transported to the Golgi apparatus, where further processing takes place before their release into the cytoplasm. However, it is worth observing which specific products are synthesized in different regions of the Golgi apparatus and the endoplasmic reticulum.

1.7.3.2. Proteins Are formed by the Granular Endoplasmic Reticulum

The granular portion of the endoplasmic reticulum is defined by a large number of ribosomes adhered to the outer surfaces of the membrane. These ribosomes are responsible for synthesizing protein molecules. While some of the synthesized protein molecules are directly released into the cytosol by the ribosomes, a significant amount is also extruded into the endoplasmic matrix through the wall of the endoplasmic reticulum and into the interior of endoplasmic vesicles and tubules.

1.7.3.3. Synthesis of Lipids by the Smooth Endoplasmic Reticulum

Lipids, particularly cholesterol and phospholipids, are also synthesized by the endoplasmic reticulum. The endoplasmic reticulum expands in size as a result of its quick incorporation into the lipid bilayer of the endoplasmic reticulum. This mostly affects the smooth region of the endoplasmic reticulum.

Small vesicles known as ER vesicles or transport vesicles continuously break away from the smooth reticulum to prevent the endoplasmic reticulum from growing beyond the needs of the cell; the majority of these vesicles then migrate rapidly to the Golgi apparatus.

Other significant functions of the endoplasmic reticulum, especially the smooth reticulum, include the following:

1. It provides the enzymes that control glycogen breakdown when glycogen is to be used for energy.
2. It provides a vast number of enzymes that are capable of detoxifying substances, such as drugs, that might damage the cell. It achieves detoxification by coagulation, oxidation, hydrolysis, conjugation with glucuronic acid, and in other ways.

1.7.3.4. Specific Functions of the Golgi Apparatus

Synthetic Functions of the Golgi Apparatus. The Golgi apparatus can synthesize certain carbohydrates that cannot be produced in the endoplasmic reticulum, despite its main function being to provide additional processing for substances already formed in the endoplasmic reticulum. This is especially true when large saccharide polymers are formed and attached to small amounts of protein; chondroitin sulfate and hyaluronic acid are two notable examples.

Hyaluronic acid and chondroitin sulfate have various roles in the body, including: (i) being major components of proteoglycans secreted in mucus and other glandular secretions; (ii) serving as major components of the ground substance outside the cells in the interstitial spaces, filling the gaps between collagen fibers and cells; (iii) being principal components of the organic matrix in both cartilage and bone; and (iv) playing important roles in numerous cell activities, such as migration and proliferation.

1.7.3.5. Processing of Endoplasmic Secretions by the Golgi Apparatus – Formation of Vesicles

The primary functions of the Golgi apparatus and endoplasmic reticulum are illustrated in Figure 1.19. When materials, particularly proteins, are synthesized in the endoplasmic reticulum, they are transported through tubules towards the regions of the smooth endoplasmic reticulum closest to the Golgi apparatus.

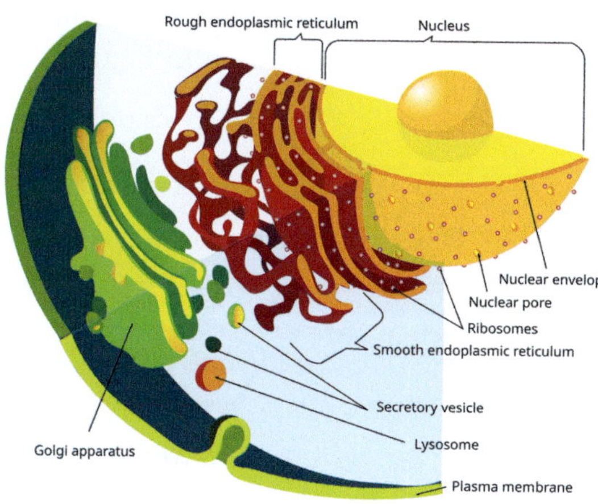

Figure 1.19. *Formation of proteins, lipids, and cellular vesicles by the endoplasmic reticulum and Golgi apparatus.*

Source: https://en.wikipedia.org/wiki/File:Endomembrane_system_diagram_en.svg.

At this stage, tiny transport vesicles derived from the smooth endoplasmic reticulum continuously detach and disperse towards the lower layer of the Golgi apparatus. These vesicles encapsulate the proteins and other products synthesized by the endoplasmic reticulum. The transport vesicles promptly merge with the Golgi apparatus and release their cargo into the vesicular spaces within the Golgi apparatus. At this point, the secretions undergo additional carbohydrate supplementation. The Golgi apparatus plays a crucial role in compacting the secretions from the endoplasmic reticulum into highly concentrated packets. This compaction and processing process continues as the secretions progress towards the outermost layers of the Golgi apparatus. Ultimately, the compacted secretory substances are transported by both large and small vesicles, repeatedly detaching from the Golgi apparatus and diffusing throughout the cell.

To indicate the timing of these processes, the following observations can be made: within a span of 3 to 5 minutes after exposure of a glandular cell to radioactive amino acids, newly synthesized radioactive protein molecules can be detected in the granular endoplasmic reticulum. The Golgi apparatus harbors nascent proteins within a mere 20 minutes, while radioactive proteins are secreted from the cell surface within a timeframe of 1 to 2 hours. Secretory vesicles and lysosomes represent two distinct types of vesicles formed by the Golgi apparatus. In highly secretory cells, the Golgi apparatus generates secretory vesicles primarily containing protein substances that are subsequently secreted through the cell membrane. Through a process known as exocytosis, these secretory vesicles initially diffuse towards the cell membrane, merge with it, and release their contents externally. In most instances, calcium ions permeate the cell and interact in an intricate manner with the vesicular membrane, leading to its fusion with the cell membrane and the subsequent initiation of exocytosis, which entails the opening of the outer surface of the membrane and the expulsion of its contents beyond the confines of the cell. Some vesicles, however, are destined for intracellular use.

1.7.3.6. Use of Intracellular Vesicles to Replenish Cellular Membranes

A portion of the intracellular vesicles generated by the Golgi apparatus merge with the cell membrane or with the membranes of intracellular organelles such as the endoplasmic reticulum and mitochondria. This process widens the membranes, replenishing them as they become depleted. For instance, the cell membrane constantly replenishes itself through the vesicular membranes of the Golgi apparatus, although it loses a significant amount of substance each time it forms a phagocytic or pinocytotic vesicle.

In conclusion, the membranous system of the endoplasmic reticulum and Golgi apparatus is a highly metabolic organ capable of creating new intracellular structures and secretory materials that can be extruded from the cell.

1.7.4. Extraction of Energy From Nutrients – Function of the Mitochondria

Carbohydrates, fats, and proteins are the main sources of energy for cells. These substances undergo chemical reactions with oxygen. The liver and digestive system convert most carbohydrates in the human body into glucose before they are absorbed by other cells. Similarly, fats are converted into fatty acids and proteins into amino acids. Glucose, fatty acids, and amino acids, along with oxygen, are all observed entering the cell. Inside the cell, food components and oxygen chemically interact with the assistance of enzymes that regulate the process and direct the released energy in the appropriate direction.

To summarize, the majority of oxidative reactions occur within the mitochondria, releasing energy to produce ATP. This high-energy compound is then utilized throughout the cell to power various metabolic processes, rather than relying solely on the original food sources.

1.7.4.1. Functional Characteristics of ATP

ATP is a nucleotide composed of adenine, ribose sugar, and three phosphate radicals. The last two phosphate radicals are connected by high-energy phosphate bonds represented by the symbol ~ in the formula. These high-energy bonds contain approximately 12,000 calories of energy per mole of ATP, which is significantly higher than the energy stored in average chemical bonds. Therefore, they are referred to as high-energy bonds. The high-energy phosphate bond can be easily broken to release energy when needed for cellular reactions, as shown in Figures 1.20 and 1.21.

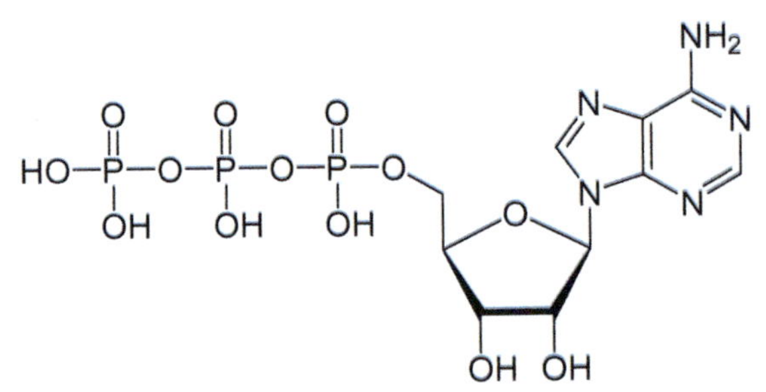

Figure 1.20. *Adenosine triphosphate.*

Source: By NEUROtiker – Own work, Public Domain, https://commons.wikimedia.org/w/index.php?curid=2194476.

After adenosine diphosphate (ADP) is created, a phosphoric acid radical is split off when ATP releases its energy. The released energy powers a variety of other processes within the cell, such as substance synthesis and muscle contraction.

$$ATP + H_2O \rightarrow ADP + P_i + Free\ energy$$

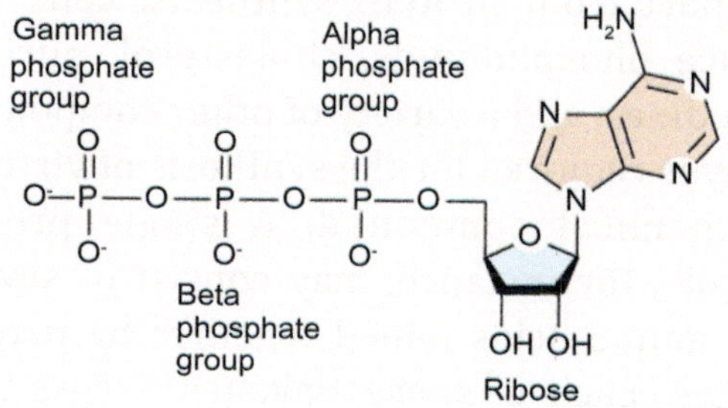

Figure 1.21. *Formation of adenosine triphosphate (ATP) in the cell, showing that most of the ATP is formed in the mitochondria. [ADP: adenosine diphosphate].*

Source: https://bio.libretexts.org/Bookshelves/Introductory_and_General_Biology/Book%3A_General_Biology_%28Boundless%29/06%3A_Metabolism/6.09%3A_ATP_-_Adenosine_Triphosphate.

Energy from cellular nutrients causes ADP and phosphoric acid to recombine, forming new ATP. This ATP is then used to replenish the cellular ATP as it is depleted. This process is repeated continuously. Due to these reasons, ATP is often referred to as the cell's energy currency. Its turnover time is short, typically just a few minutes, allowing for continuous usage and renewal.

1.7.4.2. Chemical Processes in the Formation of ATP Involve the Role of Mitochondria

Upon entering the cells, glucose undergoes glycolysis, where it is converted into pyruvic acid by cytoplasmic enzymes. The energy released during this conversion results in the production of a small amount of ATP from ADP. However, this conversion accounts for less than 5% of the cell's total energy metabolism.

Mitochondria are responsible for producing approximately 95% of the cell's ATP. In the mitochondrial matrix, carbohydrates are converted into pyruvic acid, lipids into fatty acids, and proteins into amino acids. These substances are further metabolized within the matrix by a different set of enzymes, undergoing a series of chemical reactions known as the Krebs cycle or citric acid cycle, in order to extract their energy.

During the citric acid cycle, acetyl-CoA is broken down into hydrogen atoms and carbon dioxide. The released carbon dioxide exits the mitochondria, leaves the cell, and is eventually expelled from the body through exhalation.

On the other hand, due to their high reactivity, the hydrogen atoms quickly combine with the oxygen that has also permeated the mitochondria. The mitochondria utilize the enormous amount of energy released by this process to convert a significant amount of ADP to ATP. Numerous protein enzymes that are essential components of the mitochondrial membranous shelves, extending into the mitochondrial matrix, must participate in these intricate reactions. The hydrogen atom first undergoes electron removal, transforming into a hydrogen ion. The final stage involves the reaction of hydrogen ions with oxygen to form water and the release of enormous energy to ATP synthetase, a large globular protein protruding from the mitochondrial shelf membranes like knobs. Finally, the enzyme ATP synthetase utilizes the energy from the hydrogen ions to convert ADP to ATP. The newly created ATP is transported by the mitochondria into the cytoplasm and nucleoplasm of every cell, where it is utilized as energy for various cellular processes. This entire process of ATP formation is referred to as the chemiosmotic mechanism of ATP formation.

1.7.4.3. Uses of ATP for Cellular Function

ATP is utilized for three main types of cellular processes: (i) material transport across multiple membranes within the cell; (ii) intracellular synthesis of chemical compounds; and (iii) mechanical work. Examples of these applications of ATP are shown in Figure 1.22: (a) providing energy for the translocation of sodium across the cell membrane; (b) promoting the production of new proteins by ribosomes; and (c) supplying the energy required for muscle contraction.

Apart from sodium, potassium, calcium, magnesium, phosphate, chloride, urate, hydrogen, and numerous other ions, as well as different organic substances, must be transported through membranes using energy from ATP. Membrane transport is so essential to cellular function that some cells, such as renal tubular cells, use up to 80% of their ATP synthesis just for membrane transport.

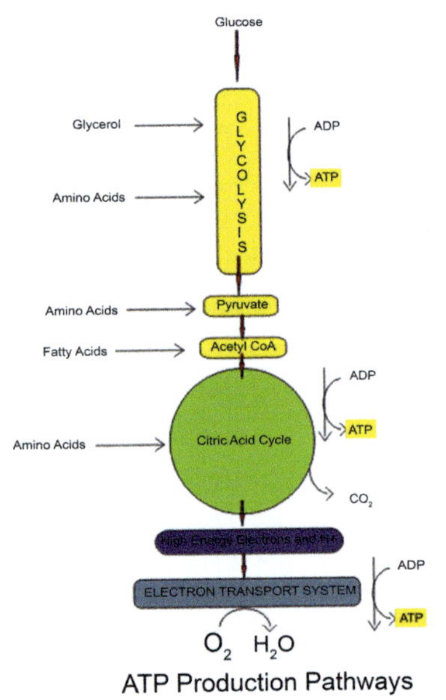

Figure 1.22. *Use of adenosine triphosphate (ATP) (formed in the mitochondrion) to provide energy for three major cellular functions: Membrane transport, protein synthesis, and muscle contraction. ADP, adenosine diphosphate.*

Source: By Boumphreyfr – Own work, CC BY-SA 3.0, https://commons.wikimedia.org/w/index.php?curid=6881456.

Apart from protein synthesis, cells also produce phospholipids, cholesterol, purines, pyrimidines, and a variety of other compounds. Energy is required for the synthesis of virtually any chemical compound. A single protein molecule, for instance, may consist of several 1,000 amino acids joined together by peptide linkages. Each of these linkages necessitates energy, which is obtained from the breakdown of four high-energy bonds. Consequently, thousands of ATP molecules must release their energy during the formation of each protein molecule. In fact, during the growth phase of cells, some cells utilize up to 75% of the ATP generated in the cell solely for the purpose of synthesizing new chemical compounds, particularly protein molecules.

The final major function of ATP is to provide power to certain cells so that they can carry out mechanical tasks. Enormous amounts of ATP energy must be expended during each muscle fiber contraction. Other cells employ different mechanisms to perform mechanical work, particularly ciliary and ameboid motion, which will be discussed later in this chapter. ATP serves as the energy source for each of these categories of mechanical labor.

In conclusion, ATP is constantly prepared to release energy wherever it is needed in the cell, doing so rapidly and almost explosively. Much slower chemical processes break down proteins, fats, and carbohydrates and utilize the energy from these breakdowns to generate new ATP and replenish the ATP that the cell utilizes. The mitochondria are commonly referred to as the "powerhouses" of the cell because they produce over 95% of the ATP that is required by the cell.

1.8. Locomotion of Cells

Since muscle cells comprise nearly half of the body's mass, the movement of skeletal, cardiac, and smooth muscle types is the most significant form of movement in the body. Other cells move in two different ways: ameboid locomotion and ciliary movement.

1.8.1. Ameboid Movement

Ameboid movement involves the movement of white blood cells through tissues. It refers to the movement of an entire cell in relation to its environment. The name is derived from the way amebae move, making them a valuable resource for studying this phenomenon.

Ameboid locomotion typically begins with a pseudopodium protruding from one end of the cell. The pseudopodium extends significantly from the cell body and anchors itself partially in a new tissue region. Subsequently, the remaining portion of the cell is drawn towards the direction of the pseudopodium. This process is depicted in Figure 1.23, which shows an elongated cell with a projecting pseudopodium at its right end. The membrane at the left end of the cell consistently follows the cell's path, while the membrane at the right end of the cell continuously moves forward.

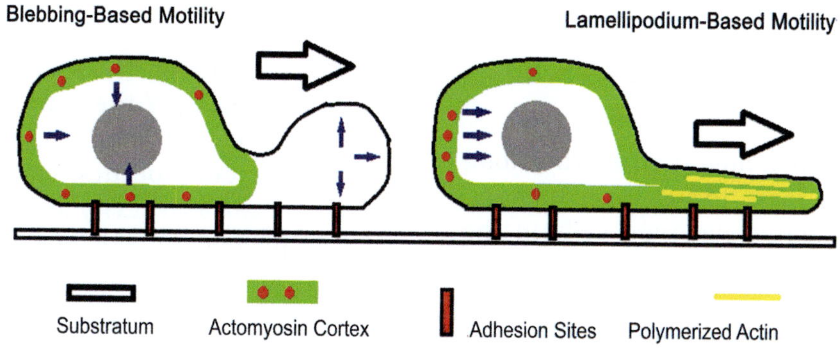

Figure 1.23. *Ameboid motion by a cell.*

Source: By Wikied007 - Own work, CC BY-SA 4.0, https://commons.wikimedia.org/w/index.php?curid=64760347.

1.8.1.1. Mechanism of Ameboid Locomotion

The general principle is depicted in Figure 1.23. Essentially, it is caused by the continuous synthesis of new cell membranes at the leading edge of the pseudopodium and the continuous absorption of that membrane in the cell's middle and posterior regions. Two additional effects are also necessary for the cell to move forward. The remaining portion of the cell body is drawn forward toward the point of attachment as the pseudopodium attaches to surrounding tissues to become fixed in its leading position. Receptor proteins lining the inside of exocytotic vesicles facilitate this attachment. The receptors now protrude to the outside and attach to ligands in the surrounding tissues as the vesicles open up to become a part of the pseudopodial membrane, allowing their interiors to shift to the outside.

The receptors separate from their ligands to form new endocytotic vesicles at the other end of the cell. These vesicles then flow inside the cell toward the pseudopodial end, where they are employed to create an additional membrane for the pseudopodium. Providing the energy needed to drag the cell body toward the pseudopodium is the second essential effect of locomotion.

The following explanation is supported by experiments: All cells have a moderate to large amount of the protein actin in their cytoplasm. A large portion of actin exists as single molecules that lack motive power; nevertheless, these molecules polymerize to create a filamentous network, which contracts when it binds to another actin-binding protein like myosin. The high-energy substance ATP powers the entire process. This is the process by which a new network of actin filaments forms inside the expanding pseudopodium of a moving cell. Additionally, contraction takes place in the cell body's ectoplasm, where a preexisting actin network is visible beneath the cell membrane.

1.8.1.2. Types of Cells That Exhibit Ameboid Locomotion

White blood cells, which migrate from the blood into the tissues to form tissue macrophages, are the most frequently observed cells in the human body to exhibit ameboid locomotion. Under certain conditions, other types of cells can also utilize ameboid locomotion to move. For instance, fibroblasts enter damaged areas to assist in repair, and even normally sessile skin germinal cells move toward a cut area to mend the opening. Additionally, cell motility plays a particularly significant role in the development of the embryo and fetus following ovum fertilization. During the development of special structures, embryonic cells often need to migrate over considerable distances from their original locations to new areas.

1.8.1.3. Control of Ameboid Locomotion – Chemotaxis

Chemotaxis is the primary process that initiates ameboid locomotion. This occurs as a result of specific chemical substances appearing in the tissues. A chemical substance is referred to as chemotactic if it induces chemotaxis. Positive chemotaxis involves the movement of most ameboid locomotor cells toward the source of a chemotactic substance or from a region of lower concentration to one of higher concentration. Negative chemotaxis, on the other hand, involves the movement of certain cells away from the source. Although the exact mechanism is unknown, it is understood that membrane alterations leading to pseudopodial protrusion occur on the side of the cell most exposed to the chemotactic substance. This suggests that chemotaxis regulates the direction of ameboid locomotion.

1.8.2. Cilia and Ciliary Movements

The whip-like movement of cilia on cell surfaces is known as ciliary movement, which is another form of cellular motion. The respiratory airways and the interior surfaces of the uterine tubes (fallopian tubes) of the reproductive tract are the exclusive sites in the human body where this phenomenon occurs. The whiplike motion of cilia in the nasal cavity and lower respiratory airways propels a layer of mucus towards the pharynx at a rate of approximately 1 cm/min, continuously clearing these passageways of mucus and particles that have become trapped. The cilia in the uterine tubes facilitate the gradual passage of fluid from the ostium of the tube into the uterus cavity, transporting the ovum from the ovary to the uterus.

A cilium extends 2 to 4 micrometers from the cell's surface and resembles a sharply pointed, straight or curved hair, as depicted in Figure 1.24. A single cell can generate a significant number of cilia; for instance, the surface of each epithelial cell in the respiratory pathways can possess up to 200 cilia. As shown in the cross-section in Figure 1.24, the cilium is supported by 11 microtubules, with 9 double tubules arranged around the cilium's periphery and 2 single tubules running through its center. The cilium is enveloped by an outcropping of the cell membrane. Each cilium originates from the basal body of the cilium, a structure located directly beneath the cell membrane.

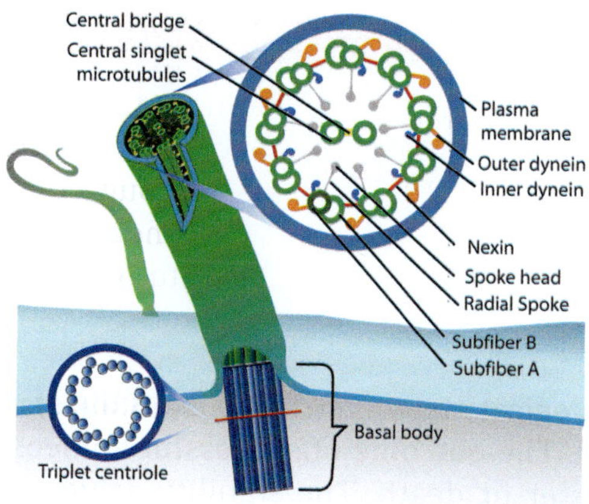

Figure 1.24. *Structure and function of the cilium.*

Source: By LadyofHats – Own work, Public Domain, https://commons.wikimedia.org/w/index.php?curid=3145956.

A sperm's flagellum and cilium are comparable in that they share many of the same structural elements and contractile mechanisms. Instead of moving like a whip, the flagellum is much longer and moves in quasi-sinusoidal waves. Around 10 to 20 times per second, the cilium moves forward in a sudden, whip-like stroke that bends sharply where it protrudes from the cell's surface. After that, it slowly returns to its starting position. The fluid next to the cell is pushed in the direction of the cilium's movement by the swift, whip-like movement thrusting forward; the slow, dragging movement in the opposite direction hardly affects the fluid's movement at all. As a result, the fluid keeps moving in the fast-forward stroke's direction. This is a useful method for transferring fluids from one area of the surface to another since the majority of ciliated cells have a large number of cilia on their surfaces and all of the cilia point in the same direction.

1.8.2.1. Mechanism of Ciliary Movement

First, it is known that the two single tubules and the nine double tubules are interconnected by a complex network of protein cross-linkages, collectively referred to as the axoneme. Despite this understanding, not all aspects of ciliary movement have been fully elucidated. Second, even after the removal of the membrane and destruction of all constituent parts except for the axoneme, the cilium can still exhibit beating motion under appropriate conditions. Third, for the axoneme to continue beating after the removal of other structures, two prerequisites must be met: (1) the availability of ATP; and (2) suitable ionic conditions, particularly the concentrations of calcium and magnesium. Fourth, the double tubules located at the front edge of the cilium slide outward towards the tip while those at the back edge remain stationary, facilitating the forward movement of the cilium. Fifth, each double tubule extends multiple protein arms towards an adjacent double tubule. These arms consist of the protein dynein, which possesses ATPase enzymatic activity.

Based on these fundamental details, it has been established that the heads of the ATPase dynein arms rapidly move along the surface of the neighboring double tubule upon ATP release. The bending of the cilium occurs as a result of the outward crawling of the front tubules while the back tubules remain fixed.

The regulation of ciliary contraction remains unknown. In certain genetically abnormal cells, the absence of the two central single tubules in their cilia prevents them from beating. This suggests that a signal, possibly of an electrochemical nature, is transmitted through these central tubules to initiate the movement of the dynein arms.

A Closer Look

Homeostasis

Homeostasis is a self-regulating process through which biological systems strive to maintain stability while adapting to conditions that are optimal for survival. The outcome of successful homeostasis is the continuation of life, while failure can lead to disaster or death. The stability achieved is a dynamic equilibrium, characterized by continuous change yet relatively consistent conditions. The concept of this self-regulating process was initially explored by French physiologist Claude Bernard in 1849, and the term "homeostasis" was coined by American neurologist and physiologist Walter Bradford Cannon in 1926.

Any system in dynamic equilibrium naturally tends to reach a steady state, a state of balance that resists external forces of change. When such a system is disrupted, inherent regulatory mechanisms respond to restore a new balance; this process is known as feedback control. All processes involving integration and coordination of functions, whether mediated by electrical circuits or by nervous and hormonal systems, exemplify homeostatic regulation.

A familiar example of homeostatic regulation in a mechanical system is the function of a room-temperature regulator or thermostat. The core component of the thermostat is a bimetallic strip that reacts to temperature changes by completing or interrupting an electric circuit. When the room cools, the circuit is completed, activating the furnace and raising the temperature. Once the preset level is reached, the circuit breaks, the furnace stops, and the temperature decreases. Biological systems are more intricate and possess regulators that are only loosely comparable to mechanical devices. However, both types of systems share the common goal of sustaining activity within a defined range, whether it is controlling the thickness of rolled steel or regulating the pressure within the circulatory system.

The control of body temperature in humans is a good example of homeostasis in a biological system. In humans, normal body temperature fluctuates around the value of 37°C (98.6°F), but various factors can affect this value, including exposure, hormones, metabolic rate, and disease, leading to excessively high or low temperatures. The body's temperature regulation is controlled by a region in the brain called the hypothalamus. Feedback about body temperature is carried through the nervous system to the brain and results in compensatory adjustments in the breathing rate, the level of blood sugar, and the metabolic rate. The circulatory system also plays important roles: its baroreceptors (pressure-sensitive receptors in the blood vessels that respond to stretching) relay blood pressure information back to the brain, and it transports hormones secreted by the hypothalamus and the thyroid gland to regulate the body's metabolism. Heat loss in humans is aided by the reduction of activity, by perspiration, and by heat-exchange mechanisms that permit larger amounts of blood to circulate near the skin surface. Heat loss is reduced by insulation, decreased circulation to the skin, and cultural modification such as the use of clothing, shelter, and external heat sources. The range between high and low body temperature levels constitutes the homeostatic plateau—the "normal" range that sustains life. As either of the two extremes is approached, corrective action (through negative feedback) returns the system to the normal range.

The concept of homeostasis has also been applied to ecological settings. First proposed by Canadian-born American ecologist Robert MacArthur in 1955, homeostasis in ecosystems is a product of the combination of biodiversity and a large number of ecological interactions that occur between species. It was thought of as a concept that could help explain the stability of an ecosystem, that is, its persistence as a particular ecosystem type over time (see ecological resilience). Since then, the concept has slightly changed to incorporate the abiotic (nonliving) parts of the ecosystem. The term has been used by many ecologists to describe the reciprocation that occurs between the living and nonliving parts of an ecosystem to maintain the status quo. The Gaia hypothesis, proposed by English scientist James Lovelock, considers the various living and nonliving parts of Earth as components of a larger system or single organism. It assumes that the collective effort of individual organisms contributes to homeostasis at the planetary level. The single-organism aspect of the Gaia hypothesis is considered controversial because it posits that living things, at some level, are driven to work on behalf of the biosphere rather than toward the goal of their own survival.

Summary

- The study of physiology covers a broad range of biological processes that are necessary for living things to function.
- The human body is a carefully designed reactor for chemical processes. The body is made up of trillions of atoms arranged in precise ways and thousands of chemical reactions that happen in a very well-organized way.
- Cells are the smallest structural and functional unit of living things. Human cells come in a wide variety of forms, yet they all share some characteristics.
- An organ is an assemblage of tissues that have been meticulously positioned to carry out specific functions. The kidneys, individual bones, liver, lungs, and stomach are a few instances of organs.
- Conversely, negative feedback mechanisms possess their own brakes due to the presence of numerous inhibitory pathways, which are an inherent component of the cycle.
- The cranial cavity and the vertebral or spinal cavity constitute the dorsal cavity, which accommodates the central nervous system.
- In general, the notions of stability, equilibrium, and balance are associated with homeostasis. It necessitates continuous observation and adjustment when circumstances change in order to maintain a stable internal environment.

References

1. Alberts, B., Johnson, A., Lewis, J., et al., (2007). *Molecular Biology of the Cell* (6th edn.). New York, Garland Science.
2. Bonifacino, J. S., & Glick, B. S., (2004). The mechanisms of vesicle budding and fusion. *Cell 116*, 153.
3. Chacinska, A., Koehler, C. M., Milenkovic, D., Lithgow, T., & Pfanner, N., (2009). Importing mitochondrial proteins: Machineries and mechanisms. *Cell, 138*, 628.
4. Cohen, A. W., Hnasko, R., Schubert, W., & Lisanti, M. P., (2004). Role of caveolae and caveolins in health and disease. *Physiol. Rev., 84*, 1341.
5. Danial, N. N., & Korsmeyer, S. J., (2004). Cell death: Critical control points. *Cell, 116*, 205.
6. Dröge, W., (2002). Free radicals in the physiological control of cell function. *Physiol. Rev., 82*, 47.
7. Edidin, M., (2003). Lipids on the frontier: A century of cell-membrane bilayers. *Nat. Rev. Mol. Cell Biol., 4*, 414.
8. Ginger, M. L., Portman, N., & McKean, P. G., (2008). Swimming with protists: Perception, motility, and flagellum assembly. *Nat. Rev. Microbiol., 6*, 838.
9. Grant, B. D., & Donaldson, J. G., (2009). Pathways and mechanisms of endocytic recycling. *Nat. Rev. Mol. Cell Biol., 10*, 597.
10. Güttinger, S., Laurell, E., & Kutay, U., (2009). Orchestrating nuclear envelope disassembly and reassembly during mitosis. *Nat. Rev. Mol. Cell Biol., 10*, 178.
11. Hamill, O. P., & Martinac, B., (2001). Molecular basis of mechanotransduction in living cells. *Physiol. Rev., 81*, 685.

12. Hock, M. B., & Kralli, A., (2009). Transcriptional control of mitochondrial biogenesis and function. *Annu. Rev. Physiol., 71*, 177.

13. Liesa, M., Palacín, M., & Zorzano, A., (2009). Mitochondrial dynamics in mammalian health and disease. *Physiol. Rev., 89*, 799.

14. Mattaj, I. W., (2004). Sorting out the nuclear envelope from the endoplasmic reticulum. *Nat. Rev. Mol. Cell Biol., 5*, 65.

15. Parton, R. G., & Simons, K., (2007). The multiple faces of caveolae. *Nat. Rev. Mol. Cell Biol., 8*, 185.

16. Raiborg, C., & Stenmark, H., (2009). The ESCRT machinery in endosomal sorting of ubiquitylated membrane proteins. *Nature, 458*, 445.

17. Ridley, A. J., Schwartz, M. A., Burridge, K., et al., (2003). Cell migration: Integrating signals from front to back. *Science, 302*, 1704.

18. Saftig, P., & Klumperman, J., (2009). Lysosome biogenesis and lysosomal membrane proteins: Trafficking meets function. *Nat. Rev. Mol. Cell Biol., 10*, 623.

19. Scarpulla, R. C., (2008). Transcriptional paradigms in mammalian mitochondrial biogenesis and function. *Physiol. Rev., 88*, 611.

20. Stenmark, H., (2009). Rab GTPases as coordinators of vesicle traffic. *Nat. Rev. Mol. Cell Biol., 10*, 513.

21. Traub, L. M., (2009). Tickets to ride: Selecting cargo for clathrin-regulated internalization, *Nat. Rev. Mol. Cell Biol., 10*, 583.

22. Vereb, G., Szollosi, J., Matko, J., et al., (2003). Dynamic, yet structured: The cell membrane three decades after the Singer-Nicolson model. *Proc. Natl. Acad. Sci. U S A., 100*, 8053.

Chapter

2

BODY TISSUES

Contents

Unit Introduction

The word "tissue" refers to a collection of cells that are present in the body collectively. Tissue cells are all descended from the same embryo. The morphological characteristics of a tissue are shared by its cells, which are arranged in a systematic way to carry out the functions of the tissue, as revealed by microscopic observation. From an evolutionary standpoint, more complex organisms have tissues. For instance, the cells of multicellular protists, which are extinct eukaryotes, are not arranged into tissues. The human body contains a wide variety of cell types, but they are generally grouped into four types of tissues: neural, muscle, connective, and epithelial. Each of these groups is distinguished by particular roles that support the body's general upkeep and health. A break in the structure indicates an illness or injury. Histology, the microscopic study of tissue appearance, organization, and function, can identify these changes.

Orientation and Directional Terms:

Term	Definition	Illustration
Epithelial tissue	Epithelial tissue is a large sheet of cells that covers the body's surfaces and lines the outside of organs.	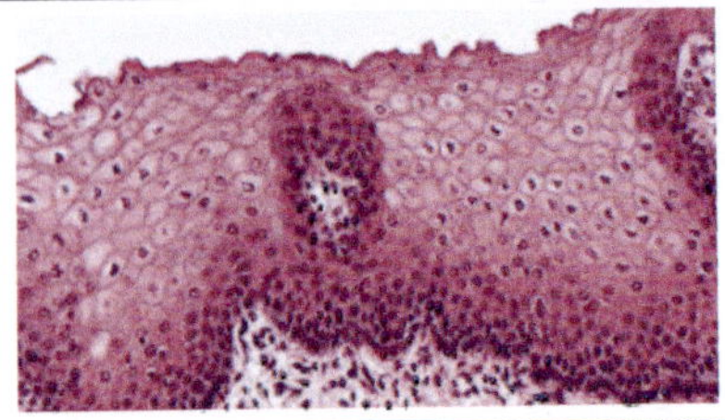
Ciliated epithelium	Ciliated epithelium is a tissue that lines certain parts of the body. It is composed of columnar cells with microscopic hairlike projections called cilia.	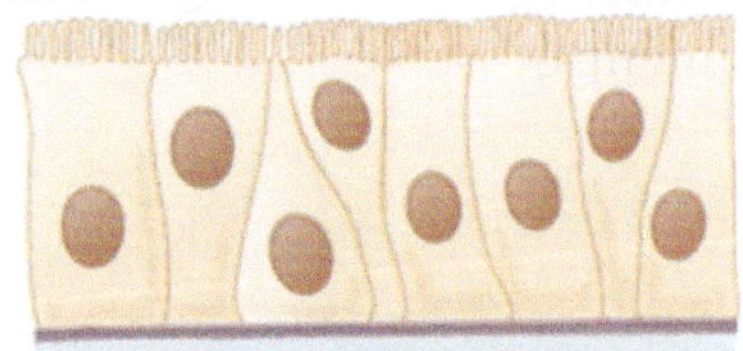 ***Ciliated Epithelium***
Adipose tissue	Adipose tissue, also known as body fat, is a connective tissue that stores energy and regulates metabolism. It is found throughout the body, including under the skin, around organs, and within bone marrow.	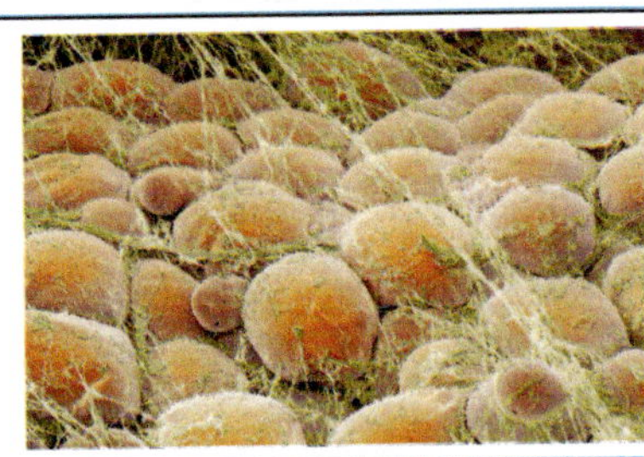
Cartilage	Cartilage is a strong and flexible connective tissue that protects your joints and bones.	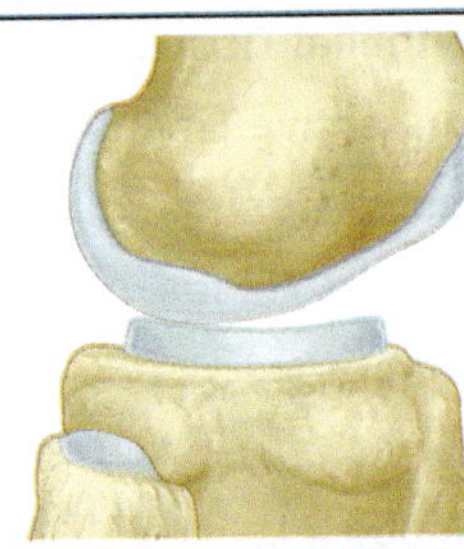
Mucous membranes	Mucous membranes, also known as mucosa, are moist tissues that line the body's canals and organs.	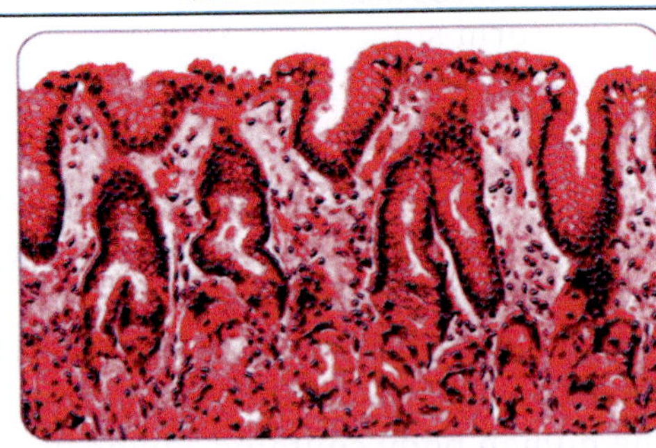 Mucous membrane

2.1. Overview of Tissues

Tissues are composed of a mixture of intercellular materials and cells in different ratios, with one component taking center stage. For instance, nerve cells predominate in nervous tissue, whereas intercellular fibrous materials predominate in connective tissues like ligaments and tendons. Therefore, one could define a tissue as being made up of cells that are similar to one another in terms of structure, function, and intercellular materials. Throughout the body's development, cells specialize before aggregating to form body tissues based on shared structural and functional characteristics. The body's high degree of organization and labor distribution is the result of this arrangement. An organ is said to be formed when different proportions of tissues are put together to create a functional entity. An organ's structure and functional capabilities are determined by the arrangement of its tissues (Figure 2.1).

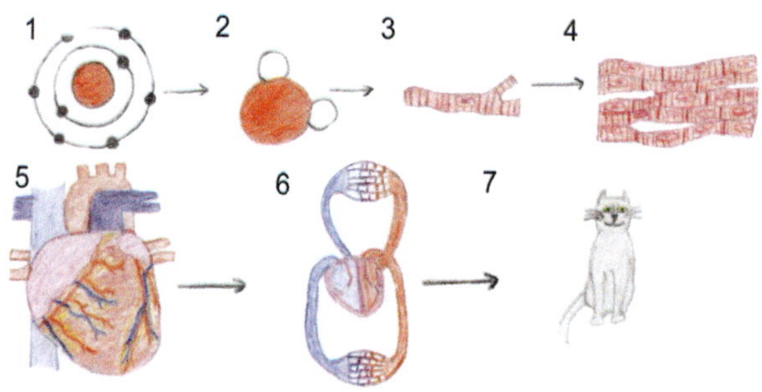

Figure 2.1. *Organization of tissues.*

Note: (1) The most basic level of anatomical organization is the atom. (2) Molecules are made up of atoms. (3) Many different molecules make up a cell (The shown cell is a cardiac muscle cell). (4) Cells make up tissue (The shown cell is cardiac muscle). (5) Tissues make up organs (The shown organ is a heart). And (6) Organs working together make up an organ system (The shown organ system is a circulatory system).

Source: https://en.wikipedia.org/wiki/File:Anatomical_Levels_of_Organization.JPG.

The sheets of cells that line the body's interior cavities and passageways, cover its external surfaces, and form some glands are collectively referred to as epithelial tissue or epithelium. As its name suggests, connective tissue serves to integrate, support, and bind the body's cells and organs together, as well as provide protection for each individual part. There are three main types of muscle tissue: smooth muscle, cardiac muscle in the heart, and skeletal (voluntary) muscle. Muscle tissue is excitable, responding to stimulation and contracting to provide movement. Additionally, excitable is nervous tissue, which facilitates the transmission of electrochemical signals in the form of nerve impulses that link various bodily parts.

2.2. Types of Tissues

The human body is composed of four primary tissue types. These are frequently referred to as the primary (basic) tissues. The body's fundamental tissues consist of the following (Figure 2.2):

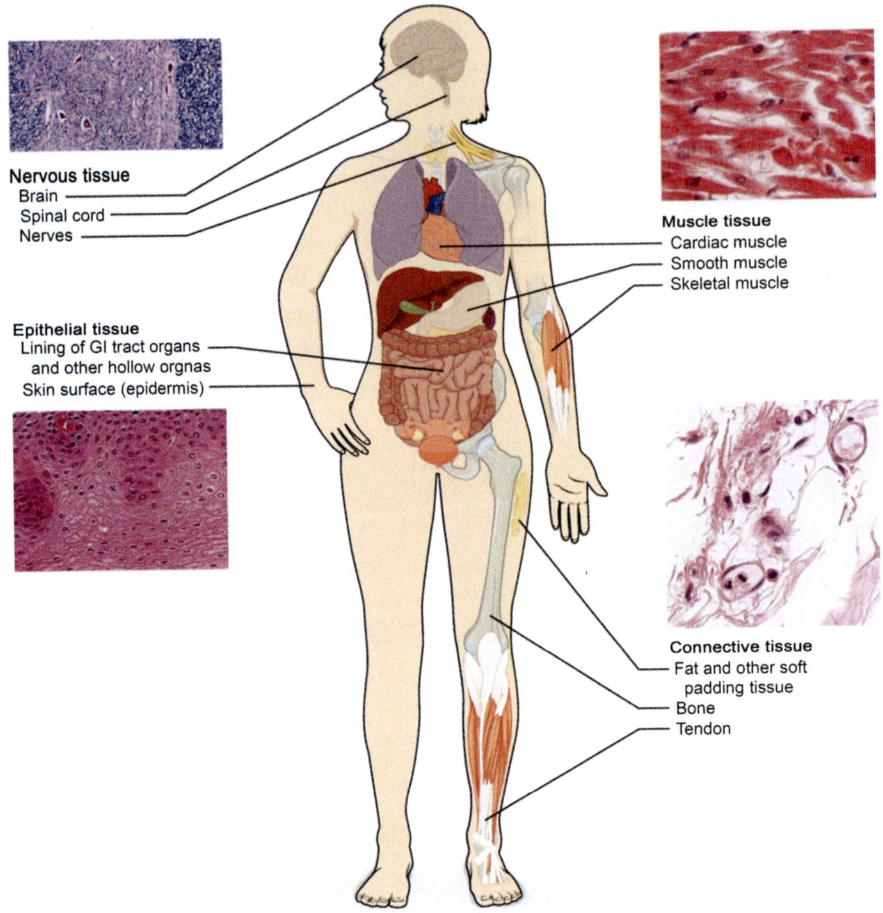

Figure 2.2. *Types of tissues.*

Source: https://courses.lumenlearning.com/suny-dutchess-ap1/chapter/animal-primary-tissues/.

2.2.1. Epithelial (Covering) Tissue

The body's cavities and tubes, as well as its exterior and interior surfaces, are covered in epithelial tissue. The epithelium contains cells in three distinct shapes.

These are:

i. Squamous (Flat) cells;

ii. Cuboidal cells; and

iii. Columnar cells.

These three cell types can be arranged in the following ways:

- A single layer to form a simple epithelium, such as the lining of the stomach (columnar epithelium).
- Several layers to form a compound (stratified) epithelium, such as the epidermis of the skin (squamous epithelium).

2.2.2. Connective Tissue

This tissue provides structural and metabolic support by connecting cells with other bodily tissues. It also serves as a conduit for waste elimination and nutrient delivery to bodily tissues and organs. Connective tissue consists of the extracellular matrix (ground substance), collagen, reticular and elastic fibers, and specialized cells called fibroblasts, as well as intercellular fibrous materials. Connective tissue is the most prevalent type of tissue in the body.

Examples of connective tissues include:

- Bones;
- Cartilage;
- Ligaments, tendons, and facial sheath;
- Areola tissue;
- Adipose (Fat) tissue;
- Blood;
- Mucous.

2.2.3. Muscle Tissue

Highly specialized contractile cells, frequently elongated in shape, constitute muscle tissue. They are responsible for coordinating the movement of body parts. Muscle fibers are the individual cells that make up muscle tissue.

Muscle tissue can be classified into four main types:

1. Smooth muscles, which line the walls of tubular structures such as blood vessels, as well as hollow organs like the stomach and urinary bladder. These muscles are under involuntary control.
2. Striated skeletal muscles, which are attached to bones and enable movement at the joints. These muscles are under voluntary control.
3. Striated non-skeletal muscles, which are not attached to bones and are also under involuntary control.
4. Striated cardiac muscles, which form the walls of the heart and are responsible for the heartbeat. These muscles are under involuntary control.

2.2.4. Nervous Tissue

This tissue is responsible for the body's ability to appropriately respond to its surroundings and be aware of both internal and external environments. It consists of specialized cells called neurons, which are highly conductive and irritable (also known as excitable). Neuroglia, which are supporting and nourishing cells for neurons, are also part of nervous tissue. The nervous system of the body is composed of nerve tissue, which includes the spinal cord, spinal nerve fibers, brain cranial nerves, and various organs and receptor cells.

2.3. Epithelial Tissue

A layer of cells that lines a bodily cavity or covers a body surface is called an epithelium, or "covering" (Figure 2.3).

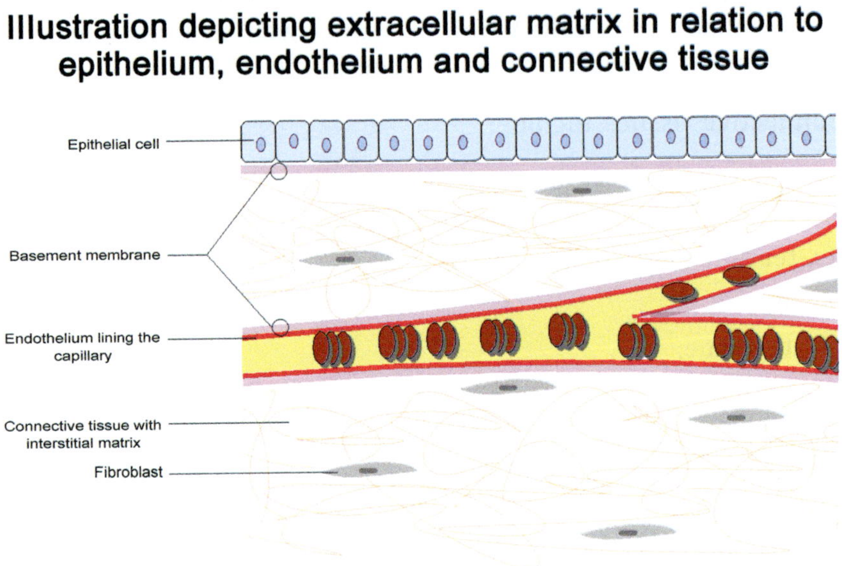

Figure 2.3. *A sheet of closely joined epithelial cells rests on connective tissue. Epithelia contain nerve endings but no blood vessels. Note the special features on the epithelial cell surfaces.*

Source: By Twooars – en:wp, Public Domain, https://commons.wikimedia.org/w/index.php?curid=4516905.

Epithelial tissue occurs in two different forms:

1. **Covering and Lining Epithelium:** It covers the outer and inner surfaces of most body organs. Examples include the outer layer of the skin, the inner lining of all hollow viscera such as the stomach and respiratory tubes, the lining of the peritoneal cavity, and the lining of all blood vessels.
2. **Glandular Epithelium:** It forms most of the body's glands. Epithelia are found where two distinct environments converge. For instance, the epidermis of the skin is situated between the interior and exterior of the body. The majority of substances that are either released from or enter the body must pass through an epithelium. Consequently, the functions of epithelial tissues are all reflective of their roles as interfaces. These functions include:
   - Protection of the underlying tissues.
   - Secretion (release of molecules from cells).
   - Absorption (uptake of small molecules into cells).
   - Diffusion (movement of molecules along their concentration gradient).
   - Filtration (passage of small molecules through a sieve-like membrane).
   - Sensory reception.

2.3.1. Special Characteristics of Epithelia

Epithelial tissues possess several characteristics that distinguish them from other tissue types (Figure 2.3):

1. **Cellularity:** Epithelia are primarily composed of cells, with minimal extracellular material. The narrow spaces between cells are mainly occupied by projections of their integral membrane proteins.
2. **Specialized Contacts:** Adjacent epithelial cells are directly joined at multiple points through special cell junctions.
3. **Polarity:** All epithelia have a free apical surface and an attached basal surface. The apical and basal surfaces differ in structure and function, exhibiting polarity. The apical surface is in contact with the open space of a cavity, tubule, gland, or hollow organ, while the basal surface rests on a thin supporting sheet called the basal lamina, which is part of the basement membrane.
4. **Support by Connective Tissue:** Epithelial sheets in the body are supported by an underlying layer of connective tissue.
5. **Avascular But Innervated:** Unlike most tissues in the body that contain blood vessels, epithelium is avascular, meaning it lacks blood vessels. Epithelial cells obtain nutrients from capillaries in the underlying connective tissue. Although blood vessels do not penetrate epithelial sheets, nerve endings do; thus, the epithelium is innervated.
6. **Regeneration:** Epithelial tissue has a high regenerative capacity. Some epithelia are exposed to friction, and their surface cells rub off. Others are destroyed by hostile substances in the external environment such as bacteria, acids, and smoke. As long as epithelial cells receive adequate nutrition, they can replace lost cells quickly by mitosis, cell division.

2.3.2. Classification of Epithelia

In the body, epithelia come in a variety of forms. The number of cell layers and the shape of the cells are the two characteristics that are used to categorize and name epithelia (Figure 2.4). The number of cell layers in an epithelium is described by the terms simple and stratified (Figure 2.4).

1. **Simple Epithelia:** These contain a single layer of cells, with each cell attached to the basement membrane.
2. **Stratified Epithelia:** These contain more than one layer of cells. The cells on the basal surface are attached to the basement membrane; those on the apical surface border an open space.

Squamous, cuboidal, or columnar cell shapes are used to characterize the appearance of the cells in section (Figure 2.4). In every instance, the nucleus's shape matches the cell's shape. When identifying different epithelial types, this is a crucial characteristic to look for.

- **Squamous Cells:** These (sqwa'mus; "scale") are flat cells with flat, disc-shaped nuclei.
- **Cuboidal Cells:** These are cube-shaped cells with spherical, centrally located nuclei.
- **Columnar Cells:** These are taller than they are wide, like columns. The nuclei of columnar cells are located near the basal surface and are commonly oval in shape, elongated from top to bottom.

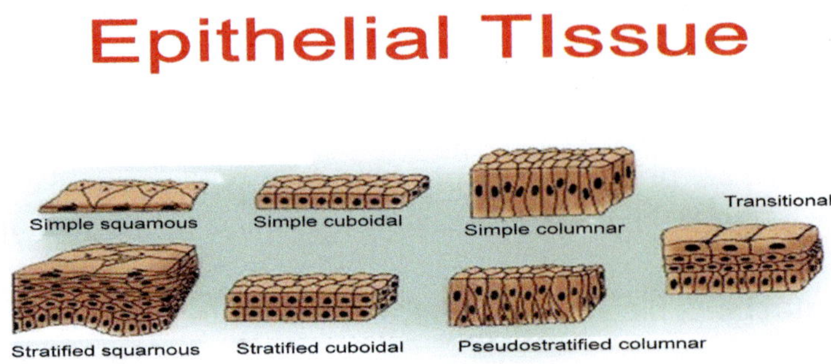

Figure 2.4. *Classification of epithelia.*

Source: By US Government – http://training.seer.cancer.gov/module_anatomy/images/illu_epithelium.jpg,which now seems to appear athttps://training.seer.cancer.gov/images/anatomy/cells_tissues_membranes/epithelium_tissue.jpgon this page: https://training.seer.cancer.gov/anatomy/cells_tissues_membranes/tissues/epithelial.html, Public Domain, https://commons.wikimedia.org/w/index.php?curid=1273805.

Table 2.1. *Function of Epithelial Tissue Related to Tissue Type*

Different Types of Epithelial Tissues		
Cell Shape	Description	Location
Squamous	Flat, irregular round shape	Simple: lung alveoli, capillaries; stratified: skin, mouth, vagina
Cuboidal	Cube shaped, central nucleus	Glands, renal tubules
Columnar	Tall, narrow, nucleus toward base; tall, narrow, nucleus along cell	Simple: digestive tract; pseudostratified: respiratory tract
Transitional	Round, simple but appear stratified	Urinary bladder

Source: https://courses.lumenlearning.com/suny-dutchess-ap1/chapter/animal-primary-tissues/.

Since all of the cells in a layer typically have the same shape, simple epithelia are simple to categorize based on cell shape. However, in stratified epithelia, the various cell layers typically have different cell shapes. Stratified epithelia are named based on the apical layer cell shape to prevent confusion. It is helpful to remember that tissue function is reflected in tissue structure (Table 2.1). The purpose of stratified epithelial tissues is protection. In regions where abrasion is frequent, the underlying connective tissues are shielded by several layers of cells. Simple epithelia show tissue function through the morphology of their cells. Because diffusion and filtration are distance-dependent processes, with the speed of the process increasing as the layer becomes thinner, squamous cells are typically found in environments where these processes play a significant role. On the other hand, organs involved in secretion and absorption are composed of columnar and cuboidal cells. These cells are larger in size due to the additional cellular machinery required for the production and packaging of secretions, as well as the energy generation needed for these processes. Ciliated epithelia are responsible for propelling mucus and other substances. When examining different types of epithelial tissue, it is important to keep these generalizations in mind. Take a close look at micrographs of various epithelium types (Figure 2.5) and make an effort to identify individual cells within each type. However, this task may not always be simple as it can be challenging to distinguish the boundaries between epithelial cells. Additionally, depending on the plane of the tissue slide, the nucleus of a specific cell may or may not be visible. Just like slices from the top and middle of a pear, tissue sections may or may not contain cells with visible nuclei, depending on the cut made.

2.3.2.1. Simple Epithelia

1. **Simple Squamous Epithelium (Figure 2.5(a)):** One layer of flat cells makes up a simple squamous epithelium. The closely fitting cells have the appearance of a tiled floor when viewed from above. They have a side-on appearance similar to fried eggs when viewed in lateral section. This kind of thin, frequently permeable epithelium develops wherever small molecules swiftly diffuse or filter through a membrane. This epithelium is the only material that makes up capillary walls, and because of its extreme thinness, waste products and nutrients are efficiently exchanged between the surrounding tissue cells and the bloodstream. This epithelium creates the slender walls of the air sacs in the lungs, which are the sites of gas exchange.

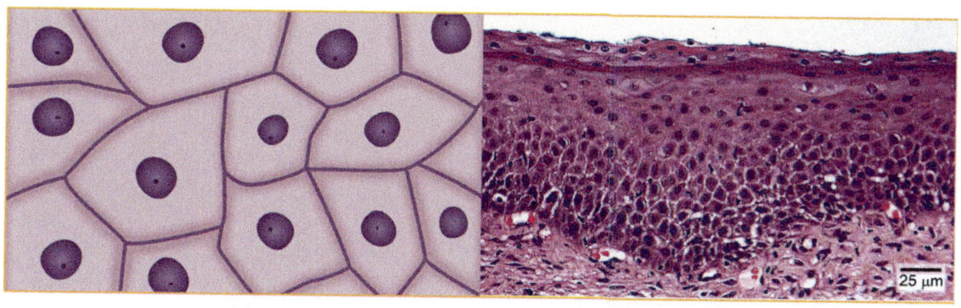

(a) (b)

Figure 2.5(a). *Simple squamous epithelium forming part of the cervix.*

Source: https://courses.lumenlearning.com/suny-dutchess-ap1/chapter/animal-primary-tissues/.

2. **Simple Cuboidal Epithelium (Figure 2.5(b)):** Simple cuboidal epithelium is composed of cube-shaped cells that are arranged in a single layer. This type of epithelium forms the walls of small gland ducts, the secretory cells of various glands, and the tubule walls of the kidneys. Its functions are similar to those of the simple columnar epithelium.
3. **Simple Columnar Epithelium (Figure 2.5(c)):** A single layer of tall cells arranged in a row, resembling soldiers, constitutes the simple columnar epithelium. This epithelium covers the tube responsible for transporting food from the stomach to the rectum. It plays a crucial role in the active transport of molecules, particularly in secretion and absorption. The structure of the simple columnar epithelium is well-suited for these functions, as it is sufficiently thick to accommodate the cellular machinery required for intricate molecular transport processes, yet thin enough to facilitate the rapid flow of a large number of molecules. Some basic columnar epithelia possess whip-like bristles known as cilia, located at the apex of the epithelial cells. These cilia beat rhythmically, facilitating the transfer of materials across specific body surfaces (*refer* Figure 2.3). The interior of the uterine tube is lined with a basic ciliated columnar epithelium. The cilia within this epithelium aid in the transportation of the ovum to the uterus.

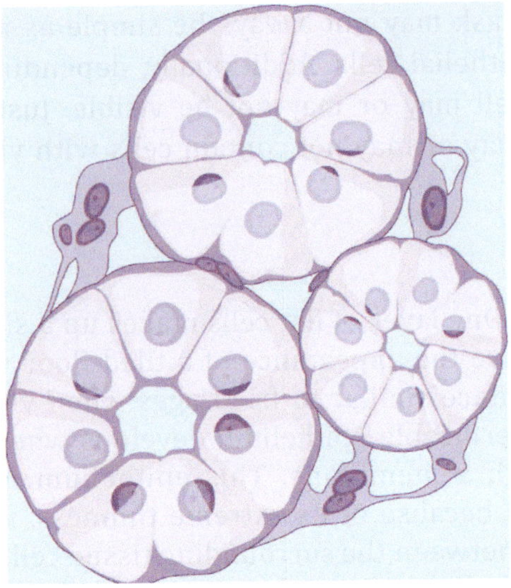

Figure 2.5(b). *Simple cuboidal epithelium in kidney tubules.*

Source: https://courses.lumenlearning.com/suny-dutchess-ap1/chapter/animal-primary-tissues/.

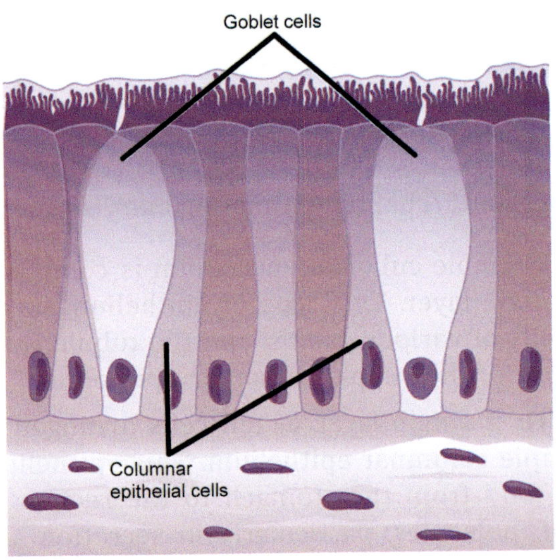

Figure 2.5(c). *Simple columnar epithelium of the small intestine.*

Source: https://courses.lumenlearning.com/suny-dutchess-ap1/chapter/animal-primary-tissues/.

4. **Pseudostratified Columnar Epithelium (Figure 2.5(d)):** The height of the pseudostratified columnar epithelium cells varies. Only the tall cells reach the apical surface of the epithelium; all other cells rest on the basement membrane. The tall cells are constantly proliferating from the undifferentiated short cells. The false impression that this epithelium is stratified is caused by the cell nuclei, which are arranged at multiple levels (pseudo = false).

   Similar to simple columnar epithelium, pseudostratified epithelium is involved in secretion or absorption. The respiratory tubes' interior is lined with ciliated type. Here, the cilia expel sheets of mucus from the lungs that trap dust.

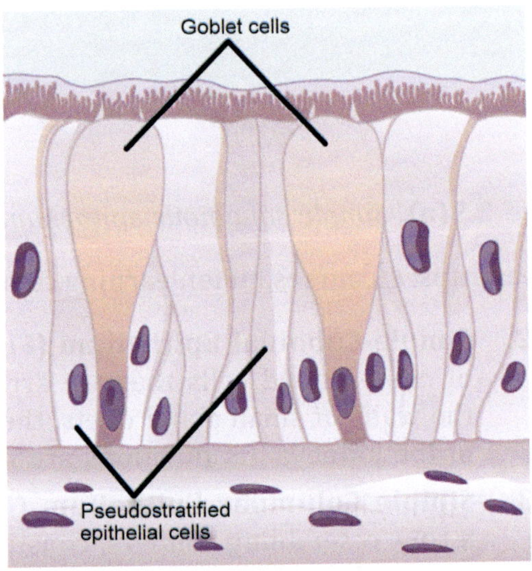

Figure 2.5(d). *Pseudostratified ciliated columnar epithelium lining the human trachea.*

Source: https://courses.lumenlearning.com/suny-dutchess-ap1/chapter/animal-primary-tissues/.

5. **Stratified Epithelia:** A stratified epithelium consists of two or more layers of cells. These layers regenerate

from the bottom, with basal cells dividing and pushing upwards to replace the older surface cells. Stratified epithelia are more resilient compared to simple epithelia, and one of their main functions, although not the only one, is defense.

6. **Stratified Squamous Epithelium (Figure 2.5(e)):** Stratified squamous epithelium, as depicted in Figure 2.5(e), is composed of multiple layers of cells with squamous surface cells, as one would expect. The deeper layers consist of columnar or cuboidal cells. This type of epithelium is the thickest and most suitable for protection among all types.

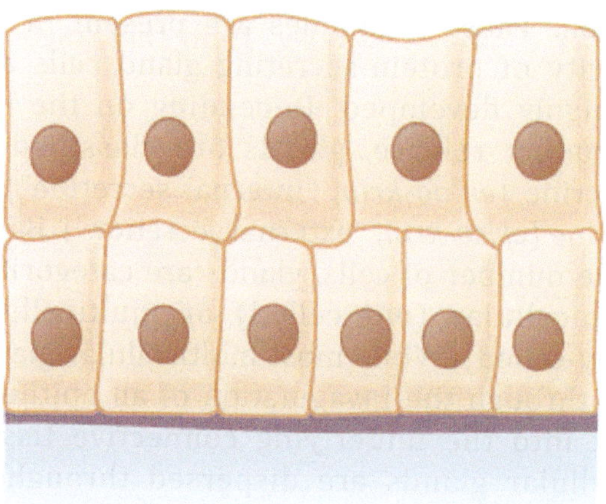

Figure 2.5(e). *Stratified squamous epithelium lining the esophagus.*

Source: By Jmarchn – File:403_Epithelial_Tissue.jpg, CC BY-SA 3.0, https://commons.wikimedia.org/w/index.php?curid=98469267.

It lines the inner surfaces of the mouth, esophagus, and vagina, as well as the epidermis of the skin, which covers the frequently abraded surfaces of our body. It is important to note that stratified squamous epithelium forms the outermost layer of the skin and extends into any bodily opening that is directly connected to the skin. The epidermis of the skin is keratinized, meaning that it contains keratin, an exceptionally durable protective protein, in its surface cells. Other stratified squamous epithelia in the body are nonkeratinized, indicating the absence of keratin.

7. **Stratified Cuboidal and Columnar Epithelia (Figures 2.5(f) and 2.5(g)):** Rare tissue types called stratified cuboidal and stratified columnar epithelia can be found in the large ducts of some glands, such as the salivary, mammary, and sweat glands. The male urethra also contains trace amounts of stratified columnar epithelium.

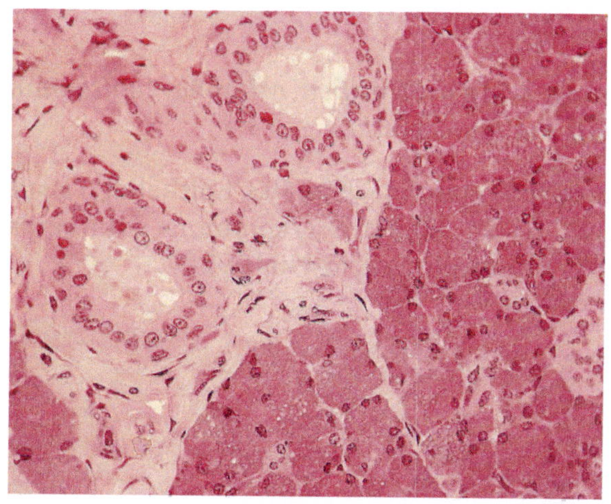

Figure 2.5(f). *Stratified cuboidal epithelium forming a salivary gland duct.*

Source: By Wbensmith – Own work, CC BY 3.0, https://commons.wikimedia.org/w/index.php?curid=2845814.

8. **Transitional Epithelium (Figure 2.5(h)):** Urinary organ hollows are lined on the inside by transitional epithelium. These organs, such as the bladder, expand when they fill with urine. The apical cells of the transitional epithelium unfold and flatten as it stretches, thinning from

roughly six to three cell layers. Parts of the apical surface invade the cell when it is relaxed, giving the surface a scalloped look. This epithelium therefore experiences "transitions" in shape. Additionally, it creates an impermeable barrier that prevents urine from penetrating the bladder wall.

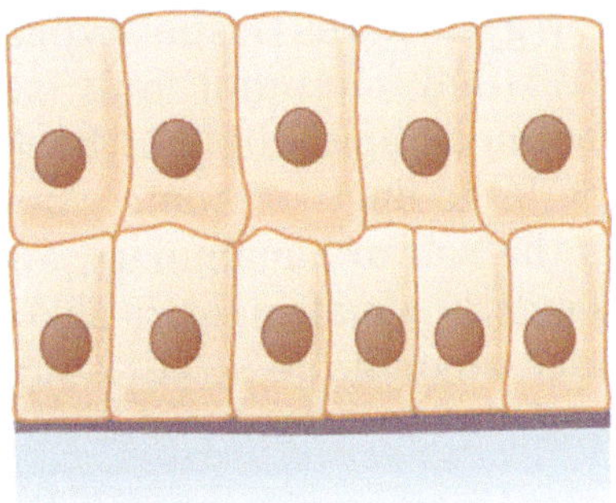

Figure 2.5(g). *Stratified columnar epithelium lining the male urethra.*

Source: By Jmarchn – File:403_Epithelial_Tissue.jpg, CC BY-SA 3.0, https://commons.wikimedia.org/w/index.php?curid=98469267.

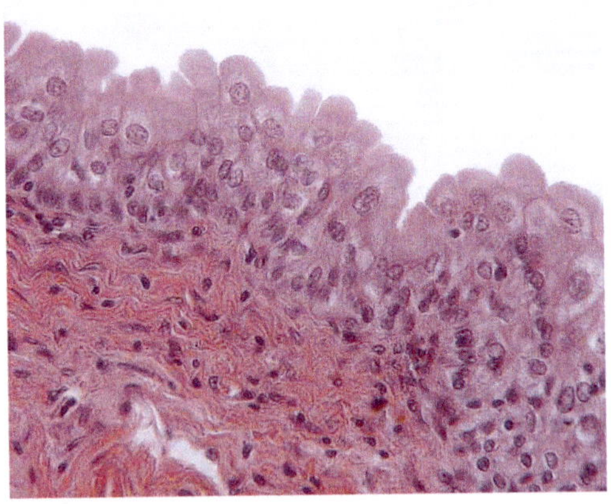

Figure 2.5(h). *Transitional epithelium lines the bladder.*

Source: By User:Polarlys – Own work, CC BY 2.5, https://commons.wikimedia.org/w/index.php?curid=988065.

Note: In its relaxed state, the cells at the surface have a bulbous, or rounded, appearance. However, when the bladder is filled with urine, these cells flatten and become elongated.

2.3.2.2. Glands

Glands are composed of epithelial cells that secrete a product. Aqueous fluids, which are produced by glands, typically contain proteins. The process by which gland cells extract necessary substances from the blood and chemically convert them into a product that is subsequently released from the cell is known as secretion. Specifically, the rough endoplasmic reticulum (ER) generates the protein product, which is then assembled into secretory granules by the Golgi apparatus and exocytosed out of the cell. These organelles are present in the majority of protein-secreting gland cells and are highly developed. Depending on the site of product release, glands are classified as endocrine (*en′do-krin*; "internal secretion") or exocrine (*ek′so-krin*; "external secretion"). Based on the number of cells, glands are categorized as unicellular (one-celled) or multicellular (many-celled). While most multicellular glands form through the invagination of an epithelial sheet into the underlying connective tissue, unicellular glands are dispersed throughout epithelial sheets.

1. **Endocrine Glands:** These are sometimes called ductless glands because they don't have ducts. They immediately release their contents into the surrounding tissue fluid. To be more precise, hormones (hor′mōnz; "exciters") are messenger molecules that are produced by endocrine glands and released into the extracellular space. The target organs for these hormones are often distant from the endocrine gland that produces them. The hormones then enter adjacent capillaries and move through the

bloodstream to reach their intended locations. Every hormone instructs the organs it targets to react in a particular way. Endocrine cells found in the intestine, for instance, secrete a hormone that instructs the pancreas to release the enzymes necessary for meal digestion. While epithelia is the source of most endocrine glands, some also originate from other tissues.

2. **Exocrine Glands:** There are numerous exocrine glands that produce a wide range of well-known products. Each exocrine gland releases its contents onto the skin or into bodily cavities, such as the digestive tube. Multicellular exocrine glands are equipped with ducts that transport their secretions to the epithelial surfaces. These secretions have localized activity, acting in close proximity to the site of release. Exocrine glands encompass a diverse group of organs, including the liver (which secretes bile), the pancreas (which secretes digestive enzymes), the mammary glands (which secrete milk), the sweat and oil glands of the skin, the salivary glands of the mouth, and many others.
3. **Unicellular Exocrine Glands:** Unicellular exocrine glands are exemplified by the goblet cell (Figure 2.6). Resembling a goblet, a drinking glass with a stem, the goblet cell is the sole noteworthy instance of a single-celled exocrine gland. Goblet cells are dispersed among columnar cells with various functions in the epithelial lining of the intestinal and respiratory tubes. They produce a glycoprotein called mucin, which is a sugar protein that dissolves in water when secreted. The resulting mucus is a viscous and slimy mixture of mucin and water. Mucus covers, protects, and lubricates numerous internal body surfaces.

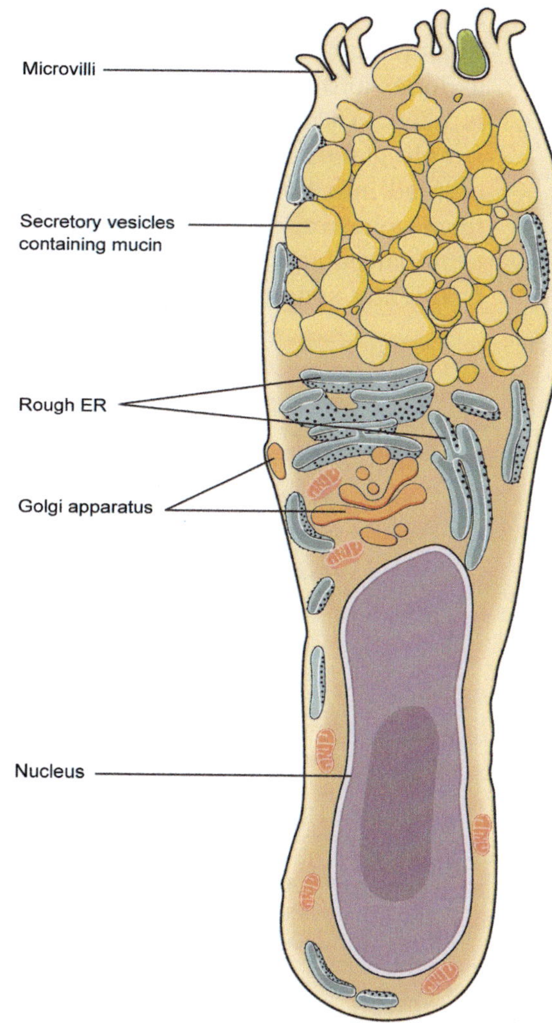

Figure 2.6. *Goblet cell (unicellular exocrine gland).*

Source: By OpenStax College – Anatomy & Physiology, Connexions Web site. http://cnx.org/content/col11496/1.6/, Jun 19, 2013., CC BY 3.0, https://commons.wikimedia.org/w/index.php?curid=30131227.

4. **Multicellular Exocrine Glands:** The two fundamental components of every multicellular exocrine gland are the secretory unit, which is composed of the secretory epithelium, and the epithelium-walled duct (Figure 2.7). Additionally, the secretory unit in all but the most basic glands is surrounded

by a supporting connective tissue that carries nerve fibers and blood vessels. The fibrous capsule that the connective tissue frequently forms divides the gland into sections known as lobes and extends into the gland proper. The ductal structure of multicellular glands is used to classify them (Figure 2.7). Compound glands have a branched duct, while simple glands have an unbranched duct. The secretory units of the glands are further divided into two groups: tubular glands, which form tubes, and alveolar glands, which form spherical sacs (an alveolus is a tiny, hollow cavity). Moreover, certain glands are tubuloalveolar, meaning they have both alveolar and tubular secretory units. Alveolar is frequently synonymous with the term acinar (as′|-nar; ı acinus = grape or berry).

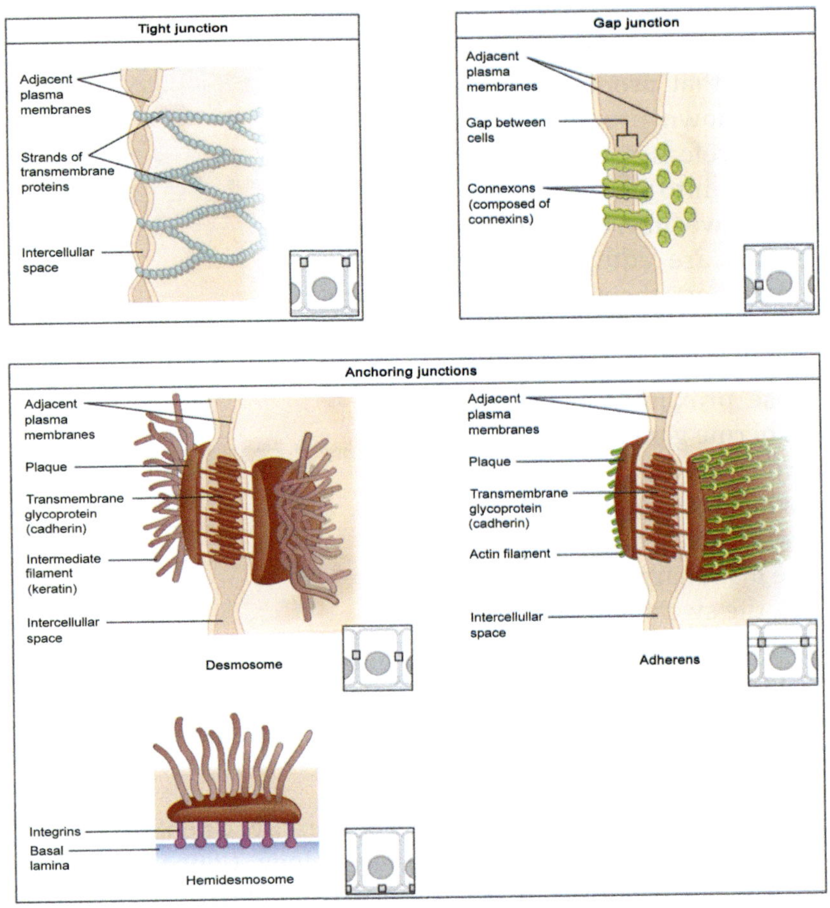

Figure 2.7. *Types of multicellular exocrine glands. Multicellular glands are classified according to the structure of their ducts (simple or compound) and the structure of their secretory units (tubular, alveolar, tubuloalveolar).).*

Source: https://courses.lumenlearning.com/suny-ap1/chapter/epithelial-tissue/.

2.3.3. Epithelial Surface Features

Numerous cells closely connected by unique cell junctions along their lateral walls make up epithelial tissues. Additionally, the apical and basal regions of epithelial tissues are unique. The underlying connective tissue and basal surface are separated by a specialized boundary; some epithelia have modifications in their apical region that are linked to particular functions.

2.3.3.1. Lateral Surface Features

1. **Cell Junctions:** Three factors act to bind epithelial cells to one another:
    - Adhesion proteins in the plasma membranes of the adjacent cells link together in the narrow extracellular space;
    - The wavy contours of the membranes of adjacent cells join in a tongue-and-groove fashion.
    - There are special cell junctions (Figure 2.8). Cell junctions, the most important of the factors, are characteristic of epithelial tissue but are found in other tissue types as well.

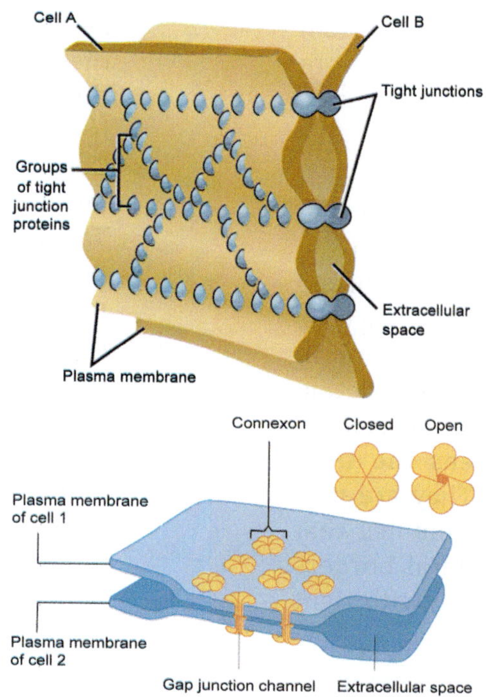

(a) Tight junctions: Impermeable junctions prevent molecules from passing through the intercellular space.

(b) Desmosomes: Anchoring junctions bind adjacent cells together and help form an internal tension-reducing network of fibers.

(c) Gap junctions: Communicating junctions allow ions and small molecules to pass from one cell to the next for intercellular communication.

Figure 2.8. *Cell junctions. An epithelial cell is shown joined to adjacent cells by three common types of cell junction.*

Source: https://courses.lumenlearning.com/suny-wmopen-biology1/chapter/the-cell-surface/.

2. **Tight Junctions:** A belt-like junction encircles the periphery of each cell in the apical region of the majority of epithelial tissues (Figure 2.8). This structure is known as a zonula occludens, which is a tight junction (pronounced "small zone that shuts off," z¯on′u-lah

o-klood'enz). Certain proteins in the plasma membranes of neighboring cells fuse together at tight junctions due to their close proximity. Tight junctions create a seal that closes off the extracellular space, preventing molecules from moving between the cells that compose the epithelium. For example, tight junctions in the epithelium lining the digestive tract prevent digestive enzymes, ions, and microbes from entering the bloodstream. It is not necessary for tight junctions to be completely impermeable; some can allow certain ions to pass through and are more prone to leakage than others.

3. **Adhesive Belt Junctions:** This also known as zonula adherens, are a type of anchoring junction located directly beneath tight junctions in epithelial tissues. Transmembrane linker proteins bind neighboring cells together by adhering to the actin microfilaments of the cytoskeleton. When the tissues are stretched, this junction strengthens the tight junctions, particularly. They are part of the tight junctional complex that surrounds the apical lateral borders of epithelial tissues, along with tight junctions.

4. **Desmosomes:** This also known as anchoring junctions, (dez'mo-s¯omz; "binding bodies"), are the main junctions that hold cells together. These adhesive patches are distributed along the adjacent cells' abutting sides. Desmosomes are complex structures with a circular plaque on the cytoplasmic face of each plasma membrane. Linker proteins bind the adjacent cell plaques together. These proteins protrude from both cell membranes and interdigitate in the extracellular space, resembling the teeth of a zipper. Moreover, intermediate filaments, which are cytoskeletal components that withstand tension, insert themselves from the inner, cytoplasmic side of each plaque. These filaments form bundles that cross the cytoplasm and attach to desmosomes on the other side of the same cell. Overall, this configuration not only keeps neighboring cells joined together but also connects the intermediate filaments of the entire epithelium into a single, uninterrupted network of strong guy-wires. Due to the even distribution of pulling forces throughout the sheet, the epithelium is less likely to tear when pulled on. Desmosomes are found in both cardiac muscle tissue and epithelial tissues. These junctions are typically observed in tissues that experience significant mechanical stress.

5. **Gap Junctions:** Anywhere along the lateral membranes of neighboring cells is where a gap junction, also known as a nexus (nek'sus; "bond"), can form. Gap junctions facilitate direct movement of small molecules between adjacent cells, which is how they work in intercellular communication. Connexons, which are hollow cylinders made of protein, connect the cells at these junctions where the adjacent plasma membranes are extremely close to one another. These cylinders allow small molecules, including ions, to move from one cell to the next. Both embryonic and adult tissues, including connective tissues, frequently contain gap junctions. They are also widely distributed in cardiac and smooth muscle, where ion transport via gap junctions synchronizes contraction.

2.4. Connective Tissue

Connective tissue, the most varied and prevalent type of tissue, is the second of the four fundamental types of tissue. Connective tissue is categorized into four primary classes and numerous subclasses.

The main classes are:

- Connective tissue proper, familiar examples of which are adipose tissue and the fibrous tissue of ligaments;
- Cartilage;
- Bone tissue;
- Blood.

The functions of connective tissues extend far beyond their role in joining the body's tissues and organs. They also serve as the building blocks of the skeleton (bone and cartilage), store and transport nutrients (blood and fat tissue), encircle all of the body's blood vessels and nerves (connective tissue proper), and spearhead the immune system's defense against infection.

2.4.1. Special Characteristics of Connective Tissues

Bone, adipose tissue, and hemoglobin are all connective tissues, notwithstanding their disparities. The fundamental structural framework of all connective tissues remains identical (Figure 2.9).

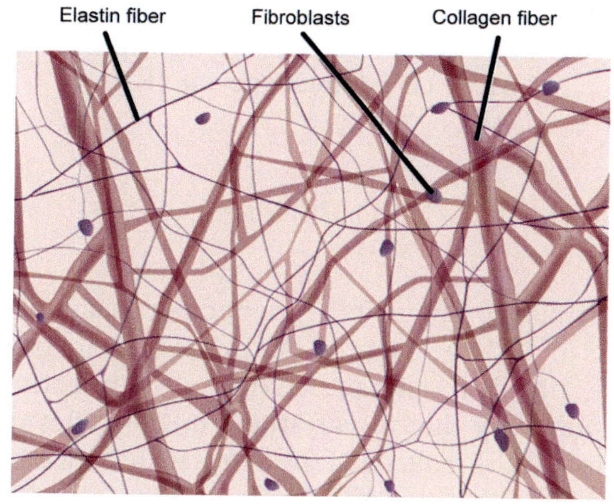

Figure 2.9. *Areolar connective tissue: A model connective tissue.*

Source: https://courses.lumenlearning.com/suny-dutchess-ap1/chapter/animal-primary-tissues/.

1. **Relatively Few Cells, Lots of Extracellular Matrix:** Connective tissues have relatively few cells but contain a significant amount of extracellular matrix. The cells in connective tissues are separated by a substantial amount of extracellular material known as the extracellular matrix. This is in contrast to epithelial tissue, where cells are closely packed together.

2. **Extracellular Matrix Composed of Ground Substance and Fibers:** The extracellular matrix is composed of ground substance and fibers, which are produced by the cells of connective tissue. The ground substance varies depending on the class of connective tissue, ranging from a soft, gel-like substance that holds tissue fluid to a hard, calcified substance in bone due to inorganic calcium salts. The fibrous portion of the matrix provides support for the connective tissue. There are three types of protein fibers found in connective tissues: collagen fibers, reticular fibers, and elastic fibers. The types, density, and distribution of these fibers are unique to each type of connective tissue. The variations in the physical properties and functions of connective tissues are attributed to differences in the composition of the extracellular matrix. The structure of the matrix will be discussed in detail for each type of connective tissue.

3. **Embryonic Origin:** Connective tissues share a common embryonic origin from a tissue called mesenchyme (Figure 2.10).

2.4.2. Structural Elements of Connective Tissues

The main components of connective tissues are cells and a large quantity of extracellular matrix. The physical characteristics of connective tissues vary due to variations in the types of cells and the makeup of the extracellular matrix. However, the structural components of cells, fibers, and ground substance are the same for all connective tissues.

2.4.2.1. Cells

Fibroblasts, also known as “fiber buds” or “fiber formers,” are the primary cell type that produces the extracellular matrix that makes up the connective tissue proper in the majority of connective tissues. Fibroblasts produce the protein building blocks of fibers, which are then secreted into the extracellular matrix and assembled into fibers. Additionally, fibroblasts secrete the molecules that form the foundation of the matrix. Chondroblasts (kon′dro-blasts; “cartilage formers”) are the cells that secrete the matrix in cartilage tissue, and osteoblasts (os′te-o-blasts′; “bone formers”) are the cells that perform the same function in bone. Once these tissue-forming cells stop actively secreting new matrix, they are referred to as fibrocytes, chondrocytes, and osteocytes (cyte = cell). Their role is to maintain and repair the tissue matrix while preserving the integrity of the tissue.

An exception to this is the cells present in blood. These cells do not contribute to the plasma matrix of blood. The cellular components of blood serve three purposes: aiding in blood clotting (platelets), fighting infections (white blood cells), and transporting respiratory gases (red blood cells). Additional cell types are found in many connective tissues (Figure 2.9):

- Adipose (ad′-|-p ˉı os) or fat cells store nutrients. The cytoplasm of fat cells is dominated by a single, enormous lipid droplet that flattens the cytoplasm and nucleus at one end of the cell. Fat cells are shaped like eggs. Mature fat cells are incapable of proliferating and are among the largest cells in the body.
- Neutrophils, lymphocytes, and eosinophils are types of white blood cells that react to and defend against infectious agents.
- Macrophages play a crucial role in phagocytosis, engulfing and consuming a wide range of foreign materials such as whole bacteria, foreign molecules, dirt particles, and dead tissue cells. They regulate inflammation and encourage recovery. Large secretory granules containing a variety of chemicals are found inside mast cells. These granules are secreted in reaction to agents that cause allergies and infections. Mast cells secrete various chemicals, such as histamine, which increases localized blood flow and capillary permeability, heparin, which interacts with other mast cell chemicals, and proteases, which are enzymes that break down proteins.

2.4.2.2. Fibers

Fibers and ground substance comprise the extracellular matrix of connective tissue (Figure 2.9). Connective tissues are composed of three types of fibers: collagen fibers, reticular fibers, and elastic fibers. While the primary function of these fibers is to provide support, each type contributes unique characteristics to the connective tissue.

Collagen fibers, depicted as thick, whitish-gray fibers in Figures 2.9 and 2.10, are the strongest and most abundant type of fiber in connective tissues. They confer strength and resistance to tension, or pulling forces. In fact, collagen fibers exhibit greater strength than steel fibers of the same size, as demonstrated by pulling tests! Under a light microscope, the observed thick collagen fibers are actually bundles of thinner collagen fibrils, which consist of even thinner strands tightly interconnected with each other. This cross-linking is responsible for the high tensile strength of collagen.

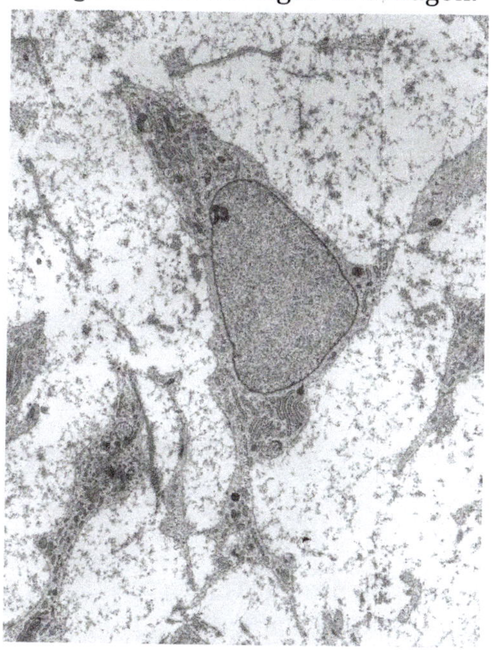

Figure 2.10(a). *Mesenchyme, an embryonic connective tissue. The matrix is composed of the fluid ground substance (clear-appearing background) and fine, sparse fibers.*

Source: By Robert M. Hunt - Own work, CC BY 3.0, https://commons.wikimedia.org/w/index.php?curid=28384153.

Reticular (re-tik'u-lar) fibers, depicted as thin blue fibers in Figures 2.9 and 2.10, are bundles of a distinct type of collagen fibril. These small fibers aggregate to form a mesh-like network (reticulum = network), which covers and supports the adjacent structures of the connective tissue. For example, reticular fibers are present in the basement membrane of epithelial tissues and form fuzzy nets within capillaries. Due to their ability to freely move across one another within the network, reticular fibers allow for greater flexibility compared to collagen fibers when subjected to pulling forces.

The ability to function like rubber bands is attributed to the presence of the rubberlike protein elastin (e-last'in) in elastic fibers (Figures 2.9 and 2.10). Rubber bands are commonly associated with stretchiness, but what really distinguishes an elastic material is its capacity to return to its initial shape after being stretched.

Before the thick, rope-like collagen fibers in connective tissue become taut, the tissue can only be stretched so far. The stretched tissue returns to its original shape as the elastic fibers recoil when the tension is released.

2.4.2.3. Ground Substance

The ground substance is the other part of the connective tissue matrix (Figure 2.9). Fibroblasts, chondroblasts, or osteoblasts—the main cell type of connective tissue—produce and secrete the molecules that make up the ground substance. Most connective tissues are made of a gel-like substance called glycosaminoglycans and proteoglycans, which are large sugar and sugar-protein molecules. These molecules have the ability to absorb liquid. The ground substance that is filled with fluid serves three purposes: it can retain the fluid that surrounds all of our cells (areolar connective tissue), cushion and protect bodily structures (connective tissue proper), or endure compressive stresses (cartilage). The calcified mineral salts embedded in the secreted ground substance of bone tissue give the matrix its hardness and aid in its ability to support the body. Again, blood is an exception in this case. The blood cells do not produce plasma, the ground substance of blood. About 90% of blood plasma is made up of water, with the remaining molecules being dissolved proteins, nutrients, ions, gases, and other substances. These molecules enter the bloodstream from an external source (water, air, and nutrients) or are produced by cells in other organs and then secreted into the blood (hormones and plasma proteins, for example).

Gelatin, jellybeans, and licorice are a few basic ingredients that can be used to construct a model of connective tissue. After dissolving the gelatin, allow it to solidify. The gelatin represents the ground substance of the connective tissue, consisting of fluid-holding proteins that are hydrolyzed collagen. This ground substance closely resembles that found in most connective tissues. Once the gelatin has thickened, which typically takes about 1.5 hours, incorporate some licorice and a few jellybeans. The licorice represents the fibers of connective tissue, while the jellybeans symbolize the cellular components. Different types of licorice can be used to represent various kinds of fibers: thin black laces for elastic fibers and thick red twists for collagen fibers. While this model provides a visual representation of the connective tissue structure, it cannot replicate the physical characteristics such as strength, elasticity, and resistance to compression that are inherent to connective tissues.

2.4.3. Classification of Connective Tissues

2.4.3.1. Connective Tissue Proper – Loose Connective Tissues

There are two subclasses of connective tissue proper: dense connective tissue (dense irregular, dense regular, and elastic) and loose connective tissue (areolar, adipose, and reticular). The density of the fibers in these subclasses is what sets them apart: in loose connective tissues, the fibers are dispersed throughout the tissue but kept apart by ground substance. Loose connective tissue comes in three varieties: reticular, adipose, and areolar.

Areolar Connective Tissue: The most common form of connective tissue proper is loose areolar connective tissue (Figures 2.9 and 2.10(b)). Nearly every epithelium in the body is supported by this tissue, which also envelops nearly every tiny blood vessel and nerve, including capillaries.

The structure of this tissue reflects its basic functions:

- Supporting and binding other tissues;
- Holding body fluids;
- Defending the body against infection;
- Storing nutrients as fat.

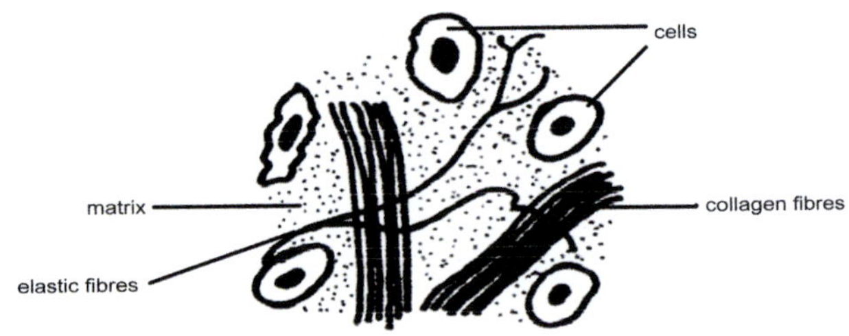

Figure 2.10(b). *Areolar connective tissue, a soft packaging tissue of the body.*

Source: By The original uploader was Sunshineconnelly at English Wikibooks. – Transferred from en.wikibooks to Commons by Adrignola using CommonsHelper. CC BY 2.5, https://commons.wikimedia.org/w/index.php?curid=13727137.

Areolar connective tissue fibers provide support. Collagen, reticular, and elastic fibers are all present in the extracellular matrix of areolar connective tissue; however, reticular fibers are not visible when using the widely used histology stains hematoxylin and eosin. The ground substance of areolar connective tissue is capable of storing fluid. Tissue fluid, also known as interstitial fluid, surrounds every cell in the body. This fluid is produced when fluid and tiny molecules from the blood leak out of the capillaries during the healing process. Through diffusion, waste molecules are removed from cells and nutrients and oxygen are supplied to the cells. Areolar connective tissue is present between the capillaries and every other cell and tissue in the body. It absorbs the fluid in the tissue like a sponge. As a result, it maintains the fluid surrounding the body's cells and facilitates the entry and exit of chemicals, gases, nutrients, and waste products in and out of the cells.

The body's first line of defense against invasive microorganisms such as bacteria, viruses, fungi, and parasites is areolar connective tissue. It is strategically positioned to eliminate microorganisms at their point of entry, before they enter the capillaries and use the vascular system to spread to other locations. Areolar connective tissue lies just beneath the epithelial tissues that line the body surfaces and surround capillaries. Within areolar connective tissue, numerous defense cells that react to infectious agents can be found (Figure 2.9). Areolar connective tissue employs various mechanisms to fend off infection, in addition to cellular defenses. The thick collagen fiber networks and viscous ground substance of the extracellular matrix hinder the growth of invasive bacteria. However, certain bacteria release digestive enzymes that rapidly degrade collagen or ground substance. These matrix-degrading bacteria are highly invasive, making it particularly challenging for the body's defenses to control their rapid spread through connective tissues. An example of this type of bacteria is the Streptococcus strain that causes strep throat. Areolar connective tissue also serves as a storage site for energy reserves in the form of fat, although this is a minor function. Within this tissue, fat cells can be found either individually or in small groups (Figure 2.9).

2.4.3.2. Adipose Tissue

In terms of structure and function, adipose tissue is comparable to areolar connective tissue, but it has a much larger capacity to store nutrients. Consequently, adipose tissue, which constitutes 90% of its mass, is densely packed with fat cells. These fat cells form large clusters known as lobules. The abundant vascularization of adipose tissue indicates its high metabolic activity. Following meals, it extracts lipids from the bloodstream and reintroduces them as needed. Without the fat reserves in our adipose tissue, we would not be able to survive for more than a few days without food. The majority of the body's adipose tissue is located in the hypodermis, the layer beneath the skin. Adipose tissue is also abundant in the mesenteries, which are serous membranes that envelop the stomach and intestines. The fat found in this area is referred to as visceral fat. Additionally, fat acts as cushioning pads behind the eyes and around the kidneys. Smaller fat depots cater to the local nutritional requirements of highly active organs, while the extensive fat beneath the skin fulfills the general nutritional needs of the entire body. These depots can be found in certain muscles, the pumping heart, lymph nodes (where immune system cells are actively fighting infection), and individual fat cells in the bone marrow (where new blood cells are produced at a rapid pace). Numerous regional depots provide unique and highly enriched lipids (Figure 2.10(c)).

White adipose tissue, or white fat, is the common type of fat that stores nutrients. Another type is known as brown adipose tissue, which consumes nutrients and generates heat. Brown fat has been found in adults, despite previously being believed to only exist in newborns to help with thermoregulation. It is located on the side of the anterior neck, on the anterior abdominal wall, and in the middle of the back, in the hypodermis between the two scapulae (shoulder blades). Compared to white fat, brown fat has even richer vascularization. Each brown-fat cell contains numerous mitochondria and lipid droplets, and these organelles use the lipid fuel to heat the bloodstream rather than produce ATP molecules.

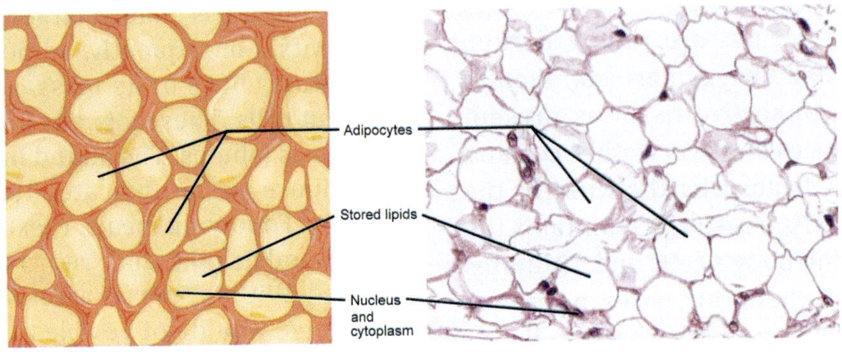

Figure 2.10(c). *Adipose tissue from the subcutaneous layer under the skin.*

Source: https://courses.lumenlearning.com/suny-dutchess-ap1/chapter/animal-primary-tissues/.

2.4.3.3. Reticular Connective Tissue

Reticular connective tissue is similar to areolar tissue, but its matrix contains only reticular fibers. These delicate fibers create a complex network resembling the frame of a house, with interconnected spaces that hold numerous free cells. Organs such as the bone marrow, spleen, and lymph nodes primarily consist of reticular connective tissue, which houses many free blood cells. Reticular cells, a type of fibroblast, are found along the reticular network of this tissue (Figure 2.10(d)).

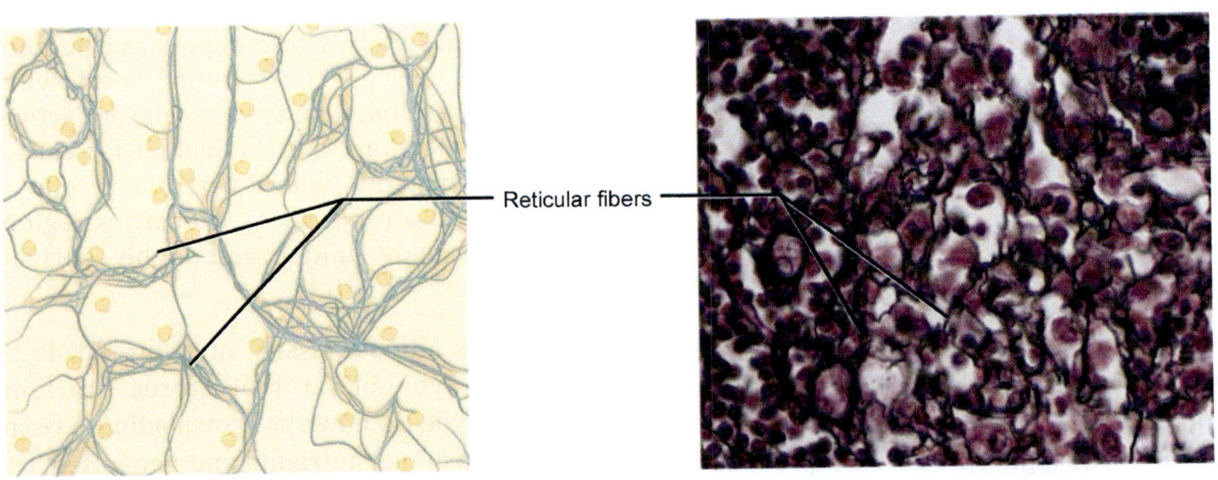

Figure 2.10(d). *Dark-staining network of reticular connective tissue fibers forming the internal skeleton of the spleen.*

Source: https://courses.lumenlearning.com/suny-ap1/chapter/connective-tissue-supports-and-protects/.

2.4.3.4. Connective Tissue Proper – Dense Connective Tissue

Compared to areolar connective tissue, dense connective tissue, also known as fibrous connective tissue, has a higher collagen content. It can withstand incredibly powerful pulling (tensile) forces thanks to its thick collagen fibers. Dense connective tissue has three varieties: elastic, regular, and irregular.

2.4.3.5. Dense Irregular Connective Tissue

Areolar tissue and dense irregular connective tissue are comparable, but the latter has substantially thicker collagen fibers. Because of the different planes in which these fibers run, the tissue is able to withstand strong tensions coming from various directions.

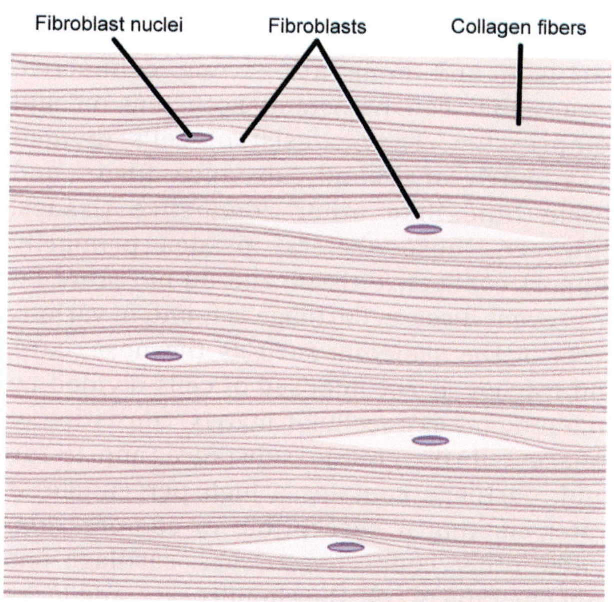

Figure 2.10(e). *Dense irregular connective tissue from the dermis of the skin.*

Source: https://courses.lumenlearning.com/suny-dutchess-ap1/chapter/animal-primary-tissues/.

This tissue predominates in the skin's leathery dermis, which is frequently pulled, stretched, and struck from different directions. This tissue also constitutes the fibrous capsules that envelop the kidneys, lymph nodes, and bones, among other organs in the body. It shares the same cellular and matrix components as areolar connective tissue. Even specialists find dense, irregular connective tissue perplexing. As one might anticipate for a tissue called "irregular," the dermis's fibers run randomly, thus it clearly lives up to its name. Nonetheless, the two layers that make up the fibrous capsules of organs are separated by a layer in which all of the fibers run perpendicular to one another but parallel to one another. In other words, a tissue can become "irregular" if it has two perpendicular "regular" layers (Figure 2.10(e)).

2.4.3.6. Dense Regular Connective Tissue

In dense regular connective tissue, the direction of all collagen fibers typically runs parallel to the pull. Rows of fibroblasts are crammed in between the collagen fibers, constantly producing the fibers and a sparse ground substance. The collagen fibers in this tissue have a slight wave to them when they are not in tension. Dense regular connective tissue lacks fat and defense cells and is poorly vascularized, in contrast to areolar connective tissue.

Dense regular connective tissue is the primary constituent of ligaments, bands, or sheets that connect bones to one another because of its exceptional tensile strength. It is also the primary tissue in aponeuroses (apo-nu-ro′s ˉes), which are sheet-like tendons, and tendons, which are cords that connect muscles to bones. Fascia (fash′e-ah; "a band") is a fibrous membrane that envelops muscles, muscle groups, large vessels, and nerves. It is also formed by dense regular connective tissue. The body is made up of numerous sheets of fascia that bind together structures much like plastic sandwich wrap. When the term fascia is used, deep fascia is what it means. Beneath the skin, the fatty hypodermis is something else entirely called superficial fascia (Figure 2.10(f)).

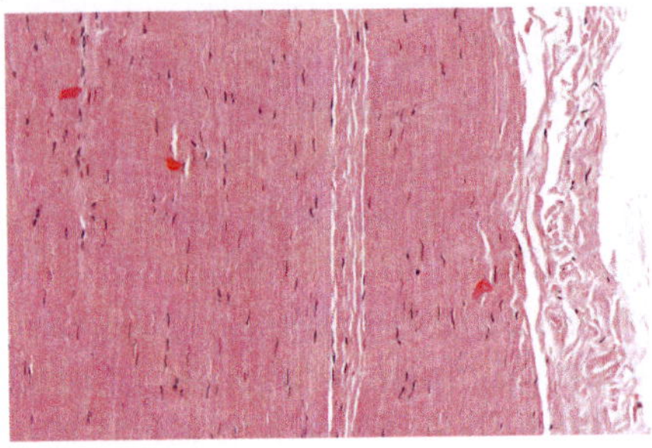

Figure 2.10(f). *Dense regular connective tissue from a tendon.*

Source: By Nephron – Own work, CC BY-SA 3.0, https://commons.wikimedia.org/w/index.php?curid=18499608.

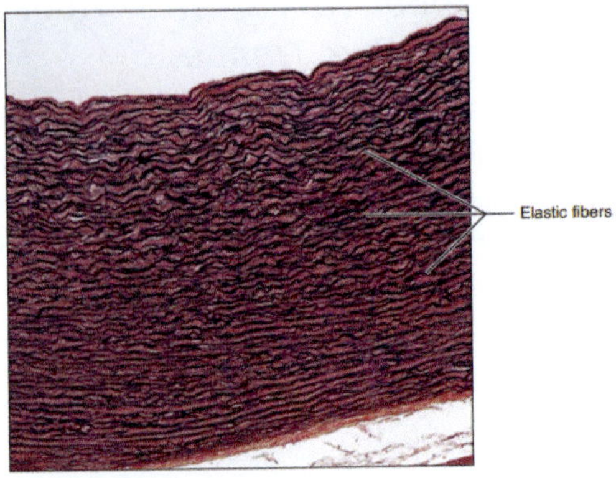

Figure 2.10(g). *Elastic connective tissue in the wall of the aorta.*

Source: By Kelvinsong – Own work, CC BY-SA 3.0, https://commons.wikimedia.org/w/index.php?curid=25179416.

2.4.3.7. Elastic Connective Tissue

Elastic fibers are the predominant type of fiber in elastic connective tissue, and their bundles outnumber those of collagen fibers. This tissue is found in places where the ability to recoil from stretching is crucial, such as the walls of arteries, the bronchial tubes in the lungs, and certain ligaments (such as the ligamentum nuchae and ligamentum flavum, which link successive vertebrae) (Figure 2.10(g)).

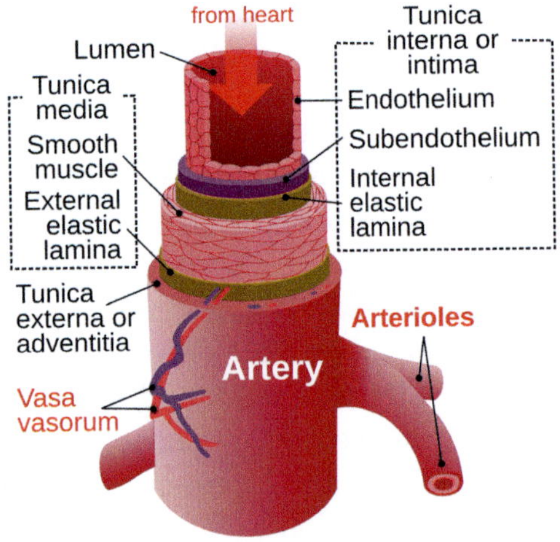

2.4.3.8. Cartilage

The connective tissue can withstand tension. Cartilage and bone are strong connective tissues that can withstand both tension and compression. They consist of cells divided by a matrix of ground substance, fibers, and tissue fluid, like other connective tissues. However, these skeletal tissues primarily support connective tissue and do not store fat or prevent disease. Cartilage is found in various parts of the skeleton, such as the nose, ears, and trachea. It is composed of cells divided by an abundant extracellular matrix, consisting of collagen fibrils, ground substance, and tissue fluid. Cartilage contains a high percentage of water, making it susceptible to compression. Unlike other connective tissues, cartilage has only one type of cell, the chondrocyte, and lacks blood vessels and nerves. Chondroblasts are immature chondrocytes that secrete the matrix during cartilage growth. There are three types of cartilage: fibrocartilage, elastic cartilage, and hyaline cartilage, each dominated by a specific type of fiber (Figure 2.10(h)).

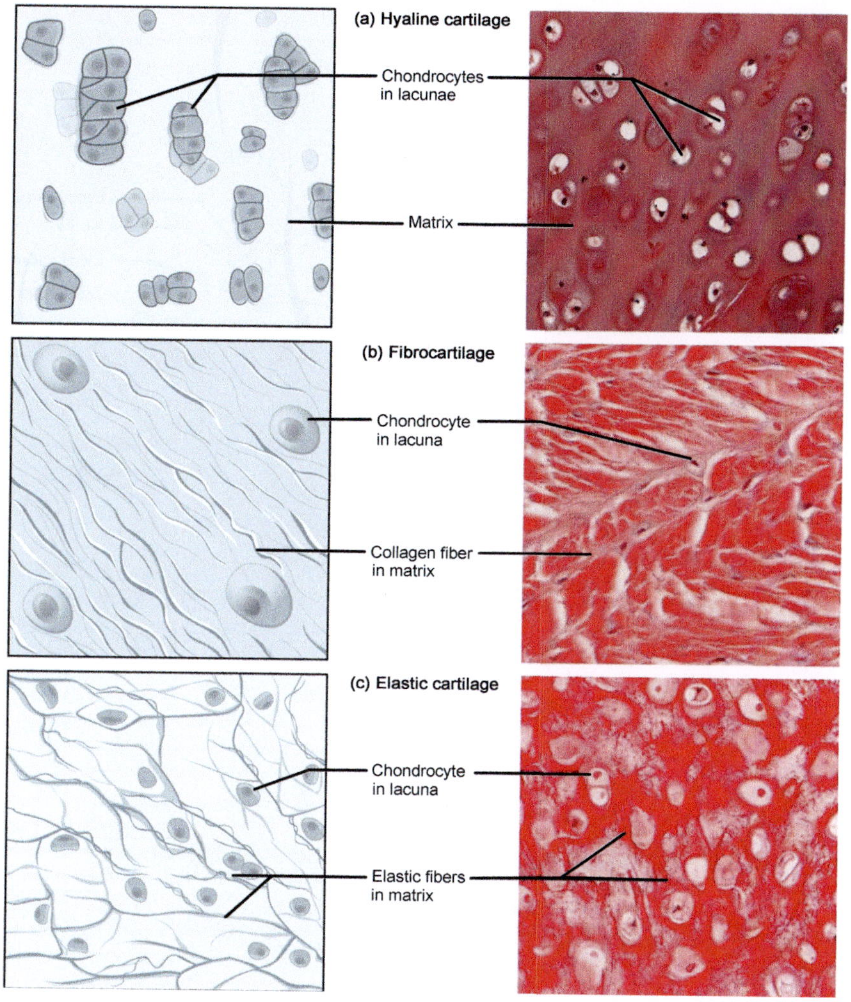

Figure 2.10(h). *Types of cartilage.*

Source: https://courses.lumenlearning.com/suny-dutchess-ap1/chapter/animal-primary-tissues/.

2.4.3.9. Bone

The extraordinary ability of bone tissue to support and shield bodily structures is a result of its hardness, akin to that of rock. Collagen fibers are abundant in the bone matrix, which allows bone to withstand strong tension, and inorganic calcium salts, which allow bone to resist compression (Figure 2.10(i)). The ground substance of the matrix and the collagen fibers are secreted by immature bone cells known as osteoblasts. The matrix is then hardened by the precipitation of calcium salts on and between the collagen fibers. The adult bone cells, known as osteocytes, live inside these hardened matrix cavities, or lacunae (plural: lacuna). Bone is a dynamic, living tissue that has an abundance of blood vessels.

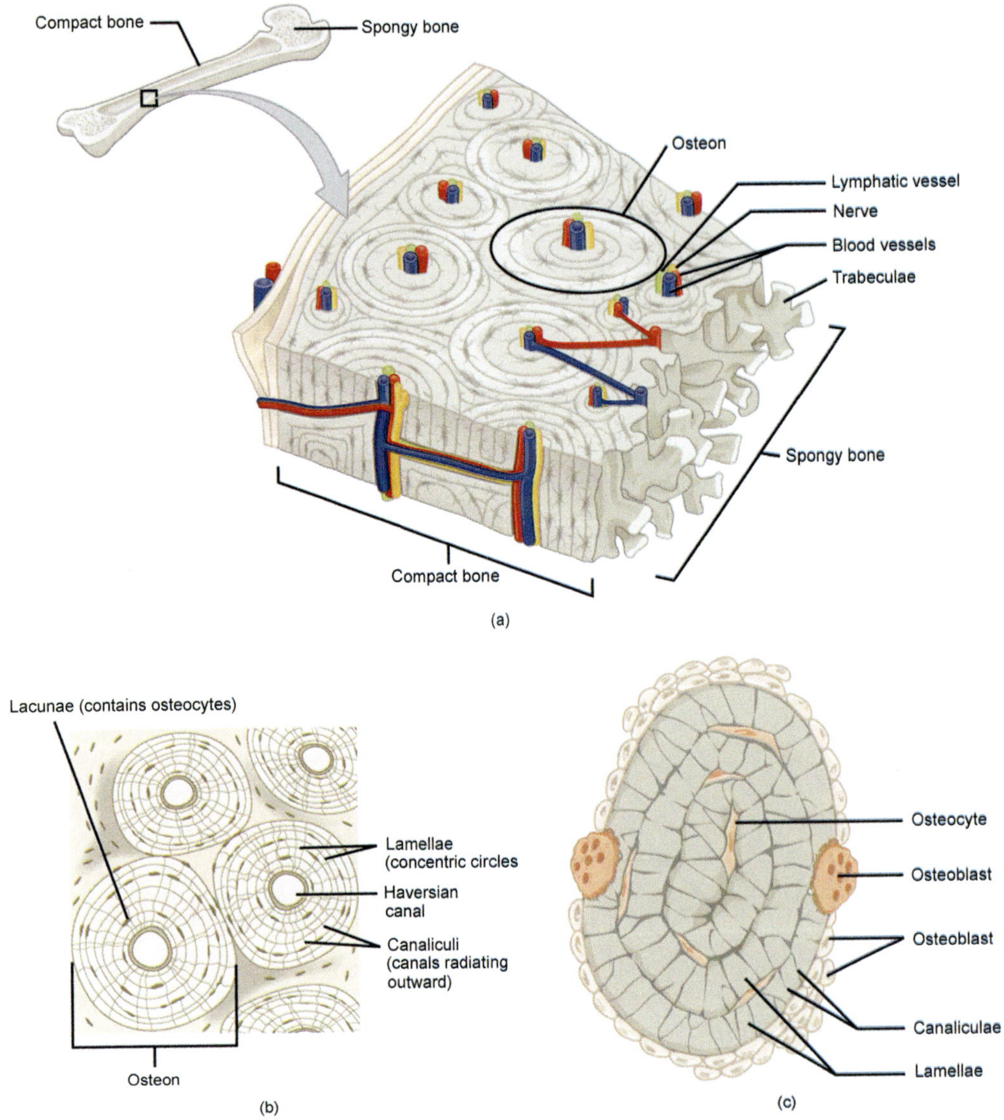

Figure 2.10(i). *Cross-sectional view of bone.*

Source: https://courses.lumenlearning.com/suny-dutchess-ap1/chapter/animal-primary-tissues/.

2.4.3.10. Blood

The fluid in the blood vessels, or blood (Figure 2.10(j)), is the most atypical connective tissue. It does not provide mechanical support or bind objects together. Because it grows from mesenchyme and is composed of blood cells encased in a nonliving matrix, liquid blood plasma, it is categorized as a connective tissue. Its matrix and cells are highly dissimilar from those found in other connective tissues. The circulatory system uses blood as a means of transportation to move nutrients, waste products, defense cells, breathing gases, and a host of other materials throughout the body. The body's most varied tissue types are connective and epithelial tissues. They are typically the hardest for students to understand as a result.

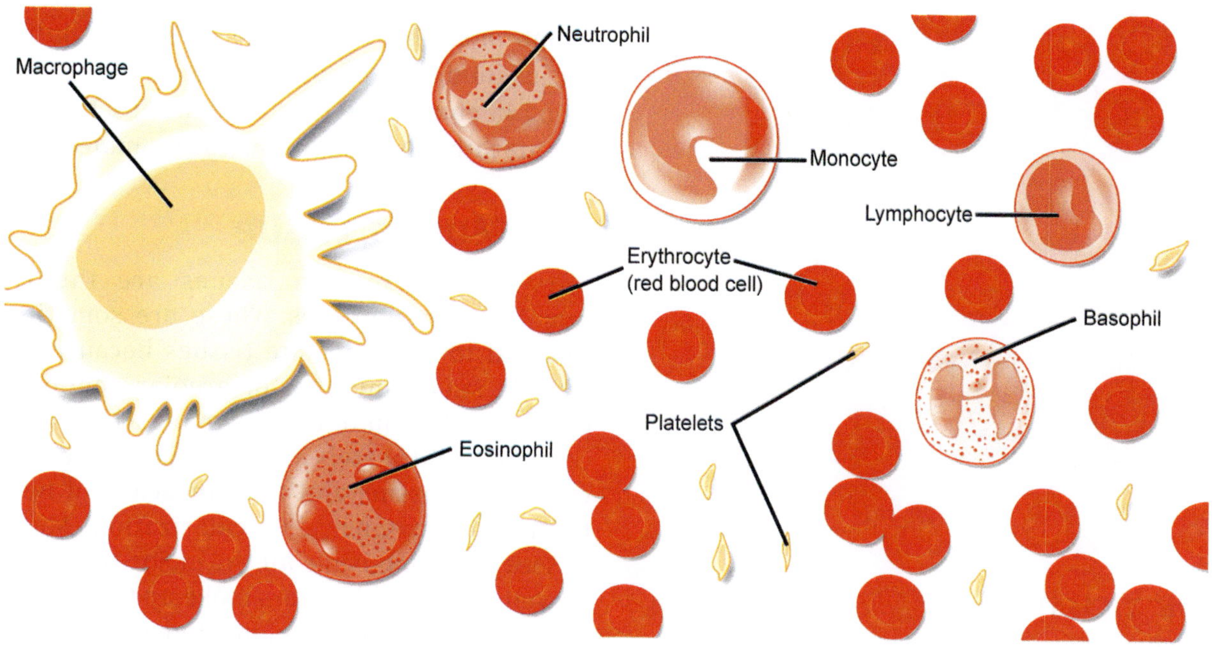

Figure 2.10(j). *Smear of human blood shows two white blood cells surrounded by red blood cells.*

Source: https://courses.lumenlearning.com/suny-dutchess-ap1/chapter/animal-primary-tissues/.

2.4.4. C Zovering and Lining Membranes

These two tissue types are combined by the covering and lining membranes (Figure 2.10). These membranes, which span large portions of the body, are composed of the underlying layer of connective tissue proper as well as an epithelial sheet.

These membranes are classified into three types: cutaneous, mucous, and serous. The cutaneous membrane (ku-ta′ne-us; "skin") refers to the skin that covers the body's exterior (Figure 2.11(a)). Its outer epithelium is formed by the thick epidermis, while the inner connective tissue is made up of the dense dermis. This membrane is dry.

Every hollow internal organ that opens to the outside of the body is lined by a mucous membrane, known as a mucosa (mu-ko′sah). Specifically, as shown in Figure 2.11(b), mucous membranes border the tubes that house the reproductive, digestive, respiratory, and urinary systems. Despite the significant variation in the types of epithelia they contain, all mucous membranes are moist. Many mucous membranes secrete mucus, as implied by their name. However, not all of them do. The lamina propria, also referred to as "one's own layer," is a layer of loose areolar connective tissue that lies directly beneath the epithelial sheet present in all mucous membranes. In the mucous membranes of the digestive system, the lamina propria is supported by a layer of smooth muscle cells.

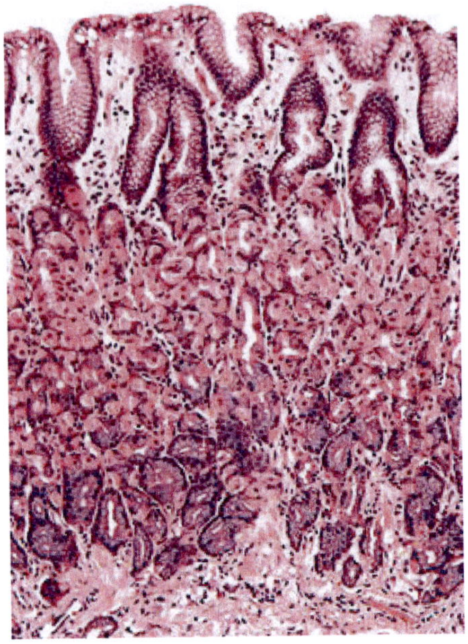

Figure 2.11(a). *Mucous membrane of the stomach.*

Source: By Nephron – Own work, CC BY-SA 3.0, https://commons.wikimedia.org/w/index.php?curid=10890698.

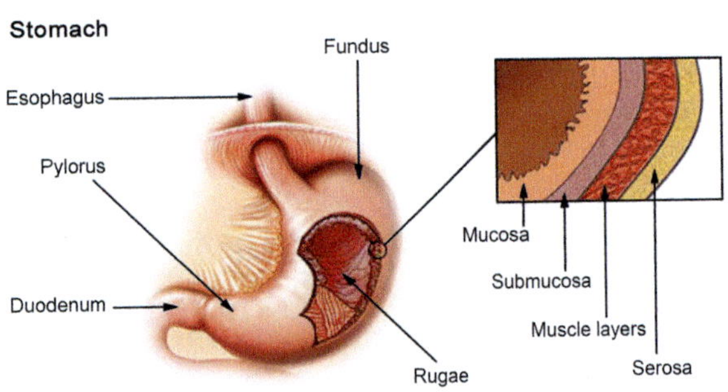

Figures 2.11(b). *Serous membranes.*

Source: By NIH / National Cancer Institute – http://training.seer.cancer.gov/anatomy/digestive/regions/stomach.html, Public Domain, https://commons.wikimedia.org/w/index.php?curid=1393218.

The slick membranes that border the closed pleural, pericardial, and peritoneal cavities are known as serous membranes, or serosae (Figure 2.11(b)). A thin layer of areolar connective tissue covers a basic squamous epithelium known as mesothelium, which makes up a serous membrane. This membrane creates a slippery serous fluid, which is first formed as a filtrate of blood in connective tissue capillaries, to which the mesothelium adds lubricating molecules.

2.5. Muscle Tissue

Nervous and muscle tissues are the two remaining tissue types. These are sometimes referred to as composite tissues because they include small amounts of areolar connective tissue in addition to their own muscle or nerve cells. All blood vessels are surrounded by areolar connective tissue, and both muscle and nerve tissue have extensive vascularization. Muscle tissues are responsible for the majority of bodily movements. Muscle fibers make up the majority of muscle cells. Their elongated shape causes them to contract forcefully as they shorten. These cells contain numerous myofilaments, also known as "muscle filaments," which are cellular organelles packed with actin and myosin filaments that cause contraction in all cell types.

There are three types of muscle tissue: skeletal, cardiac, and smooth. Skeletal muscle tissue is the main component of the organs known as skeletal muscles, which pull on bones to produce body movements (Figure 2.12). The long, large cylinders that form skeletal muscle cells are filled with nuclei. Their distinct banded or striated appearance indicates a highly organized arrangement of myofilaments.

Heart wall tissue includes cardiac muscle (Figure 2.12(b)). To force blood through the blood vessels, it contracts. Heart muscle cells are striated, just like skeletal muscle cells. They differ, though, in two respects: (i) there is only one nucleus in each cardiac cell; and (ii) cardiac cells branch and join at unique cellular junctions known as intercalated (in-ter'kah-lah-ted) discs.

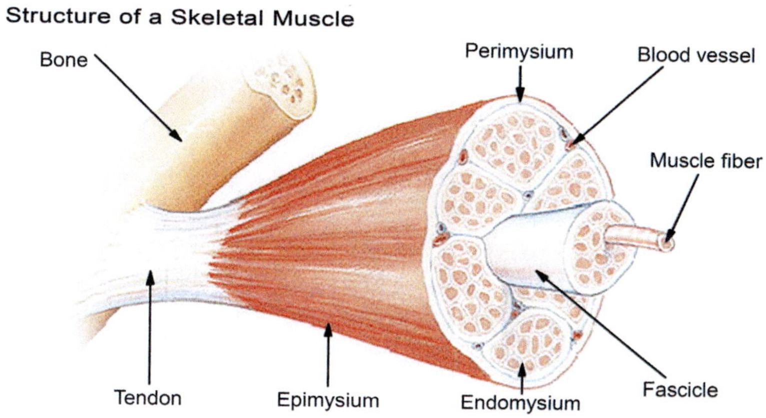

Figure 2.12(a). *Skeletal muscle. Notice the obvious banding pattern and the fact that these large cells are multinucleate.*

Source: https://courses.lumenlearning.com/wm-biology2/chapter/the-muscular-system/.

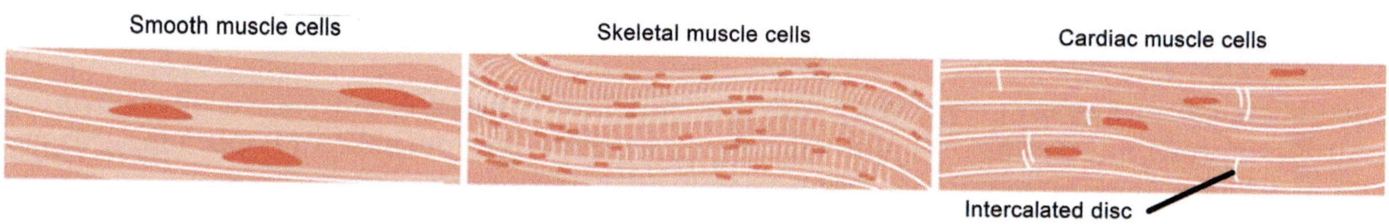

Figure 2.12(b). *Cardiac muscle and smooth muscle.*

Source: https://courses.lumenlearning.com/wm-biology2/chapter/the-muscular-system/.

Smooth muscle tissue is distinguished by its absence of visible striations in cells. The cells are elongated with tapered ends and contain a solitary nucleus positioned in the center. Smooth muscle is predominantly present in the walls of hollow organs such as the gastrointestinal and urinary tracts, uterus, and blood vessels. Its principal function is to propel substances through these organs by contracting and relaxing alternately.

2.6. Nervous Tissue

The primary constituent of the nervous organs—the brain, spinal cord, and nerves—that govern and control bodily functions is nervous tissue. It contains two types of cells: neurons and supporting cells. Neurons are highly specialized nerve cells (Figure 2.13) that generate and conduct electrical impulses. They have extensions, or processes, that allow them to transmit impulses over substantial distances within the body.

Dendrites are cell processes that extend from the cell body of a neuron, like branches of a tree. The dendrites, the receptive region of the neuron, transmit signals toward the cell body. A neuron also has a singular, long cell process extending from its cell body, the axon, that generates nerve impulses and transmits them away from the cell body. The supporting cells, called neuroglia, are nonconducting cells that nourish, insulate, and protect the delicate neurons.

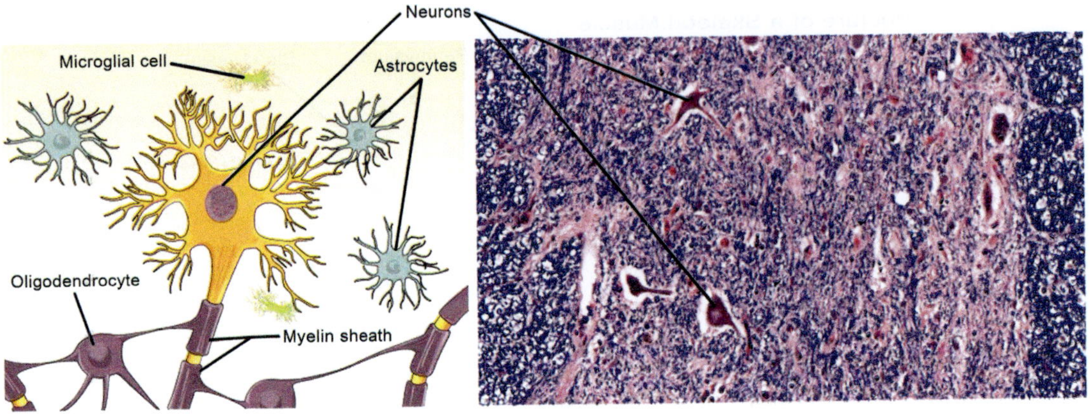

Figure 2.13. *Neurons.*

Source: hhttps://courses.lumenlearning.com/suny-ap1/chapter/nervous-tissue-mediates-perception-and-response/.

2.7. Membranes

Tissue sheets called membranes cover, border, or divide organs or organ parts (lobes) from one another. Numerous membranes secrete substances with distinct purposes. Membranes classified into two main groups are connective tissue membranes and epithelial membranes.

2.7.1. Epithelial Membranes

Mucous and serous epithelial membranes are two distinct types found in specific parts of the body, each secreting a fluid. These fluids are known as mucus and serous fluid.

2.7.1.1. Serous Membranes

Serous membranes, composed of simple squamous epithelium (Figure 2.14), cover organs within closed body cavities. The pleural membranes are the serous membranes of the thoracic cavity. The lungs are covered by the visceral pleura, while the chest wall is lined by the parietal pleura. It is important to note that "cover" refers to the outside, while "line" refers to the inside. These terms cannot be used interchangeably. The pleural membranes secrete serous fluid, which prevents friction between the lungs during breathing. The thoracic cavity, which houses the heart between the lungs, also has its own unique set of serous membranes. The fibrous pericardium, a connective tissue membrane, is lined by the parietal pericardium, while the epicardium (or visceral pericardium) is located on the surface of the heart muscle. Serous fluid is produced to reduce friction as the heart beats.

The serous membrane that lines the abdominal cavity is called the peritoneum. The abdominal organs are covered by the mesentery, also known as the visceral peritoneum. Here, as the stomach and intestines contract and rub against other organs, the serous fluid reduces friction.

2.7.1.2. Mucous Membranes

Mucous membranes encircle the bodily tracts, or systems, that possess apertures to external surroundings. The reproductive, digestive, urinary, and respiratory systems are among them. The mucosa, or mucous membrane, has distinct epithelium depending on the organs involved. The stomach mucosa is columnar epithelium, the trachea's mucosa is ciliated epithelium, and the esophageal and vaginal mucosas are stratified squamous epithelium.

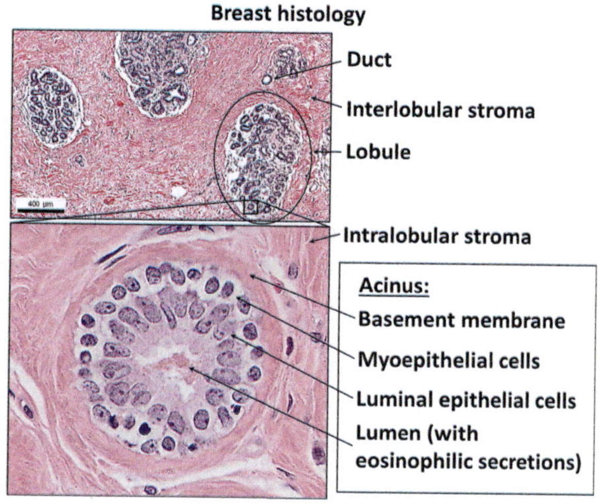

Figure 2.14. *Epithelial membranes in the breast, as an example.*

Source: By Mikael Häggström, M. D. Author info – Reusing images – Conflicts of interest: None Mikael Häggström, M. D. Consent note: Consent from the patient or patient's relatives is regarded as redundant, because of absence of identifiable features (List of HIPAA identifiers) in the media and case information (See also HIPAA case reports guidance).The image integrates a source image by de Bel, T., Litjens, G., Ogony, J., Stallings-Mann, M., Carter, J. M., & Hilton, T. Own work. Source images: Breast lobules. By: de Bel, T., Litjens, G., Ogony, J., Stallings-Mann, M., Carter, J. M., Hilton, T. (Attribution 4.0 International License) Normal breast acinus (own work), CC BY 4.0, https://commons.wikimedia.org/w/index.php?curid=127049680.

These membranes secrete mucus, which keeps the lining epithelial cells moist. It is important to note that these are living cells and they will perish if they dry out. Mucus also lubricates the surface of the digestive tract, facilitating the easy passage of food. In the respiratory tract, mucus captures dust and bacteria, which are then transported to the pharynx by ciliated epithelium.

A Closer Look

Adipose Tissue

Adipose tissue is a type of connective tissue that primarily consists of fat cells, known as adipocytes. These cells are specialized in synthesizing and storing large globules of fat within a structural network of fibers. Adipose tissue is predominantly found beneath the skin, but it can also be found in deposits between muscles, in the intestines and their folds, around the heart, and in other areas of the body. Additionally, it is present in the bone marrow, giving it a yellow color, with yellow marrow being most abundant in adults. The fat stored in adipose tissue can come from dietary fats or be produced within the body.

Mammals possess two distinct types of adipose tissue: white adipose tissue and brown adipose tissue. White adipose tissue, being the most common type, provides insulation, serves as an energy reserve during times of starvation or intense physical activity, and forms protective pads between organs. When muscles and other tissues require energy, specific hormones bind to adipose cells, triggering the hydrolysis of triacylglycerol. This process releases energy-rich fatty acids and glycerol, a phenomenon known as lipolysis. The enzyme responsible for this hydrolysis is lipase, which is present in the blood, certain gastrointestinal juices, and adipose tissue. Lipase is activated by hormones such as epinephrine, norepinephrine, glucagon, and adrenocorticotropin, all of which bind to adipocytes. White adipose tissue is also a source of numerous hormones that play various roles in metabolism and endocrine function. Adiponectin, leptin, and resistin, which are hormones produced by adipose tissue, are involved in energy metabolism. Additionally, plasminogen activator inhibitor-1 prevents the dissolution of blood clots.

Brown adipose tissue, primarily found in newborn animals, generates heat and consumes energy. However, in humans, the percentage of brown adipose tissue decreases with age. In contrast, other animals, particularly those that hibernate such as grizzly bears and black bears, have brown adipose tissue in adulthood, which plays a crucial role in their survival. Hibernating species experience a decrease in body temperature and a slowdown in metabolism during winter dormancy, enabling them to conserve energy. Brown adipose tissue releases heat by consuming energy, which is essential for awakening and emerging from dormancy. It is typically tan to red in color, a characteristic imparted by the abundance of mitochondria, the energy-producing organelles, found in brown fat cells. The distribution of adipose tissue in the human body can vary depending on sex. Generally, men tend to accumulate fat around the waist, while women tend to accumulate more fat around the hips than the waist. Geneticists have identified specific regions in the human genome associated with fat distribution, and several genes appear to have a greater impact on the waist-to-hip ratio in women compared to men. Understanding the precise functions of these genes, as they regulate the activities of fat cells, could provide valuable insights into the biological mechanisms underlying obesity, diabetes mellitus, and cardiovascular disease.

Summary

- The term "tissue" denotes an aggregation of cells that exist collectively within the body. Tissue cells all originate from the same embryo.
- Tissues are comprised of a blend of intercellular substances and cells in varying proportions, with one constituent assuming prominence.
- Epithelial tissue covers the body's cavities, tubes, as well as its external and internal surfaces.
- Stratified epithelia are designated based on the cellular shape of the apical layer to avoid any potential confusion. It is beneficial to bear in mind that tissue function is reflected in tissue structure.
- The simple cuboidal epithelium consists of cuboid-shaped cells arranged in a solitary layer. This epithelium forms the linings of the smallest glandular ducts, the secretory cells of various glands, and the tubular walls of the kidney.
- Glands are composed of epithelial cells that excrete a substance. Aqueous (water-based) fluids, which are generated by glands, generally contain proteins.
- Endocrine glands are sometimes referred to as ductless glands because they lack ducts. Instead, they release their contents directly into the surrounding tissue fluid.
- Adhesive belt junctions, also known as zonula adherens, are a type of anchoring junction found directly beneath tight junctions in epithelial tissues.
- Connective tissue, the most diverse and widespread type of tissue, is the second of the four fundamental types of tissue. Connective tissue is classified into four main categories and numerous subcategories.
- Reticular connective tissue is akin to areolar tissue, but its matrix comprises solely of reticular fibers. These fragile fibers form an intricate network resembling the framework of a house, with interconnected spaces that house numerous free cells.

References

1. Bodolay, E., Csiki, Z., Szekanecz, Z., Ben, T., Kiss, E., Zeher, M., Szücs, G., et al., (2003). Five-year follow-up of 665 Hungarian patients with undifferentiated connective tissue disease (UCTD). *Clin. Exp. Rheumatol., 21*(3), 313–320.
2. Calderon, L. M., & Pope, J. E., (2021). Scleroderma epidemiology update. *Curr. Opin. Rheumatol., 33*(2), 122–127.
3. Carstens, P. O., & Schmidt, J., (2014). Diagnosis, pathogenesis, and treatment of myositis: Recent advances. *Clin. Exp. Immunol., 175*(3), 349–358.
4. Cui, D., (2011). *Atlas of Histology with Functional and Clinical Correlations*. Wolters Kluwer Health/Lippincott Williams & Wilkins.
5. Davies, J. E., Walker, J. T., & Keating, A., (2017). Concise review: Wharton's jelly: The rich, but enigmatic, source of mesenchymal stromal cells. *Stem Cells Transl. Med., 6*(7), 1620–1630.
6. Durcan, L., O'Dwyer, T., & Petri, M., (2019). Management strategies and future directions for systemic lupus erythematosus in adults. *Lancet, 393*(10188), 2332–2343.

7. Edwards, D. A., (1946). The blood supply and lymphatic drainage of tendons. *J. Anat., 80*, 147–152.
8. Franchi, M., Trirè, A., Quaranta, M., Orsini, E., & Ottani, V., (2007). Collagen structure of tendon relates to function. *Scientific World Journal, 7*, 404–420.
9. Gartner, L. P., & Hiatt, J. L., (2009). *Color Atlas of Histology* (5th edn.). Wolters Kluwer Health/ Lippincott Williams & Wilkins.
10. Human Tissue Authority: Directions given under the Human Tissue Act 2004 to establishments licensed under the Quality and Safety Regulations. , available at https://www.hta.gov.uk/guidance-professionals/codes-practice-standards-and-legislation/legal-directions
11. Kannus, P., (2000). Structure of the tendon connective tissue. *Scand J. Med. Sci. Sports, 10*(6), 312–320.
12. Kardas, T., Wielosz, E., & Majdan, M., (2022). Methods of assessment of joint involvement in various systemic connective tissue diseases. *Reumatologia., 60*(1), 53–62.
13. Kierszenbaum, & Abraham, L., (2007). *Histology and Cell Biology: An Introduction to Pathology* (2nd edn.). Mosby Elsevier.
14. Kyriakidis, N. C., Kapsogeorgou, E. K., & Tzioufas, A. G., (2014). A comprehensive review of autoantibodies in primary Sjögren's syndrome: Clinical phenotypes and regulatory mechanisms. *J. Autoimmun, 51*, 67–74.
15. Lee, C. T., & Strek, M. E., (2021). The other connective tissue disease-associated interstitial lung diseases: Sjogren's syndrome, mixed connective tissue disease, and systemic lupus erythematosus. *Curr. Opin. Pulm. Med., 27*(5), 388–395.
16. LeRoy, E. C., Maricq, H. R., & Kahaleh, M. B., (1980). Undifferentiated connective tissue syndromes. *Arthritis Rheum, 23*(3), 341–343.
17. Light, N., & Champion, A. E., (1984). Characterization of muscle epimysium, perimysium, and endomysium collagens. *Biochem J., 219*(3), 1017–1026.
18. Liu, Q., Wang, X., & Yi, S., (2018). Pathophysiological changes of physical barriers of peripheral nerves after injury. *Front Neurosci., 12*, 597.
19. Martin, C. L., & Pope, J. E., (2022). Precursors to systemic sclerosis and systemic lupus erythematosus: From undifferentiated connective tissue disease to the development of identifiable connective tissue diseases. *Front Immunol., 13*, 869172.
20. Pepmueller, P. H., (2016). Undifferentiated connective tissue disease, mixed connective tissue disease, and overlap syndromes in rheumatology. *Mo. Med., 113*(2), 136–140.
21. Rose, J., (2022). Autoimmune connective tissue diseases: Systemic lupus erythematosus and rheumatoid arthritis. *Emerg. Med. Clin. North Am., 40*(1), 179–191.
22. Smolen, J. S., Aletaha, D., & McInnes, I. B., (2016). Rheumatoid arthritis. *Lancet, 388*(10055), 2023–2038.
23. Statutory Instrument 2007 No. 1523 The Human Tissue (Quality and Safety for Human Application) Regulations 2007, and subsequent amendments. Available at www.legislation.gov.uk
24. Ushiki, T., (2002). Collagen fibers, reticular fibers, and elastic fibers. A comprehensive understanding from a morphological viewpoint. *Arch. Histol. Cytol., 65*(2), 109–126.

25. Vaz, C. C., Couto, M., Medeiros, D., Miranda, L., Costa, J., Nero, P., Barros, R., et al., (2009). Undifferentiated connective tissue disease: A seven-center cross-sectional study of 184 patients. *Clin. Rheumatol., 28*(8), 915–921.

26. Weatherholt, A. M., Fuchs, R. K., & Warden, S. J., (2012). Specialized connective tissue: Bone, the structural framework of the upper extremity. *J. Hand Ther., 25*(2), 123–131. quiz 132.

27. Yang, G., Rothrauff, B. B., & Tuan, R. S., (2013). Tendon and ligament regeneration and repair: Clinical relevance and developmental paradigm. *Birth Defects Res C Embryo Today, 99*(3), 203–222.

Chapter

THE INTEGUMENTARY SYSTEM

3

Contents

Unit Introduction

The integumentary system is composed of the skin, the subcutaneous tissue beneath the skin, hair, nails, and various glands. The primary function of the integumentary system is to provide protection for underlying tissues. The skin acts as a barrier against harmful substances and prevents fluid loss. The subcutaneous tissue connects the skin to underlying tissues, such as muscles. Hair on the scalp serves to protect the head from cold temperatures. The hair on our lashes and eyebrows helps to keep dust and sweat out of our eyes, while the hair in our nostrils prevents dust from entering our nasal cavities. The presence of hair on the rest of our bodies is considered an evolutionary artifact rather than a functional feature. Nails protect the tips of our fingers and toes from mechanical harm and aid in picking up small objects. The integumentary system includes four types of glands: sebaceous glands, ceruminous glands, mammary glands, and sudoriferous glands. Sudoriferous glands, also known as sweat glands, play a crucial role in regulating body temperature. Sebaceous glands produce oil that helps fight bacteria, waterproofs the skin, and prevents dryness of the skin and hair. Ceruminous glands produce earwax, which keeps the outer surface of the eardrum pliable and prevents it from drying out. Mammary glands produce milk.

Orientation and Directional Terms:

Term	Definition	Illustration
Arterioles	Arterioles are small blood vessels that carry blood away from the heart and connect arteries to capillaries.	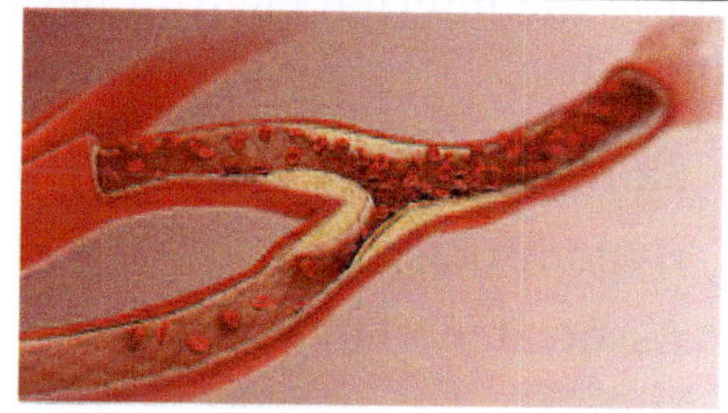
Dermis	The dermis is a connective tissue layer sandwiched between the epidermis and subcutaneous tissue. It is a fibrous structure composed of collagen, elastic tissue, and other extracellular components that include vasculature, nerve endings, hair follicles, and glands.	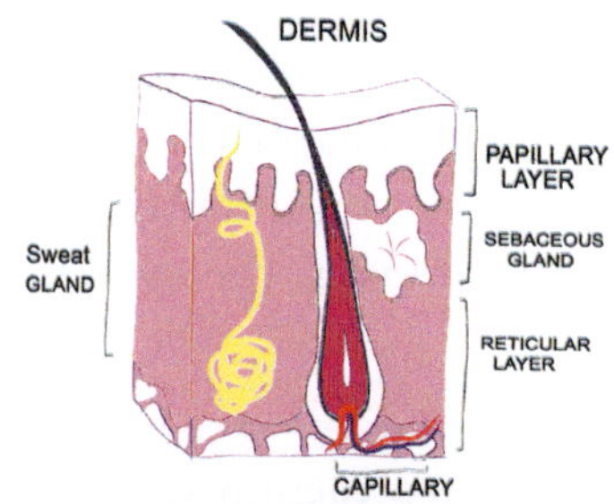
Epidermis	The epidermis is the most superficial layer of the skin and provides the first barrier of protection from the invasion of substances into the body.	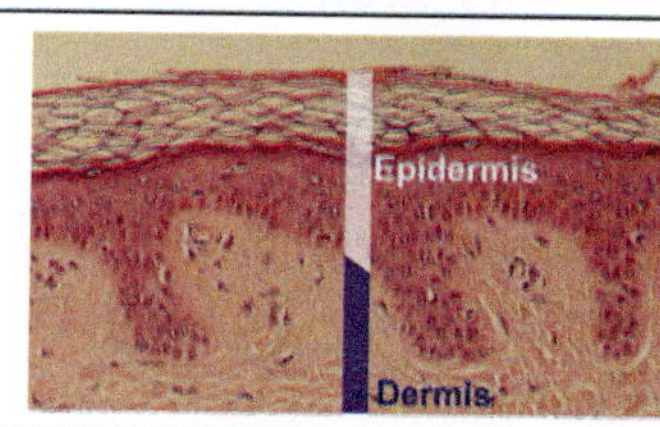
Hair follicle	The hair follicle is a tube-like structure that surrounds the root and strand of a hair. It is located in the top two layers of the skin, beginning at the surface of the epidermis.	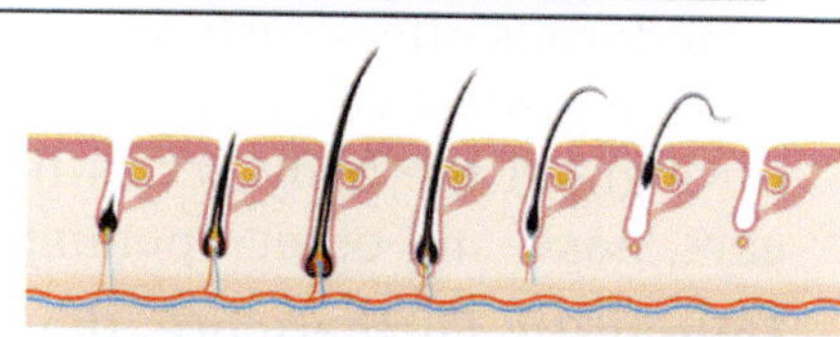
Receptors	Receptors are proteins, typically cell surface receptors, that bind to ligands and induce responses in the immune system, encompassing cytokine receptors, growth factor receptors, and Fc receptors.	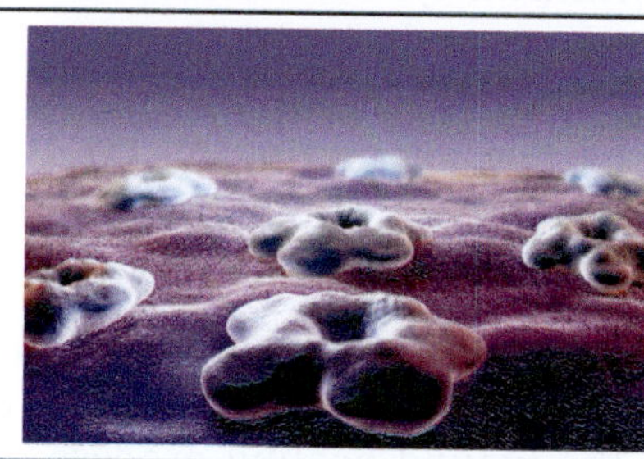

3.1. Understand the Integumentary System

The integumentary system, which is the body's largest organ, acts as a physical barrier to protect and preserve the internal environment by separating it from the outside world. The integumentary system includes:

- Skin (epidermis, dermis);
- Hypodermis;
- Associated glands;
- Hair;
- Nails.

Apart from its barrier role, this system carries out numerous complex tasks such as controlling body temperature, maintaining cell fluid, synthesizing vitamin D, and identifying stimuli. To accomplish these tasks, the system's numerous parts cooperate with one another.

3.1.1. General Function

The integumentary system serves multiple functions and purposes.

1. **Physical Protection:** One of its primary roles is physical protection, as it acts as a covering for the human body. The skin, composed of tightly knit cells, provides strength and resilience. The outermost layer of the epidermis, consisting of layers of dead keratin, can withstand the wear and tear of the external environment. The dermis, in addition to supplying blood to the epidermis, contains nerves that alert us to potential dangers. The hypodermis offers cushioning against mechanical trauma through adipose storage. Glands secrete protective films throughout the body, while nails protect the digits. Hairs located throughout the body act as filters, preventing harmful particles from entering the eyes, ears, nose, and other openings.
2. **Immunity:** Furthermore, the integumentary system plays a crucial role in immunity. It serves as the body's first line of defense, acting as a physical barrier against the direct entry of pathogens. Antimicrobial peptides (AMPs) and lipids on the skin act as a biomolecular barrier, disrupting bacterial membranes. The skin also houses resident immune cells, including myeloid and lymphoid cells. Certain cells, such as Langerhans cells or dermal dendritic cells, can travel to the periphery and activate the broader immune system.
3. **Wound Healing:** Additionally, the integumentary system is involved in wound healing. When the body experiences trauma and sustains an injury, the integumentary system coordinates the wound healing process, which includes hemostasis, inflammation, proliferation, and remodeling.
4. **Thermoregulation:** The skin has a large surface area that is highly vascularized, allowing it to conserve and release heat through vasoconstriction and vasodilation, respectively.
5. **Vitamin D Synthesis:** The primary sources of vitamin D are sun exposure and oral intake, which are crucial for bone health.
6. **Sensation:** Skin innervation is provided by various types of sensory nerve endings that discriminate pain, temperature, touch, and vibration. Each type of receptor and nerve fiber varies in its adaptive and conductive speeds, resulting in a wide range of signals

that can be integrated to create an understanding of the external environment and help the body react appropriately.

3.2. Skin

Skin is an organ of the integumentary system, comprising a layer of tissues that protect underlying muscles and organs, according to zoology and dermatology. Its function as the interface with the environment makes it the most crucial barrier against infections. Its other primary roles include sensation, temperature regulation, insulation, and the synthesis of vitamins D and B. One of the most vital organs in the body is the skin.

Melanocytes produce melanin, which gives skin its pigmentation and helps it absorb some of the potentially harmful solar radiation. Additionally, it has DNA repair enzymes that counteract UV damage; skin cancer is highly prevalent in those who lack the genes for these enzymes. Malignant melanoma, which is primarily caused by UV light, is one type that is extremely invasive, spreads swiftly, and frequently has fatal consequences. Population differences in skin pigmentation are quite noticeable. This has occasionally resulted in the skin color of the person or people being classified. When skin is damaged, it will attempt to heal by producing scar tissue, which frequently results in skin discoloration and depigmentation.

The skin is often known as "the largest organ in the human body." This applies to an exterior surface, as it covers the body, appearing to have the largest surface area of all the organs. Moreover, it applies to weight, as it weighs more than any single internal organ, accounting for about 15% of body weight. For the average adult human, the skin has a surface area of between 1.5–2.0 square meters, most of it is between 2–3 mm thick. The average square inch of skin holds 650 sweat glands, 20 blood vessels, 60,000 melanocytes, and more than a 1,000 nerve endings. Throughout many cultures, the appearance of the face and skin conditions (like pore control and blackhead cleansing) are treated with natural or synthetic cosmetics.

3.2.1. Layers

The skin is composed of two main layers, each consisting of distinct tissues and serving different purposes. The dermis and the epidermis together make up the skin. Below these layers lies the hypodermis, also known as the subcutaneous adipose layer, which is not typically considered a part of the skin.

Beneath the stratified squamous keratinizing epithelium that forms the outermost layer of the epidermis, there is a basement membrane. This membrane is nourished by diffusion from the dermis and does not contain blood vessels. The primary cell types found in the epidermis are melanocytes, Langerhans cells, and keratinocytes. The outermost layer of the epidermis can be further divided into the following strata: corneum, lucidum, granulosum, spinosum, and basale. Mitosis occurs in the innermost layers, leading to the formation of new cells. As these cells differentiate, they move up through the strata, undergoing changes in composition and shape, and expressing new types of keratin genes. Eventually, when they reach the corneum, they are shed off through a process called desquamation. This process, known as keratinization, takes approximately 30 days. The main function of this layer of skin is to prevent infections and the entry of harmful substances into the body, while also retaining water.

Beneath the epidermis, there are blood capillaries that connect to venules and arterioles. Arterial shunt vessels can bypass the fingertips, nose, and ears. Numerous structures, including blood vessels, nerves, hair follicles, smooth muscle, glands, and lymphatic tissue, are found in the dermis, which is located beneath the epidermis. It is composed of loose connective tissue, also known as areolar connective tissue, which contains reticular fibers, elastin, and collagen. Goose bumps are caused when the erector muscles, situated between the hair papilla and epidermis, contract, pulling the hair fiber upright. Fibroblasts, adipocytes (cells that store fat), and macrophages are the three primary cell types. Sebaceous glands are exocrine glands that secrete a mixture of lipids and waxy substances known for their lubricating, waterproofing, softening, and antibacterial properties. Sweat glands emerge from the skin through a pore and a duct.

Collagen and elastin fibers constitute the asymmetric fibrous connective tissue that forms the dermis. It is divided into two sections: the reticular and papillary layers. The outermost layer is called the papillary layer, and it extends into the epidermis to provide blood vessels. It is composed of loosely arranged fibers. The lines on our hands that form our fingerprints are made up of papillary ridges. The reticular layer is continuous with the hypodermis and has a higher density. Most structures, including sweat glands, are located there. The reticular layer is resistant to stretching due to its erratic fiber arrangement.

The hypodermis is located beneath the dermis and is not a component of the skin. Its function is to supply the skin with blood vessels and nerves, as well as to attach the skin to the underlying muscle and bone. It is made up of elastin and loose connective tissue. The primary cell types are adipocytes, macrophages, and fibroblasts (half of body fat is found in the hypodermis). The body uses fat as insulation and cushioning.

The outer epidermis and the inner dermis are the two main layers of skin. These layers are composed of various tissues and serve distinct purposes.

3.2.2. Epidermis

The stratified squamous keratinizing epithelial tissue that makes up the epidermis is thickest on the palms and soles. There are no capillaries between the most prevalent cells, which are referred to as keratinocytes. Two of the epidermis's sublayers—the innermost stratum germinativum and the outermost stratum corneum—are the most significant, despite the fact that the epidermis can be further divided into four or five sublayers (Figure 3.1).

3.2.2.1. Stratum Germinativum

Another name for the stratum germinativum is the stratum basale. Every name provides information about this layer. To germinate is to "grow" or "sprout." "Basal" refers to the "lowest part" or "base." The base of the epidermis, or the innermost layer where mitosis occurs, is called the stratum germinativum. Older cells are pushed toward the surface of the skin by the constant production of new cells. These cells die as they move farther from the dermal capillaries and produce the protein keratin. Lower layer cells replace dead skin cells as they wear away from the skin's surface. Merkel cells, also referred to as Merkel discs, are distinct cells that are dispersed among the keratinocytes of the stratum germinativum and serve as touch receptors (Figure 3.2).

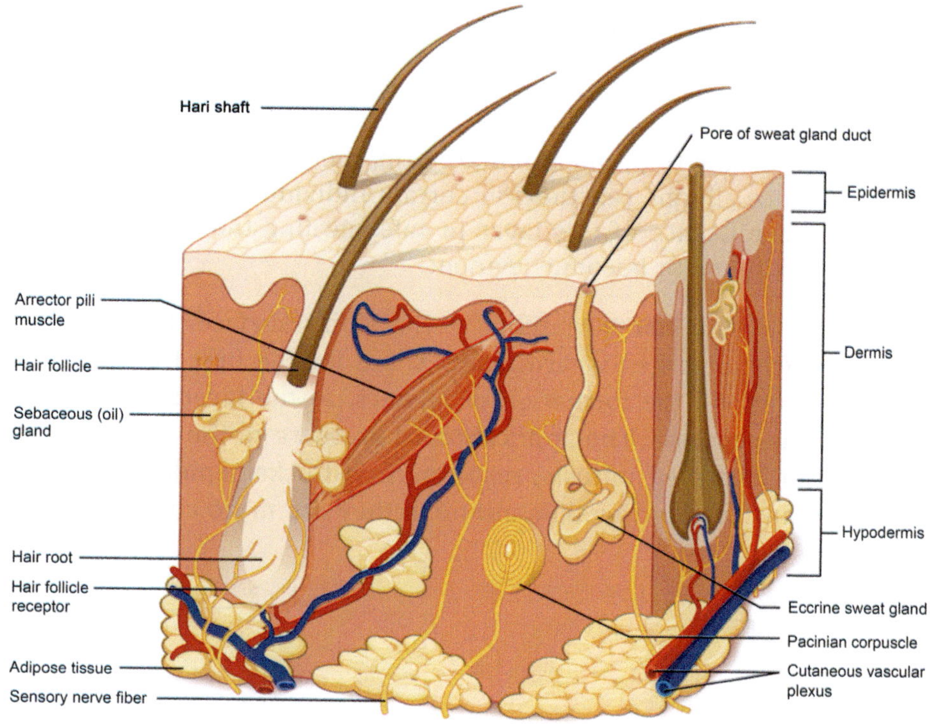

Figure 3.1. *Structure of the skin and subcutaneous tissue.*

Source: https://courses.lumenlearning.com/suny-wmopen-biology2/chapter/structure-and-function-of-skin/.

Defensins are antimicrobial peptides that can be synthesized by living keratinocytes. The process of inflammation that follows any skin injury involves the production of these and other chemicals. Defensins break the pathogens' membranes, allowing bacteria and other pathogens to enter through skin breaks.

The living layer of the epidermis also produces a vitamin: when exposed to UV light, the cells' form of cholesterol is converted to vitamin D, which is subsequently processed by the liver and kidneys into the most active form, known as 1,25-D, or calcitriol, which is regarded as a hormone. Because of this, vitamin D is sometimes called the "sunshine vitamin." Individuals who do not receive enough sunlight are more likely to rely on fortified milk and other dietary sources of vitamin D. However, the best way to obtain vitamin D is most likely to be outside, and 15 minutes a day, a few times a week is usually sufficient. It has long been known that vitamin D plays a crucial role in the small intestine's ability to absorb calcium and phosphorus from food. However, according to recent studies, vitamin D is also necessary for insulin function, the maintenance of muscle strength, particularly in older adults, and certain immune responses, which may protect against some cancers.

3.2.2.2. Stratum Corneum

The outermost layer of the skin, known as the stratum corneum, is composed of multiple layers of dead cells containing keratin. This protein is hydrophobic, aiding in the prevention of body water evaporation and acting as a barrier against water infiltration. Moreover, the stratum corneum functions as a protective shield against pathogens and chemicals, with the majority of microorganisms unable to penetrate the skin. The shedding of dead skin cells and the presence of fatty acids in sebum also contribute to the elimination of microorganisms and the inhibition of their growth. While most chemicals are unable to permeate intact skin, there are exceptions, such as the sap of poison ivy, which can induce allergic reactions in certain individuals. When the stratum corneum is disrupted or lost, the significance of this layer in safeguarding the body from external threats and maintaining overall skin health becomes evident.

You may be familiar with minor variations in the skin's surface. For instance, the skin of the foot may experience friction when wearing new shoes for the first time. This can lead to the accumulation of tissue fluid and the formation of blisters, as the layers of the epidermis or the epidermis from the dermis separate. The application of pressure to the skin prompts the stratum germinativum to undergo increased mitosis, resulting in a thicker epidermis known as a callus. Calluses can develop on any area of the skin, although they are more commonly observed on the palms and soles.

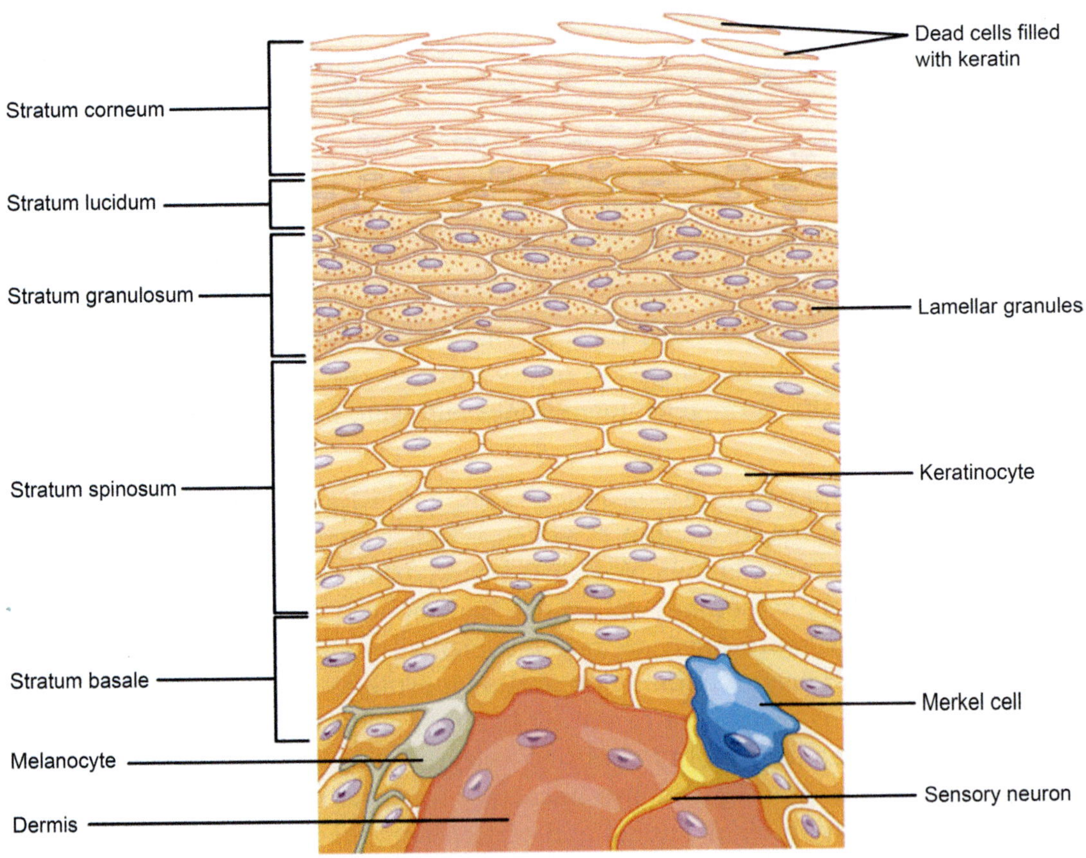

Figure 3.2. *The epidermis, showing the different kinds of cells present and the blood supply in the upper dermis.*

Source: https://courses.lumenlearning.com/suny-wmopen-biology2/chapter/structure-and-function-of-skin/.

3.2.2.3. Langerhans Cells

Langerhans cells, also known as dendritic cells due to their branched appearance during movement, are found within the epidermis. These highly mobile cells originate in the red bone marrow. They have the ability to phagocytize foreign substances, including bacteria that enter the body through breaks in the skin. Once these pathogens are engulfed, the Langerhans cells migrate to lymph nodes where they present the pathogen to lymphocytes, a subset of white blood cells. This triggers an immune response that involves the production of antibodies, which are proteins that tag foreign objects for elimination. While many details of this process remain unknown, the skin plays a significant role in the body's defense mechanisms due to its close proximity to the external environment.

3.2.2.4. Melanocytes

The melanocyte, which is also depicted in Figure 3.2, is another type of cell present in the lower epidermis. Melanocytes produce melanin, a pigment, and another protein. The quantity of melanocytes in individuals of similar sizes is generally the same, but the activity level of these cells varies. Melanocytes in individuals with dark skin constantly produce a significant amount of melanin, while those with lighter skin produce less melanin. Melanocyte activity is genetically controlled, as skin color is an inherited trait.

UV rays, which are a component of sunlight and can be harmful to living cells, stimulate the production of melanin in the skin of all individuals. As a result, the epidermal cells migrate towards the surface and absorb more melanin. This leads to a darker skin tone and provides greater protection to the living stratum germinativum against UV radiation. Individuals with lighter skin are not as well-protected from the harmful effects of UV radiation as those with darker skin. Additionally, melanin not only has a protective effect on the hair on the head, but also contributes to hair color. Melanin is responsible for the color of the iris and the inner layer of the eyeball known as the choroid. Table 3.1 provides a list of the cells that comprise the skin.

Table 3.1. Cells of the Skin

Named Tissue and Associated Cell Groups	Cell Count	Aggregate Cell Mass (g)	Percent of Total Mass
Skin total	6.1E+11	846.7	100%
Adipocyte	7.3E+08	291.9	34.5%
Endothelial cell (EnCs)	1.5E+10	6.16	0.7%
Epithelial cells (EpC)	4.1E+11	313.9	37.1%
Eccrine gland	1.7E+11	105	12.4%
Epidermal keratinocytes	1.1E+11	85.5	10.1%
Hair follicle	1.3E+11	119.9	14.2%
Mechanoreceptors	4.9E+09	3.6	0.4%
Epithelial cells (EpC); non-nucleated	7.2E+10	28.2	3.3%

Fibroblasts	4.3E+10	94.6	11.2%
Myocytes	2.6E+07	0.08	0.01%
Neuroglia	8.5E+09	12.8	1.5%
Perivascular cells / pericytes / mural	1.5E+09	0.56	0.07%
Stem cells; epithelial (EpSC)	3.6E+09	1.50	0.2%
White blood cells	5.4E+10	97.1	11.5%
Granulocytes (mast cell)	2.2E+10	32.6	3.8%
Lymphoid	1.3E+10	1.6	0.2%
Monocyte-macrophage series	1.9E+10	62.9	7.4%

Source: "Human Cell Data." humancelltreemap.mis.mpg.de: https://en.wikipedia.org/wiki/Human_skin#cite_note-19.

3.2.3. Dermis

The fibrous connective tissue that comprises the dermis is irregular, indicating that its fibers run in multiple directions rather than parallel. Fibroblasts are the cells responsible for producing elastin and collagen fibers. It is important to note that elastin fibers have the ability to contract back to their original state after being stretched, whereas collagen fibers possess great strength. The dermis possesses two key characteristics: elasticity and strength. However, as individuals age, their skin gradually loses its elasticity due to the degradation of elastin fibers. Consequently, the development of a few wrinkles is an anticipated outcome of the aging process.

The papillary layer refers to the irregular junction between the dermis and epidermis (*refer* Figure 3.1). This region contains numerous capillaries that provide support to the stratum germinativum and the dermis. The blood supply delivers oxygen and nutrients to the lower, living cells in the epidermis, which lacks its own capillaries.

The dermis houses various auxiliary skin structures, including hair and nail follicles, sensory receptors, and different types of glands. While their active components reside in the dermis, some of these structures extend through the epidermis and reach the surface of the skin.

3.3. Hair Follicles

Since epidermal tissue comprises hair follicles, the growth of hair and the epidermis are highly similar processes. The hair root, situated at the base of a follicle, houses the matrix cells where mitosis takes place (Figure 3.3). The newly formed cells produce keratin, acquire melanin for coloration, undergo cell death, and merge with the hair shaft, which is drawn towards the skin's surface. Every day, we remove dead, keratinized hair cells through brushing and combing. The average rate of hair growth is between 0.3 to 0.4 inches per month, equivalent to 8 to 10 mm.

Humans possess less hair compared to other mammals, and human hair serves limited practical purposes. The hairs inside the nostrils help prevent dust from entering the nasal cavities, while the eyebrows and eyelashes aid in keeping sweat and dust away from the eyes. The hair on the scalp contributes to keeping the head warm during winter. Although the hair on our bodies no longer serves this purpose, we still retain evolutionary remnants of it. The pilomotor or arrector pili muscle, a small smooth muscle attached to each hair follicle, causes the hair follicles to stand upright when stimulated by cold or strong emotions such as fear. This response would trap air and enhance insulation for a furry animal. In humans, this mechanism only results in "goose bumps" since we lack thick fur.

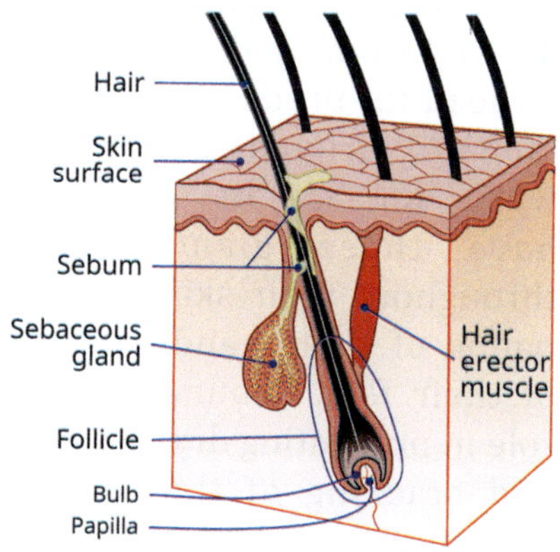

Figure 3.3. *Structure of a hair follicle.*

Source: By National Institutes of Health – This file has been extracted from another file, Public Domain, https://commons.wikimedia.org/w/index.php?curid=6910143.

3.4. Nail Follicles

Nail follicles, located on the tips of fingers and toes, produce nails in a similar manner to hair follicles. Mitosis occurs at the base of the nail, in the nail root, as depicted in Figure 3.4. The newly formed cells eventually die after producing keratin, a more potent form of this protein compared to that found in hair. The nail bed, despite being composed of keratinized dead cells, consists of living epidermis and dermis. This explains why cutting a nail too short can be quite painful. Nails not only provide greater dexterity and protection against mechanical harm, but also facilitate the grasping of small objects with the fingertips. Fingernails also serve as a useful tool for scratching. This has more significance than initially perceived. An itchy area could indicate the presence of fleas, ticks, mosquitoes, or lice. With the exception of ticks, these parasites are insects that feed on blood and have the ability to transmit diseases caused by bacteria, viruses, or protozoa. A swift and forceful scratch can eliminate the arthropod or, at the very least, dislodge it, preventing the spread of illness. Fingernails grow at a rate of approximately 0–12 inches (3 mm) per month, with slightly faster growth during the summer.

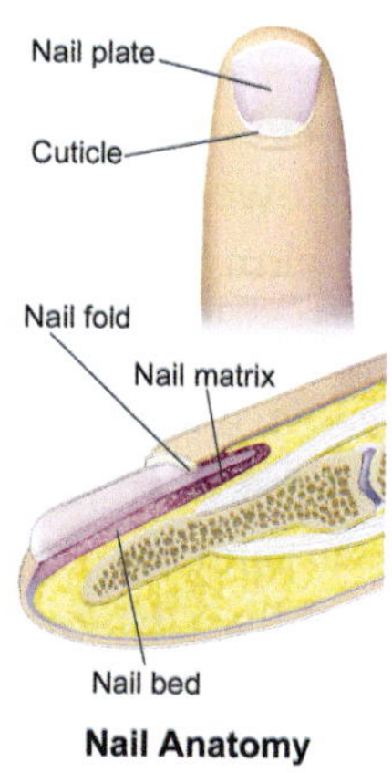

Figure 3.4. *Structure of a fingernail.*

Source: By BruceBlaus. When using this image in external sources, it can be cited as: Blausen.com staff (2014). "Medical gallery of Blausen Medical 2014." WikiJournal of Medicine, 1(2). doi: 10.15347/wjm/2014.010.ISSN 2002-4436. – Own work, CC BY 3.0, https://commons.wikimedia.org/w/index.php?curid=30871436.

3.5. Receptors

The dermis contains the majority of the sensory receptors for the cutaneous senses (nerve endings and Merkel cells are located in the stratum germinativum). The five senses of the skin are pain, pressure, heat, and cold. There is a specific kind of receptor—a structure that can recognize a specific change—for every kind of sensation. The receptors are free nerve endings that respond to pain, heat, and cold. The receptors for pressure and touch are referred to as encapsulated nerve endings, indicating that the sensory nerve ending is surrounded by a cellular structure. These receptors and feelings serve to convey information about the external environment and its impact on the skin to the central nervous system. This knowledge could prompt actions like cleaning a sore cut finger, picking at an insect bite, or putting on a sweater in response to feeling cold.

The quantity of receptors in a skin area determines its sensitivity. For example, the skin on the fingertips has many receptors per square inch, making it extremely sensitive to touch. Because there are fewer touch receptors per square inch on the skin of the upper arm, it is less sensitive.

Nerve impulses are sent by receptors that identify changes to the brain, which interprets the impulses as a specific sensation. Thus, sensation is essentially a brain function.

3.6. Glands

Tissue called epithelium makes up glands. The dermis contains the secretory parts of the skin's exocrine glands.

1. **Sebaceous Glands:** These ducts can open directly onto the skin's surface or into hair follicles. Sebum, a lipid substance that is commonly referred to as oil, is what they secrete. As previously mentioned, sebum prevents bacteria from growing on the surface of the skin. Protecting the skin and hair from drying out is one of sebum's other roles. It is important to note that dry skin is more prone to cracking, which can allow bacteria to enter the skin through even the smallest of cracks. Another effect of aging is decreased sebum production, resulting in dry and more delicate skin, which is common in the elderly.

   Overactive sebaceous glands can be problematic for adolescents. Excessive sebum production can lead to minor infections by trapping bacteria in hair follicles. Young people often experience pimples around their mouth and nose due to the higher concentration of sebaceous glands in these areas.

   Mammals possess sebaceous glands in their skin, which are responsible for secreting sebum, an oily substance derived from lipids and the remnants of dead fat-producing cells. The term "sebum" originates from the Latin words for "fat" or "tallow." Humans have these glands distributed throughout their skin, except for the palms of their hands and the soles of their feet. Sebum plays a crucial role in preventing dryness, brittleness, and cracking of the skin and hair by acting as a waterproofing agent. Additionally, it exhibits antimicrobial properties, inhibiting the growth of microorganisms on the skin.

   Sebaceous glands are typically found in areas covered by hair and are connected to hair follicles. They secrete sebum onto the hairs, which then travels along the hair shaft and reaches the surface of the skin. The structure composed of hair, hair follicles, and sebaceous glands is referred to as the pilosebaceous unit. Sebaceous glands are also present in non-haired regions such as the lips, eyelids, penis, labia minora, and nipples. Ducts allow the sebum to be released from these glands and reach the skin's surface. These glands are classified as holocrine glands since sebum is produced within specialized cells within the glands and is released upon cell rupture (Figure 3.5).

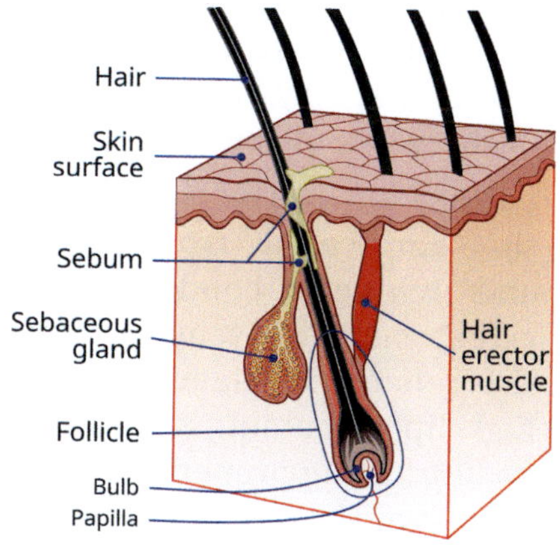

Figure 3.5. *Schematic view of a hair follicle and a sebaceous gland.*

Source: By National Institutes of Health – This file has been extracted from another file, Public Domain, https://commons.wikimedia.org/w/index.php?curid=6910143.

Sebum is odorless, but its bacterial breakdown can produce odors. Sebum is the cause of some individuals experiencing "oily" hair if it is not washed for several days. Earwax and mucopurulent discharge, the dry substance accumulating in the corners of the eye after sleeping, both contain sebum.

Different species have varying compositions of sebum. In humans, the lipid content consists of approximately 25% wax monoesters, 41% triglycerides, 16% free fatty acids, and 12% squalene. During puberty, elevated androgen levels lead to increased activity of the sebaceous glands.

Skin conditions such as keratosis pilaris and acne are associated with sebaceous glands. A blocked sebaceous gland can result in the formation of a sebaceous cyst. Isotretinoin, a prescription medication used to treat acne, significantly reduces sebum secretion by the sebaceous glands. Bodybuilders who excessively use anabolic steroids (up to 10 times the recommended dosage) in an attempt to prevent weight loss often stimulate their sebaceous glands, which can lead to acne.

The sebaceous glands of a human fetus in utero secrete a substance called Vernix caseosa, a "waxy" or "cheesy" white substance that coats the skin of newborns.

Mice and rats have large modified sebaceous glands called preputial glands, which produce pheromones.

2. **Ceruminous Glands:** The dermis of the ear canals contains these glands. Cerumen, also known as ear wax, is the term for their secretion, which also contains sebum secreted in the ear canals. Cerumen prevents drying and maintains the eardrum's outer surface pliable, but too much of it can build up in the ear canal and press against the eardrum. This may cause the eardrum to vibrate less properly, which could reduce hearing acuity.

   The yellowish-waxy substance called earwax, or cerumen in medical parlance, is secreted in the ear canals of humans and many other mammals. It is essential to the human ear canal's function, helping to lubricate and clean it while offering some defense against germs, fungi, and insects. Roeser and Ballachanda provide a thorough analysis of the physiology and pathophysiology of cerumen. Hearing loss may result from excessive cerumen or cerumen that has lodged against the eardrum, obstructing the external auditory canal.

3. **Production, Composition, and Different Types:** Cerumen is produced in the outer third of the human ear canal's cartilaginous portion. It is a blend of less viscous secretions from modified apocrine sweat glands and viscous secretions from sebaceous glands.

   There are two different genetically determined types of earwax: the recessive dry type and the dominant wet type. Caucasians and Africans are more likely to have the wet type of cerumen, which is honey-brown to dark-brown and moist. On the other hand, Asians and Native Americans are more likely to have the dry type, which is gray and flaky. Anthropologists have utilized cerumen type to trace human migration patterns, including those of the Inuit people.

   The difference in cerumen type has been traced back to a single base change, specifically a single nucleotide polymorphism, in a gene known as the "ATP-binding cassette C11 gene." This mutation not only affects cerumen type but also reduces sweat production. The researchers hypothesize that the decrease in sweat production was advantageous to the ancestors of East Asians and Native Americans, who are believed to have inhabited cold climates.

4. **Function:** In terms of function, the process of epithelial migration, often referred to as the "conveyor belt" process, is facilitated by jaw movement and serves to clean the ear canal. The cells located centrally in the tympanic membrane move outward from the umbo towards the walls of the ear canal at a rate comparable to the growth of fingernails. Eventually, they reach the entrance of the canal. Additionally, any dirt, dust, or other particles that may have accumulated in the canal are carried out by the cerumen. Jaw movement enhances the likelihood of extrusion by dislodging debris that may have become trapped in the walls of the ear canal.

   Lubrication prevents the skin inside the ear canal from drying out and itching, a condition known as asteatosis. The sebum secreted by the sebaceous glands, which has a high lipid content, is responsible for its lubricating properties. These lipids consist of alcohols, various long-chain fatty acids, squalene, and cholesterol, particularly in wet-type cerumen.

   Studies conducted prior to the 1960s provided limited evidence of cerumen's antibacterial properties. However, more recent research has demonstrated that cerumen does offer some bactericidal defense against specific strains of bacteria. It has been discovered that cerumen is effective in reducing the viability of various bacteria, including *Haemophilus influenzae, Staphylococcus aureus*, and several variations of *Escherichia coli*, sometimes by as much as 99%. Human cerumen has also been found to significantly inhibit the growth of two fungi commonly found in otomycosis. The main contributors to these antimicrobial properties are the presence of lysozyme, saturated fatty acids, and, most importantly, the relatively low pH of cerumen, which is typically around 6.1 in healthy individuals.

5. **Sweat Glands:** There are two types of sweat glands: apocrine and eccrine. Apocrine glands are most abundant in the genital and axillary (underarm) regions, and they become most active

during stressful and emotional events. Their secretions do have an odor, although not one that is noticeable to others. Dogs, however, are able to distinguish between individuals easily due to their unique scents. Allowing apocrine secretions to accumulate on the skin leads to the breakdown of chemicals in perspiration by bacteria, resulting in the production of waste products with distinct odors that many people find unpleasant.

6. **Eccrine:** Though they are present throughout the body, eccrine glands are particularly abundant on the forehead, upper lip, palms, and soles. The secretory section of these glands is a dermal coiled tube. The duct of this tube runs to the surface of the skin, where it opens into a pore.

   Sweat, produced by eccrine glands, plays a critical role in regulating body temperature. In warm environments or during physical activity, more sweat is released onto the skin to help cool the body through evaporation. Due to water's high heat of vaporization, a small amount of sweat can dissipate a significant amount of heat. While this method effectively aids in cooling down the body, excessive sweating can potentially lead to dehydration, especially in situations such as heat exhaustion or intense exercise on hot and humid days. It is essential to increase fluid intake when sweating excessively to prevent dehydration.

   Regular exercisers are aware of the need to replenish both salt and water. Sweat also contains trace amounts of urea, a nitrogenous waste product of amino acid metabolism, and sodium chloride. However, the skin's excretory function is minimal, as the kidneys are primarily responsible for eliminating waste from the blood and maintaining the body's ideal salt-to-water ratio.

   The majority of human eccrine sweat is composed of water, with various salts and organic compounds mixed in. It contains trace amounts of urea, other waste products, and fatty materials. Sodium concentrations range from 35 to 65 mmol/l, with individuals acclimated to hot climates having lower concentrations. Sweat composition differs in other species.

7. **Apocrine:** These glands appear between the ages of 15 and 20 during the early to mid-puberty stage. They release more sweat than usual for about a month before regulating and releasing normal sweat levels after a predetermined amount of time. Sweat from apocrine sweat glands contains fatty substances. The activity of these glands, primarily found in the armpits and surrounding the genital area, is primarily responsible for sweat odor due to the bacteria that break down the organic compounds in the sweat. Stress can cause the apocrine glands to produce more sweat or squeeze out the sweat already present in the tubule, resulting in increased sweating. Apocrine sweat glands essentially function as scent glands.

   However, in certain parts of the body, such as the cerumen (or "wax") of the outer ear, these sweat glands are modified to secrete completely different substances. Other glands, like the mammary glands, undergo significant enlargement and modification to produce milk.

8. **Mammary Glands:** These found in female mammals, are responsible for producing milk to nourish the young.

These exocrine glands, which are enlarged and modified sweat glands, are a defining feature of mammals.

- **Structure:** The mammary gland's structure consists of alveoli, which are hollow cavities lined with milk-secreting epithelial cells surrounded by myoepithelial cells. These alveoli combine to form lobules, groups of alveoli connected to lactiferous ducts that empty into nipple openings. Similar to muscle cells, myoepithelial cells can contract, allowing milk to be forced from the alveoli through the lactiferous ducts and into the nipple, where it collects in the duct widenings known as sinuses. Essentially, a baby extracts milk from these sinuses by sucking (Figure 3.6).

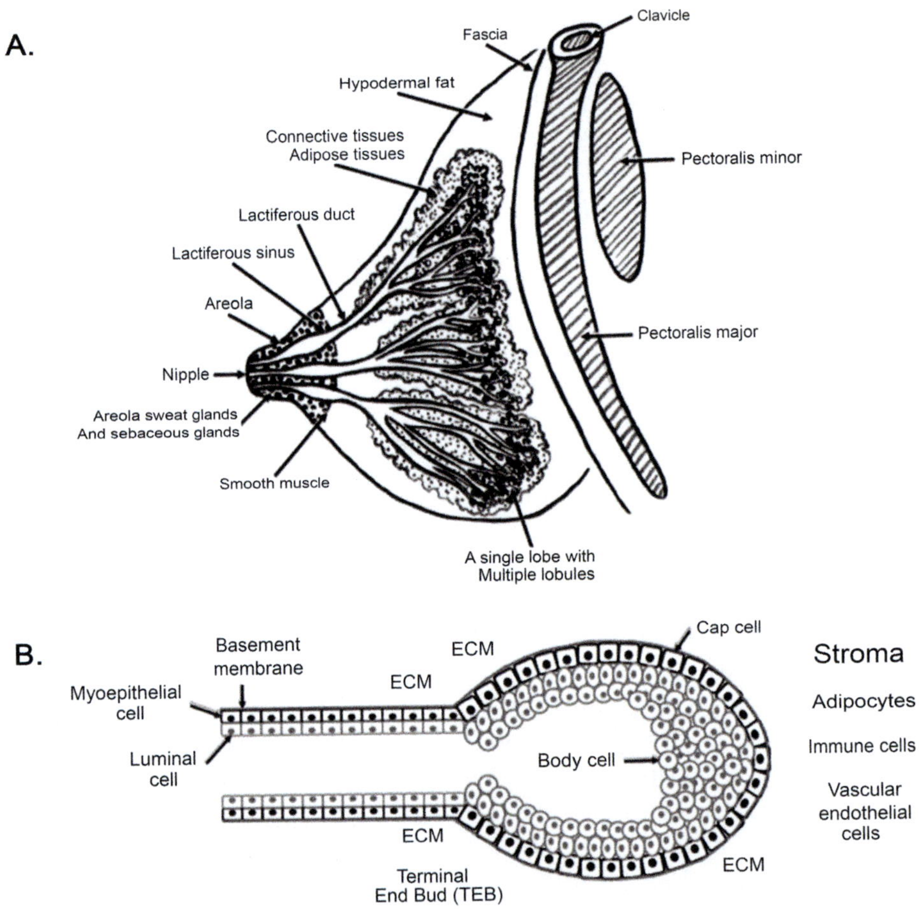

Figure 3.6. *Cross section of the breast of a human female.*

Source: Biswas, S. K., Banerjee, S., Baker, G. W., Kuo, C. Y., & Chowdhury, I., (2022). The mammary gland: Basic structure and molecular signaling during development. International Journal of Molecular Sciences, 23(7), 3883. https://doi.org/10.3390/ijms23073883.

A simple mammary gland is composed of all the milk-secreting tissue that leads to a single lactiferous duct. Conversely, a complex mammary gland is composed of all the simple mammary glands that serve a single nipple.

Typically, humans possess two intricate mammary glands – one in each breast. Each of these mammary glands is composed of 10-20 smaller simple glands. If an individual has more than two nipples, it is referred to as polythelia, and if they have more than two complex mammary glands, it is known as polymastia (Figure 3.7).

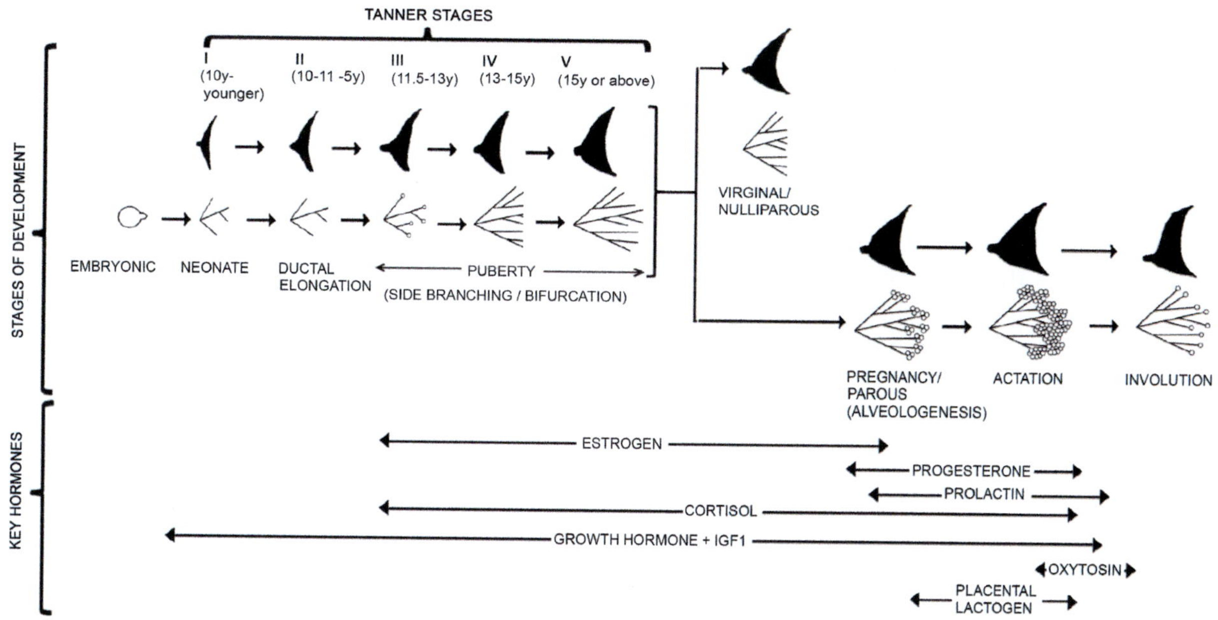

Figure 3.7. *Dissection of a lactating breast.*

Source: Biswas, S. K., Banerjee, S., Baker, G. W., Kuo, C. Y., & Chowdhury, I., (2022). The mammary gland: Fundamental structure and molecular signaling during development. International Journal of Molecular Sciences, 23(7), 3883. https://doi.org/10.3390/ijms23073883.

3.6.1. Development and Hormonal Control

Hormones regulate the development of mammary glands. Both sexes have mammary glands, but until puberty, when females begin to develop them in response to ovarian hormones, they are in a primitive state. A woman's breast tissue undergoes changes during menstruation. Testosterone inhibits its formation, while estrogen encourages it.

At birth, infants lack alveoli but possess lactiferous ducts. Before puberty, ovarian estrogens promote the branching differentiation of the ducts into spherical masses of cells, which eventually become alveoli. During this stage, there is minimal branching. True secretory alveoli only form during pregnancy, due to increased adipose tissue, enhanced blood flow, and additional branching and differentiation of the duct cells, triggered by rising estrogen and progesterone levels.

In the final stages of pregnancy and the initial days following childbirth, colostrum is secreted. A few days later, true milk secretion (lactation) begins as prolactin is present and progesterone levels have dropped. The hormone oxytocin is released during breastfeeding, causing the contraction of myoepithelial cells.

3.6.2. Breast Cancer

Hormones can easily trigger the cells of mammary glands to grow and multiply. If this growth becomes unmanageable, cancer may occur. The majority of breast cancer cases start in the lobules or ducts of the mammary glands (Figure 3.8).

Types of breast cancer are as follows:

- DCIS: Ductal carcinoma *in situ*;
- LCIS: Lobular carcinoma *in situ*;
- Invasive ductal carcinoma;
- Invasive lobular carcinoma;
- Inflammatory breast cancer;
- Paget's disease.

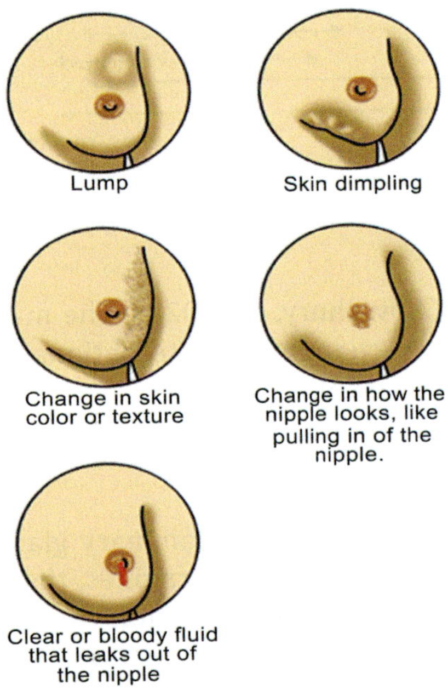

Figure 3.8. *Early signs of breast cancer.*

Source: By Morning2k – http://www.4woman.gov/faq/cancer-illustrations-with-t.gif, Public Domain, https://commons.wikimedia.org/w/index.php?curid=37747125.

3.6.3. Other Mammals

Mammals differ greatly in the number of simple and complex mammary glands they possess. The two milk lines, which run roughly parallel along the front of the body, are where the nipples and glands can appear. On dogs or cats, they are easy to observe, with three to five pairs of nipples that correspond to the milk lines. Along these lines, most mammals develop their mammary glands in pairs, roughly equal to the number of offspring that are typically born at a time.

With the exception of a few species, all male mammals have simple mammary glands and nipples. For instance, male mice are sterile, while male horses are not.

Given that mammary glands serve as protein factories, several companies have created transgenic animals, primarily goats and cows, to produce proteins for medical use. Genetically modified bacteria are incapable of producing complex glycoproteins such as antithrombin or monoclonal antibodies, and producing them in live mammals is much more cost-effective than in mammalian cell cultures.

3.7. Blood Vessels

The arterioles are additional blood vessels of significant importance in addition to the dermal capillaries. Small arteries called arterioles can dilate (open) or constrict (close) due to the smooth muscle in their walls. This is crucial for maintaining body temperature because heat is a type of energy carried by the blood.

In a warm environment, the arterioles widen to increase blood flow through the skin and release excess heat to the environment. This is known as vasodilation. Conversely, in a cold environment, the arterioles narrow to conserve body heat, known as vasoconstriction. This adjustment is crucial for maintaining internal balance, or homeostasis. The nervous system regulates the size of the arterioles in response to temperature changes. These changes are more noticeable in light-skinned individuals, who may experience flushing in warm weather and paleness in cold weather. However, in individuals with dark skin, these changes are less visible due to the presence of melanin in the skin.

Stressful circumstances can also cause vasoconstriction in the dermis. Stress typically required our ancestors to react physically, either by fighting or by fleeing to safety. We refer to this as the "fight or flight response." Our neurological systems are still wired to react as though engaging in physical activity would be essential to handle the stressful circumstance. Blood will be redirected, or shunted, to more important organs like the heart, brain, and muscles when the dermis becomes vasoconstricted. The skin is a relatively insignificant organ that can temporarily function with little blood flow when under stress. The phrase "broke out in a cold sweat" is undoubtedly familiar to you, and you may have experienced it yourself during a tense moment. Because of the dermis's vasoconstriction, which keeps the skin relatively cool, this type of sweating feels cold.

Prolonged pressure on the skin can disrupt blood flow in the dermis. A decubitus ulcer, also known as a pressure ulcer or pressure sore, may occur, for instance, in a hospital patient who is unable to turn over on their own. Between an external object, like a bed, and an internal bony prominence, like the lower back's sacrum or heel bone, the skin is compressed. The skin dies when its blood supply is cut off, and the dead tissue can become infected with bacteria (Figure 3.9).

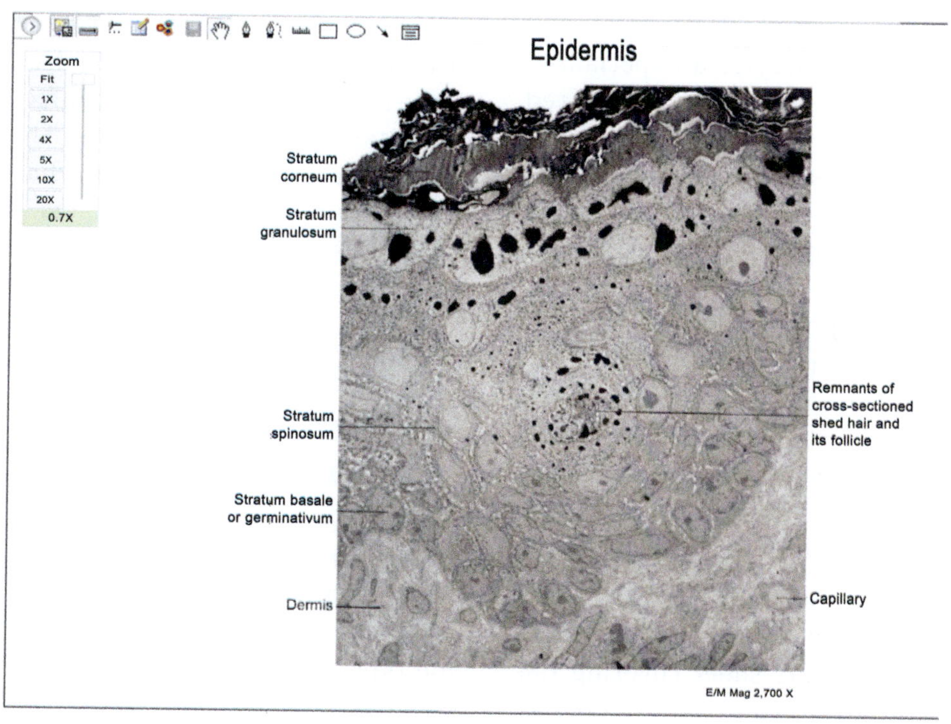

Figure 3.9. *Cells of the epidermis.*

Source: https://courses.lumenlearning.com/suny-wmopen-biology2/chapter/structure-and-function-of-skin/.

3.8. Subcutaneous Tissue

The superficial fascia, a connective tissue membrane, is another name for the subcutaneous tissue. The superficial fascia, which connects the dermis to the underlying muscles, is composed of adipose and areolar connective tissue.

Areolar connective tissue, also known as loose connective tissue, contains collagen, elastin, and a significant number of white blood cells that have escaped from their capillaries and are present in the tissue fluid between the skin and muscles. These migrating white blood cells help eliminate pathogens that enter the body through skin breaks. Mast cells, specialized connective tissue cells, are also found in the areolar tissue. In response to damage, the body produces histamine, leukotrienes, and other chemicals that cause inflammation.

Adipose tissue, or adipocytes, are specialized cells that store fat. Excess nutrients are stored as potential energy in our subcutaneous layer of fat. Additionally, this layer provides some insulation against the cold and cushions bony prominences during activities such as sitting. However, compared to animals like whales and seals, humans do not have a thick layer of fat, so this function is relatively insignificant. Adipose tissue also produces cytokines, which are chemicals that activate white blood cells and play a role in inflammation. It is also involved in regulating the initiation and cessation of eating, as well as the body's utilization of insulin.

Subcutaneous tissue is a continuous layer, albeit an internal one, much like the epidermis which forms a continuous sheet covering the body. Subcutaneous tissue can be considered as a secondary line of defense against pathogens, if we consider the epidermis as the first line of defense. However, there is a notable anatomical distinction. The cells and protein fibers of subcutaneous tissue are more widely spaced, and there is a greater volume of tissue fluid, compared to the cells of the epidermis, which are densely packed together. If the epidermis is analogous to a four-lane highway with heavy traffic during rush hour, the superficial fascia can be likened to the same highway at three in the morning, when it is less congested and vehicles can travel much more quickly. While this is clearly advantageous for the white blood cells migrating, it could also work against them because some bacterial pathogens can spread even more quickly through subcutaneous tissue once they are established.

Necrotizing fasciitis, for instance, is caused by Group A streptococcus. Necrotizing is defined as "to cause death," and fasciitis is the inflammation of a fascia, in this case, the deep fasciae surrounding muscles and the superficial fascia. Necrotizing fasciitis is a highly dangerous infection that requires surgical treatment to attempt to halt the bacteria from spreading. This may involve removing infected tissue or potentially amputating a limb. The "looseness" of areolar connective tissue, which is typically an anatomical advantage, has been turned against us and transformed into a disadvantage, overwhelming the body's defenses.

3.9. Age-Related Physiological Changes in the Integumentary System

The effects of aging on the integumentary system are often highly noticeable. The repair process for even minor breaks or cuts is slowed down as fibroblasts in the dermis die and are not replaced, resulting in thinning and increased fragility of both skin layers. Wrinkles appear as collagen and elastin fibers in the dermis break down. The skin becomes dry, sebaceous glands and sweat glands become less active, and regulating body temperature in hot weather becomes more challenging. Hair loss occurs on the body and scalp as hair follicles become dormant. The melanocytes that remain die and are not replenished, causing the remaining hair to turn white. Additionally, subcutaneous tissue tends to have less fat in older individuals, making them more susceptible to the cold. It is important for elderly individuals (and their caregivers) to be aware of the potential dangers of extreme temperatures and to take extra safety precautions during periods of extreme heat or cold.

Since it deals with the skin, hair, and nails, this system has undergone the most visible changes. Elderly individuals are more susceptible to skin tears and shearing injuries due to the loss of elasticity and moisture in their skin. The nails become brittle and thick, while the hair loses its pigmentation. In addition to the aforementioned integumentary changes, there is a gradual loss of muscle and subcutaneous fat. Consequently, elderly individuals often exhibit muscle atrophy, a "double" chin, skin wrinkles, and sagging earlobes and eyelids. Breasts may sag and lose firmness in women as they age. As subcutaneous fat diminishes, so does one's tolerance to cold temperatures. Teaching about health promotion can encompass topics such as safeguarding the skin from sun damage with protective clothing and sunscreen, maintaining skin health through proper nutrition and hydration, and avoiding harsh detergents and abrasive textures.

Being the first line of defense against the external environment requires significant effort. A day in the life of our skin would reveal the numerous threats it encounters from harmful chemicals, bacteria, viruses, and pollutants. Let us examine the changes that occur in our largest defense mechanism, our skin, from infancy to old age. It is truly remarkable how resilient our skin is, even after a lifetime of exposure to these assailants.

3.9.1. Infants: The Armor as Soft as Angels

Everyone wishes their skin could be as delicate and soft as that of a newborn. Its dewy moisture creates the illusion that you are touching the skin of a cherub. Nevertheless, an infant's skin is not immune to the unwanted daily visitors that land on the delicate surface, just like the majority of people who are now exposed to the dangers of the earth. Compared to children and adults, an infant's skin is more water-rich, but they lose extra water more quickly.

In the first year of life, an infant's skin barrier reaches maturity, making the early months of life more vulnerable to skin conditions. Physiologic jaundice is another common occurrence for an infant's skin. If a baby's skin turns yellowish two or three days after birth, parents shouldn't freak out. Additionally, they might have vernix caseosa, a white, cheesy substance covering their skin, and milia, tiny white nodules scattered across their face.

A peculiarity of an infant's skin is that bathing can harm it as well. A baby as young as a few weeks old who is bathed with a washcloth loses more water and has dehydrated skin. Using a washcloth causes almost no damage compared to simply submerging the baby in water. Even though an infant's skin may seem perfect, it needs to be handled with extreme caution, and only products that have been prescribed by a pediatrician should be used on it. Much for the flawless, kind skin of a cherub, which is as smooth as a piece of cotton.

3.9.2. Children: The Armor in Molding

There is no doubt that the likelihood of skin damage increases as we age and focus solely on having fun and playing games. Children never seem to run out of energy; as long as they are enjoying themselves, they can play all day long in any kind of environment. The fun never seems to end until an adult forcibly removes them from their playgrounds and assesses the day's damages. For children, from toddlers to school-age, maintaining skin integrity is of utmost importance because they are more exposed to their surroundings compared to infants.

Apart from its moisture content and maturity, a child's skin shares many characteristics with that of an infant. A child's skin barrier begins to develop in their first year of life. It contains less water and is tougher than an infant's skin. Although not as impermeable as an adult's, it still provides some level of protection. The thickness of its stratum corneum is slightly better than that of an infant, but it remains highly susceptible to drug toxicity. The volume of vellus hair follicles is increased, and the surface volume ratio is higher. A child's skin absorbs more through the skin than an adult's, making them more vulnerable to environmental irritants such as dust, sebum, sweat, and bacteria.

Vellus hair grows on the majority of a person's body during childhood and is short, fine, light-colored, and hardly noticeable. Children's skin integrity is compromised because they are also more likely to have accidents. Falls are one of the main reasons why skin integrity is disturbed. The majority of wounds resulting from these damages are abrasions and open wounds, so it is important to monitor the potential for pathogen entry. When caring for a child with impaired skin integrity, it can be difficult to overcome their fear of being mutilated; in these situations, reassurance and cautious handling are necessary. As long as your child's safety is guaranteed and illnesses are far off, you can allow them to engage in whatever behavior they choose if they are bursting with energy.

3.9.3. Adolescents: The Armor in Training

Adolescents are arguably the most conscious individuals, as they are concerned about the condition of their skin. They have every right to feel this way, as puberty brings about significant physical changes in the body. These changes in our skin are primarily caused by hormonal fluctuations. Although our skin does not regenerate its layers as frequently as a child's, it remains resilient and robust. This resilience protects our skin from harmful toxins, allergies, and physical damage.

One of the most noticeable changes that occur during puberty is the increased activity of sweat and oil glands. The maturation of these glands is primarily triggered by the surge of sex hormones. These hormones also contribute to the growth of body hair.

As we approach puberty, we may begin to experience acne breakouts. This can be attributed to the increased activity of sweat and oil glands, which are now functioning at full capacity. Adolescents must prioritize good personal hygiene practices to maintain the health of their skin.

3.9.4. Adults: The Armor That Is at the Height of Life's Battles

The protective layers of our skin fully develop by the time we reach adulthood. They become much more impermeable and tougher. If appropriately maintained, our skin can tolerate the daily abrasions and damages it faces. It is crucial to take good care of our skin because it serves as our body's first line of defense. It can already regulate our body temperature better than the skin of newborns and small children. Sebum secretion is more pronounced in adult skin compared to teenage skin. Our skin has reached the peak of its ability to produce and absorb vitamin D, and its receptors are now more responsive to stimuli.

Despite the perception that our skin is as resilient as armor, it still has vulnerabilities. Skin disorders affecting adult skin are more challenging to treat. The gentle attention we give to a baby's delicate, sensitive skin is still necessary for an adult's skin. Precautions against harm and infection should still be taken. Maintaining proper hydration helps prevent dryness and reduces the risk of injury. Although our skin will inevitably age with us, we can still preserve its appearance and functionality.

3.9.5. Elderly: The Armor That Has Wrinkled Through Time

Dry, wrinkled skin is often associated with the aging process. The skin of the elderly is as delicate as that of a newborn and should be treated with great care. Due to decreased water content, it has already lost much of its elasticity and is more susceptible to injuries, as falls and accidents are common among the elderly. The reduced activity of sweat and sebaceous glands is the cause of dryness in the skin. Additionally, you may notice flaky and dry skin with decreased turgor. Melanotic freckles, which are flat, tan-colored macules, are commonly observed on the skin's surface.

Given that the skin of the elderly is just as sensitive as that of a newborn, it is crucial that they increase their water intake and receive close supervision. The use of lotions and moisturizers can help alleviate dryness. Just as we treat our own babies with care and tenderness, we should extend the same level of care to our elderly loved ones, recognizing their fragility and sensitivity.

Perhaps we have taken the small things in life for granted. Throughout our lives, our skin remains by our side, supporting us in both good and bad times, and protecting us when it senses danger. Only by providing our body's largest organ with the meticulous and compassionate care it deserves, before reaching a point where it would rather be shed than continue serving as our personal armor, can we truly appreciate this simple yet vital service.

A Closer Look

Burns

Burns of the skin may be caused by flames, hot water or steam, sunlight, electricity, or corrosive chemicals. The severity of burns ranges from minor to fatal, and the classification of burns is based on the extent of damage.

- **First-Degree Burn:** A first-degree burn refers to a burn that only affects the superficial epidermis. It is painful but does not result in blistering. In individuals with light-colored skin, the affected area will appear red due to localized vasodilation. Vasodilation is part of the inflammatory response that brings more blood to the injured site.
- **Second-Degree Burn:** Deeper layers of the epidermis are affected. Another aspect of inflammation is that damaged cells release histamine, which increases capillary permeability. This leads to the leakage of plasma from the capillaries, resulting in the accumulation of tissue fluid at the burn site and the formation of blisters. The burned skin is often highly painful.
- **Third-Degree Burn:** The entire epidermis is charred or burned away, and the burn may extend into the dermis or subcutaneous tissue. Initially, such burns may not be painful if the dermal receptors have been destroyed.

Extensive third-degree burns pose a potentially life-threatening risk due to the loss of the stratum corneum. Without this natural barrier, living tissue is exposed to the environment, making it susceptible to infection and dehydration.

Bacterial infection is a serious concern for burn patients, as pathogens can enter the bloodstream (septicemia) and rapidly spread throughout the body. Dehydration can also be fatal if not promptly addressed. The sequence of events includes the evaporation of tissue fluid from the burned surface, leading to the pulling of more plasma from the capillaries into the tissue spaces. As more plasma is lost, blood volume and pressure decrease, resulting in circulatory shock. Eventually, the heart becomes unable to pump an adequate amount of blood, leading to heart failure and death. To prevent these severe consequences, third-degree burns are covered with donor skin or artificial skin until skin grafts using the patient's own skin can be performed.

Summary

- The dermis, the subcutaneous tissue beneath the dermis, hair, nails, and various glands constitute the integumentary system.
- The integumentary system comprises four distinct types of glands: sebaceous, ceruminous, mammary, and sudoriferous glands. Sweat-producing glands are referred to as sudoriferous glands.
- Skin is an organ of the integumentary system, encompassing a layer of tissues that safeguards underlying muscles and organs, as per the fields of zoology and dermatology.
- Defensins are antimicrobial peptides that can be synthesized by living keratinocytes. The process of inflammation that ensues any skin injury involves the production of these and other chemicals.
- The fibrous connective tissue that constitutes the dermis is irregular, signifying that its fibers ran in all directions rather than parallel.
- Nail follicles, which are situated on the tips of fingers and toes, generate nails in the same manner that hair follicles accomplish.
- The dermis encompasses the majority of the sensory receptors for the cutaneous senses (nerve endings and Merkel cells are situated in the stratum germinativum).
- Sebaceous gland ducts have the ability to open directly onto the skin's surface or into hair follicles. Sebum, a lipid substance commonly referred to as oil, is the substance that they secrete.
- The dermis of the ear canals harbors these glands. Cerumen, also known as ear wax, is the term used to describe their secretion, which also contains sebum secreted within the ear canals.
- A rudimentary mammary gland consists of the entirety of the milk-producing tissue that has led to a solitary lactiferous duct; conversely, an intricate mammary gland is comprised of all the rudimentary mammary glands that serve a solitary nipple.
- The arterioles are supplementary blood vessels of considerable significance in conjunction with the dermal capillaries.

References

1. Abbasi, N. R., Shaw, H. M., Rigel, D. S., Friedman, R. J., McCarthy, W. H., Osman, I., Kopf, A. W., & Polsky, D., (2004). Early diagnosis of cutaneous melanoma: Revisiting the ABCD criteria. *JAMA, 292*(22), 2771–2776.
2. Abraira, V. E., & Ginty, D. D., (2013). The sensory neurons of touch. *Neuron., 79*(4), 618–639.
3. Arsic, A. V. S., Milobratovic, D., Barac, A. M., Vekic, B., Marinkovic, J., & Kostic, V. S., (2014). A laboratory-based study on patients with Parkinson's disease and seborrheic dermatitis: The presence and density of Malassezia yeasts, their different species and enzymes production. *BMC Dermatol., 14*, 5.
4. Boguniewicz, M., & Leung, D. Y., (2011). Atopic dermatitis: A disease of altered skin barrier and immune dysregulation. *Immunol. Rev., 242*(1), 233–246.

5. Brannon, H., (2006). "*Nail Anatomy.*" About, Inc., A part of The New York Times Company.
6. Breitkopf, T., Leung, G., Yu, M., Wang, E., & McElwee, K. J., (2013). The basic science of hair biology: What are the causal mechanisms for the disordered hair follicle? *Dermatol. Clin., 31*(1), 1–19.
7. Brown, T. M., & Krishnamurthy, K., (2022). *StatPearls* [Internet]. StatPearls Publishing; Treasure Island (FL). Histology, Dermis.
8. Buffoli, B., Rinaldi, F., Labanca, M., Sorbellini, E., Trink, A., Guanziroli, E., Rezzani, R., & Rodella, L. F., (2014). The human hair: From anatomy to physiology. *Int. J. Dermatol., 53*(3), 331–341.
9. De Jong, E. M., Seegers, B. A., Gulinck, M. K., Boezeman, J. B., & Van De, K.P. C., (1996). Psoriasis of the nails associated with disability in a large number of patients: Results of a recent interview with 1,728 patients. *Dermatology, 193*(4), 300–303.
10. Ellis, J. A., Sinclair, R., & Harrap, S. B., (2002). Androgenetic alopecia: Pathogenesis and potential for therapy. *Expert Rev. Mol. Med., 4*(22), 1–11.
11. Faergemann, J., Bergbrant, I. M., Dohsé, M., Scott, A., & Westgate, G., (2001). Seborrhoeic dermatitis and pityrosporum (*Malassezia*) folliculitis: Characterization of inflammatory cells and mediators in the skin by immunohistochemistry. *Br. J. Dermatol., 144*(3), 549–556.
12. Gleeson, M., (1998). Temperature regulation during exercise. *Int. J. Sports Med., 19*(Suppl 2), S96–99.
13. Gollnick, H., Cunliffe, W., Berson, D., Dreno, B., Finlay, A., Leyden, J. J., Shalita, A. R., & Thiboutot, D., (2003). Global alliance to improve outcomes in acne. management of acne: A report from a global alliance to improve outcomes in acne. *J. Am. Acad. Dermatol., 49*(1 Suppl), S1–37.
14. Graaff, V. De., (2002). *Human Anatomy* (6th edn.). New York: McGraw-Hill.
15. Grover, C., & Khurana, A., (2012). Onychomycosis: Newer insights in pathogenesis and diagnosis. *Indian J. Dermatol. Venereol. Leprol., 78*(3), 263–270.
16. Haneke, E., (2015). Anatomy of the nail unit and the nail biopsy. *Semin. Cutan. Med. Surg., 34*(2), 95–100.
17. Hay, R. J., & Baran, R., (2011). Onychomycosis: A proposed revision of the clinical classification. *J. Am. Acad. Dermatol., 65*(6), 1219–1227.
18. Hoover, E., Alhajj, M., & Flores, J. L., (2019). *Physiology, Hair*. InStatPearls [Internet]. StatPearls Publishing. Available from: https://www.ncbi.nlm.nih.gov/books/NBK499948/ (accessed on 30 March 2024).
19. Kasumagic-Halilovic, E., & Prohic, A., (2009). Nail changes in alopecia areata: Frequency and clinical presentation. *J. Eur. Acad. Dermatol. Venereol., 23*(2), 240–241.
20. Kim, J. Y., & Dao, H., (2020). *Physiology, Integument.* InStatPearls [Internet] Feb 17. StatPearls Publishing. Available from: https://www.ncbi.nlm.nih.gov/books/NBK554386/ (accessed on 30 March 2024).
21. Kuo, I. H., Yoshida, T., De Benedetto, A., & Beck, L. A., (2013). The cutaneous innate immune response in patients with atopic dermatitis. *J. Allergy Clin. Immunol., 131*(2), 266–278.
22. Lips, P., (2006). Vitamin D physiology. *Prog. Biophys Mol. Biol., 92*(1), 4–8.
23. Liu, C., Bayer, A., Cosgrove, S. E., Daum, R. S., Fridkin, S. K., Gorwitz, R. J., Kaplan, S. L., et al., (2011). Infectious Diseases Society of America. Clinical practice guidelines by the infectious

diseases society of America for the treatment of methicillin-resistant *Staphylococcus aureus* infections in adults and children. *Clin. Infect. Dis., 52*(3), e18–55.

24. Lonsdale-Eccles, A., Leonard, N., & Lawrence, C., (2003). Axillary hyperhidrosis: Eccrine or apocrine? *Clin. Exp. Dermatol., 28*(1), 2–7.
25. Mader, S. S., (2004). *Human Biology.* New York: McGraw-Hill.
26. Martini, F. H., & Nath, J. L., (2009). *Fundamentals of Anatomy and Physiology* (8th edn.) Pearson. San Francisco: Benjamin Cummings.
27. Merola, J. F., Li, T., Li, W. Q., Cho, E., & Qureshi, A. A., (2016). Prevalence of psoriasis phenotypes among men and women in the USA. *Clin. Exp. Dermatol., 41*(5), 486–489.
28. Mertens, D. M., Jenkins, M. E., & Warden, G. D., (1997). Outpatient burn management. *Nurs. Clin. North Am., 32*(2), 343–364.
29. Nguyen, A. V., & Soulika, A. M., (2019). The dynamics of the skin's immune system. *Int. J. Mol Sci., 20*(8).
30. Nunez, L. O., Cambiaso-Daniel, J., Branski, L. K., Norbury, W. B., & Herndon, D. N., (2017). Predicting and managing sepsis in burn patients: Current perspectives. *Ther. Clin. Risk Manag., 13*, 1107–1117.
31. O'Neill, A. M., & Gallo, R. L., (2018). Host-microbiome interactions and recent progress into understanding the biology of acne vulgaris. *Microbiome, 6*(1), 177.
32. *Overview of the Integumentary System Image* – © Kenhub https://www.kenhub.com/en/study/anatomy-of-integumentary-system (accessed on 30 March 2024).
33. Pellegrini, C., Maturo, M. G., Di Nardo, L., Ciciarelli, V., García-Rodrigo, C. G., & Fargnoli, M. C., (2017). Understanding the molecular genetics of basal cell carcinoma. *Int. J. Mol. Sci., 18*(11)
34. Picardo, M., Ottaviani, M., Camera, E., & Mastrofrancesco, A., (2009). Sebaceous gland lipids. *Dermatoendocrinol., 1*(2), 68–71.
35. Raff, A. B., & Kroshinsky, D., (2016). Cellulitis: A review. *JAMA, 316*(3), 325–337.
36. Riciputo, R. M., Oliveri, S., Micali, G., & Sapuppo, A., (1996). Phospholipase activity in Malassezia furfur pathogenic strains. *Mycoses, 39*(5, 6), 233–235.
37. Sandilands, A., Sutherland, C., Irvine, A. D., & McLean, W. H., (2009). Filaggrin in the frontline: Role in skin barrier function and disease. *J. Cell Sci., 122*(Pt 9), 1285–1294.
38. Sato, K., Kang, W. H., Saga, K., & Sato, K. T., (1989). Biology of sweat glands and their disorders. I. Normal sweat gland function. *J. Am. Acad. Dermatol., 20*(4), 537–563.
39. Sato, K., Kang, W. H., Saga, K., & Sato, K. T., (1989). Biology of sweat glands and their disorders. II. Disorders of sweat gland function. *J. Am. Acad. Dermatol., 20*(5 Pt 1), 713–726.
40. Schneider, M. R., Schmidt-Ullrich, R., & Paus, R., (2009). The hair follicle as a dynamic miniorgan. *Curr. Biol., 19*(3), R132–142.
41. Sorrentino, S. A., (2004). *Mosby's Textbook for Nursing Assistants* (6th edn.) St. Louis, Missouri: Mosby.
42. Spicknall, K. E., Zirwas, M. J., & English, J. C., (2005). Clubbing: An update on diagnosis, differential diagnosis, pathophysiology, and clinical relevance. *J. Am. Acad. Dermatol., 52*(6), 1020–1028.

43. Stevens, D. L., Bisno, A. L., Chambers, H. F., Dellinger, E. P., Goldstein, E. J., Gorbach, S. L., Hirschmann, J. V., et al., (2014). Infectious Diseases Society of America. Practice guidelines for the diagnosis and management of skin and soft tissue infections: 2014 update by the Infectious Diseases Society of America. *Clin. Infect. Dis., 59*(2), e10–52.

44. Stevens, D. L., Bisno, A. L., Chambers, H. F., Dellinger, E. P., Goldstein, E. J., Gorbach, S. L., Hirschmann, J. V., et al., (2014). Practice guidelines for the diagnosis and management of skin and soft tissue infections: 2014 update by the infectious diseases society of America. *Clin. Infect. Dis., 59*(2), 147–159.

45. Strazzulla, L. C., Wang, E. H. C., Avila, L., Lo Sicco, K., Brinster, N., Christiano, A. M., & Shapiro, J., (2018). Alopecia areata: Disease characteristics, clinical evaluation, and new perspectives on pathogenesis. *J. Am. Acad. Dermatol., 78*(1), 1–12.

46. Van, L. E., & Coreno, A., (1992). Inhaled albuterol powder for pulmonary function testing. *Chest, 101*(4), 985–988.

47. Waldman, A., & Schmults, C., (2019). Cutaneous squamous cell carcinoma. *Hematol. Oncol. Clin. North Am., 33*(1), 1–12.

48. Zouboulis, C. C., Picardo, M., Ju, Q., Kurokawa, I., Törőcsik, D., Bíró, T., & Schneider, M. R., (2016). Beyond acne: Current aspects of sebaceous gland biology and function. *Rev. Endocr. Metab. Disord., 17*(3), 319–334.

Chapter 4

NERVOUS SYSTEM

Contents

Unit Introduction

The brain, spinal cord, sensory organs, and all of the nerves that connect these organs to the rest of the body constitute the nervous system. These organs collaborate to regulate the body and facilitate communication between its components. Decisions are made and information is analyzed in the central nervous system (CNS), which comprises the brain and spinal cord. The peripheral nerve system (PNS) sensory nerves and organs monitor conditions both internally and externally and transmit this information to the CNS. The PNS's efferent nerves convey signals to the muscles, glands, and organs from the control center to regulate their various functions.

Orientation and Directional Terms:

Term	Definition	Illustration
Synapses	Synapses refer to the points of contact between neurons where information is passed from one neuron to the next. Synapses most often form between axons and dendrites, and consist of a presynaptic neuron, synaptic cleft, and a postsynaptic neuron.	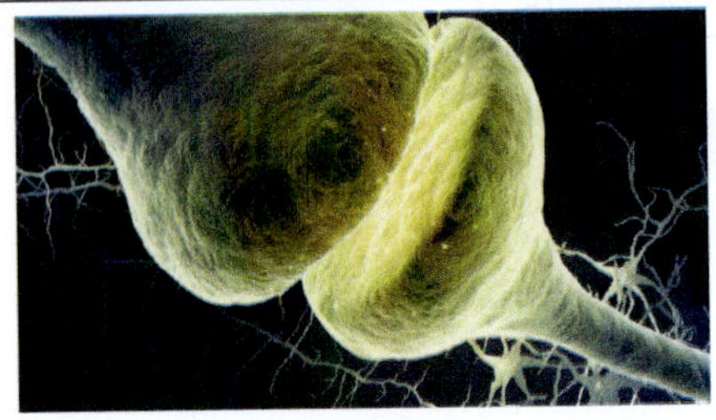
Spinal nerves	Spinal nerves are pairs of nerve fibers that originate from the spinal cord. They are made up of both sensory and motor fibers. Spinal nerves act as an intermediary between the central nervous system (CNS) and the periphery.	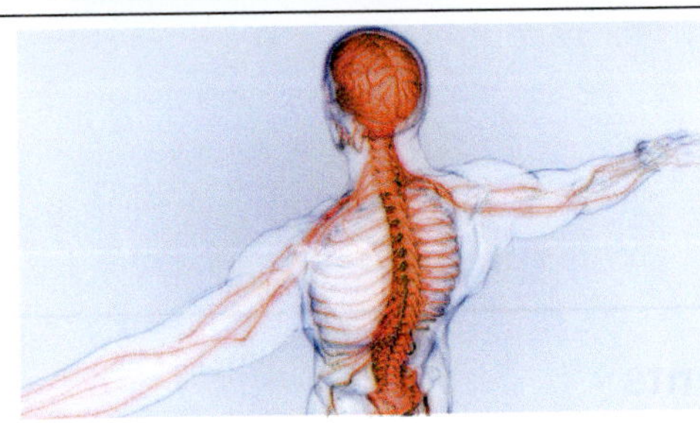
Ventricles	Ventricles of the brain are a communicating network of cavities filled with cerebrospinal fluid (CSF) and located within the brain parenchyma.	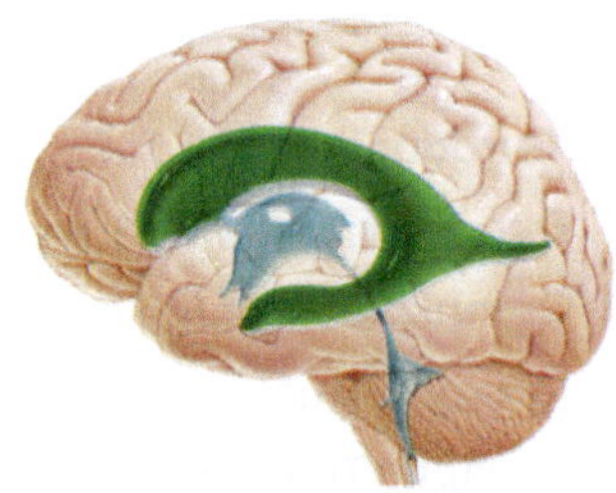
Medulla	Medulla oblongata, also known as the medulla, is the bottom part of the brainstem. It connects the brain to the spinal cord and is essential for survival.	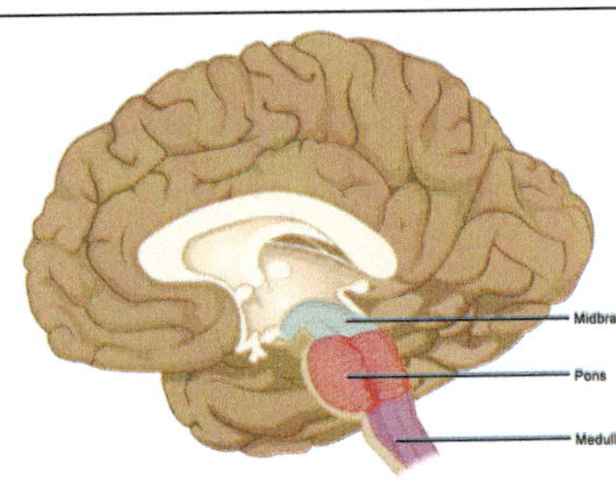
Hypothalamus	The hypothalamus is a small but crucial part of the brain. It controls functions such as sleep and growth.	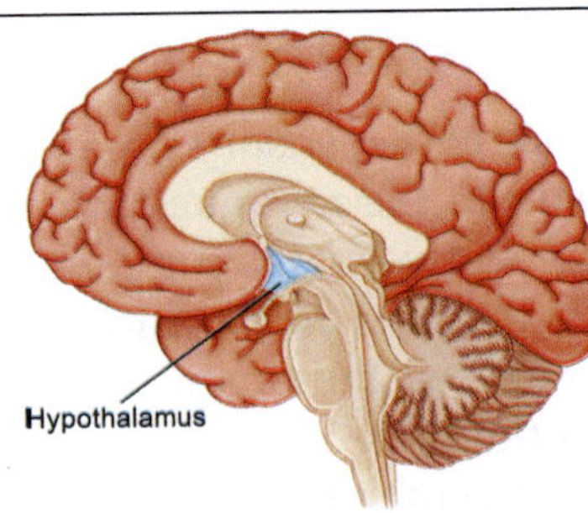

4.1. Overview of the Entire Nervous System

The nervous system performs three primary tasks: motor output, data integration, and sensory input. The body uses neurons, glia, and synapses to gather information or data through sensory input. The nervous system is composed of excitable nerve cells called neurons and the synapses that connect them to other neurons or to other centers in the body. Nerve cells can vary in size and location, but their ability to communicate with each other determines how these neurons function. They can be either excited or inhibited. These nerves transmit impulses from sensory receptors to the brain and spinal cord. The next step in data processing is data integration, which can only occur in the brain. Motor output is the process by which impulses are sent from the brain and spinal cord to muscles and glands after the brain has processed the information. Tissue-resident glia cells assist in extracellular fluid, myelination, and ionic regulation. They are non-excitable (Figure 4.1).

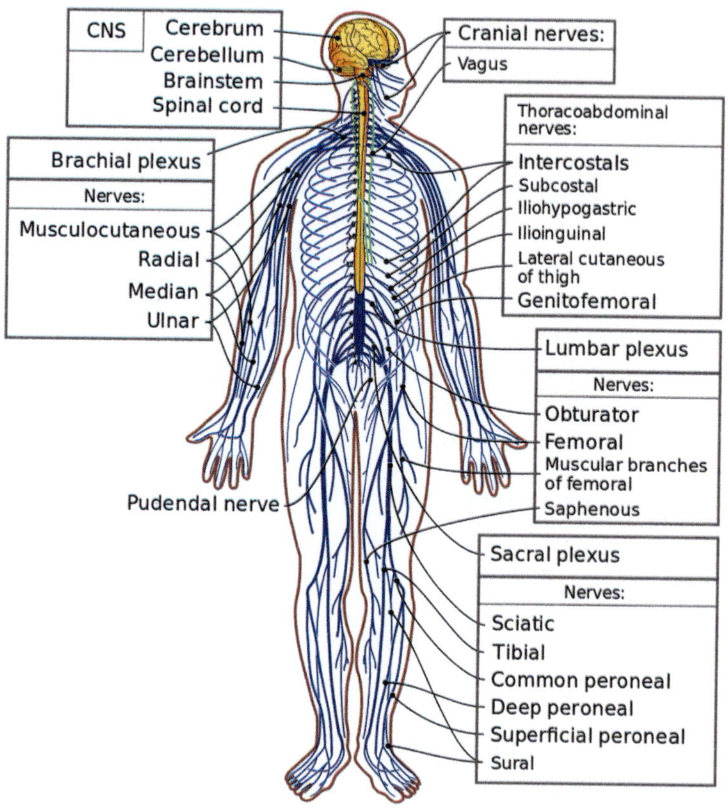

Figure 4.1. *Nervous system.*

Source: https://courses.lumenlearning.com/wm-biology2/chapter/nervous-system/.

The central nervous system (CNS) and the peripheral nervous system (PNS) are the two main components, or subdivisions, of the nervous system. The brain and spinal cord are parts of the central nervous system (CNS). The CNS serves as the "control center" of the body, carrying out sensory, motor, and data integration through various centers. These centers can be further categorized into Higher centers that communicate with the brain through effectors, and Lower centers, which include the brain stem and spinal cord. The PNS, connected to the brain and spinal cord, forms an extensive network of cranial and spinal nerves. It contains sensory receptors that assist in processing internal and external environmental changes. Afferent sensory nerves transmit this data to the central nervous system. The PNS is further divided into the autonomic nervous system and the somatic nervous system. The autonomic nervous system controls smooth muscles, cardiac muscles, blood vessels, and internal organs involuntarily. The somatic nervous system, on the other hand, controls the skin, bones, joints, and skeletal muscles voluntarily. The two systems work in tandem through the integration of PNS neurons into the CNS and vice versa.

4.2. Organization of the Nervous System

There are two main sections of the nervous system. Each component is made up of billions of neurons, also known as nerve cells. Your body uses these unique cells to transmit and receive electrical signals that instruct it what to do.

The main parts of the nervous system are:

- Central nervous system;
- Peripheral nervous system.

4.2.1. Central Nervous System (CNS)

The CNS is comprised of the brain and spinal cord. The brain communicates with the body through nerves. Myelin serves as a protective layer for each nerve, facilitating signal transmission.

4.2.2. Peripheral Nervous System (PNS)

The peripheral nervous system is composed of numerous nerves that emerge from the central nervous system and extend throughout the body. This system allows for the transmission of information from the brain and spinal cord to the arms, legs, fingers, and toes.

The peripheral nervous system consists of two main divisions:

i. The somatic nervous system, which governs voluntary movements.
ii. The autonomic nervous system, which controls involuntary activities.

4.3. Neuron Structure and Function

4.3.1. Types of Neurons

In terms of neuron structure and function, there is a wide variety due to their sheer quantity, much like the diverse species found on Earth. However, there are five major forms of neurons, each combining different elements of the basic neuron shape:

1. **Multipolar Neurons:** These neurons have a single axon and symmetrical dendrites extending from it. They are the most common type of neuron in the central nervous system.
2. **Unipolar Neurons:** Typically found in invertebrate species, these neurons have a single axon.
3. **Bipolar Neurons:** These neurons have two extensions extending from the cell body. One side contains the axon, while the other side has the dendrites. Bipolar neurons are primarily found in the retina of the eye but can also be present in parts of the nervous system related to the nose and ear function.
4. **Pyramidal Neurons:** These neurons have one axon but several dendrites, forming a pyramid-type shape. They are the largest neuron cells and are predominantly found in the cortex, which is responsible for conscious thoughts.

5. **Purkinje Neurons:** These have multiple dendrites that fan out from the cell body. These neurons are inhibitory neurons, meaning they release neurotransmitters that prevent other neurons from firing.

Based on their roles, the neurons found in the human nervous system can be divided into three classes: sensory neurons, motor neurons, and interneurons.

i. **Sensory Neurons:** These receive information about internal and external stimuli and transmit it to the central nervous system (CNS) for processing. For example, if you were to touch a hot coal, sensory neurons in your fingertips would relay the information to the CNS, indicating the high temperature.

ii. **Motor Neurons:** On the other hand, receive information from other neurons and transmit commands to muscles, organs, and glands. In the case of touching a hot coal, motor neurons innervating the muscles in your fingers would prompt your hand to release the object.

iii. **Interneurons:** This which are exclusively found in the CNS, establish connections between different neurons. They receive information from other neurons, such as sensory neurons or interneurons, and transmit it to other neurons, including motor neurons or interneurons.

For instance, if you were to touch a hot coal, the signal from the sensory neurons in your fingertips would reach the interneurons in your spinal cord. Some of these interneurons would transmit the signal up the spinal cord to neurons in the brain, where it would be interpreted as pain. Others would send a signal to the motor neurons that control your finger muscles, compelling you to release your grip.

Interneurons, being the most common type of neurons, play a crucial role in information processing within both simple reflex circuits, like those activated by hot objects, and more complex brain circuits. Your brain's interneurons would collaborate to help you recognize that objects resembling hot coals should not be touched, and ideally retain that knowledge for future reference.

4.3.2. The Basic Functions of a Neuron

It is possible to draw the generalization that all neurons perform the same three primary tasks if you consider the roles of the three classes of neurons.

These are to: receive signals (or information), integrate incoming signals (to determine whether or not the information should be passed along), and communicate signals to target cells (other neurons or muscles or glands). These neuronal functions are reflected in the anatomy of the neuron.

4.3.3. Anatomy of a Neuron

Similar to other cells, neurons have a cell body known as the soma. The soma contains the neuron's nucleus. A large number of proteins are required by neurons, and the majority of these proteins are also produced in the soma.

From the cell body, different processes (appendages or protrusions) emerge. These consist of several short, branching processes called dendrites and an additional process called an axon that is usually longer than the dendrites.

4.3.3.1. Dendrites

Receiving and processing incoming information are typically the first two neuronal functions that occur in the dendrites and cell body. One of two types of incoming signals is excitatory, which means that it tends to cause the neuron to fire (create an electrical impulse), or inhibitory, which tends to prevent the neuron from firing. Most neurons' dendritic trees are filled with numerous input signals. A single neuron can receive thousands of input signals and have multiple sets of dendrites. A neuron's ability to fire an impulse is determined by the total amount of excitatory and inhibitory signals it receives. The nerve impulse, also known as the action potential, is carried down the axon in the event that the neuron fires (Figure 4.2).

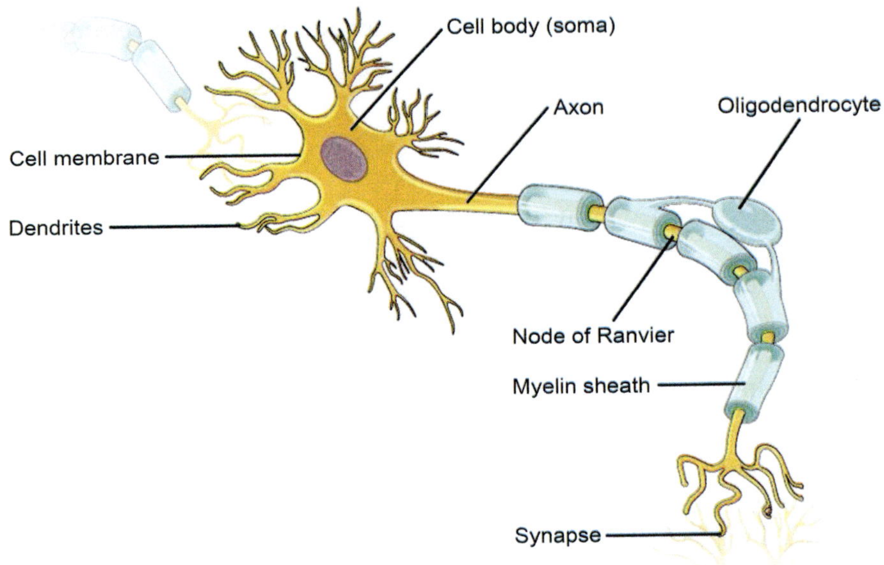

Figure 4.2. *Neuron structure.*

Source: https://courses.lumenlearning.com/adolescent/chapter/brain-basics/.

4.3.3.2. Other Important Parts

1. **Nissl Granules:** A large granular body found in neurons is called a Nissl body, also referred to as a Nissl substance or Nissl material. Nissl bodies are responsible for the synthesis and release of amino acids and proteins.
2. **Schwann Cells:** For the peripheral nervous system (PNS) to remain functional, the Schwann cell is essential. There are two types of Schwann cells: myelinating and non-myelinating. Schwann cells are derived from neural crest cells. Both are essential for the preservation and regeneration of the PNS's neurons' axons. They are primarily needed to provide nutrition and insulation (myelinating) to the PNS neurons' individual nerve fibers, or axons.
3. **Myelin Sheath:** An insulating layer, or sheath, called myelin develops around nerves, including the spinal cord and brain. It is composed of fatty and protein components. Electrical impulses can travel along nerve cells with speed and efficiency thanks to the myelin sheath.
4. **Node of Ranvier:** The term "Node of Ranvier" refers to a recurring opening in the myelin sheath (insulating layer) of some neurons, which allows nerve impulses to pass through

more quickly. The high concentration of ion channels in the unmyelinated nodes of Ranvier compels the current to flow down the nerve fiber.

5. **Axon Terminal:** The somewhat enlarged axon endings, which are frequently club- or button-shaped, are referred to as axon terminals. The portion of a nerve cell called an axon terminal is responsible for creating synaptic connections with other nerve cells.
6. **Synaptic Knobs:** With the aid of neurotransmitters, synaptic knobs are crucial in the transfer of impulses between neurons across synapses.
7. **Synapses:** These are the cellular junctions or connections that occur between two neurons, nerve cells, or between a neuron and a muscle or gland cell. A synapse is a tiny opening at the end of a neuron that permits signal transmission between neurons. Where nerve cells meet other nerve cells is called a synapse.
8. **Axons:** These differ from dendrites in several ways:
   - The dendrites tend to taper and are often covered with little bumps called spines. In contrast, the axon tends to stay the same diameter for most of its length and doesn't have spines.
   - The axon arises from the cell body at a specialized area called the axon hillock.
   - Finally, many axons are covered with a special insulating substance called myelin, which helps them convey the nerve impulse rapidly. Myelin is never found on dendrites.

   The axon ends in numerous branches and develops bulbous swellings called axon terminals (also known as nerve terminals). On target cells, these axon terminals form connections.
9. **Cell Body:** The central region of a neuron is called the cell body, or soma for short. The cell body supplies energy to power activities, preserves the structure of the neuron, and houses genetic information. The soma of a neuron has specialized organelles and a nucleus, just like other cell bodies. It is shielded from harm and able to communicate with its immediate environment thanks to a membrane surrounding it.

4.3.4. Neurons Function

Action potentials are used by neurons to send signals. An action potential is a change in the potential electric energy of a neuron brought on by charged particles entering and exiting the neuron's membrane. An action potential is produced and travels to a presynaptic ending via the axon.

Chemical and electrical synapses can both be triggered by action potentials. Neurons can communicate electrically and chemically with one another at synapses. A postsynaptic ending, a synaptic cleft, and a presynaptic ending comprise a synapse.

1. **Chemical Synapses:** Chemical messengers, known as neurotransmitters, are released by the neuron at a chemical synapse. These substances attach to receptors in the postsynaptic ending of a dendrite after crossing the synaptic cleft. The postsynaptic neuron can respond to neurotransmitters by generating its own action potential. Alternatively, they can inhibit the firing of the postsynaptic neuron, preventing it from producing an action potential.
2. **Electrical Synapses:** On the other hand, electrical synapses can only generate firing. These synapses are formed when two neurons are connected by a gap junction. This gap,

which is much smaller than a chemical synapse, consists of ion channels that facilitate the transmission of positive electrical signals.

Due to the nature of their transmission, signals travel much faster across electrical synapses compared to chemical synapses. However, these signals may become weaker as they pass from one neuron to the next, making them less efficient in transmitting repeated signals.

3. **Transmission and Communication between Neurons:** Neurons exchange signals chemically and electrically. Electrical signals are produced from sensory stimuli. Electrical signals that travel through neurons are called action potentials. Chemical or electrical connections called synapses enable electrical signals to travel from neurons to neighboring cells. Movement and contraction of muscles are mediated by electrical signals. A synapse's function can be improved or diminished by variations in the level of activity there. Neuronal communication can be influenced by an individual's lifestyle choices, including exercise, stress management, and drug use. Combinations of signals between neurons produce all perceptions, thoughts, and actions.

4.4. Synaptic Transmission

4.4.1. Synapses

Other neurons' dendrites and cell bodies are the sites of neuron-to-neuron connections. Information is transferred from the first neuron, the presynaptic neuron, to the target neuron, the postsynaptic neuron, at these connections, also referred to as synapses. Neuromuscular junctions are the synaptic connections made by neurons with skeletal muscle cells, and neuroeffector junctions are the connections made by neurons with smooth muscle cells or glands. Neurotransmitters are chemical messengers that carry information between synapses and junctions. Neurotransmitter is released from the presynaptic cell when an action potential travels down an axon and reaches the axon terminal. Neurotransmitter molecules transmit an excitatory or inhibitory signal by crossing the synapse and attaching to membrane receptors on the postsynaptic cell (Figure 4.3).

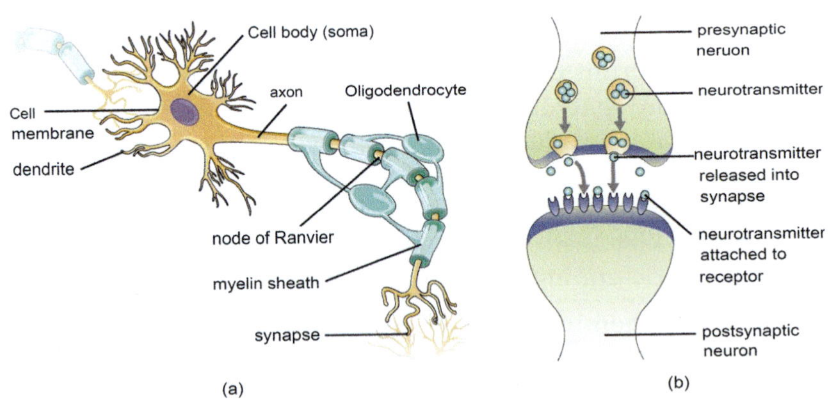

Figure 4.3. *A diagram outlining how a presynaptic neuron's axon terminals form synapses with the postsynaptic neuron's dendrites.*

Source: https://courses.lumenlearning.com/suny-microbiology/chapter/anatomy-of-the-nervous-system/.

Thus, the axon and axon terminals perform the third fundamental neuronal function, which is information transmission to target cells. A single neuron can form synaptic connections on multiple postsynaptic neurons via various axon terminals, just as it can receive inputs from multiple presynaptic neurons.

4.4.2. Variations on the Neuronal Theme

While most neurons have a similar overall structure, each neuron's structure is unique and tailored to the particular task that neuron (or class of neurons) must perform. Because the nervous system is so complex and has so many different functions, it makes sense that different types of neurons exhibit a great diversity in size and shape (Figure 4.4).

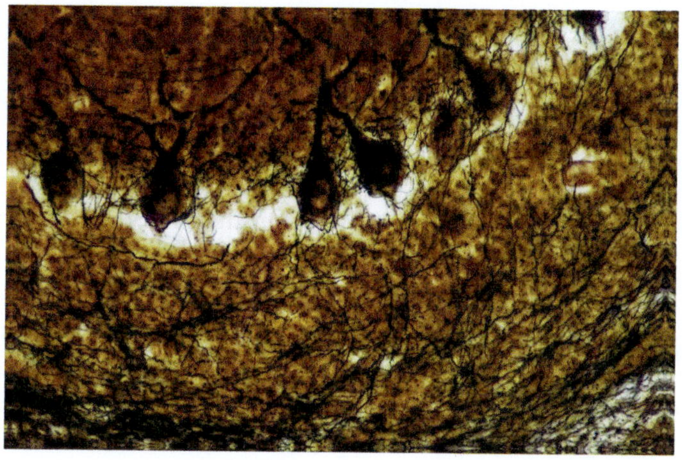

Figure 4.4. *Purkinje cells.*

Source: By Lazar.zenit – Own work, CC BY-SA 4.0, https://commons.wikimedia.org/w/index.php?curid=65160778.

For example, the cerebellum, a part of the brain, contains specialized neurons known as Purkinje cells. As demonstrated above, Purkinje cells have an extremely intricate dendritic tree that enables them to receive and process a vast array of synaptic inputs. The unique shapes of other neuronal subtypes in the cerebellum can also be used to identify them.

Neurons also vary greatly in length. Motor neurons that extend from the spinal cord to innervate the toes can reach a meter or longer, while many neurons are small in size. Examples of individuals with long axons include basketball players such as Michael Jordan, LeBron James, and Yao Ming.

The distinction between axons and dendrites can be blurry in sensory neurons, highlighting the diversity in their structure. In these neurons, a myelinated process emerges from the cell body and splits into two branches. One branch transmits information to the spinal cord, while the other branch connects to peripheral sensory receptors to receive information.

4.4.3. Neurons Form Networks

The function relies on networks of cooperating neurons, as an individual neuron has limited capabilities on its own. Neurons form circuits that process incoming information and generate responses by connecting with other neurons to either stimulate or inhibit their activity. Simple neural circuits with a small number of neurons can exist, as well as more complex neural networks.

4.4.3.1. The Knee-Jerk Reflex

One example of a basic neuronal circuit is the knee-jerk reflex, which is triggered by a hammer blow to the patellar tendon below the knee. When pressure is applied to the tendon, stretching the quadriceps muscle of the thigh, the sensory neurons that innervate it are activated.

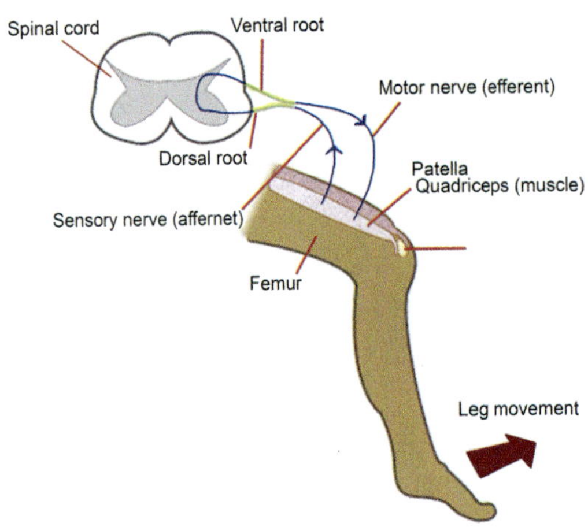

Figure 4.5. *The knee-jerk reflex.*

Source: By ChristinaT3 at English Wikipedia, CC BY-SA 3.0, https://commons.wikimedia.org/w/index.php?curid=13404902.

These sensory neurons transmit signals down the spinal cord to motor neurons, which then innervate the quadriceps through connections. The motor neurons are stimulated by excitatory signals from the sensory neurons, causing the quadriceps to contract and straighten the knee. The knee-jerk reflex is a reflex in which a muscle contracts after being stretched because the motor neurons innervating that muscle are directly connected to the sensory neurons of the same muscle (Figure 4.5).

The muscle that opposes or antagonizes the quadriceps, the hamstring, relaxes as a result of a circuit that includes sensory neurons from the quadriceps. The hamstring would contract as a result, making it more difficult for the quadriceps to contract, so it would not make sense for the sensory neurons in the quadriceps to activate the motor neurons in the hamstring. Rather, an inhibitory interneuron mediates an indirect connection between the motor neurons of the hamstring and the sensory neurons of the quadriceps. The hamstring muscle relaxes as a result of the interneuron's activation, which inhibits the motor neurons that innervate it.

Not only do the quadriceps sensory neurons take part in this reflex circuit, but they also communicate with the brain, informing it that a hammer was used to tap a tendon and possibly triggering an action. "Why did you do that?" Although very basic behaviors like the knee jerk reflex can be mediated by spinal cord circuits, conscious perception of sensory stimuli and all other higher functions of the nervous system rely on the more intricate neuronal networks found in the brain.

4.4.4. Glial Cells

The nervous system is composed of two different types of cells: glia and neurons. While neurons serve as the primary functional unit of the nervous system, glia play a supporting role. Glia are essential for the operation of the nervous system, much like supporting actors are crucial to the success of a film. In fact, the brain contains a significantly higher number of glial cells compared to neurons.

In the adult vertebrate nervous system, glial cells are classified into four major types. Three of these types are unique to the central nervous system (CNS) and are known as astrocytes, oligodendrocytes, and microglia. The fourth type of cell, called Schwann cells, is found only in the peripheral nervous system (PNS).

Let's explore the different types of glia and their functions:

1. **Astrocytes:** These are the most abundant type of glial cell, making them the most numerous cells in the brain. Astrocytes come in different forms and have various functions. They help regulate blood flow in the brain, maintain the composition of the fluid surrounding neurons, and facilitate communication between neurons at the synapse. During development, astrocytes assist neurons in finding their proper destinations and contribute to the formation of the blood-brain barrier, which protects the brain from potentially harmful substances in the blood.
2. **Microglia:** These are similar to the macrophages of the immune system and act as scavengers, removing dead cells and other debris.
3. **Oligodendrocytes:** Both oligodendrocytes in the CNS and Schwann cells in the PNS share a similar function. These types of glial cells produce myelin, an insulating substance that forms a sheath around the axons of many neurons. Myelin significantly increases the speed at which an action potential travels down the axon and plays a crucial role in the functioning of the nervous system (Figure 4.6).

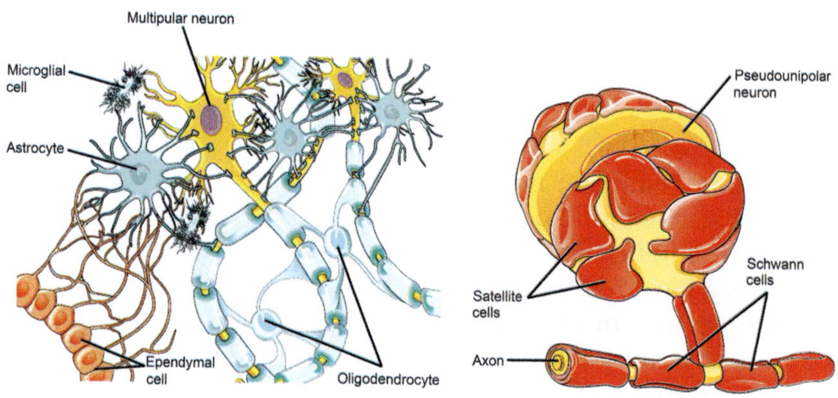

Figure 4.6. *Glial cells.*

Source: https://courses.lumenlearning.com/wm-biology2/chapter/glial-cells/.

4. **Satellite Glial Cells:** These cover the cell bodies of neurons in the PNS ganglia. Satellite glial cells are thought to support the function of the neurons and might act as a protective barrier, but their role is still not well-understood.
5. **Ependymal Cells:** These which line the ventricles of the brain and the central canal of the spinal cord, have hairlike cilia that beat to promote circulation of the cerebrospinal fluid found inside the ventricles and spinal canal.

4.4.5. Membrane Polarization

Now that we know that neurons possess long-range axons and dendrites that transmit signals both to and from other cells, let's examine a portion of a neuron's dendrite to see how these signals are actually transmitted.

The dendrite is said to be in its resting state when it is not sending out any signals. In this condition, the cell's exterior has a net positive charge and the interior has a net negative charge. Because there are positive and negative charges on opposing sides of the membrane, it is referred to as polarized.

The neuron actively maintains the polarized state of the membrane by means of sodium-potassium pumps. For every two positively charged potassium ions that these sodium-potassium pumps pump into the cell, three positively charged sodium ions are pumped out of it. The polarization increases slightly with each pump cycle. Furthermore, by diffusion, potassium ions seep back through the membrane and exit the cell, increasing the negative charge inside the cell and the positive charge outside.

4.4.6. Membrane Depolarization

A neuron's depolarization, or reduction in the difference in charge across the membrane, occurs as a result of the opening of sodium channels in the membrane. This allows a localized influx of positive sodium ions into the cell in response to a signal. A cascade effect is initiated when the localized depolarization also triggers the opening of adjacent sodium channels, leading to the depolarization of the nearby membrane. Consequently, more sodium channels open and depolarize the membrane further away.

Beginning at the dendrite that received the signal, depolarization propagates across the membrane in the form of a wave that travels towards, across, and eventually away from the cell down the axon. Depolarization can be likened to spectators rising to perform the wave in a football stadium. As the wave reaches seated individuals,

it prompts them to stand up, which in turn causes the individuals sitting next to them to stand up, and so on, allowing the wave to continue throughout the stands. Subsequently, the membrane repolarizes by closing sodium channels and activating sodium-potassium pumps to restore the charge differential across the membrane. At this stage, the neuron is ready to transmit another signal, much like the spectators who resume their seats.

4.5. Central and Peripheral Nervous System

For the sake of description, the nervous system is divided into two main sections: the peripheral nervous system, which consists of the cranial and spinal nerves along with their ganglia, and the central nervous system (Figure 4.7), which comprises the brain and spinal cord.

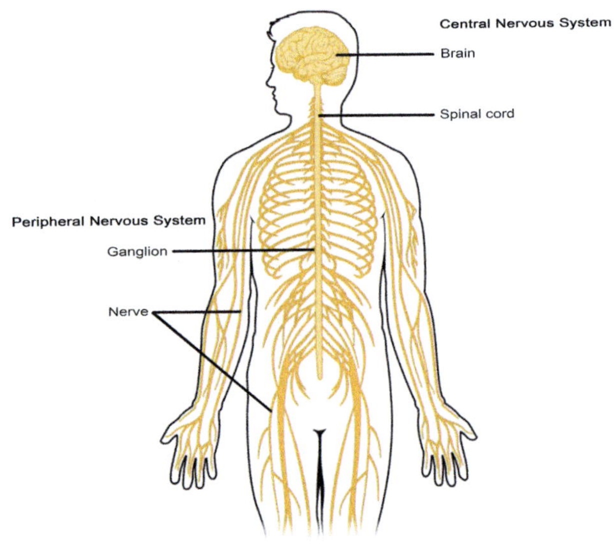

Figure 4.7. *The main divisions of the central nervous system. and the peripheral nervous system.*

Source: https://courses.lumenlearning.com/suny-ap1/chapter/the-nervous-system-and-nervous-tissue/.

The brain and spinal cord are the principal sites in the central nervous system where correlation and integration of nerve information occur. The meninges, a system of membranes, envelop the brain and spinal cord and are suspended in the cerebrospinal fluid. The skull and vertebral column offer supplementary safeguarding for the brain and spinal cord (Figure 4.8).

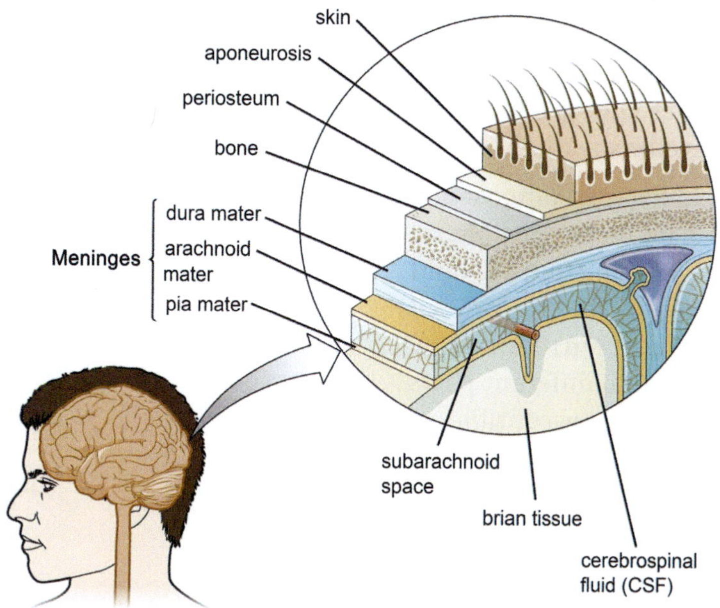

Figure 4.8. *Protective coverings of the CNS.*

Source: https://courses.lumenlearning.com/suny-microbiology/chapter/anatomy-of-the-nervous-system/.

Large numbers of excitable nerve cells and their processes, known as neurons, make up the central nervous system. These neurons are supported by specialized tissue known as neuroglia (Figure 4.9). Axons, also known as nerve fibers, are lengthy processes of a nerve cell.

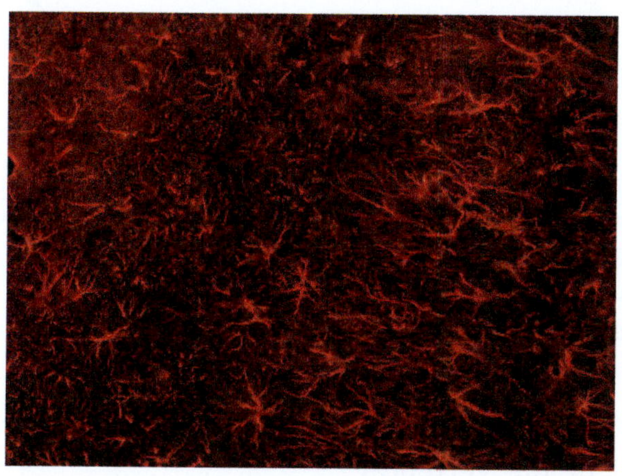

Figure 4.9. *Photomicrograph of several large nerve cells with surrounding neuroglia.*

Source: By ArizonaLifeScience – Own work Orchinik Lab, Arizona State University, Public Domain, https://commons.wikimedia.org/w/index.php?curid=10018500.

Gray and white matter constitute the interior of the CNS. Gray matter, which is gray in color, consists of nerve cells embedded in neuroglia. White matter, on the other hand, is composed of nerve fibers embedded in neuroglia, with many of these fibers containing lipid material in their myelin sheaths.

The cranial and spinal nerves, composed of bundles of axons, form part of the peripheral nervous system. These nerves transmit and receive information to and from the central nervous system. Despite being surrounded by fibrous sheaths as they travel to different parts of the body, these nerves are susceptible to damage due to their relatively exposed nature.

4.5.1. Autonomic Nervous System

The autonomic nervous system, present in both the central and peripheral nervous systems, is responsible for innervating the body's involuntary structures, such as the heart, smooth muscles, and glands. Both the sympathetic and parasympathetic branches of the autonomic nervous system contain afferent and efferent nerve fibers. The sympathetic activity of the autonomic nervous system prepares the body for emergencies, while the parasympathetic branch works to conserve and replenish energy.

4.5.2. Divisions of the Central Nervous System

It is crucial to comprehend the primary characteristics of the brain and spinal cord as well as their general relationships before diving into a detailed description of these structures.

4.5.2.1. Spinal Cord

Within the vertebral canal of the vertebral column, the dura mater, arachnoid mater, and pia mater are the three meninges that encircle the spinal cord. The cerebrospinal fluid, which envelops the spinal cord in the subarachnoid space, offers additional defense. Roughly cylindrical in shape, the spinal cord starts superiorly at the skull's foramen magnum and continues into the brain's medulla oblongata (Figures 4.10 and 4.11).

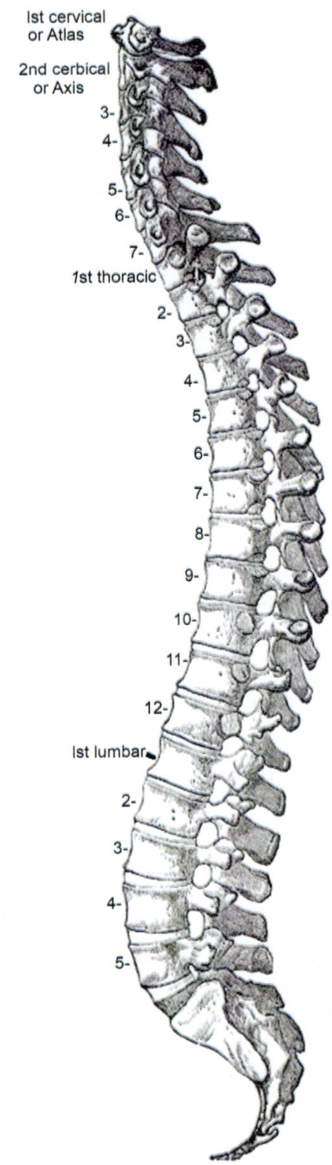

Figure 4.10. *The spinal cord.*

Source: https://courses.lumenlearning.com/suny-ulster-ap1/chapter/spinal-cord/.

It ends in the lumbar area inferiorly. The filum terminale, a prolongation of the pia mater, descends from the apex of the conus medullaris, where the spinal cord tapers off below to attach to the back of the coccyx.

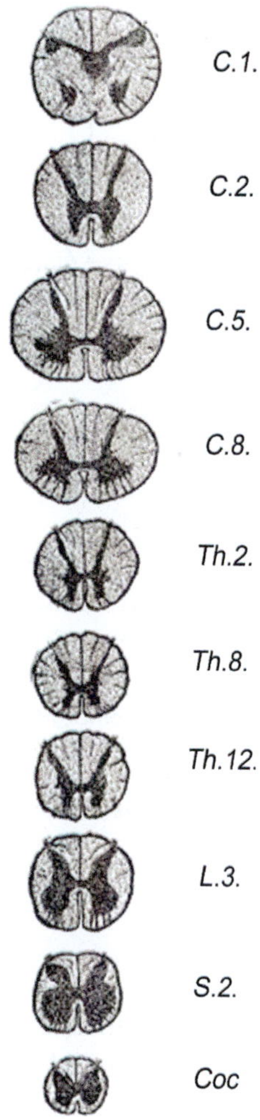

Figure 4.11. *Brain spinal nerves.*

Source: https://courses.lumenlearning.com/suny-ulster-ap1/chapter/spinal-cord/.

Around 31 pairs of spinal nerves, the anterior or motor roots and the posterior or sensory roots, are connected along the entire length of the spinal cord (Figures 4.11 and 4.12). A set of rootlets that run the entire length of the corresponding segment of the cord connects each root to the cord. Peripheral and central nerve fibers originate from the cells of the posterior root ganglion, which is present in every posterior nerve root.

4.5.2.2. Structure of the Spinal Cord

The spinal cord is composed of an outer layer of white matter that surrounds an inner core of gray matter (Figure 4.12). A thin gray commissure, which contains the small central canal, connects the anterior and posterior gray columns, or horns, that constitute the gray matter. In cross section, the gray matter appears as an H-shaped pillar. For descriptive purposes, the white matter can be divided into anterior, lateral, and posterior white columns (Figure 4.12).

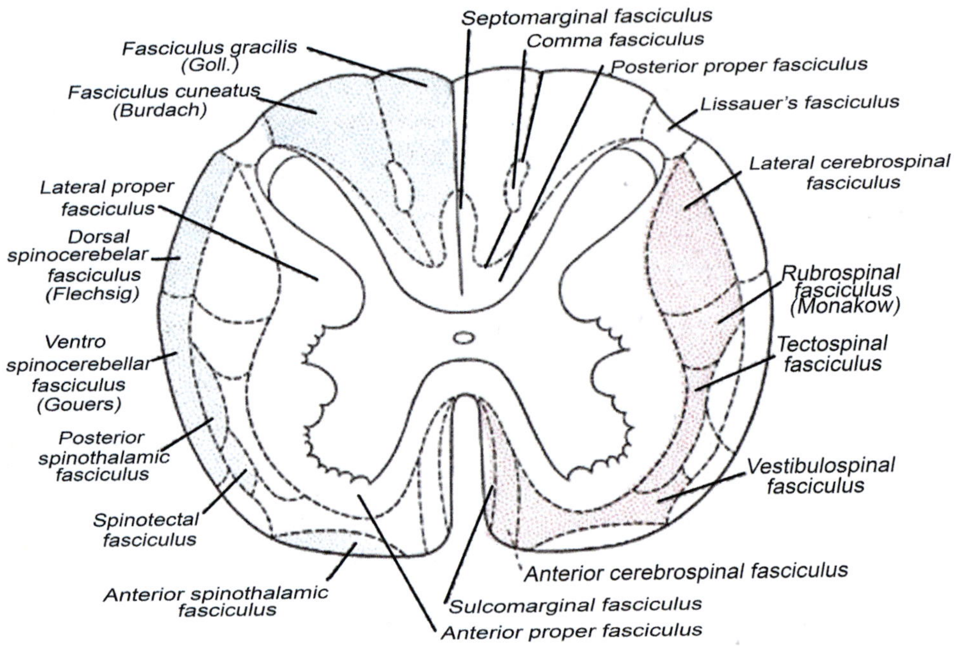

Figure 4.12. *Transverse section through the spinal cord.*

Source: https://courses.lumenlearning.com/suny-ulster-ap1/chapter/spinal-cord/.

4.5.2.2. Brain

The central nervous system (Figure 4.13 – through the foramen magnum) connects to the spinal cord and is situated in the cranial cavity (Figure 4.11(A)).

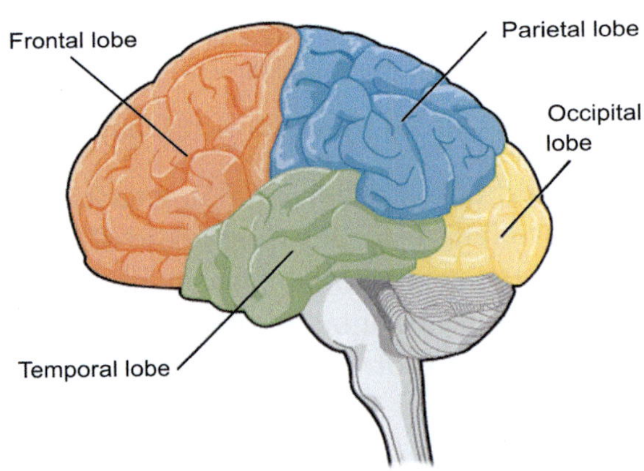

Figure 4.13. *Lateral view of the brain within the skull.*

Source: https://courses.lumenlearning.com/waymaker-psychology/chapter/reading-parts-of-the-brain/.

The dura mater, arachnoid mater, and pia mater are the three meninges that encompass it; they are continuous with the corresponding meninges of the spinal cord. The subarachnoid space encloses the brain and is filled with cerebrospinal fluid. There are three primary divisions in the brain according to conventional wisdom. These are the forebrain, midbrain, hindbrain, and spinal cord in ascending order. The medulla oblongata, the pons, and the cerebellum are potential divisions of the hindbrain. The diencephalon, or "between brain," which is the central region of the forebrain, and the cerebrum are additional divisions of the forebrain. The portion of the brain that remains after the removal of the cerebral hemispheres and cerebellum is referred to as the brainstem, which is a collective term for the medulla oblongata, pons, and midbrain.

4.5.2.3. Hindbrain

1. **Medulla Oblongata:** The pyramidal-shaped medulla oblongata connects the spinal cord inferiorly to the pons superiorly (Figure 4.14). It functions as a conduit for ascending and descending nerve fibers and contains numerous clusters of neurons, or nuclei.

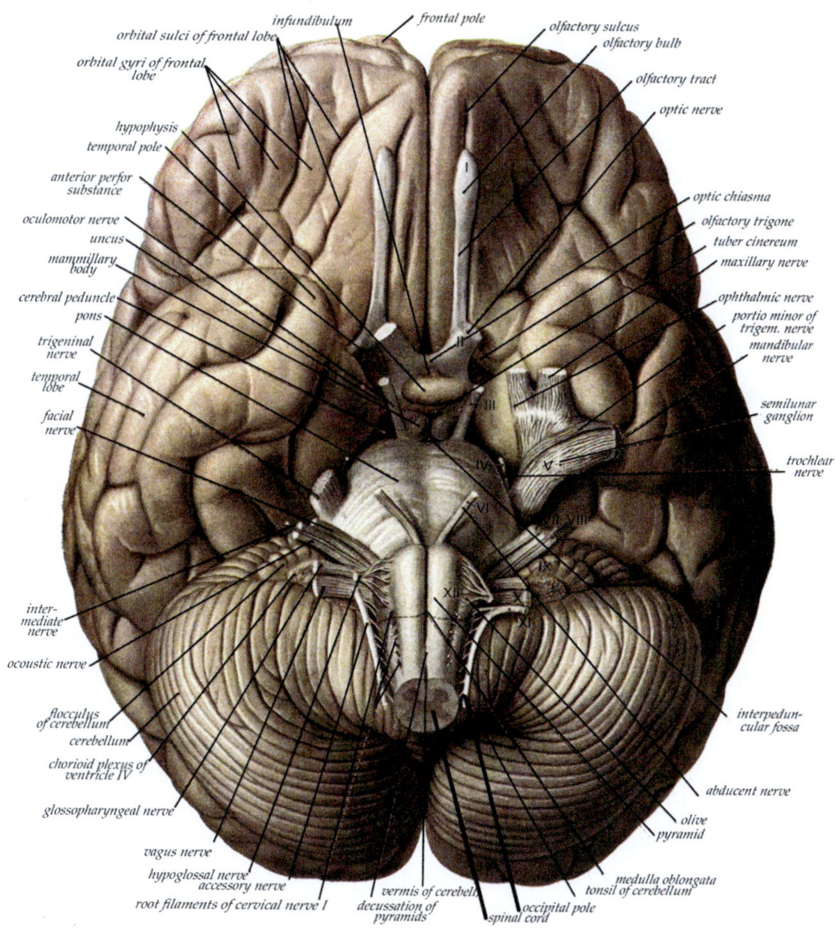

Figure 4.14. *Inferior view of the brain.*

Source: By Dr. Johannes Sobotta – Atlas and Textbook of Human Anatomy Volume III vascular system, lymphatic system, nervous system and sense organs, public domain. https://commons.wikimedia.org/w/index.php?curid=29135453.

2. **Pons:** It is located on the anterior surface of the cerebellum, positioned above the medulla oblongata and below the midbrain (Figures 4.14 and 4.15). Its name is derived from the numerous transverse fibers that connect the two cerebellar hemispheres on its anterior aspect, also known as the bridge. In addition to various nuclei, the pons contains ascending and descending nerve fibers.

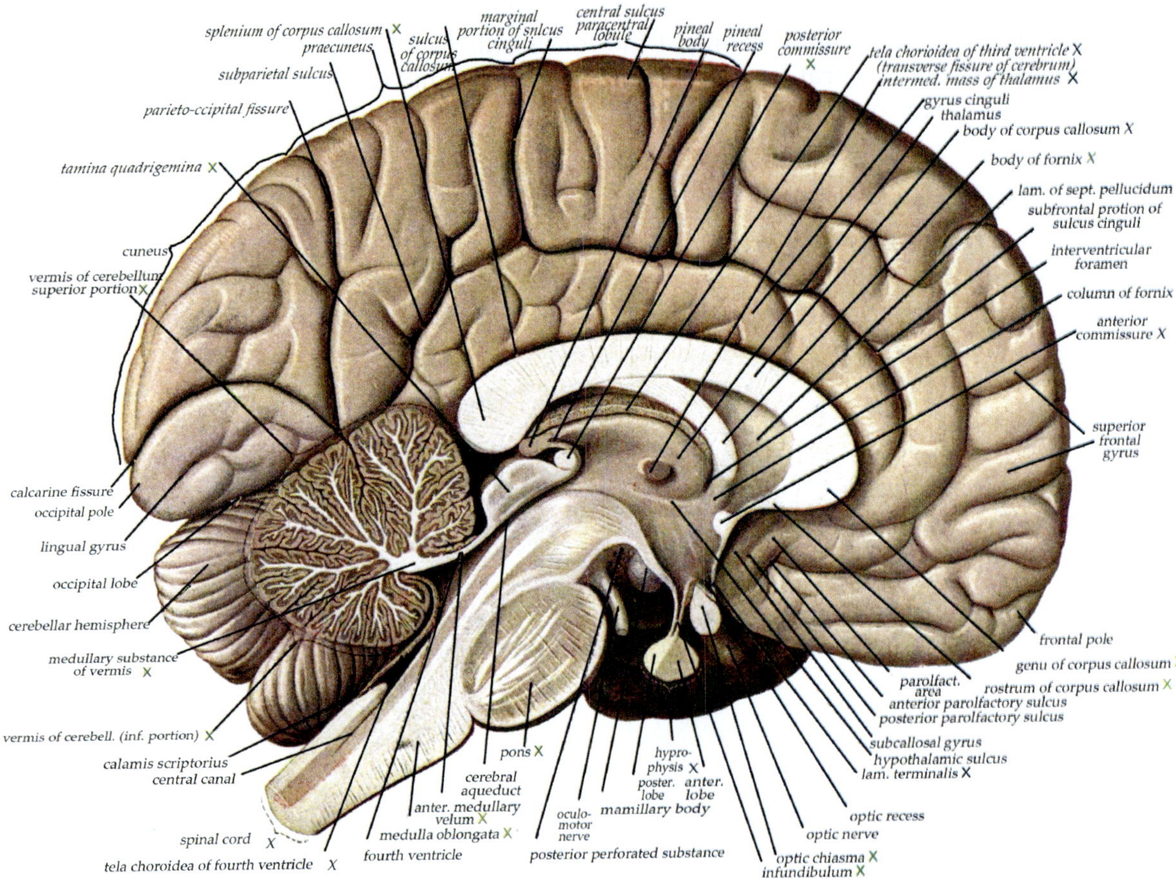

Figure 4.15. *Brain viewed from its right lateral aspect.*

Source: By Dr. Johannes Sobotta – Atlas and Textbook of Human Anatomy Volume III vascular system, lymphatic system, nervous system and sense organs, public domain. https://commons.wikimedia.org/w/index.php?curid=29135452.

3. **Cerebellum:** It is situated in the posterior cranial fossa of the skull (Figures 4.13–4.15), is positioned behind the medulla oblongata and the pons. It consists of two hemispheres laterally joined by the vermis, which acts as a median. The superior cerebellar peduncles connect the cerebellum to the midbrain, the middle cerebellar peduncles connect to the pons, and the inferior cerebellar peduncles connect to the medulla. The peduncles are composed of large bundles of nerve fibers that link the cerebellum to the rest of the nervous system. The cortex, which is the surface layer of each cerebellar hemisphere (Figure 4.17), is made up of gray matter. The cerebellar cortex is divided into folds called folia, separated by closely spaced transverse fissures. The largest gray matter mass,

known as the dentate nucleus, is located within the cerebellum and is embedded in the white matter. The medulla oblongata, pons, and cerebellum surround a cavity called the fourth ventricle, which is filled with cerebrospinal fluid. The cerebral aqueduct connects the fourth ventricle superiorly to the third ventricle, and it is continuous inferiorly with the central canal of the spinal cord (Figures 4.16 and 4.17). The roof of the fourth ventricle has three apertures through which it communicates with the subarachnoid space. These apertures allow the cerebrospinal fluid of the central nervous system to reach the subarachnoid space.

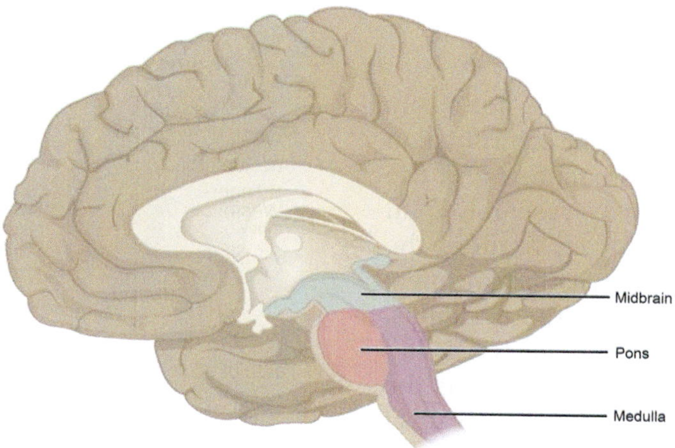

Figure 4.16. *Median sagittal section of the.*

Source: https://courses.lumenlearning.com/suny-ulster-ap1/chapter/brain/.

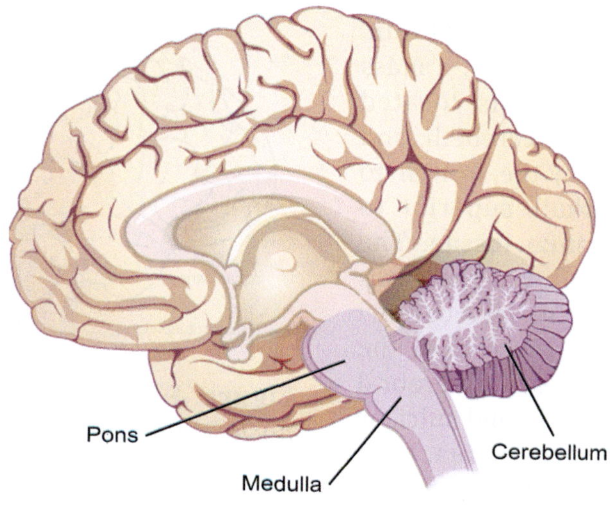

Figure 4.17. *Sagittal section through the brainstem and the cerebellum.*

Source: https://courses.lumenlearning.com/waymaker-psychology/chapter/reading-the-limbic-system-and-other-brain-areas/.

4.5.2.4. Midbrain

The small region of the brain that joins the forebrain and hindbrain is known as the midbrain. The midbrain contains the cerebral aqueduct, a narrow cavity that connects the third and fourth ventricles. Within the midbrain, there are numerous nuclei and bundles of ascending and descending nerve fibers.

4.5.2.5. Diencephalon

Moving on to the diencephalon, it is not easily visible from the brain's surface. The diencephalon consists of the ventral hypothalamus and the dorsal thalamus. The thalamus, resembling an egg-shaped mass of gray matter, borders the third ventricle. The interventricular foramen, located at the posterior end of the thalamus, forms the connection between the third and lateral ventricles. The hypothalamus forms the floor and lower portion of the lateral wall of the third ventricle.

4.5.2.6. Cerebrum

The two cerebral hemispheres that compose the cerebrum, the largest part of the brain, are connected by the corpus callosum, a mass of white matter. The cerebrum is located posteriorly above the tentorium cerebelli, and each hemisphere extends from the frontal to the occipital bones in the skull, superior to the anterior and middle cranial fossae. The longitudinal fissure, a deep cleft that separates the hemispheres, is where the falx cerebri protrudes. Gray matter forms the cortex, the outer layer of each hemisphere. The cerebral cortex is divided into gyri, or folds, and sulci, or fissures, which increase the surface area. Each hemisphere is divided into lobes by large sulci. The lobes are named after the cranial bones beneath them. The basal nuclei or ganglia, a central core of white matter, contain multiple masses of gray matter within each hemisphere. The corona radiata, a group of nerve fibers resembling a fan, travels through the white matter to the brainstem and from the cerebral cortex. The corona radiata converges on the basal nuclei and moves between them as the internal capsule. The caudate nucleus is the tailed nucleus located on the medial side of the internal capsule, and the term "lentiform nucleus" refers to the lens-shaped nucleus on the lateral side of the internal capsule.

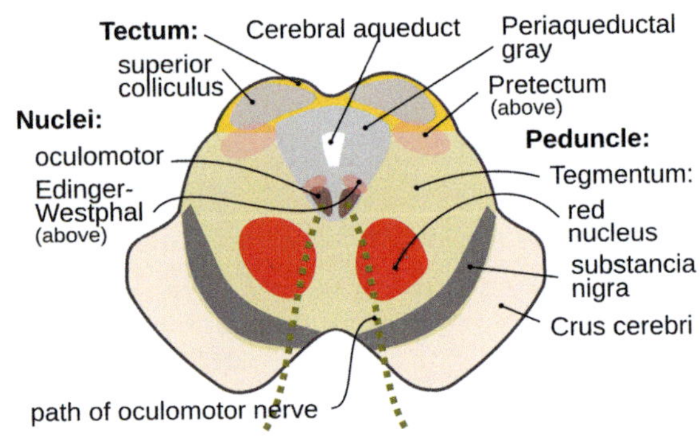

Figure 4.18. *The crus cerebri.*

Source: By Jmarchn – Own work, CC BY-SA 3.0, https://commons.wikimedia.org/w/index.php?curid=133426787.

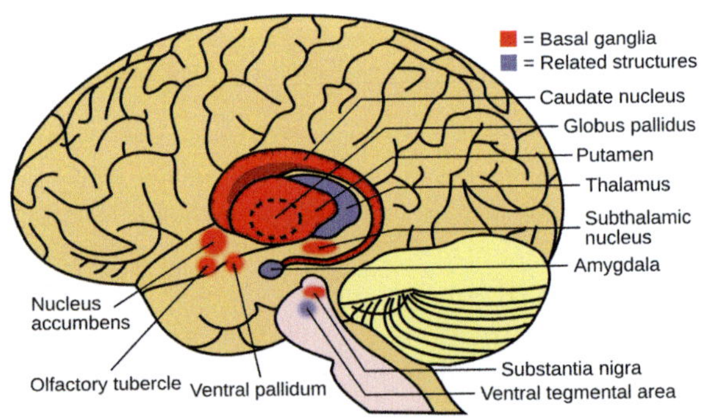

Figure 4.19. *Diagram showing the caudate nucleus, and the thalamus.*

Source: By File:BrainCaudatePutamen.svg: User:LeevanjacksonDerivative work: User:SUM1 – Derivative work based on File:BrainCaudatePutamen.svg, CC BY-SA 4.0, https://commons.wikimedia.org/w/index.php?curid=85845448.

The lateral ventricle is the hollow space within each cerebral hemisphere. The lateral ventricles and the third ventricle exchange information through the interventricular foramina. The cerebrum expands significantly during development and extends beyond the diencephalon, midbrain, and hindbrain (Figures 4.18 and 4.19).

4.5.2.7. Structure of the Brain

The brain is composed of an outer layer of gray matter surrounding an inner core of white matter, in contrast to the spinal cord. However, as previously mentioned, there are certain significant gray matter masses situated deep within the white matter. For example, the gray cerebellar nuclei are found in the cerebellum, and the gray thalamic, caudate, and lentiform nuclei are located in the cerebrum.

4.5.3. Divisions of the Peripheral Nervous System

The cranial and spinal nerves, along with the ganglia that support them, constitute the peripheral nervous system.

4.5.3.1. Cranial and Spinal

4.5.3.1.1. Nerves

The bundles of nerve fibers that form the cranial and spinal nerves are held in place by connective tissue. The cranial nerves are organized into 12 pairs (Figure 4.14), which exit the brain and travel through cranial foramina. The spinal nerves exit the spinal cord through intervertebral foramina in the vertebral column, totaling 31 pairs. The spinal nerves are categorized as 8 cervical, 12 thoracic, 5 lumbar, 5 sacral, and 1 coccygeal, corresponding to the respective regions of the vertebral column they are associated with. It is important to note that there is one coccygeal nerve and four coccygeal vertebrae, and that there are eight cervical nerves but only seven cervical vertebrae.

There are two roots that connect each spinal nerve to the spinal cord: the anterior root and the posterior root. Bundles of nerve fibers that carry nerve impulses away from the central nervous system make up the anterior root. These nerve cells are referred to as efferent fibers. Motor fibers are those efferent fibers that travel to the skeletal muscles and induce contractions in them. The anterior gray horn of the spinal cord contains their original cells.

Nerve fiber bundles known as afferent fibers, which transmit nerve impulses to the central nervous system, make up the posterior root. These fibers are referred to as sensory fibers because they are involved in transmitting information about touch, pain, temperature, and vibration sensations. The posterior root ganglion is a swelling on the posterior root that houses the cell bodies of these nerve fibers.

After leaving the spinal cord at the level of each of their individual intervertebral foramina, the spinal nerve roots combine to form a spinal nerve. A spinal nerve is composed of a mixture of motor and sensory fibers because this is where the motor and sensory fibers combine. The length of the roots gradually increases from above downward due to the vertebral column's disproportionate growth in length during development compared to that of the spinal cord (Figure 4.20). The spinal nerve roots in the upper cervical region are short and nearly horizontal, but the lumbar and sacral nerve roots form a vertical nerve leash around the filum terminale below the level of the cord's termination (lower border of the adult lumbar vertebra). The cauda equina refers to the collective name for these lower nerve roots.

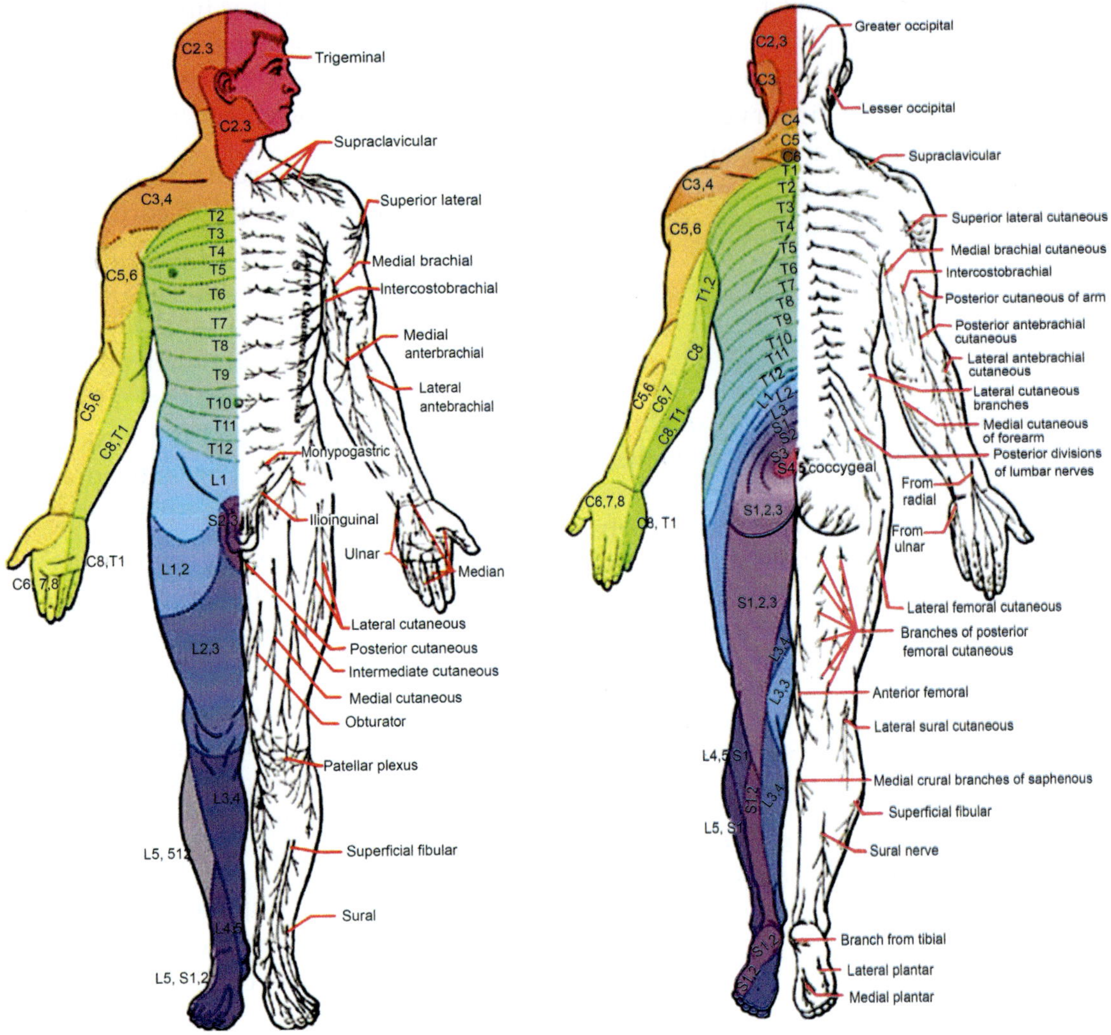

Figure 4.20. *Anterior and posterior views of the spinal cord showing the origins of the roots of the spinal nerves and their relationship to the different vertebrae.*

Source: https://courses.lumenlearning.com/suny-dutchess-anatomy-physiology/chapter/spinal-nerves-and-plexuses/.

Each spinal nerve, which contains both motor and sensory fibers, splits into a large anterior ramus and a smaller posterior ramus as soon as it emerges from the intervertebral foramen. The posterior ramus supplies the muscles and skin of the back by encircling the vertebral column posteriorly.

The anterior ramus, which continues anteriorly, supplies all the muscles and skin of the limbs, as well as the muscles covering the anterolateral body wall. Complex nerve plexuses are formed at the root of the limbs where the anterior rami unite. The cervical and brachial plexuses are located at the base of the upper limbs, while the lumbar and sacral plexuses are found at the base of the lower limbs.

4.5.3.2. Ganglia

Ganglia can be further subdivided into autonomic ganglia, cranial nerves, and posterior root ganglia of the spinal nerves.

4.5.3.3. Sensory Ganglia

Fusiform swellings on the posterior root of each spinal nerve, immediately proximal to the junction with the corresponding anterior root, are known as sensory ganglia or posterior root ganglia. Similar ganglia are also present along the course of cranial nerves V, VII, VIII, IX, and X.

4.5.3.4. Autonomic Ganglia

Located along the path of efferent nerve fibers in the autonomic nervous system are the often asymmetrical autonomic ganglia. They are located in the paravertebral sympathetic chains in the vicinity of or embedded in the walls of different viscera, as well as at the base of the great visceral arteries in the abdomen.

A Closer Look

Lumbar Puncture

A lumbar puncture, also known as a spinal tap, is a diagnostic procedure used to assess the pressure and composition of cerebrospinal fluid. The procedure involves the removal of cerebrospinal fluid using a syringe, typically from the lumbar area. Since the spinal cord terminates between the 1st and 2nd lumbar vertebrae, the needle is usually inserted between the 4th and 5th lumbar vertebrae. The meningeal sac, which contains cerebrospinal fluid, extends to the end of the lumbar vertebrae, allowing access to the fluid with minimal risk of spinal cord damage.

Cerebrospinal fluid (CSF) is a circulating fluid that normally has a pressure of 70 to 200 mmH2O. Abnormal pressure readings often indicate circulation obstruction, which can be caused by infection, tumors, or mechanical injury. Further diagnostic tests are required to determine the precise cause.

One of the most common reasons for performing a lumbar puncture is suspected meningitis, which can be caused by various types of bacteria. In cases of meningitis, the cerebrospinal fluid appears cloudy instead of clear, and it is examined for the presence of bacteria and an increased number of white blood cells. It is normal to find a few white blood cells in CSF, as they are present in all tissue fluids.

Another abnormal finding in cerebrospinal fluid is the presence of red blood cells, which indicates bleeding within the central nervous system. There can be numerous causes for this, and additional testing is necessary to determine the underlying cause.

Summary

- The brain, spinal cord, sensory organs, and all of the nerves that link these organs to the rest of the body make up the nervous system.
- The nervous system performs three primary tasks: motor output, data integration, and sensory input.
- The central nervous system (CNS) and the peripheral nervous system (PNS) are the two main components, or subdivisions, of the nervous system.
- Bipolar neurons possess two extensions emanating from the cell body. At the termination of one side lies the axon, while the dendrites are situated on the opposing side.
- Purkinje neurons exhibit multiple dendrites that radiate from the cell body. These neurons function as inhibitory neurons, signifying their release of neurotransmitters that prevent the firing of other neurons.
- The dendritic trees of most neurons are replete with numerous input signals. A solitary neuron can receive thousands of input signals and possess multiple sets of dendrites.
- Chemical agents referred to as neurotransmitters are discharged by the neuron at a chemical synapse.
- Neurons also exhibit significant variations in length. A meter or longer can be observed in the axons of the motor neurons that departed from the spinal cord to provide innervation to your toes, despite the fact that numerous neurons are minuscule in size.
- The nervous system is comprised of two distinct types of cells: glial cells and neurons. While neurons function as the primary unit of the nervous system, glial cells play a supportive role.
- The depolarization of a neuron, or the reduction in the electrical potential difference across the membrane, occurs due to the activation of sodium channels in the membrane. This allows for a localized influx of positively charged sodium ions into the cell in response to a signal.
- The diencephalon is nearly indiscernible from the brain's surface. It consists of the ventral hypothalamus and the dorsal thalamus.
- The brain is composed of an outer layer of gray matter encircling an inner core of white matter, in contrast to the spinal cord.
- Nerve fiber bundles referred to as afferent fibers, which transmit nerve impulses to the central nervous system, constitute the posterior root.
- Ganglia can be further subdivided into autonomic ganglia, cranial nerves, and posterior root ganglia of the spinal nerves.

References

1. Adams, W. K. M., Nelson, B. R., Stencel-Baerenwald, J. E., Studholme, C., Kapur, R. P., Armistead, B., & Rajagopal, L., (2018). Congenital Zika virus infection as a silent pathology with loss of neurogenic output in the fetal brain. *Nature Medicine, 24*(3), 368–374. doi:10.1038/nm.4485
2. Alexander, G. E., DeLong, M. R., & Strick, P. L., (1986). Parallel organization of functionally segregated circuits linking basal ganglia and cortex. *Annu. Rev. Neurosci., 9*, 357–381.
3. Anegroaie, P., Frasch, M. G., Rupprecht, S., Antonow-Schlorke, I., Muller, T., Schubert, H., & Schwab, M., (2016). Development of somatosensory-evoked potentials in foetal sheep: Effects of betamethasone. *Acta Physiology (Oxf)*. doi:10.1111/apha.12795
4. Bult, H., Boeckxstaens, G. E., Pelckmans, P. A., Jordaens, F. H., Van, M. Y. M., & Herman, A. G., (1990). Nitric oxide as an inhibitory non-adrenergic non-cholinergic neurotransmitter. *Nature, 345*(6273), 346–347.
5. Canedo, A., (1997). Primary motor cortex influences on the descending and ascending systems. *Prog. Neurobiol., 51*(3), 287–335.
6. DeMaagd, G., & Philip, A., (2015). Parkinson's disease and its management: Part 1: Disease entity, risk factors, pathophysiology, clinical presentation, and diagnosis. *P T., 40*(8), 504–532.
7. Flament-Durand, J., (1980). The hypothalamus: Anatomy and functions. *Acta Psychiatr. Belg., 80*(4), 364–375.
8. Fridriksson, J., Fillmore, P., Guo, D., & Rorden, C., (2015). Chronic Broca's aphasia is caused by damage to Broca's and Wernicke's areas. *Cereb. Cortex., 25*(12), 4689–4696.
9. Fung, S., Cherry, A. E., Xu, C., & Stella, N., (2015). Alkylindole-sensitive receptors modulate microglial cell migration and proliferation. *Glia, 63*(10), 1797–1808. doi:10.1002/glia.22845
10. Galli, R., Gritti, A., Bonfanti, L., & Vescovi, A. L., (2003). Neural stem cells: An overview. *Circ. Res., 92*(6), 598–608.
11. Gottschalk, A., Van, A. H., Zenz, M., & Standl, T., (2011). Is anesthesia dangerous? *Dtsch Arztebl. Int., 108*(27), 469–474.
12. Harvey, A. M., & Macintosh, F. C., (1940). Calcium and synaptic transmission in a sympathetic ganglion. *J. Physiol., 97*(3), 408–416.
13. Henn, F. A., Haljamäe, H., & Hamberger, A., (1972). Glial cell function: Active control of extracellular K + concentration. *Brain Res., 43*(2), 437–443.
14. Herculano-Houzel, S., (2009). The human brain in numbers: A linearly scaled-up primate brain. *Frontiers in Human Neuroscience, 3*, 31.
15. Imitola, J., Raddassi, K., Park, K. I., Mueller, F. J., Nieto, M., Teng, Y. D., Frenkel, D., et al., (2004). Directed migration of neural stem cells to sites of CNS injury by the stromal cell-derived factor 1alpha/CXC chemokine receptor 4 pathway. *Proc. Natl. Acad. Sci. U S A., 101*(52), 18117–18122.
16. Katz, B., & Miledi, R., (1967). A study of synaptic transmission in the absence of nerve impulses. *J. Physiol., 192*(2), 407–436.
17. Kennea, N. L., & Mehmet, H., (2002). Neural stem cells. *J. Pathol., 197*(4), 536–550.

18. Lanciego, J. L., Luquin, N., & Obeso, J. A., (2012). Functional neuroanatomy of the basal ganglia. *Cold Spring Harb. Perspect. Med., 2*(12), a009621.

19. Luengo-Sanchez, S., Bielza, C., Benavides-Piccione, R., Fernaud-Espinosa, I., DeFelipe, J., & Larrañaga, P., (2015). A univocal definition of the neuronal soma morphology using Gaussian mixture models. *Frontiers in Neuroanatomy, 9*, 137.

20. McLachlan, N. M., & Wilson, S. J., (2017). The contribution of brainstem and cerebellar pathways to auditory recognition. *Front Psychol., 8*, 265.

21. Mehndiratta, M. M., Mehndiratta, P., & Pande, R., (2014). Poliomyelitis: Historical facts, epidemiology, and current challenges in eradication. *Neurohospitalist., 4*(4), 223–229.

22. Miller, M. A., & Zachary, J. F., (2017). Mechanisms and morphology of cellular injury, adaptation, and death. *Pathologic Basis of Veterinary Disease*, 2.

23. Nattie, E., & Li, A., (2012). Central chemoreceptors: Locations and functions. *Compr. Physiol., 2*(1), 221–254.

24. Phelps, E. A., & LeDoux, J. E., (2005). Contributions of the amygdala to emotion processing: From animal models to human behavior. *Neuron, 48*(2), 175–187.

25. Raghavendra, T., (2002). Neuromuscular blocking drugs: Discovery and development. *J R Soc. Med., 95*(7), 363–367.

26. Rajmohan, V., & Mohandas, E., (2007). The limbic system. *Indian J. Psychiatry., 49*(2), 132–139.

27. Schachter, A. S., & Davis, K. L., (2000). Alzheimer's disease. *Dialogues Clin. Neurosci., 2*(2), 91–100.

28. Scoville, W. B., & Milner, B., (2000). Loss of recent memory after bilateral hippocampal lesions. 1957. *J. Neuropsychiatry Clin. Neurosci., 12*(1), 103–113.

29. Shipp, S., (2007). Structure and function of the cerebral cortex. *Curr. Biol., 17*(12), R443–449.

30. Siegel, J. H., & Relkin, E. M., (1987). Antagonistic effects of perilymphatic calcium and magnesium on the activity of single cochlear afferent neurons. *Hear. Res., 28*(2, 3), 131–147.

31. Snyder, S. H., (1980). Brain peptides as neurotransmitters. *Science, 209*(4460), 976–983.

32. Stiles, J., & Jernigan, T. L., (2010). The basics of brain development. *Neuropsychol. Rev., 20*(4), 327–348.

33. Tziridis, K., Dicke, P. W., & Thier, P., (2012). Pontine reference frames for the sensory guidance of movement. *Cereb. Cortex, 22*(2), 345–362.

34. Vrselja, Z., Brkic, H., Mrdenovic, S., Radic, R., & Curic, G., (2014). Function of circle of willis. *J. Cereb. Blood Flow Metab., 34*(4), 578–584.

35. Zola-Morgan, S., Squire, L. R., & Amaral, D. G., (1986). Human amnesia and the medial temporal region: Enduring memory impairment following a bilateral lesion limited to field CA1 of the hippocampus. *J. Neurosci., 6*(10), 2950–2967.

Chapter

CARDIOVASCULAR SYSTEM

5

Contents

Unit Introduction

The circulatory system, also known as the cardiovascular system, is composed of the heart, a muscular pump, and a closed network of blood vessels including capillaries, veins, and arteries. As the name implies, the blood within the circulatory system is continuously pumped by the heart through a closed circuit of vessels as it circulates throughout the body.

Similar to adults, the survival of a developing embryo relies on blood circulation to maintain homeostasis and create an optimal cellular environment. The cardiovascular system begins to develop early in embryonic development and becomes functional well before other major organ systems, in response to this necessity. Remarkably, the primitive heart starts beating regularly as early as the fourth week after conception.

Thousands of miles of capillaries penetrate every tissue and reach every cell in the body, and the steady and regulated flow of blood through them is crucial for the cardiovascular system's vital role in maintaining homeostasis. Microscopic capillaries perform the primary transport function of blood. As waste products are removed, nutrients and other essential substances are transferred from the capillary blood into the fluids surrounding the cells.

The many components of the cardiovascular system work together to integrate and regulate various functions, including the delivery of blood to different parts of the body as needed. These systems ensure that every body cell maintains a consistent internal environment, even in the face of varying nutritional needs or waste product production.

Orientation and Directional Terms:

Term	Definition	Illustration
Arteriole	An arteriole is a small blood vessel that branches off from an artery and carries blood from the heart to tissues and organs.	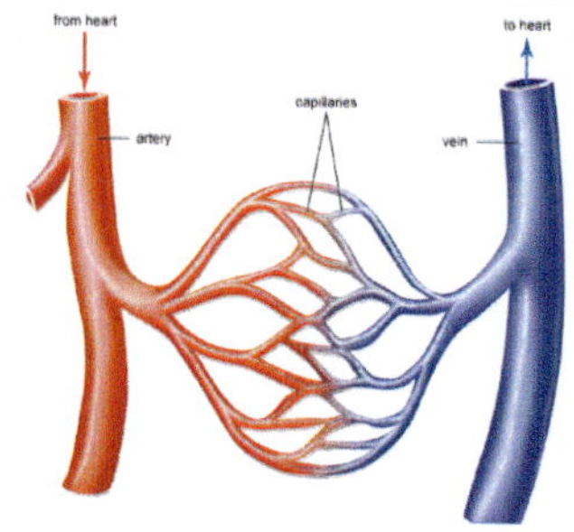
Ductus arteriosus	The ductus arteriosus is a blood vessel that connects the fetal pulmonary artery to the aorta. It is a temporary opening that is necessary before birth for a baby's blood flow.	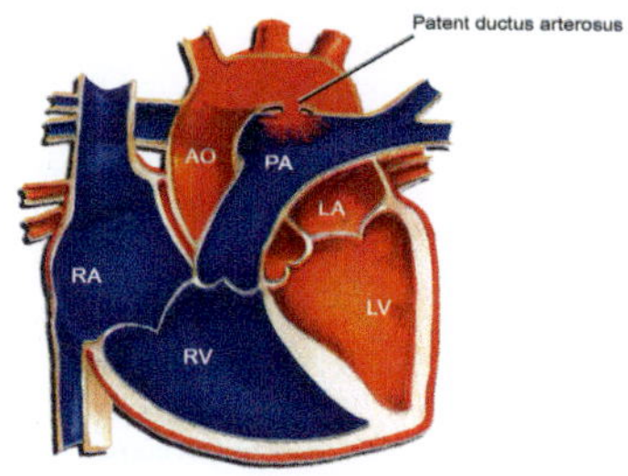
Foramen ovale	A foramen ovale is a small opening between the upper chambers of the heart in an unborn baby.	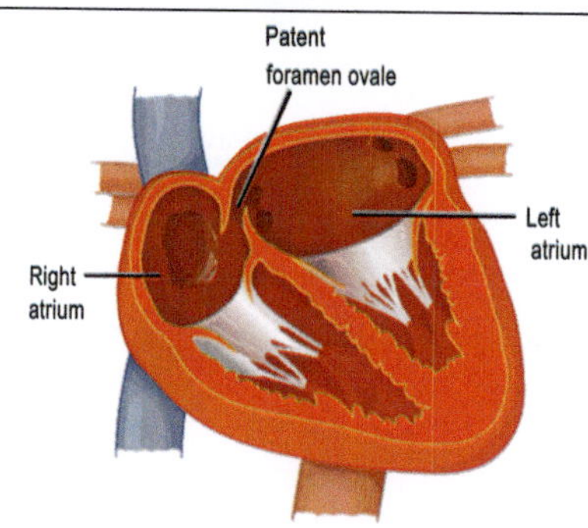
Sinusoid	A sinusoid is a small blood vessel that is a type of capillary similar to a fenestrated endothelium.	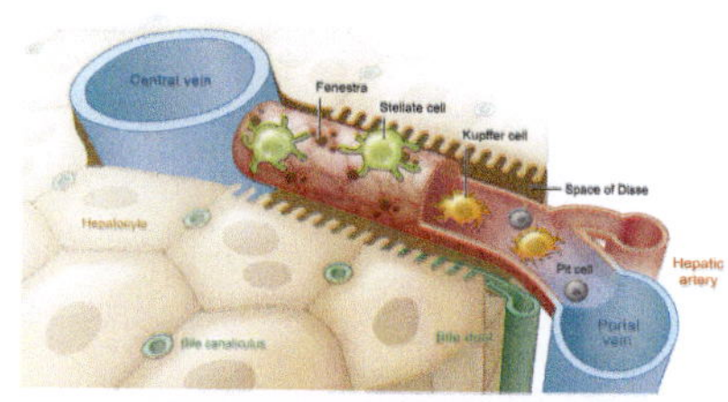
Venule	A venule is any of the small vessels that collect blood from the capillary plexuses and join to form veins.	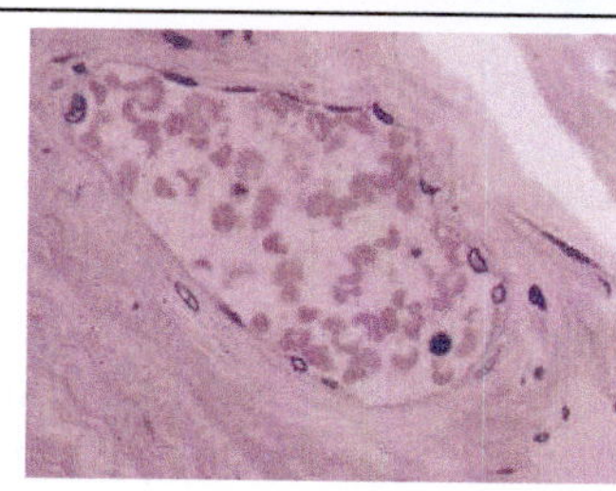

5.1. Overview of the Cardiovascular System

The circulatory system in humans is an organ system that transports blood via vessels to and from every area of the body, supplying tissues with nutrients and oxygen while expelling waste products like carbon dioxide. It is a closed tubular system with a muscular heart that pumps blood. There are two circuits made up of arterial, capillary, and venous components: the pulmonary and the systemic.

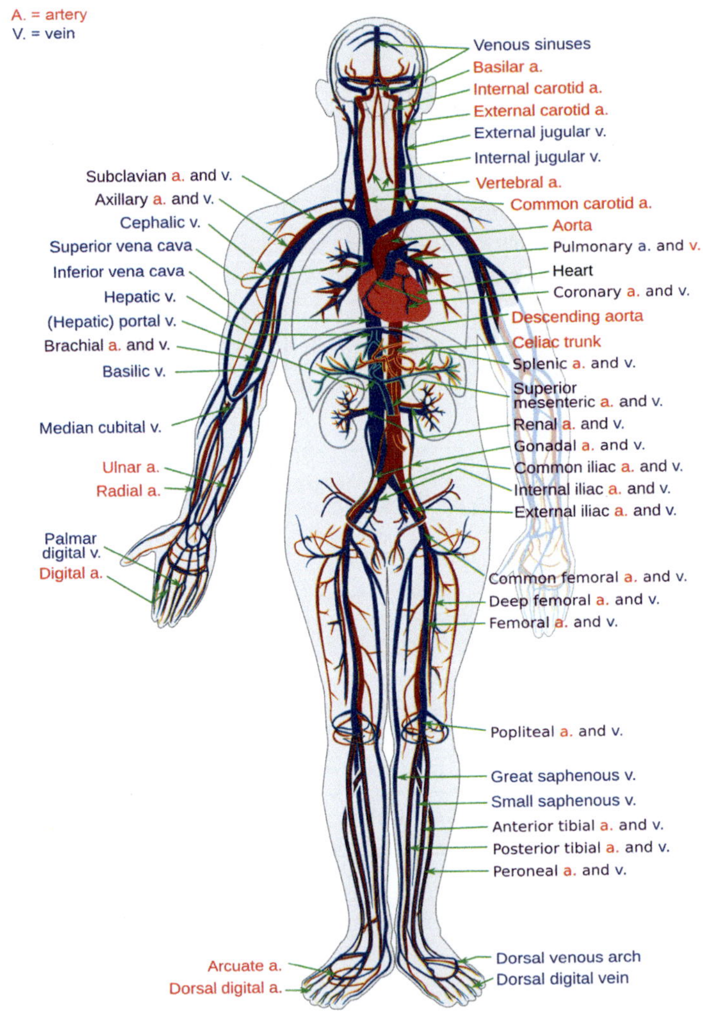

Figure 5.1. *Cardiovascular system.*

Source: By Lady of Hats, Mariana Ruiz Villarreal – Did myself based in the information and diagrams found in: "gray's anatomy "36th Edition by Williams & Warwick." Sobotta Atlas der Anatomie des menschen, volumes 1 and 2. Auflage by Urban & Schwarzenberg. Atlas fotografico de anatomia del cuerpo humano. 3a edicion by Yokochi, Rohen & Weinrebmultiple websites included: [1–6], and others., Public Domain, https://commons.wikimedia.org/w/index.php?curid=6698231.

The main role of the heart is to act as a strong pump that moves blood through vessels to all parts of the body. Arteries have thick walls composed of elastic tissue and muscle cells, receiving blood at high pressure and conducting it throughout the body. The branching system of arteries ends in arterioles, small muscular vessels that lead to capillaries. Capillaries allow for the exchange of nutrients and waste products. Blood then moves to venules, small vessels that converge to form veins, carrying blood back to the heart (Figure 5.1).

5.1.1. Functions of Cardiovascular System

The cardiovascular system performs three main roles: transportation of materials, defense against pathogens, and maintenance of the body's internal balance.

1. **Transportation:** The cardiovascular system is responsible for transporting blood to nearly all of the body's tissues. Blood carries essential nutrients and oxygen, while removing waste products and carbon dioxide for processing or elimination. Hormones are also transported throughout the body via the liquid plasma in the blood.
2. **Protection:** The cardiovascular system provides protection through its white blood cells. These cells clean up cellular debris and combat pathogens that have entered the body. Platelets and red blood cells form scabs to seal wounds and prevent pathogens from entering the body, as well as to prevent fluids from leaking out. Additionally, blood carries antibodies that offer specific immunity to pathogens that the body has previously encountered or has been vaccinated against.
3. **Regulation:** The cardiovascular system plays a crucial role in maintaining homeostatic control of various internal conditions. Blood vessels help regulate body temperature by controlling blood flow to the skin's surface. During overheating, blood vessels near the skin dilate, allowing hot blood to release heat into the surroundings. Conversely, in cases of hypothermia, these blood vessels constrict to prioritize blood flow to vital organs in the body's core. Blood also contributes to balancing the body's pH levels due to the presence of bicarbonate ions, which act as a buffer solution. Lastly, the albumins in blood plasma help maintain an isotonic environment, ensuring the osmotic concentration of the body's cells remains balanced.

5.1.2. Components of Cardiovascular System

The system responsible for circulating blood to various parts of the body is known as the cardiovascular system. It consists of the following organs and tissues:

- **Heart:** A muscular pump that propels blood throughout the body.
- A closed network of blood vessels, including:
  - **Arteries:** Vessels that carry blood away from the heart.
  - **Veins:** Vessels that return blood back to the heart.
  - **Capillaries:** Tiny vessels that branch off from arteries to deliver blood to all body tissues.

5.2. Heart Structure and Function

The heart is the organ responsible for pushing blood through blood vessels. It directly pumps blood into arteries, particularly the pulmonary or aortic arteries. The heart pumps oxygenated blood out of the left ventricle and into the aorta to begin systemic circulation.

After the blood has supplied cells throughout the body with oxygen and nutrients, it returns deoxygenated blood to the right atrium of the heart.

The deoxygenated blood flows down from the right atrium to the right ventricle. The heart then pumps it out of the right ventricle and into the pulmonary arteries to begin pulmonary circulation.

The blood moves to the lungs, exchanging carbon dioxide for oxygen, and then returns to the left atrium. From there, the oxygenated blood is propelled to the left ventricle below, initiating systemic circulation once again. Each half of the heart consists of a receiving chamber called the atrium and a pumping chamber called the ventricle.

In humans, cardiac output typically ranges from 5–6 L/min at rest to over 35 L/min in elite athletes during exercise. The weight of the heart is approximately 300g. Two thin-walled atria are separated by an interatrial septum. Two thick-walled ventricles are separated by an interventricular septum (Figure 5.2).

LV: Left Ventricle

RV: Right Ventricle

LA: Left Atrium

RA: Right Atrium

LV → RA → RV → lungs → LA → LV

LV → Aortic valve → Aorta → Sup. & Inf. Vena Cava → RA → Tricuspid valve → RV → Pulmonary valve → Pulmonary artery → lungs →Pulmonary vein → LA → Mitral valve → LV.

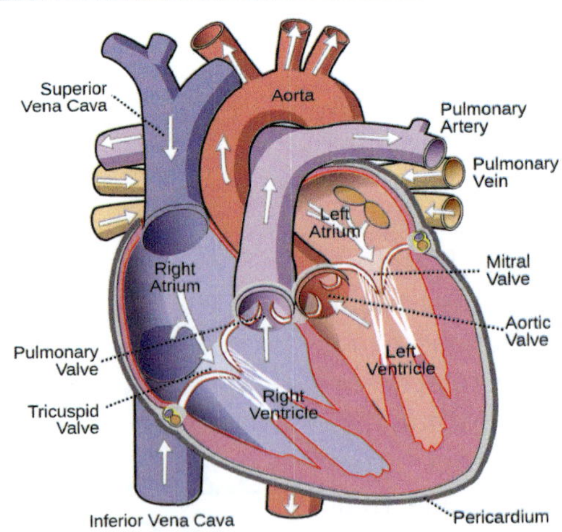

Figure 5.2. *Structure of heart.*

Source: https://upload.wikimedia.org/wikipedia/commons/thumb/e/e5/Diagram_of_the_human_heart_%28cropped%29.svg/917px-Diagram_of_the_human_heart_%28cropped%29.svg.png.

1. **Location of the Heart:** The heart, situated in the center of your chest, is connected to blood vessels that spread throughout your body to supply oxygen and nutrients to all parts and remove waste from cells.

2. **Pericardium:** A membranous sac of its own, suspends the heart. The diaphragm below, the mediastinal pleura on the side, and the sternum in front are all securely attached to the robust outer part of the sac, known as the fibrous pericardium. It eventually melds with the pulmonary (lung) arteries and veins that lead to and from the heart, as well as the coverings of the superior vena cava. The mediastinal pleura, a continuation of the membrane lining the chest, borders the mediastinum, the area between the lungs. The main vein that carries venous blood from the head, neck, arms, and chest is the superior vena cava.

   The fibrous pericardium is lined with a smooth, serous (moisture-exuding) membrane that bends back to cover the heart. The membrane covering the heart is referred to as the visceral serous layer (also known as the epicardium or visceral pericardium), and it is called the parietal serous layer (parietal pericardium).

   Merely 10 to 15 milliliters (0.06 to 0.09 cubic inches) of pericardial fluid, secreted by the serous membranes, typically divide the two layers of the serous membrane. The pericardial cavity is the name given to the tiny opening made by the separation. Every heartbeat lubricates the two membranes as their surfaces pass over one another. This fluid is called pericardial fluid. Both the visceral and parietal pericardia filter fluid into the pericardial space.

3. **Chambers of the Heart:** The heart is divided into two chambers, the right and left halves, which are separated by partitions called septa. The ventricles, the lower chambers, are divided from the atria, the upper chambers, by the interventricular septum and the interatrial septum, respectively. The atria receive blood from different areas of the body and then send it to the ventricles. The ventricles, in turn, pump blood to the lungs and the rest of the body.

   The right atrium, also known as the right superior portion of the heart, is a narrow chamber that receives blood from all body parts except the lungs. It is supplied by three veins: the coronary sinus, which drains blood from the heart itself, and the superior and inferior vena cavae, which bring blood from the upper and lower limbs of the body, respectively. The right atrium then supplies blood to the right ventricle. The right ventricle, located in the right inferior section of the heart, pumps blood to the lungs through the pulmonary artery.

   On the other hand, the left atrium, the left superior chamber of the heart, has a thicker wall and is slightly smaller than the right atrium. It receives oxygen-enriched blood from the lungs through the four pulmonary veins. The left atrium then sends the blood to the left ventricle. The left ventricle, the inferior left chamber of the heart, has walls that are three times thicker than those of the right ventricle. It pumps blood to all body parts, except the lungs, through the aorta.

4. **External Surface of the Heart:** Shallow grooves, known as interventricular sulci, can be observed on the anterior and posterior surfaces of the heart,

demarcating the separation between the ventricles. These grooves contain blood vessels and serve to segregate the various chambers of the heart. The external surface of the heart features two primary grooves: the atrioventricular groove, situated at the junction of the right atrium and right ventricle, which accommodates a branch of the right coronary artery, and the anterior interventricular sulcus, running between the right and left ventricles, housing a branch of the left coronary artery. Both of these grooves play a crucial role in supplying blood to the cardiac muscle.

The division between the right and left ventricles is indicated on the posterior aspect of the heart surface by a groove referred to as the posterior longitudinal sulcus, which also contains an additional branch of the coronary artery. Additionally, there exists a fourth groove that houses the coronary sinus, a venous blood channel, positioned between the left atrium and ventricle.

5. **Origin and Development:** The pharyngeal, or throat, region of the embryo is where the heart starts to form. The undifferentiated mesoderm, which is in the middle of the embryo's three primary layers, is where the embryonic heart first becomes visible as a thickening of invasive cells. A tube of flattened cells known as the endocardial (lining) tube then forms, and it keeps differentiating until a young tube with anterior and posterior forked ends emerges. This primordial tube starts to fold upon itself as differentiation and growth proceed, and constrictions along its length result in the formation of four main chambers. These are known as the sinus venosus, atrium, ventricle, and truncus arteriosus, in order from posterior to anterior. The ventricle swings first to the right and then behind the atrium due to the tube's characteristic bending, with the truncus falling in between the atrium's sideways dilations. These are the developmental and growth stages when the heart's first beats occur.

   The single opening between the ventricle and the atrium is "pinned" into two sections by endocardial cushions, which are local thickenings of the endocardium, or heart lining. The two atrioventricular valves, or the valves between the atria and ventricles, which control the direction of blood flow through the heart, are also formed as a result of these cushions.

   Initially, a primary partition with a septum primum divides the atrium into its right and left halves. Later, a secondary partition with a large opening in its lower part called the foramen ovale separates the two halves. Blood continues to flow through the two openings, from the right atrium to the left, despite their slight spatial mismatch. At birth, the primary partition is pushed against the secondary one due to increased blood pressure in the left atrium, blocking the two openings and causing complete separation of the atria. Eventually, the two partitions merge.

   At the apex of the ventricle, the myocardium, or heart muscle, forms an indentation that partially divides the ventricle into two chambers. This developing partition consists mainly of muscle, with the addition of membranous connective tissue that forms simultaneously with the division of the truncus arteriosus into two channels: the pulmonary artery and the aorta for systemic circulation. At this stage, the left chambers of the heart are positioned posteriorly to the right chambers, and the heart undergoes leftward and clockwise rotation to reside in the left thorax. The ductus arteriosus, a blood vessel that connects the pulmonary artery and the aorta, returns most of the blood that passes through the right side of the heart in the fetus to the systemic circulation. This duct's muscular wall contracts forcefully at birth, closing it off. The blood from the right side of the heart is then propelled to the left side of the heart for ejection into the systemic circulation after passing through the pulmonary arteries to the lungs for oxygenation. The external division of the ventricle into the right and left chambers is indicated by a distinct median furrow at the apex of the ventricles.

5.2.1. Structure of Heart

The heart is composed of two upper chambers known as "atria" and two lower chambers known as "ventricles." The atria and ventricles are separated by a wall, or "septum." Blood flow among the various chambers is regulated by valves.

Blood follows the following path through the heart:

- Blood lacking oxygen returns from the body and enters the right atrium (upper right chamber) via the inferior vena cava and superior vena cava veins.
- Blood flows through the tricuspid valve and enters the right ventricle (lower right chamber).
- The right ventricle pumps blood through the pulmonary valve and out of the heart via the main pulmonary artery.
- The blood then flows through the left and right pulmonary arteries into the lungs. Here, the process of respiration draws oxygen into the blood and removes carbon dioxide. As a result, the blood is now rich in oxygen.
- The blood returns to the heart and flows into the left atrium (upper left chamber) via four pulmonary veins.
- Blood flows through the mitral valve and enters the left ventricle (lower left chamber).
- The left ventricle pumps the blood through the aortic valve into a large artery called the "aorta." This artery delivers blood to the rest of the body.

The average dimensions and weight of an adult human heart are approximately 13 × 9 × 6 cm (5 × 3.5 × 2.5 inches) and 300 grams, respectively. The heart is typically slightly larger than a closed fist. It is shaped like a cone, with the wide base pointing upward and to the right and the apex pointing leftward and downward. It is situated in the space between the lungs and above the diaphragm, which is the muscular wall that separates the chest and abdominal cavities, in the chest (thoracic cavity), behind the sternum, in front of the windpipe (trachea), the esophagus, and the descending aorta. The heart is located to the left of the midline in roughly two-thirds.

5.2.1.1. Valves of the Heart

The heart has valves that allow blood to flow in only one direction in order to prevent blood from flowing backward.

There are two types of valves located in the heart:

1. Atria-Ventricular Valve (AV Valve)
   - Tricuspid valve;

- Mitral valve.

2. Semilunar Valve:
   - Pulmonary valve;
   - Aortic valve.

Between the atria and the ventricles lie thin, leaf-like structures known as atrioventricular valves. The right atrioventricular opening is protected by the tricuspid valve, which consists of three irregularly shaped cusps or flaps. The endocardium, which lines the heart, is folded into leaflets that are reinforced by a thin layer of dense connective tissue. The central supporting flat plate and the dense connective tissue of the ridge surrounding the openings merge at the base of the leaflets.

The middle supporting layer on the ventricular surface of each leaflet is connected to tendinous cords of dense tissue called chordae tendineae. These cords are covered by a thin layer of endocardium and originate from the papillary muscles, which resemble nipples. The chordae tendineae and papillary muscles restrict the extent to which the valve portions near their free margin can bulge towards the atria. The left atrioventricular opening is guarded by the mitral valve, also known as the bicuspid valve due to its two flaps. The mitral valve is attached in the same manner as the tricuspid valve, but it is thicker and stronger due to the left ventricle being a more powerful pump that operates at higher pressure.

The tricuspid and mitral valves propel blood through them when the atria contract. Blood is forced backward when the ventricles contract, passing between the flaps and the walls. Consequently, the flaps are forced upward until they come together to form a whole partition that separates the ventricles and the atria. The chordae tendineae and papillary muscles prevent the expanded flaps of the valves from opening into the atria.

The pulmonary artery and aorta exit the ventricles at the location of the semilunar valves, which are pocket-like structures. The opening that connects the pulmonary artery and the right ventricle is protected by the pulmonary valve. The opening that connects the left ventricle to the aorta is shielded by the aortic valve. The aortic semilunar valve's three leaflets and the pulmonary valve's two leaflets are both thinner than the atrioventricular valve's leaflets, but they share the same general structure aside from the absence of chordae tendineae.

The heartbeat, an audible sound, is connected to the closure of the heart valves. The closure of the tricuspid and mitral valves produces the first sound, and the closure of the pulmonary and aortic semilunar valves produces the second. It has been discovered that the major vessels surrounding the heart and the walls of the heart vibrate, producing these distinctive heart sounds. When the ventricles contract and there is a sudden backflow of blood, the valves close and the ventricles bulge back, producing the low-frequency first heart sound. The blood then returns to each ventricle according to the elasticity of the valves. The ventricle walls vibrate as a result of this action, and the vibrations move away from the valves. With the use of a stethoscope, sound waves that are produced when the vibrations reach the chest wall where the wall and the heart are in contact can be heard.

As the blood reverberates back and forth between the walls of the arteries and the valves following the sudden closure of the pulmonary and aortic semilunar valves, vibrations are generated in the walls of the aorta, the ventricles, and the pulmonary artery. These vibrations cause the second heart sound. The chest wall then converts these vibrations into sound waves, which are audible as a high-frequency sound. There is a brief pause before the second heart sound occurs. The start of the subsequent cycle is followed by a pause that is roughly twice as long as the first sound. There is no sound when the valves open.

5.2.1.2. Wall of the Heart

The myocardium, which is the middle layer, the endocardium, which is the inner layer, and the epicardium, which is the outer layer, make up the heart's wall. Coronary vessels enter the myocardium after passing through the epicardium to deliver arterial blood to the heart. This outer layer, also known as the visceral pericardium, is made up of flattened epithelium (covering) cells that are supported by connective tissue (Figure 5.3).

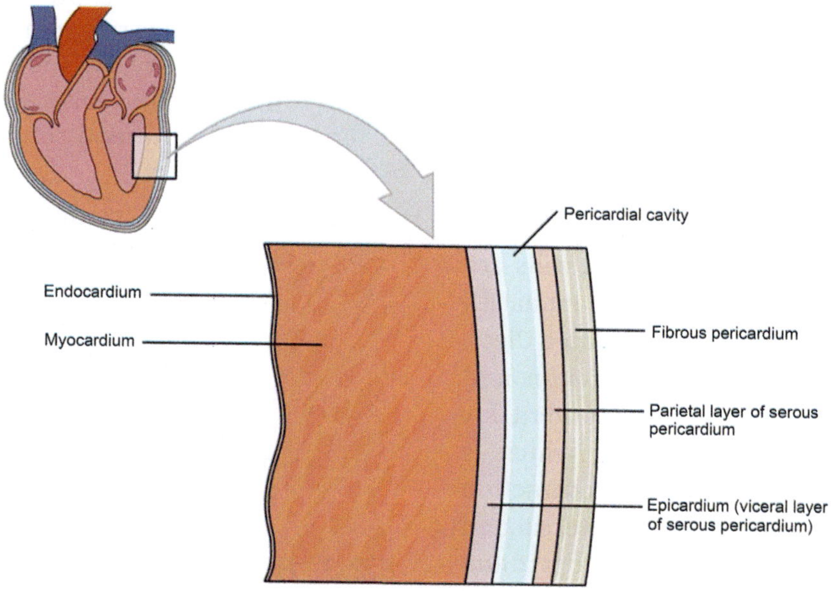

Figure 5.3. *Wall of the heart.*

Source: https://courses.lumenlearning.com/suny-ap2/chapter/heart-anatomy/.

The heart's contractile components are located in the myocardial layer. The myocardium's bundles of striated muscle fibers are grouped in a branching pattern that creates a wringing motion that effectively draws blood from the heart with each beat. The thickness of the myocardium is determined by the pressure needed to pump blood to its destination. The right ventricle's myocardium, responsible for propelling blood to the lungs, is moderately thickened, while the atrial walls are relatively thin. Consequently, the left ventricle's myocardium, which must forcefully pump blood into the systemic circulation, is the thickest.

Muscle fibers, composed of cardiac muscle cells, constitute the portion of the myocardium that undergoes contraction. Within each cell, smaller fibers called myofibrils house highly organized contractile units known as sarcomeres. Sarcomere-derived mechanical function is generated by distinct contractile proteins called myosin and actin, also referred to as thick and thin filaments, respectively. The sarcomere, located between two Z lines (also known as Z discs) in a muscle fiber, is comprised of two populations of actin filaments that project from opposing Z lines in an antiparallel manner and surround thick myosin filaments. As actin slides along cross bridges that periodically protrude from myosin filaments, every myosin comes into contact with a neighboring myosin filament. This process leads to muscle contraction by shortening the muscle fiber.

Numerous biological processes that are generally connected to the concentration of calcium within the cell control the interaction between actin and myosin. Large amounts of energy and calcium are needed for actin to slide over myosin. The mitochondria make up about 25% of the cardiac cell volume and supply the energy required for contraction, while the contractile machinery occupies approximately 70% of the cell volume. Heart muscle cells are connected to one another and to their boundaries by special junctions known as intercalated discs, or gap junctions, which enable calcium and energy conductance. The primary conduit for cardiac cell-to-cell communication, which is necessary for coordinated muscle contraction and circulation maintenance, is the intercalated disc. A thin lining known as the endocardium forms the inner surface of the myocardial wall. This layer is continuous with the lining membrane of the large blood vessels and lines the cavities of the heart, as well as the valves and small muscles involved in valve opening and closing.

5.2.2. Function of Heart

The purpose of the cardiovascular system is to ensure that the body receives the necessary oxygen, nutrients, and other substances, and eliminates them. The heart beats continuously, even during sleep, pumping blood throughout the body. This is why a doctor can hear the heartbeat, as it indicates normal heart function. The heart circulates approximately 2,000 gallons of blood daily. Blood is transported to the heart through specific blood vessels called veins, and away from the heart through other blood vessels called arteries. Additionally, blood vessels remove waste products, such as carbon dioxide, from the cells. The heart always pumps blood along the same path, and valves ensure that the blood flows in the correct direction.

5.2.2.1. Types of Circulation

1. **Pulmonary Circulation:** Blood without oxygen enters the right side of your heart and is transported to the lungs to acquire oxygen and eliminate carbon dioxide. Subsequently, the oxygenated blood returns through the left side of your heart.
2. **Systemic Circulation:** Blood that has just received oxygen from the lungs and returned through the left side of your heart is then propelled to the cells throughout your body, providing them with oxygen and nutrients. The cycle begins anew when deoxygenated blood reaches the right side of your heart.

5.2.3. Regulations of Heartbeat

Since there are no nerves within the heart and no external regulatory mechanisms are required to stimulate the muscle to contract rhythmically, the heart beats regularly due to the intrinsic rhythmicity of cardiac muscle. Observing cardiac development in the embryo provides evidence that these rhythmic contractions originate in the cardiac muscle; cardiac pulsations start before adequate development of nerve fibers. Furthermore, even pieces of cardiac muscle in tissue culture have been shown to exhibit rhythmic contractions in the lab. Moreover, the heart's muscle fibers do not contract to a varying degree, which would be predicted if they were primarily controlled by the nervous system.

Nevertheless, the heart cannot work effectively merely because it possesses this intrinsic ability. The heart's complex conducting system, which is primarily composed of two small, specialized masses of tissue called nodes from which impulses originate and nerve-like conduits for impulse transmission with terminal branches extending to the inner surface of the ventricles, maintains coordination, which is necessary for proper function.

An electrical impulse that moves from the top of the heart, in the atria, to the bottom, in the ventricles, is the source of rhythmic cardiac contractions. Propagation of the impulse occurs as a wave that moves between cells. The membrane that envelops the muscle fiber, the sarcolemma, has voltage-sensitive protein channels on its surface that facilitate current flow in relation to the flow of specific ions (ion-specific channels). The voltage sensed on the outer and inner sides of the sarcolemma, where a difference in electrical potential exists, determines the opening and closing of these voltage-sensitive channels. An excess of negative ions immediately inside the sarcolemma and an equal excess of positive ions outside the sarcolemma (also referred to as the resting potential) combine to form an electrical potential gradient. Muscle cell contraction results from depolarization, which is brought on by positive ions entering the cell in response to a nerve impulse that opens ion channels.

The sole ions that enter the cardiac cell while it is at rest are positively charged potassium ions, which gradually permeate into the cell. The negative resting potential rhythmically moves towards the positive threshold potential in specific pacemaking cells situated in the sinoatrial node. Ion channels open and permit sodium and calcium to enter the cell when the threshold potential is surpassed, inducing the cell to depolarize. This sudden increase in cardiac membrane potential triggers a wave of depolarization that functions as the operational representation of the heart's excitation signal. It is transmitted from cell to cell. A slower dispersion of the signal occurs in the ventricular muscle cells after it rapidly travels down conduction tissue via specialized atrial cells, the atrioventricular node, and the bundles of His and Purkinje cells. One notable factor influencing heart rate is the rate of spontaneous depolarization.

Drugs that may alter the carriers or channels associated with these ions, as well as changes in the ion concentration of the extracellular and intracellular fluid, can impact both the excitation and propagation mechanisms. Following the initial depolarization event, heart muscle cells undergo a series of channel openings and closures, ultimately leading to the restoration of the transmembrane potential to its resting state. The cardiac action potential is the result of a meticulously orchestrated interplay between multiple voltage-sensitive channels and subsequent transmembrane voltage fluctuations.

In the cardiac muscle cell, the depolarization event also opens a calcium channel, allowing calcium to enter the myocardium. The process of "excitation-contraction coupling," which occurs when cardiac depolarization (excitation) and contraction are linked, is largely mediated by calcium. The concentration of free calcium ions in the heart muscle cell is typically very low. The sarcoplasmic reticulum, an internal membrane system that sequesters calcium ions, is responsible for maintaining this low concentration. When the cell is excited and depolarized, the calcium channel opens and permits a small amount of calcium to enter, which is associated with the change in the membrane potential. In response to this minute quantity of calcium, the calcium-sensitive channels of the sarcoplasmic reticulum release more calcium, increasing the cellular calcium concentration by nearly 100-fold. When the heart repolarizes, the sarcoplasmic reticulum reabsorbs the excess calcium, returning the cellular calcium concentration to its previous low level and allowing the heart muscle to relax. The reuptake of cellular calcium mediated by the sarcoplasmic reticulum is crucial because it inhibits the onset of tense muscles. When muscles are at rest, two proteins known as troponin and tropomyosin attach to actin molecules and prevent actin and myosin from interacting, thereby preventing muscle contraction. Actin is capable of binding with myosin when the concentration of calcium increases during depolarization, leading to a conformational change in troponin and tropomyosin. The myocardial cell relaxes as the sarcoplasmic reticulum once again absorbs calcium. Heart function is significantly influenced by factors that regulate the fluctuation of calcium concentrations in the cardiac muscle cell.

5.2.3.1. Electrocardiogram

An electrocardiogram is capable of analyzing and characterizing the electrical impulse generated by the heart during each depolarization event. This diagnostic tool has proven to be highly valuable in the clinical assessment of cardiac conditions. By applying leads or wires to the arms, legs, and chest, researchers in the early 20th century were able to measure the minute voltage variations that coincide rhythmically with cardiac stimulation. The investigation of potential variations among different lead sets is conducted throughout the cardiac cycle. Ultimately, the readout of the electrocardiogram provides an explanation of how the heart is electrically activated.

The P wave represents the recorded impulse when a wave of depolarization crosses the atria, while it is recognized as the QRS complex as it passes through the ventricles. The T wave is generated by currents produced during ventricular repolarization. Approximately 0.25 seconds after depolarization, the ventricular muscle undergoes the repolarization process. Consequently, the electrocardiogram displays both repolarization and depolarization waves. The larger QRS wave masks the atrial repolarization wave, which occurs simultaneously with ventricular depolarization. When evaluating cardiac electrical function and diagnosing heart disease, the relative timing, size, and direction of these waves are all crucial factors to consider.

5.2.3.2. Nervous Control of the Heart

Both the sympathetic and parasympathetic fibers in the vagus nerve, which are parasympathetic, maintain nervous control over the heart. The sympathetic nerves act as cardiac excitors, while the vagus nerve functions as a cardiac inhibitor. By slowing down the rate of impulse formation and atrial contractility, stimulation of the vagus nerve reduces cardiac output and slows the heart rate. In cases of heart diseases, parasympathetic stimulation can lead to varying degrees of impaired impulse formation or heart block. In a total heart block, the ventricles and atria beat separately. On the other hand, the sympathetic nervous system is stimulated to increase the contractility of the ventricles and atria.

The cardiac cycle, which consists of a diastolic phase of relaxation and a systolic period of contraction, is defined as the duration from the end of one heart contraction to the end of the subsequent contraction. Throughout the cycle, the arteries maintain pressure, although it fluctuates during the two periods. The normal diastolic pressure ranges between 60 and 80 millimeters of mercury, while the normal systolic pressure ranges between 90 and 120 millimeters of mercury.

5.3. Blood Vessels

The blood vessels form a complex network of closed tubes that transport blood from the heart to all parts of the body. The structure and function of these vessels are closely intertwined, as is the case with any biological system, making it impossible to discuss one without considering the other.

The heart's pumping action generates high pressure in the arteries, which is utilized to deliver blood to the body's tissues. The heart forcefully propels blood into these flexible tubes, causing them to recoil and continue pumping blood in pulsating waves. Therefore, in order to ensure rapid and efficient blood flow to the tissues, the vessels must possess strong and elastic walls.

An artery's wall consists of three layers. The innermost layer, known as the tunica intima, is composed of an elastic tissue surface that covers a smooth endothelium inner surface. The middle layer, or tunica media, is comprised of smooth muscle cells intermingled with elastic fibers, and it is thicker in arteries, particularly the larger ones. Elastic fibers and muscle cells surround the vessel. In larger vessels, elastic fibers make up the majority of the tunica media. As arteries decrease in size, smooth muscle fibers become more predominant while elastic fibers decrease. Among the three layers, the outermost layer, tunica adventitia, is the strongest. It consists of elastic and collagenous fibers. Collagen is a protein found in connective tissue. The tunica adventitia provides a protective barrier against excessive expansion of the vessel. Another characteristic of this layer is the presence of tiny blood vessels called the vasa vasorum, which supply the walls of larger arteries and veins. Meanwhile, as blood is transported, diffusion provides nourishment to the inner and middle layers. Arteries can expand and contract with each pulse, returning to their original size due to their thicker and more elastic walls.

A gradual thinning of the vessel wall and a reduction in lumen size, or passageway, are the hallmarks of the transition from artery to arteriole. The tunica media in arterioles is composed of a single layer of circular or spiral smooth muscle fibers and no longer contains elastic fibers. The tunica intima is still present in arterioles as a lining covered by a layer of thin longitudinal fibers. The components of connective tissue make up the tunica adventitia.

Blood is released into the capillaries via control valves found in the arterioles and small arteries. The robust muscle wall has the ability to completely obstruct the passageway or allow it to expand to multiple times its original dimensions, significantly altering the way blood flows to the capillaries. This mechanism directs blood flow to the tissues that require it the most. The three layers become less distinct as the arterioles become smaller; the smallest arterioles are essentially composed of a layer of smooth muscle encircling the endothelium, or lining. The innermost lining cells of arteries and veins continue as a single layer of endothelium in the microscopic capillary tubules.

Small venules are formed as the capillaries converge, and their function is to collect blood from the capillary beds (i.e., the capillary networks). The venules consist of an endothelial tube supported by a small amount of collagenous tissue and a few smooth muscle fibers in the larger venules. The wall structure of venules, although much thinner than that of arteries, becomes more apparent as they increase in size.

The tunica media, which contains less muscle and elastic tissue compared to the arterial wall, surrounds the endothelial lining of veins that transport blood from the peripheral tissues to the heart. The primary component of the outermost layer, known as the tunica adventitia, is connective tissue. In contrast to the arterial system, the blood pressure in these vessels is remarkably low, and the blood must exit at an even lower pressure. Consequently, a unique system is necessary to maintain blood flow as it returns to the heart. To achieve this, many veins possess a specialized valve system. These valves, which exist in pairs and consist of semilunar folds in the tunica intima, regulate blood flow towards the heart, particularly when it is flowing upward. As blood moves towards the heart, the valve flaps flatten against the vein wall. When the pressure from the blood and surrounding tissues fills the valve pocket, the flaps expand to obstruct the opening. The veins in the extremities have a higher number of these valves compared to other areas of the body (Figure 5.4).

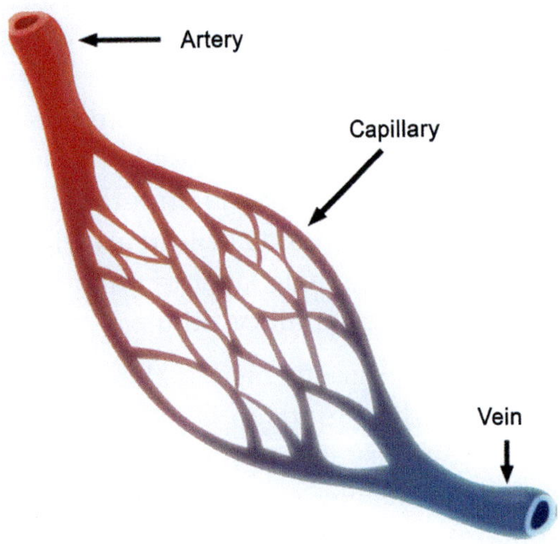

Figure 5.4. *Blood vessels.*

Source: https://upload.wikimedia.org/wikipedia/commons/f/f6/Capillary_system_CERT.jpg.

Veins are more malleable than arteries due to the composition of their walls, allowing them to expand and contract. This contractility plays a significant role in reducing the cardiovascular system's capacity by causing constriction in the peripheral vessels in response to insufficient blood pumping by the heart.

Despite being more abundant, veins often run parallel to arteries in the body. They have thinner walls and larger channels compared to arteries. Typically, veins contain around 40% of the blood volume, while the remaining 60% circulates through the systemic circulation. The pulmonary circuit consists of the right ventricle, the pulmonary artery and its branches, the arterioles, capillaries, and venules in the lungs, and the pulmonary veins that empty into the left atrium.

The upper surface of the right ventricle gives rise to the pulmonary trunk, which serves as the common stem of the pulmonary arteries. Beyond this point, the pulmonary arteries divide into the left and right pulmonary arteries, supplying the lungs approximately four to five centimeters further. The pulmonary valve protects the aperture between the pulmonary trunk and the right ventricle. It has two leaflets, or cusps. The walls of the trunk are roughly twice as thick as the vena cava and one-third that of the aorta, making it relatively thin for an artery. Despite their short length, the diameter of the left and right pulmonary arteries is comparatively large. This allows the vessels to stretch and accommodate the stroke volume of the right ventricle, which is an essential function equivalent to that of the left ventricle.

The pulmonary trunk crosses the aortic route and ascends diagonally to the left. It then splits into the right and left pulmonary arteries, which enter the lungs between the fifth and sixth thoracic vertebrae (roughly at the level of the bottom of the breastbone). After entering the lungs, the branches of the pulmonary arteries divide, with the capillaries being the last branch to form. These capillaries surround the alveoli, or air sacs, in the lungs. They facilitate the exchange of oxygen and carbon dioxide.

The capillaries carrying oxygenated blood merge with progressively larger vessels, eventually reaching the pulmonary veins. These veins transport oxygenated blood from the lungs to the left atrium of the heart.

5.3.1. Arteries

Blood vessels known as arteries are responsible for transporting blood from the heart. As blood leaves the lungs and travels to the body's tissues, it typically carries a high oxygen content. However, this rule does not apply to the pulmonary trunk and arteries of the pulmonary circulation loop. These particular arteries transport deoxygenated blood from the heart to the lungs, where it is then oxygenated.

Due to the forceful pumping action of the heart, arteries are subjected to elevated blood pressure. To withstand this pressure, the walls of arteries are thicker, more muscular, and more elastic compared to other blood vessels. The elastic nature of arterial tissue allows it to stretch and accommodate the pressure exerted by the heart.

Smaller arteries have a more muscular structure in their walls. These arteries contain smooth muscles that contract and expand, thereby regulating blood flow through their lumen. This mechanism enables the body to control the amount of blood that reaches different body parts in various situations. Additionally, the regulation of blood flow also influences blood pressure. As blood flows through smaller arteries, it increases the pressure exerted on the arterial walls (Figure 5.5).

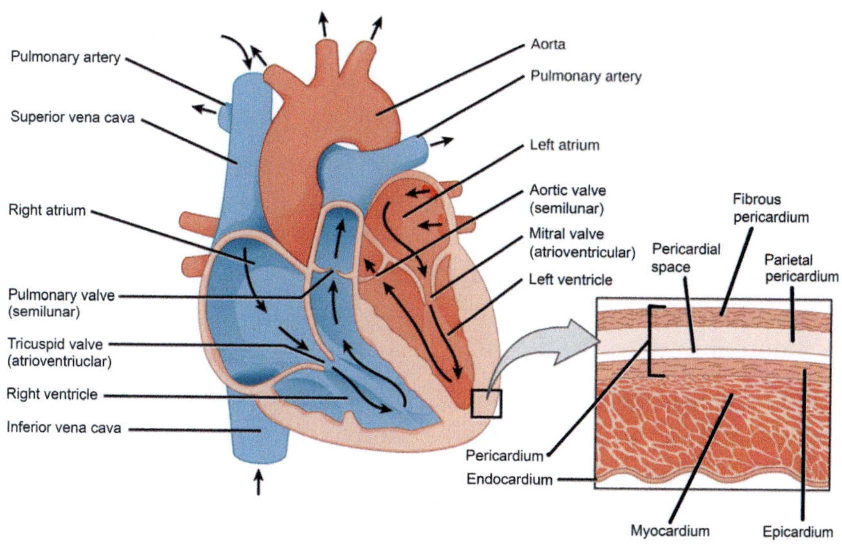

Figure 5.5. *Heart arteries.*

Source: https://courses.lumenlearning.com/suny-wmopen-biology2/chapter/the-mammalian-heart/.

5.3.1.1. Aorta

The left ventricle gives rise to the aorta, which is the largest vessel in the systemic circuit. The ascending aorta, the aortic arch, and the descending aorta—which can be further divided into the thoracic and abdominal aortas—are the three regions that comprise this structure.

The ascending segment of the aorta gives rise to the right and left coronary arteries, which supply oxygen-rich blood to the heart. Three significant arteries, namely the innominate, left common carotid, and left subclavian, emerge from the arch of the aorta, numbered in that order from the heart. The blood in these three branches provides oxygen to the head, neck, and arms. The innominate artery, also known as the brachiocephalic artery, bifurcates into the right subclavian and right common carotid arteries as it ascends towards the clavicle, or collarbone. At the top of the thyroid cartilage, the primary cartilage in the larynx, or voice box, the two common carotid arteries extend in parallel on either side of the neck. Here, they divide to become the internal and external carotid arteries. The internal carotid arteries supply the anterior part of the brain, the eye and its appendages, the forehead and nose, while numerous branches of the external carotid arteries supply the head and neck.

The basilar artery, which divides into the posterior cerebral arteries, is formed at the base of the brain by the fusion of the two vertebral arteries, one of which originates as a branch of the innominate artery and the other as a branch of the left subclavian artery. The circle of Willis is composed of the two internal carotid arteries, the two vertebral arteries, and the connecting arteries between them, and it is responsible for the majority of the blood supply to the brain.

The left subclavian artery and the continuation of the innominate artery on the right supply the arms. These blood vessels are referred to as the axillary artery at the border of the first rib. As the artery travels down the upper arm, it becomes the brachial artery. At the level of the elbow, the brachial artery divides into the radial and ulnar arteries. The radial artery descends on the distal (thumb) side of the forearm, while the ulnar artery passes along the medial side. The hand and wrist receive blood supply from connections (anastomoses) between these two arteries, with branches at the level of the palm.

The thoracic (chest) section of the descending aorta gives rise to parietal branches, which supply the walls surrounding the thoracic cavity, and visceral branches, which supply the organs. The visceral branches provide blood to the pericardium, lungs, bronchi, lymph nodes, and esophagus. The parietal vessels supply blood to the membrane lining the thoracic cavity, the spinal cord, the vertebral column, and part of the diaphragm. They also supply blood to the intercostal muscles (the muscles between the ribs) and the muscles of the thoracic wall.

The aorta produces both visceral and parietal branches as it passes through the diaphragm, referred to as the abdominal aorta. Examples of visceral vessels include the renal, testicular or ovarian, and celiac, superior and inferior mesenteric arteries. The celiac artery emerges from the aorta just below the diaphragm and quickly splits into the hepatic artery (supplying the liver), the splenic artery (supplying the stomach, pancreas, and spleen), and the left gastric artery (supplying part of the stomach and esophagus).

Below the celiac artery in the abdominal aorta, the superior mesenteric artery originates. Its branches supply the small intestine and a portion of the large intestine. The inferior mesenteric artery arises a few centimeters above the aortic end and divides to supply the lower portion of the colon. The renal arteries reach the kidneys, while the ovarian or testicular arteries supply the female ovaries and male testes, respectively.

The inferior phrenic artery, which supplies the lumbar and middle sacral arteries, as well as the suprarenal (adrenal) glands, is one of the parietal branches originating from the abdominal aorta. The muscles in the abdominal wall, the skin, the lumbar vertebrae, the spinal cord, and the meninges (which cover the spinal cord) are all provided with blood by the four pairs of lumbar arteries. The common iliac arteries, which descend laterally and give rise to external and internal branches, branch off from the abdominal aorta. After passing through the inguinal region, the right and left external iliac arteries, which are a direct continuation of the common iliacs, are referred to as the femoral arteries. These arteries supply the lower extremities and abdomen with various branches.

The femoral artery continues as the popliteal artery just above the knee, from which the anterior and posterior tibial arteries emerge. The popliteal artery is directly continued by the posterior tibial artery, which travels down the lower leg to supply structures in the posterior leg and foot.

The peroneal artery arises from the posterior tibial artery just below the knee. It branches off to supply the muscles in the lower leg and the fibula, which is the smaller of the two lower leg bones. The branches of the peroneal artery terminate in the foot. The dorsalis pedis artery, responsible for supplying the foot, is formed when the anterior tibial artery descends the lower leg to the ankle.

5.3.1.2. Pulse

An artery that is close to the skin's surface can be palpated to feel the pulse. The heartbeat causes the arterial wall to alternately expand and contract, resulting in the pulse. When the heart pumps blood into the aorta and it strikes the elastic walls, a pressure wave is generated along the arteries. This wave is the pulse. While every artery pulsates, it is easiest to detect at locations where the vessel is closest to the body's surface.

The pulse can be easily detected at the following locations: (i) the wrist, where the radial artery is close to the surface; (ii) the side of the jaw, where the external maxillary (facial) artery crosses; (iii) the temple above and to the outer side of the eye, near the temporal artery; (iv) the side of the neck, from the carotid artery; (v) the inner side of the biceps, from the brachial artery; (vi) the groin, from the femoral artery; (vii) behind the knee, from the popliteal artery; (viii) the upper side of the foot, from the dorsalis pedis artery.

The most commonly used method for checking the pulse is through the radial artery. A few fingers are placed on the artery near the wrist. It is preferred to use multiple fingertip placements to have a larger, more sensitive surface area to feel the pulse wave. While examining the pulse, certain information is noted, such as the quantity and regularity of beats per minute, the force and intensity of the beat, and the tension provided by the finger's artery. The time interval between beats is typically consistent in length.

5.3.2. Veins

Venules gather blood from sinusoids, or blood channels, and capillaries. They then join to form veins that progressively increase in size until they reach the great veins, also known as venae cavae. In the extremities, there are both deep and superficial veins. The deep veins are named after the principal arteries of the extremities, while the superficial veins are located just beneath the skin and drain the skin and superficial fasciae (sheets of fibrous tissue). Connections between the deep and superficial veins are often present.

There are three routes through which venous blood enters the right atrium: the coronary sinus, which originates from the heart muscle; the superior vena cava, which originates from the upper body; and the inferior vena cava, which originates from the lower body (Figure 5.6).

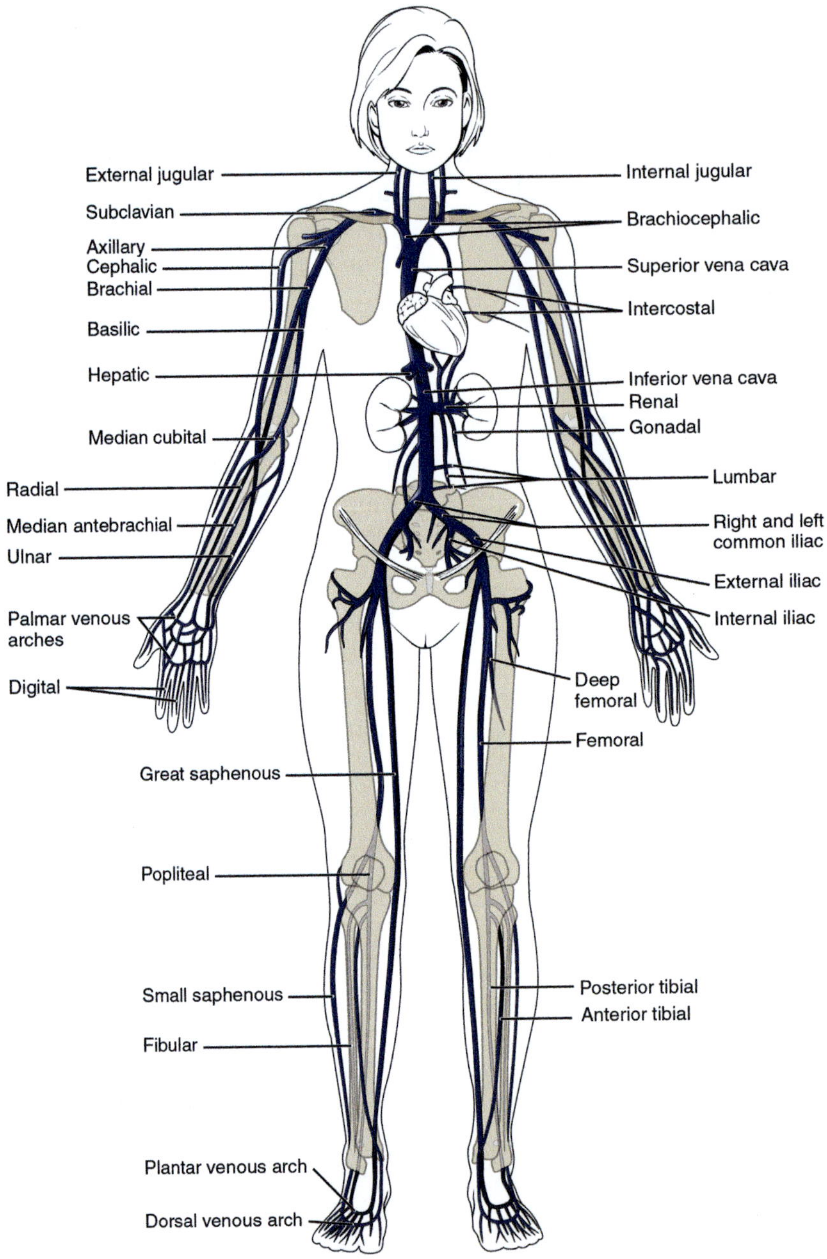

Figure 5.6. *Veins.*

Source: https://courses.lumenlearning.com/suny-ap2/chapter/circulatory-pathways/.

5.3.2.1. Superior Vena Cava and Its Branches

The superior vena cava is constituted by the fusion of branches from the cranium and cervix, the upper limbs, and a segment of the thorax. The dura mater, the external covering of the brain, is partitioned into two layers by venous channels recognized as venous sinuses. These channels lack valves. These sinuses and connecting veins influence the cerebral venous drainage. This system continues downwards through the neck and receives blood from various regions of the visage, neck, and brain into the internal jugular vein. Each unites with the corresponding side's subclavian vein at the level of the clavicle to form the innominate veins.

The junction of its branches, close to the mandibular angle, forms the external jugular vein. It empties into the innominate vein on the same side as the subclavian, draining portions of the head and neck structures in the process. The subclavian vein on that side receives blood from all of the veins in the arm. They have valves and can be found in both shallow and deep waters. The majority of the deep veins are paired and have cross connections amongst them.

The superficial venous drainage of the hand is achieved by tiny anastomosing (interconnecting) veins that combine to form the basilic vein, which runs up the ulnar side of the forearm and receives blood from the hand, forearm, and arm, and the cephalic vein, which runs up the radial (thumb) side of the forearm. The radial veins, which are deep anastomosing veins of the hand and wrist, and the ulnar veins, which run parallel to the corresponding artery, are two examples of the forearm's deep veins. The brachial vein, which is formed at the elbow by the radial and ulnar veins joining, merges with the basilic vein at the level of the shoulder to form the axillary vein. The axillary vein changes into the subclavian vein at the outer edge of the first rib, marking the end of the upper extremity's venous system.

The innominate vein is formed when the subclavian, external, and internal jugular veins converge. The superior vena cava, which opens into the upper posterior region of the right atrium, is where the right and left innominate veins come to an end.

Apart from the innominate veins, the azygous vein and tiny veins from the pericardium and mediastinum (the space between the two lungs) also supply blood to the superior vena cava. The majority of blood from the back, chest, and abdominal walls flows into veins that are next to the vertebral bodies, which are the parts of the vertebrae that support weight. Together, these veins make up the so-called azygous system, which connects the inferior and superior vena cava. This system's azygous, hemiazygous, and accessory hemiazygous veins are its terminal veins. The right ascending lumbar vein continues upward as the azygous vein at the level of the diaphragm. The right intercostal veins, which drain the muscles of the intercostal spaces, are the principal branches of this vein. Along with the pericardium, right lung, lymph nodes, and esophagus as branches, it enters the superior vena cava approximately at the level of the fourth thoracic vertebra.

The left side of the azygous system differs widely between people. The hemiazygous vein typically begins as a continuation of the left ascending lumbar vein just below the diaphragm and ends in the azygous vein. The esophagus, the intercostal muscles, and a section of the mediastinum are drained by the hemiazygous branches. With branches from the left intercostal spaces and the left bronchus, the accessory hemiazygous typically extends downward as a continuation of the fourth intercostal space's vein. It empties just above the hemiazygous entrance into the azygous vein.

5.3.2.2. Inferior Vena Cava and Its Branches

Blood is received by the inferior vena cava, a large venous trunk with no valves, from the back, the legs, the walls, and the contents of the abdomen and pelvis. The dorsal venous arch, which passes over the top of the foot not far from the base of the toes, is primarily responsible for draining the foot. Veins draining the sole are connected to the arch. The large and small saphenous veins, which are extensions of the dorsal venous arch, superficially drain the lower leg. The popliteal vein is typically where the small saphenous vein ends after extending up the back of the lower leg. There is some correspondence between the great saphenous vein and deep veins. The longest vein in the body, the latter one, originates from the dorsal venous arch and travels up the inside of the lower leg and thigh. It ends in the femoral vein after taking venous branches from the knee and thigh region.

The deep veins carry the majority of the blood returning from the lower extremities. These comprise the veins that accompany the anterior and posterior tibial and peroneal arteries, as well as the femoral and popliteal veins. The popliteal vein, which is formed at the knee by the union of the anterior and posterior tibial veins at the level of the foot, eventually becomes the femoral vein as it extends through the thigh.

The femoral vein becomes known as the external iliac vein at the level of the inguinal ligament, which is at the anterior, diagonal border between the trunk and the thigh. This vein then joins the internal iliac vein to form the common iliac vein. The pelvic walls, viscera, external genitalia, buttocks, and a portion of the thigh are all drained by the internal iliac vein. Most of the pelvis and legs are drained by the paired common iliac veins. The inferior vena cava is formed by the union of the two common iliacs at a level above the coccyx, the lowest bone in the spine. The inferior vena cava draws blood from the lumbar, renal, suprarenal, hepatic, and common iliac veins as it travels upward through the abdomen and empties into the right atrium. The ascending lumbar vein, a vertical connecting vein, unites the pairs of lumbar veins on either side, draining blood from the abdominal walls and loins; the left ascending lumbar vein becomes the hemiazygous, and the right ascending lumbar vein becomes the azygous. Normally, these veins enter the inferior vena cava independently.

The renal veins are located in front of the corresponding renal artery; the left renal vein receives blood from various organs, while the right renal vein receives branches only from the kidney. Both the right phrenic and right suprarenal veins end directly in the inferior vena cava, above the gonadal vein. A diaphragm allows the inferior vena cava, which is emptied into the inferior vena cava by two or three short hepatic trunks.

5.3.2.3. Portal System

One way to conceptualize the portal system is as a distinct region within the systemic circulatory system. The portal system, despite originating from capillaries, is unique because it terminates in the liver's capillary-like vascular bed. Prior to reaching the heart, blood from the pancreas, intestine, spleen, and stomach passes through the liver. The liver receives 20% of its blood supply from the hepatic artery and 80% from the portal vein. Blood exiting the liver flows through the hepatic vein and empties into the inferior vena cava. The hepatic artery supplies the liver with the necessary oxygen. The portal vein carries blood from the abdominal viscera, particularly the intestinal tract, to the liver. Within the liver, substances present in the portal blood are broken down (refer to the human digestive system).

5.3.2.4. Venous Pulmonary System

The oxygenated blood in veins is collected from the pulmonary capillaries, where blood absorbs oxygen and exhales carbon dioxide. It then moves through venules, gradually larger veins, and four pulmonary veins, two from each lung's hilum. On each lung, the bronchus, blood vessels, and nerves enter through the hilum. After that, these veins flow into the left atrium, where the heart receives their contents.

5.3.3. Capillaries

The extensive network of approximately 10,000,000,000 microscopic capillaries serves as a mechanism for facilitating the exchange of waste products, nutrients, and fluids between the tissues and the bloodstream. Despite their minute size—the largest capillary having a diameter of about 0.2 mm, roughly equivalent to the width of a pin—the vast capillary network functions as a reservoir that typically holds one-sixth of the circulating blood volume. Capillaries in active tissues such as muscle, liver, kidney, and lungs are more abundant compared to those in tendons or ligaments. Furthermore, capillaries are absent in the epidermis, hyaline cartilage (a translucent cartilage found in joints), and the cornea.

In addition to their diminutive size, the network of capillaries into which the arterioles empty is remarkably thin, with walls that consist of only a single cell layer. These vessels essentially serve as tubular extensions of the inner lining cells of larger vessels. Typically, they exhibit a circular shape and vary in size from three to four endothelial cells, except for the venous terminations where they slightly widen to a circumference of four to six cells. These cells are enveloped by a thin membrane called the basement membrane, which provides structural integrity to the vessel (Figure 5.7).

An average capillary unit is composed of a network of vessels that branch off and connect (anastomose), with each vessel ranging in length from 0.5 to 1 millimeter. Due to the thinness of the capillary wall, it acts as a semipermeable membrane that allows the passage of substances with small molecules, such as water, fatty acids, glucose, carbon dioxide, oxygen, and ketones. At the arteriolar end of the capillary unit, oxygen and nutrients enter the tissues through the wall, while waste materials and carbon dioxide enter the vessel at the venous end of the capillary bed through the membrane. The primary mechanism that regulates blood flow into the capillaries is the dilation and constriction of the arterioles. However, the capillary unit's muscular gatekeepers, known as sphincters, function to direct the flow to the areas that require it the most.

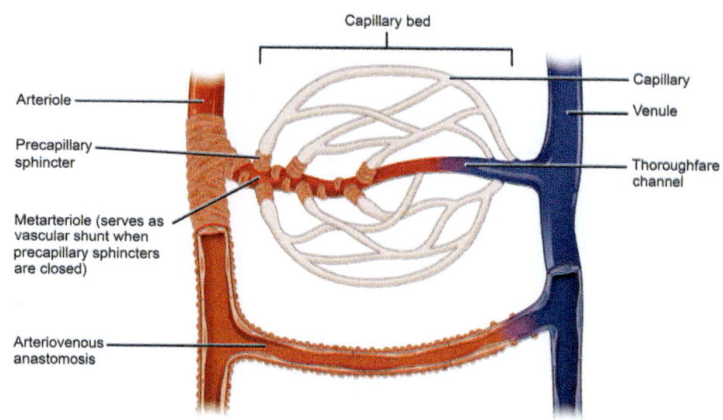

Figure 5.7. *Capillaries.*

Source: https://courses.lumenlearning.com/suny-ap2/chapter/structure-and-function-of-blood-vessels/.

The capillary wall's cellular membrane is crossed in three different ways. Substances soluble in the capillary cells' lipid (fatty) membrane can pass directly through them via a process called diffusion. Through a process called ultrafiltration, certain substances that are required by the tissues and soluble in water but completely insoluble in the lipid membrane are able to pass through small water-filled passageways, or pores, in the membranes. These pores make up only 1/1,000th of the capillaries' surface area. Specific endothelium receptors are responsible for the transportation of other substances, such as cholesterol.

5.4. Blood Flow

The passage of blood through a tissue, organ, or vessel is referred to as blood flow, and it is typically measured in terms of blood volume per unit of time. The heart's ventricles contract first, initiating the process. Blood is forced into the major arteries by ventricular contraction, causing blood to flow from high-pressure areas to low-pressure areas as it passes through capillaries, venules, and veins in the venous system, as well as smaller arteries and arterioles (Figure 5.8).

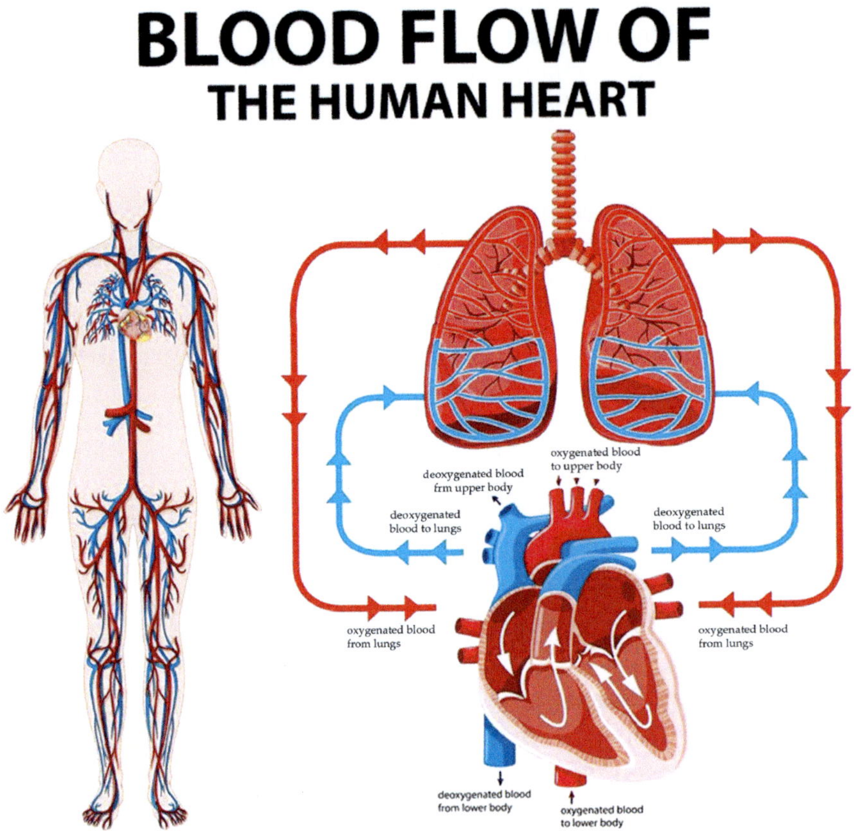

Figure 5.8. *Blood flow of the human heart.*

Source: https://img.freepik.com/free-vector/diagram-showing-blood-flow-human_1308-100957.jpg?size=626&ext=jpg&ga=GA1.1.290185697.1710060024&semt=ais.

5.4.1. Cardiac Cycle

The heart undergoes a sequence of pressure changes known as the cardiac cycle. Blood flows through the various heart chambers and throughout the body as a result of these pressure variations (Figure 5.9).

Systole, or the contraction phase, and diastole, or the relaxation phase, are the two main phases of the cardiac cycle.

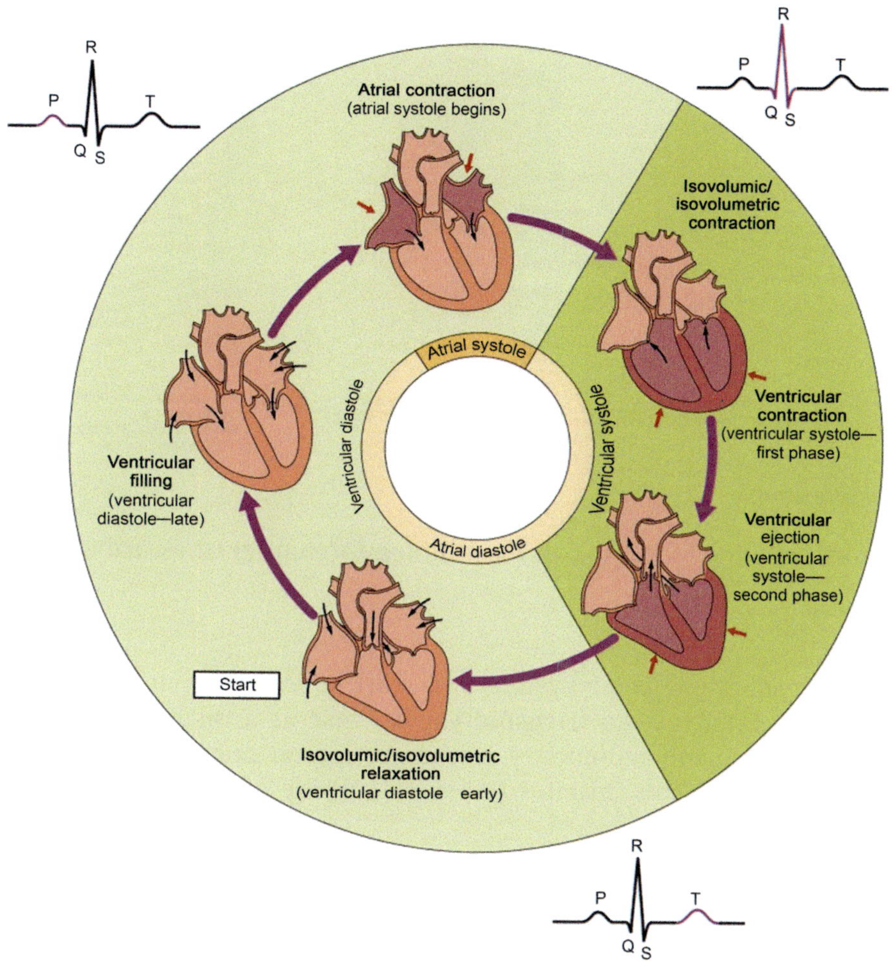

Figure 5.9. *The cardiac cycle.*

Source: https://courses.lumenlearning.com/suny-ap2/chapter/cardiac-cycle/.

5.4.1.1. Diastole

During diastole, all of the heart's muscles relax. This allows blood to enter the heart and fill the ventricles and atria. The mitral and tricuspid valves open in response to a decrease in ventricle pressure, allowing blood from the atria to enter the left and right ventricles, respectively (Figure 5.10).

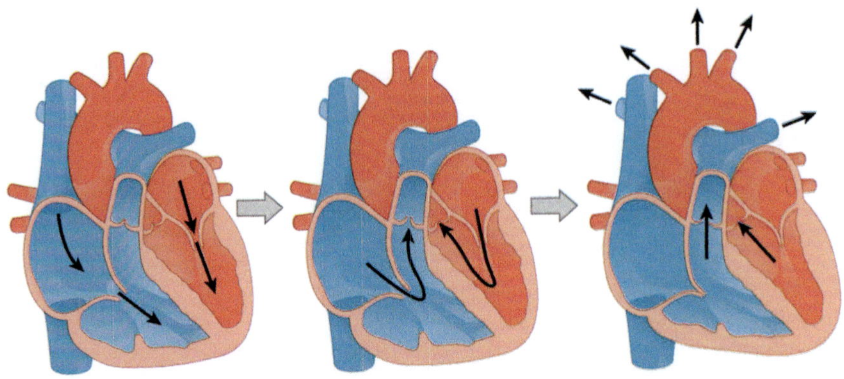

Figure 5.10. *Diastole phase.*

Source: https://courses.lumenlearning.com/wm-biology2/chapter/the-cardiac-cycle/.

5.4.1.2. Systole

When the ventricles reach ventricular systole and start contracting on their own, another wave of contraction begins. The mitral and tricuspid valves close as a result of the increased pressure in the ventricles. The aortic and pulmonary valves are forced open by this pressure. The image below illustrates this process. This initiates the systole phase of the cycle (Figure 5.11).

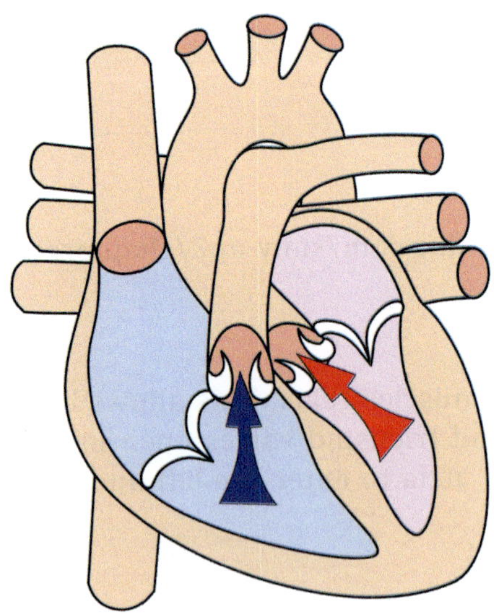

Figure 5.11. *Systole.*

Source: By Wapcaplet, Reytan, Mtcv – Image:Diagram of the human heart (cropped).svg, CC BY-SA 3.0, https://commons.wikimedia.org/w/index.php?curid=4158464.

5.5. Blood Pressure

The force or pressure of blood within your arteries is measured by your blood pressure. Your heart pumps blood into the arteries that distribute blood throughout your body with each beat. This occurs 60–100 times every minute, every day of the year. Your body needs oxygen and nutrients from arteries in order to function. Blood pressure can be influenced by a wide range of factors, including hormones, stress, exercise, diet, sitting, and standing. One-way valves, smooth muscle, blood vessel size, and blood pressure all work together to control how much blood moves through the body.

The amount of pressure that blood applies to vessels during a heartbeat is measured by the systolic blood pressure. Systolic blood pressure of 120 mmHg is ideal. The pressure inside the vessels in between heartbeats is measured by diastolic blood pressure. About 80 mmHg is the ideal diastolic blood pressure (Figure 5.12).

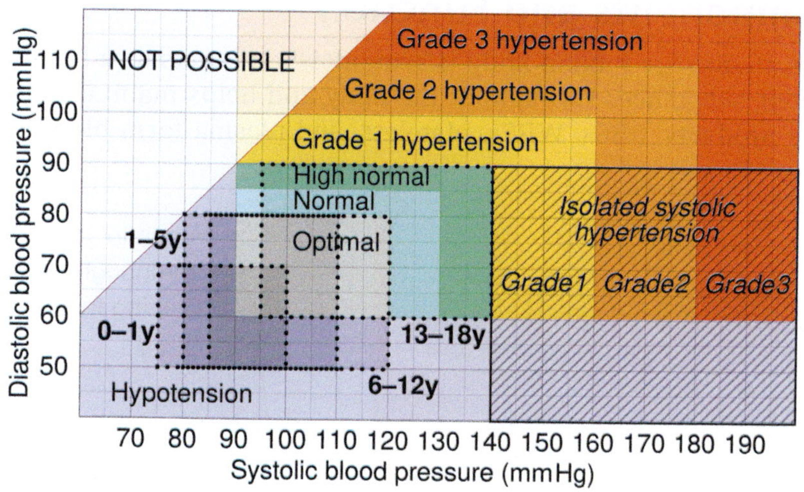

Figure 5.12. *Blood pressure.*

Source: By Cmglee – Own work, CC BY-SA 4.0, https://commons.wikimedia.org/w/index.php?curid=130430576.

5.5.1. Blood Pressure Measured

Blood pressure is measured in millimeters of mercury (mmHg):

Systolic pressure – the pressure when the heart pushes blood out.

Diastolic pressure – the pressure when the heart rests between beats.

For example, if your blood pressure is "140 over 90," or 140/90 mmHg, it means that your diastolic pressure is 90 mmHg and your systolic pressure is 140 mmHg.

As a general guide:

- Ideal blood pressure is considered to be between 90/60 mmHg and 120/80 mmHg.
- High blood pressure is considered to be 140/90 mmHg or higher.

- Low blood pressure is considered to be below 90/60 mmHg.

5.5.1.1. High Blood Pressure

Several unhealthy lifestyle choices, such as smoking, excessive drinking, being overweight, and lack of exercise, are associated with high blood pressure. If left untreated, high blood pressure can increase the risk of coronary heart disease and other long-term health issues. Additionally, it can potentially damage the blood vessels in the kidneys or eyes.

5.5.1.2. Low Blood Pressure

Low blood pressure is less common. It can be a side effect of certain medications or caused by dehydration and heart failure, among other underlying conditions.

5.6. Blood Components and Function

The blood volume in an average human body is around 4-5 L. It acts as a liquid connective tissue that transports various substances throughout the body and helps maintain the balance of gases, nutrients, and waste products. RBCs, WBCs, platelets, and plasma form blood (Figure 5.13).

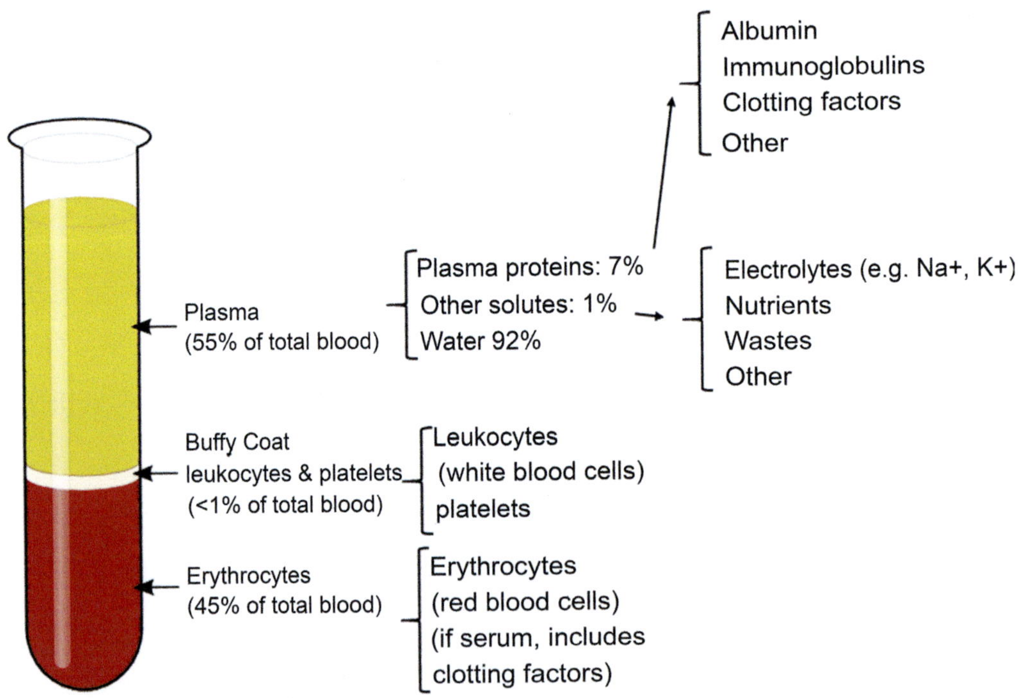

Figure 5.13. *Components of blood.*

Source: https://commons.wikimedia.org/wiki/File:Components_of_blood.png.

5.6.1. Components of Blood

There are four components of blood are:

- Plasma;
- Red blood cells;
- White blood cells;
- Platelets.

5.6.1.1. Red Blood Cells

Erythrocytes, also known as red blood cells, constitute approximately 45% of the blood volume and are the most abundant type of blood cell. Stem cells in the red bone marrow produce erythrocytes at an astonishing rate of around 2 million cells per second. Erythrocytes have a biconcave shape, meaning they are disc-shaped with a concave curve on both sides, with the thinnest part in the center. This unique shape allows erythrocytes to have a high surface area to volume ratio and enables them to fold and fit into narrow capillaries. The nucleus of immature erythrocytes contributes to their distinctive shape and flexibility, but it is expelled upon maturation. Due to the absence of a nucleus, red blood cells lack DNA and cannot repair themselves when damaged.

Erythrocytes carry oxygen throughout the blood via the red pigment hemoglobin. The iron and proteins present in hemoglobin enhance the oxygen-carrying capacity of erythrocytes. The high surface area to volume ratio of erythrocytes facilitates the efficient transport of oxygen from the lungs to the cells in systemic tissues and vice versa through capillaries.

5.6.1.2. White Blood Cells

Leukocytes, also known as white blood cells, comprise a relatively small portion of all blood cells but play vital roles in the body's immune system. There are two main categories of white blood cells: granular leukocytes and agranular leukocytes:

1. **Granular Leukocytes:** The three types of granular leukocytes are neutrophils, eosinophils, and basophils. Each type is distinguished by the presence of chemical-filled vesicles in their cytoplasm, which contribute to their specific functions. Neutrophils contain digestive enzymes that neutralize invading bacteria. Eosinophils possess specialized digestive enzymes for breaking down viruses that have been bound by antibodies in the blood. Basophils release histamine to enhance allergic reactions and aid in protecting the body against parasites.
2. **Agranular Leukocytes:** The two major classes of agranular leukocytes are lymphocytes and monocytes. Lymphocytes consist of T cells and natural killer cells, which combat viral infections, and B cells, which produce antibodies against pathogens. Monocytes develop into macrophages, which engulf and ingest pathogens as well as dead cells resulting from wounds or infections.

5.6.1.3. Platelets

Platelets, which are tiny cell fragments also referred to as thrombocytes, are responsible for blood clotting and scab formation. Platelets originate in the red bone marrow from large megakaryocyte cells that periodically burst and release thousands of membrane fragments, which eventually become platelets. Due to the absence of a nucleus, platelets can only survive in the body for a week or less before being taken up and broken down by macrophages.

5.6.1.4. Plasma

About 55% of the volume of blood is composed of plasma, which is the non-cellular or liquid component of the blood. Plasma is a mixture of dissolved materials, proteins, and water.

Water constitutes approximately 90% of plasma, although the exact percentage may vary depending on the individual's level of hydration. Plasma contains various proteins, including albumins and antibodies. Antibodies, a component of the immune system, attach themselves to antigens on the surface of pathogens that invade the body. Albumins help maintain the osmotic balance of the organism by providing body cells with an isotonic solution. Additionally, plasma contains a diverse range of substances dissolved in it, such as glucose, oxygen, carbon dioxide, electrolytes, nutrients, and waste products from cells. These substances circulate throughout the body using plasma as a means of transportation.

5.6.2. Functions of Blood Cells

Blood has many different functions, including:

- Transporting oxygen and nutrients to the lungs and tissues.
- Forming blood clots to prevent excess blood loss.
- Carrying cells and antibodies that fight infection.
- Bringing waste products to the kidneys and liver, which filter and clean the blood.
- Regulating body temperature.

5.7. Cardiovascular Disease

The World Health Organization reports that the leading cause of death worldwide is cardiovascular disease. Cardiovascular disease encompasses heart and blood vessel problems, including coronary artery disease, stroke, hypertension, and heart failure.

1. **Aging/Hypertension:** Aging and hypertension are closely linked. Persistently elevated blood pressure in the arteries, also known as high blood pressure, is associated with the development of disorders such as atherosclerosis, heart attack, stroke, and kidney damage.
   - As individuals age, there is a decrease in arterial compliance due to a loss of elasticity, particularly in the aorta.
   - This is accompanied by an increase in fibrotic changes, characterized by an increase in collagen fibers and their cross-linking.
   - Consequently, higher blood pressure becomes more prevalent in older age.
   - The pathophysiology of hypertension involves factors such as diabetes, hypercholesterolemia, and cigarette smoking, all of which contribute to arteriosclerotic changes.
2. **Coronary Artery Disease:** Also known as heart disease, occurs when the coronary arteries, which supply blood directly to the heart muscle, become narrowed or blocked. Complete blockage of blood flow in these arteries can lead to a heart attack.
3. **Stroke:** It is the death of brain cells (neurons) due to the lack of blood supply.
4. **Heart Failure:** It occurs when the heart is unable to adequately supply enough blood to the body tissues. This condition can be caused by various factors, including hypertension, heart disease, and cardiomyopathy (a chronic disease affecting the heart muscle).
5. **Vessel Aneurysm:**
   - With the loss or defect of elastic components in a vessel, the outward transmural

pressure (distension) can become unbalanced, resulting in an inadequate tension force that allows for the formation of an aneurysm, which is susceptible to rupture.

- The rupture of an aneurysm in the brain leads to a life-threatening subarachnoid hemorrhage.
- Atherosclerosis:
- Atherosclerosis is a form of arteriosclerosis characterized by the deposition of atheromatous plaques containing cholesterol and lipids on the innermost layer of the walls of large and medium-sized arteries.

6. **Dissection:** It is the abnormal and usually abrupt formation of a tear along the inside wall of an artery. As the tear becomes larger, it forms a small pouch called a "false lumen." The accumulation of blood inside this false lumen can generate blood clots or otherwise block blood flow, leading to a stroke.

A Closer Look

Hypertension

Hypertension, also known as high blood pressure, refers to a resting systemic pressure consistently above the normal range of 90 to 120/60 to 80 mmHg. Clinicians now classify 125 to 139/85 to 89 mmHg as prehypertension. A systolic reading of 140 to 159 mmHg or a diastolic reading of 90 to 99 mmHg may be categorized as stage 1 hypertension, while a systolic reading above 160 mmHg or a diastolic reading above 100 mmHg may be classified as stage 2 hypertension.

The term "essential hypertension" indicates that no specific cause can be determined, with most cases falling into this category. However, for some individuals, an overproduction of renin by the kidneys is the underlying cause of their hypertension. Excess renin leads to increased production of angiotensin II, which in turn raises blood pressure. Although hypertension often presents no symptoms, its long-term consequences can be severe. Chronic hypertension primarily affects the arteries and the heart.

Despite the strength of arterial walls, hypertension weakens them and contributes to arteriosclerosis. Weakened arteries are prone to rupture or the development of aneurysms, which can lead to a cerebrovascular accident (CVA) or kidney damage.

Hypertension impacts the heart by requiring the left ventricle to pump blood against the higher arterial pressure. As a result, the left ventricle works harder and undergoes enlargement, known as left ventricular hypertrophy. However, this abnormal growth of the myocardium does not correspondingly increase the number of coronary capillaries, potentially compromising the blood supply to the left ventricle in certain situations. For instance, during exercise, the heart faces additional demands, and the individual may experience angina due to oxygen deficiency or even a myocardial infarction in cases of severe oxygen deprivation.

Although several different kinds of medications (diuretics, vasodilators) are used to treat hypertension, individuals with moderate hypertension may reduce their reliance on medications by adhering to specific guidelines:

1. Refrain from smoking, as nicotine stimulates vasoconstriction, leading to elevated blood pressure. Smoking also damages arteries, contributing to arteriosclerosis.
2. If overweight, strive to lose weight. Even a modest weight loss of 10 pounds can lower blood pressure. Additionally, a diet rich in fruits and vegetables may help lower blood pressure for certain individuals.
3. Reduce salt intake by half. While salt consumption may not be the direct cause of hypertension, decreasing salt intake can assist in lowering blood pressure by reducing blood volume.
4. Engage in regular exercise. Moderate aerobic exercise, such as a daily half-hour walk, benefits the entire cardiovascular system and may also aid in weight loss.

Summary

- The circulatory system in humans is an organ system that transports blood via vessels to and from every area of the body, supplying tissues with nutrients and oxygen while expelling waste products like carbon dioxide.
- The cardiovascular system transports blood to almost all of the body's tissues. The blood delivers essential nutrients and oxygen and removes wastes and carbon dioxide to be processed or removed from the body.
- The fibrous pericardium is lined with a smooth, serous (moisture-exuding) membrane that bends back to cover the heart.
- The right atrium, also referred to as the right superior portion of the heart, is a narrow chamber that propels blood from all body parts other than the lungs.
- The pharyngeal, or throat, region of the embryo is where the heart initiates its formation. The undifferentiated mesoderm, situated in the middle of the embryo's three primary layers, is where the embryonic heart initially becomes visible as a thickening of invasive cells.
- The ventricular surface of each leaflet's middle supporting layer is connected to tendinous cords of dense tissue (chordae tendineae) that are covered in a thin layer of endocardium and originate from the papillary muscles that resemble nipples.
- Sarcoplasmic reticulum-mediated cellular calcium reabsorption is crucial because it inhibits the onset of tense muscles.
- The cardiac cycle, which consists of a diastolic phase of relaxation and a systolic period of contraction, is defined as the duration from the end of one heart contraction to the end of the subsequent contraction.

References

1. Elkin, H. K., & Winter, A., (2018). Grounding patients with hypertension improves blood pressure: A case history series study. *Altern. Ther. Health Med., 24*(6), 46–50.
2. Expert Panel on Detection, Evaluation, and Treatment of High Blood Cholesterol in Adults. (2001). Executive summary of the third report of the National Cholesterol Education Program (NCEP) expert panel on detection, evaluation, and treatment of high blood cholesterol in adults (Adult Treatment Panel III). *JAMA.*
3. Grundy, S. M., Bazzarre, T., Cleeman, J., et al., (2000). Writing Group I. Prevention Conference V. Beyond secondary prevention: Identifying the high-risk patient for primary prevention. Medical Office Assessment. *Circulation.*
4. Gruzdeva, O. V., Borodkina, D. A., Belik, E. V., Akbasheva, O. E., Palicheva, E. I., & Barbarash, O. L., (2019). Ghrelin physiology and pathophysiology: Focus on the cardiovascular system. *Kardiologiia., 59*(3), 60–67.
5. Hayden, M., Pignone, M., Phillips, C., et al., (2002). Aspirin for the primary prevention of cardiovascular events: A summary of the evidence for the U.S. Preventive Services Task Force. *Ann Intern Med.*

6. Huang, Y., Hu, D., Huang, C., & Nichols, C. G., (2019). Genetic discovery of ATP-sensitive K^+ channels in cardiovascular diseases. *Circ. Arrhythm. Electrophysiol., 12*(5), e007322.
7. National Heart Lung and Blood Institute Fact Book, Fiscal Year 2006, (2006). Bethesda, Md: National Heart Lung and Blood Institute, National Institutes of Health.
8. Park, S., Nguyen, N. B., Pezhouman, A., & Ardehali, R., (2019). Cardiac fibrosis: Potential therapeutic targets. *Transl. Res., 209*, 121–137.
9. Polak-Iwaniuk, A., Harasim-Symbor, E., Gołaszewska, K., & Chabowski, A., (2019). How hypertension affects heart metabolism. *Front Physiol., 10*, 435.
10. Rosamond, W., Flegal, K., Furie, K., et al., (2008). Heart disease and stroke statistics—2008 update: A report from the American Heart Association Statistics Committee and Stroke Statistics Subcommittee. *Circulation*.
11. Rossignol, P., Hernandez, A. F., Solomon, S. D., & Zannad, F., (2019). Heart failure drug treatment. *Lancet, 393*(10175), 1034–1044.
12. Seo, D. Y., Kwak, H. B., Kim, A. H., Park, S. H., Heo, J. W., Kim, H. K., Ko, J. R., et al., (2020). Cardiac adaptation to exercise training in health and disease. *Pflugers Arch., 472*(2), 155–168.
13. Tsibulnikov, S. Y., Maslov, L. N., Gorbunov, A. S., Voronkov, N. S., Boshchenko, A. A., Popov, S. V., Prokudina, E. S., et al., (2019). A review of humoral factors in remote preconditioning of the heart. *J. Cardiovasc. Pharmacol. Ther., 24*(5), 403–421.

Chapter

HUMAN SKELETAL SYSTEM

6

Contents

Unit Introduction

The skeletal system is a part of the body made up of bones, ligaments, cartilage, and other tissues that serve the body's vital purposes. Osseous tissue, also known as bone tissue, is a tough, dense connective tissue that makes up the majority of the adult skeleton, which is the body's internal support structure. The human skeleton serves six main purposes: endocrine regulation, blood cell production, mobility, protection, and mineral storage.

For a moment, let us consider a world in which skeletons were nonexistent. The first thing that probably comes to mind is that, similar to a jellyfish out of water, each of us would be a little heap on the ground. This illustration accurately demonstrates the primary purpose of the skeleton, which is to support the body. Despite serving as the body's framework, the skeleton differs greatly from the wooden beams supporting a house. As living organs, bones actively participate in preserving the body's internal environment.

The skeletal system is composed of bones, along with additional structures that provide support to the joints of the skeleton. There are three distinct types of tissue: cartilage, bone tissue, and fibrous connective tissue, which forms the ligaments that connect one bone to another.

Orientation and Directional Terms:

Term	Definition	Illustration
Diaphysis	The diaphysis is the main or midsection of a long bone. It is a tube-like shaft composed of compact bone that encloses a central marrow cavity.	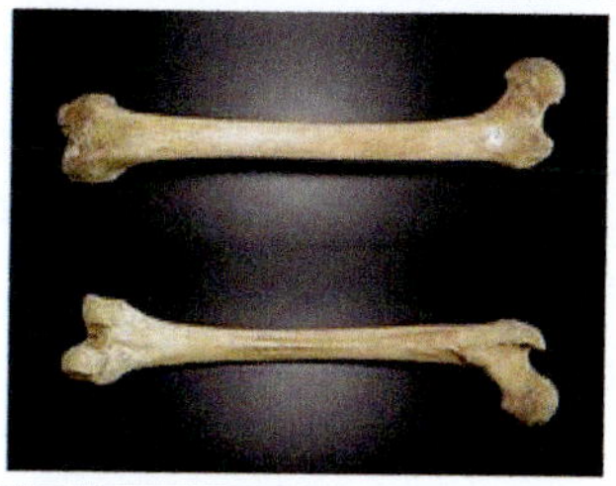
Epiphyzeal disc	An epiphyzeal disc, also known as a growth plate or physa, is a disc of cartilage that is found between the middle and end of long bones. Most long bones have one growth plate at each end.	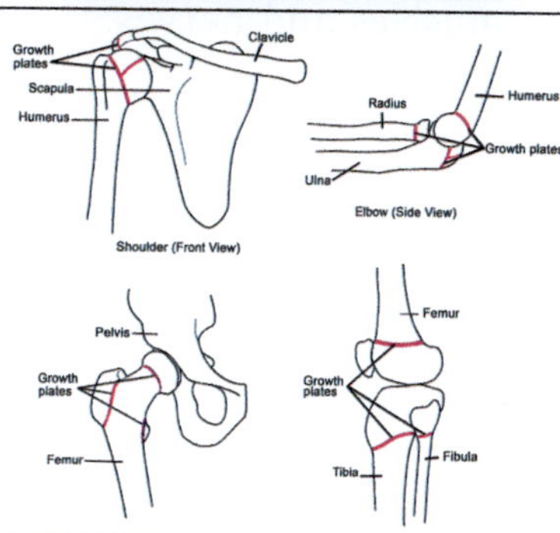
Fontanel	Fontanel is a membrane-covered gap in the skull where sutures intersect but don't touch completely.	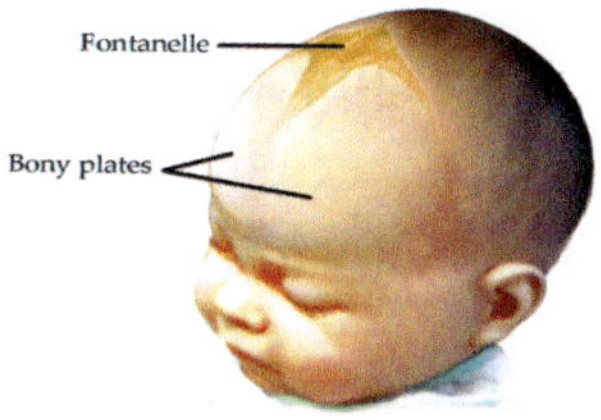
Haversian system	The Haversian system is a system of longitudinal canals in compact bone that are connected by transverse canals.	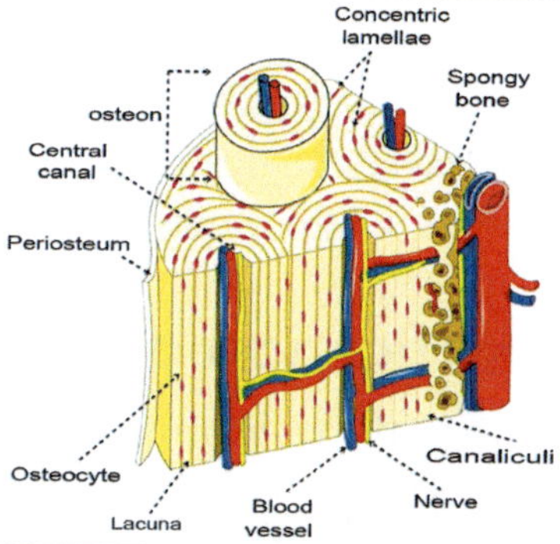
Ossification	Ossification (also called osteogenesis or bone mineralization) in bone remodeling is the process of laying down new bone material by cells named osteoblasts.	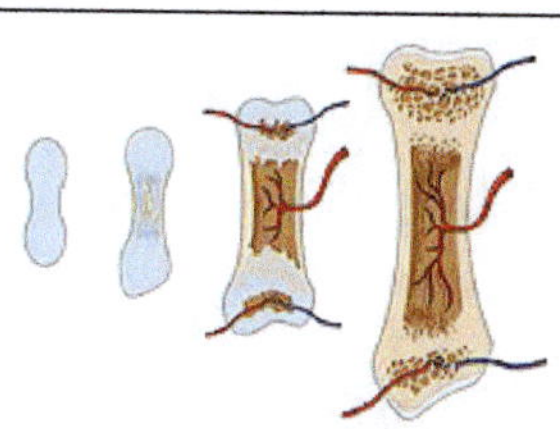

6.1. Functions of the Skeleton

1. Provides a framework that supports the body; the muscles that are attached to bones move the skeleton.
2. Protects some internal organs from mechanical injury; the rib cage protects the heart and lungs, for example.
3. Contains and protects the red bone marrow, the primary hemopoietic (blood-forming) tissue.
4. Provides a storage site for excess calcium. Calcium may be removed from bone to maintain a normal blood calcium level, which is essential for blood clotting and proper functioning of muscles and nerves.

6.2. Types of Bone Tissue

Remember that collagen and calcium salts make up the matrix of bone, and that the cells that make up bone are known as osteocytes. The calcium salts, calcium phosphate ($Ca_3(PO_4)^2$) and calcium carbonate ($CaCO_3$), provide bone with the strength needed to carry out its protective and supporting roles. Although the bone matrix is not alive, it is always changing as calcium from the diet replaces that which is taken from the bone and enters the bloodstream. Normally, there is an equal amount of calcium deposited to replace the calcium that is removed. Osteocytes are responsible for controlling the quantity of calcium deposited in or removed from the bone matrix.

There are two different types of bone tissue in the organ of bone (Figure 6.1). Though it appears solid, compact bone is incredibly well-structured. Osteons or haversian systems, which are microscopic cylinders of bone matrix with osteocytes arranged in concentric rings around central haversian canals, are the building blocks of compact bone. There are blood vessels in the haversian canals, and through microscopic channels called canaliculi in the matrix, the osteocytes are in contact with both these blood vessels and each other.

Spongy bone, which has visible holes or cavities, does resemble a sponge. This is the second type of bone tissue. Although they are present, the blood vessels, matrix, and osteoblasts are not organized in Haversian systems. Red bone marrow, which generates platelets, red blood cells, and the five types of white blood cells, is frequently found in the cavities in spongy bone.

6.3. Classification of Bones

Long bones are the bones of the arms, legs, hands, and feet (excluding the wrists and ankles). The shaft of a long bone is called the diaphysis, while the ends are referred to as epiphyses (*refer* Figure 6.1). The diaphysis consists of compact bone and has a hollow structure, forming a canal within the shaft. This canal, known as the marrow canal or medullary cavity, contains yellow bone marrow, which is primarily composed of adipose tissue. The epiphyses are composed of spongy bone covered by a thin layer of compact bone. While red bone marrow is present in the epiphyses of children's bones, it is largely replaced by yellow bone marrow in adult bones.

Short bones are found in the wrists and ankles. Flat bones include the ribs, shoulder blades, hip bones, and cranial bones. Irregular bones consist of the vertebrae and facial bones.

All bones, whether short, flat, or irregular, are composed of spongy bone that is thinly coated in compact bone. Inside the spongy bone, there is red bone marrow. The joint surfaces of bones are covered by articular cartilage, which provides a smooth surface. The remaining portion of the bone is covered by the periosteum, a fibrous connective tissue membrane. The periosteum's collagen fibers combine with those of the tendons and ligaments attached to the bone. These structures are held in place by the periosteum, which also houses the blood vessels that supply the bone and the osteoblasts that become active in the event of a bone fracture.

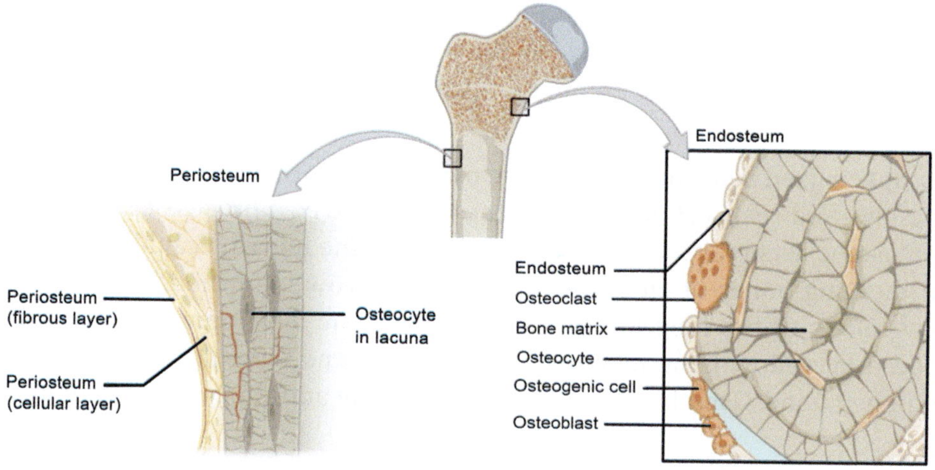

Figure 6.1. *Bone tissue.*

Source: https://courses.lumenlearning.com/suny-ap1/chapter/bone-structure/.

6.4. Embryonic Growth of Bone

The skeleton is initially composed of cartilage and fibrous connective tissue during embryonic development, which are progressively replaced by bone. Osteoblasts—the word "bone" comes from the Greek word "osteo," which means "growing" or "producing"—are the cells that make up bone matrix. Osteoblasts distinguish themselves from fibroblasts in the embryonic model of the skeleton. Each bone has a center of ossification where the process of creating bone matrix, or ossification, starts.

The initial constituent of the cranial and facial bones is fibrous connective tissue. Fibroblasts, or spindle-shaped connective tissue cells, specialize and differentiate into osteoblasts, which make bone matrix, in the third month of fetal development. As calcium salts are deposited in the collagen of each ossification center, bone growth expands outward from the model of the bone. There is still fibrous connective tissue in some places between the baby's skull bones at birth, indicating that this process is not finished. Fontanels are the term for these (Figure 6.2), which allow the head of the newborn to be compressed without breaking the cranial bones, which are still very thin. Additionally, the fontanels allow the brain to grow after birth. Fontanels are what are known as "soft spots," as you may have heard. Because a baby's skull is so delicate, it needs to be shielded from harm. After all of the fontanels have solidified by the time the child reaches two years old, the skull serves as a more reliable barrier for the developing brain.

Ossification in the long bones begins during the third month of gestation, while the embryonic skeleton is primarily composed of cartilage. Osteoblasts create bone matrix in the central region of short, flat, and irregular bones, as well as in the diaphysis of long bones. Over time, the original cartilage is gradually replaced by bone matrix (Figure 6.3).

Similarly, centers of ossification develop in the epiphyses of long bones. Ossification starts at birth and continues throughout childhood. Growth occurs at the epiphyseal discs, where each epiphysis and the diaphysis join. These discs consist of cartilage, and as more cartilage forms on the epiphysis side, the bone lengthens (*see* Figure 6.3). On the diaphysis side, osteoblasts create bone matrix to replace the cartilage. Between the ages of 16 and 25 (depending on testosterone or estrogen levels), all cartilage in the epiphyseal discs is replaced by bone. This marks the closure of the epiphyseal discs.

Osteoclasts, specialized cells known as "destroying" cells, are also present in bones. They have the ability to dissolve and reabsorb minerals in the bone matrix, a process called resorption. In the diaphysis center, osteoclasts reabsorb bone matrix to form the marrow canal. These osteoclasts are highly active in the long bones of embryos. Red bone marrow is formed, and blood vessels grow into the marrow canals of the long bones during embryonic development. After birth, red bone marrow is replaced by yellow bone marrow. In short, flat, and irregular bones, red bone marrow remains in the spongy bone. Osteoblasts and osteoclasts play additional roles in bone development.

6.5. Factors That Affect Bone Growth and Maintenance

1. **Heredity:** With genes from both parents, each person has a genetic potential for height, or a maximum height. There are numerous genes at play, and little is known about how they interact. Given that this is how bones grow, some of these genes most likely correspond to the enzymes that produce cartilage and bone.
2. **Nutrition:** It plays a crucial role in bone development. Bones are formed of raw materials called nutrients, such as protein, phosphorus, and calcium, which are incorporated into the bone matrix itself. For the small intestine to effectively absorb calcium and phosphorus, vitamin D is required. Additionally, vitamins A and C, although not directly part of bone, are essential for the ossification process, which creates the bone matrix. Without these and other nutrients, bones cannot develop correctly. In the case of undernourished children, their growth in height may be stunted as they grow very slowly, unable to reach their full genetic potential.
3. **Hormones:** This also play a significant role in bone growth. Endocrine glands produce hormones that stimulate specific effects in certain cells.

Numerous hormones have a significant impact on the formation and maintenance of bones. These include insulin, thyroxine, parathyroid hormone, and growth hormone, which support the regulation of energy production, protein synthesis, cell division, and calcium metabolism. The sex hormones testosterone and estrogen contribute to the cessation of bone formation. Table 6.1 lists the hormones and their respective functions.

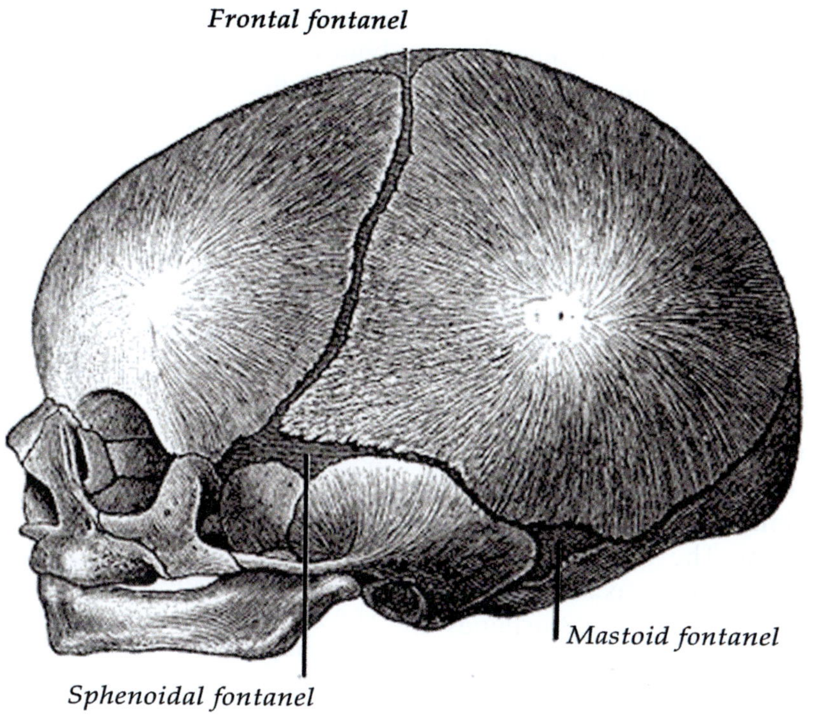

Figure 6.2. *Infant skull with fontanels.*

Source: By Henry Vandyke Carter – Henry Gray (1918) Anatomy of the Human Body (See "Book" section below)Bartleby.com: Gray's Anatomy, Plate 198, Public Domain, https://commons.wikimedia.org/w/index.php?curid=792102.

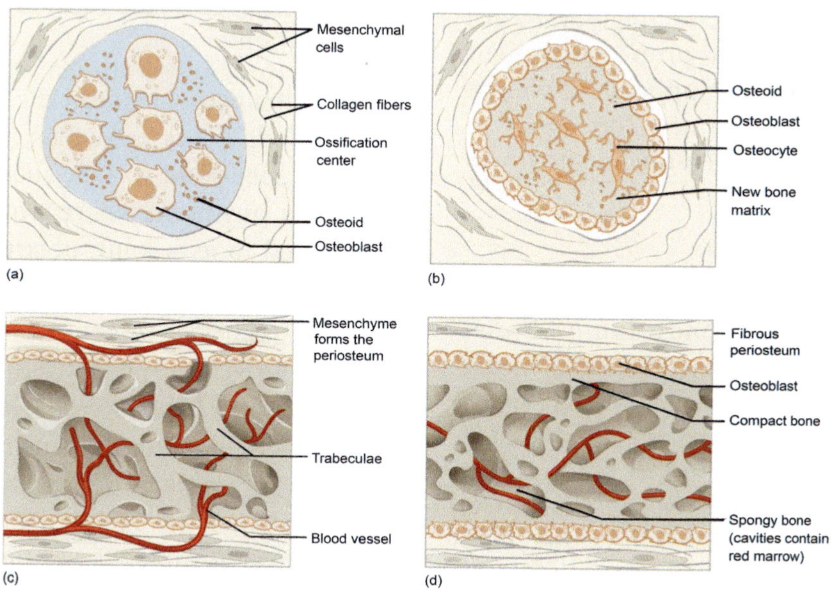

Figure 6.3. *The ossification process in a long bone.*

Source: https://courses.lumenlearning.com/suny-ap1/chapter/bone-formation-and-development/.

Exercise or "stress"—Exercise for bones involves bearing weight, which is precisely what they are designed to do. Without this natural stress, bones will lose calcium more quickly than they can reabsorb it. Walking for daily tasks counts as a form of exercise that does not have to be very intense. Patients confined to bed, for example, will experience a decrease in bone mass and a greater degree of fragility.

6.6. The Skeleton

The axial skeleton, which forms the body's axis, and the appendicular skeleton, which supports the appendages or limbs, are the two divisions of the human skeleton. The rib cage, spinal column, and skull make up the axial skeleton. The appendicular skeleton consists of the bones in the arms, legs, shoulder, and pelvic girdles. Ligaments, which are robust cords or sheets of fibrous connective tissue, connect many bones to other bones across joints. A sprained joint makes the significance of ligaments very clear. A sprain is when a joint's ligaments stretch or even tear, leaving the joint flimsy and unstable even though the bones are still in place. Although we don't give ligaments much thought, they are essential to maintaining the proper alignment of our bones so that we can support our weight and remain upright. There are 206 bones in total, and the complete skeleton is shown in Figure 6.4.

6.6.1. Skull

There are eight cranial bones and 14 facial bones in the skull. The hyoid bone, which supports the base of the tongue, and the three tiny bones in each middle ear cavity are also located in the head. The brain, eyes, and ears are enclosed and shielded by the braincase, which is made up of cranial bones and lined with meninges. You'll recognize some of these bones by name because they share the same names as the terms used to describe different parts of the head. The frontal bone, two parietal bones, two temporal bones, and one occipital bone are these. The orbits (sockets) for the eyes and the floor of the braincase are made up of the sphenoid and ethmoid bones. The forehead and the anterior region of the skull's top are formed by the frontal bone. The word parietal refers to "wall," and the posterior top and most of the side walls of the skull are formed by the two large parietal bones. The middle ear cavity, the inner ear labyrinth, and the external auditory meatus (ear canal) are located in each temporal bone on the side of the skull. The posterior, lower portion of the braincase is formed by the occipital bone. Its two condyles, or rounded projections, on either side articulate with the atlas, the first cervical vertebra, and its foramen magnum, a sizable opening for the spinal cord. The greater wing is visible on the side of the skull between the frontal and temporal bones, and the sphenoid bone is said to have a bat-like shape. The pituitary gland is housed in a depression on the bat's body known as the sella turcica. The cranial meninges are anchored by the crista galli, also known as the "rooster's comb," a vertical projection on the ethmoid bone. The roof, upper walls, and upper portion of the nasal septum are formed by the remaining ethmoid bone.

The joints that connect the cranial bones are all immobile joints known as sutures. Although it might seem odd to talk about a joint that is immobile, any point where two bones converge is referred to as a joint, or articulation.

A suture is where the serrated edges of adjacent bones fit together to prevent shifting if the skull is impacted. Examples include the coronal suture between the frontal and parietal bones, the squamosal suture between the parietal and temporal bones, and the lambdoidal suture between the occipital and parietal bones. The sagittal suture, where the parietal bones meet at the top of the skull, is not visible (Figure 6.5).

Table 6.1. *Hormones Involved in Bone Growth and Maintenance*

Hormones	Author	Study design/ Experimental model	Subjects and number	Results	Year
Thyroxine	Ursomanno et al. (2020)	Retrospective study	Patient N = 635	Patients with HT have a decreased rate of bone loss	2020
	Feitosa dda et al. (2008)	animal experiment	Wistar rat N = 43	Osseointegration ↑healing process in the cortical bone around titanium implants	2008
Estrogen	August et al. (2001)	Retrospective study	Patient N = 526	Estrogen deficiency may be risk factors for maxillary implant failure	2001
	Pan et al. (2000)	animal experiment	female Wistar rats N = 18	The bone mass around the implant and the BIC in the cancellous bone area ↓	2000
	Duarte et al. (2003)	animal experiment	female Wistar rats N = 30		2003
Androgen	Maus et al. (2013)	animal experiment	SD rats N = 20	Dihydrotrophil 2 promotes cobalt-chromium implant bone bonding	2013
Growth hormone	Tresguerres et al. (2002)	animal experiment	New Zealand rabbits N = 8	(topical application) Periimplant bone reaction and mineralization of osteoid ↑	2002
	Stenport et al. (2001)	animal experiment	New Zealand rabbits N = 16	(Systematic administration) Improving Initial implant stability	2001
	Calvo-Guirado et al. (2011)	animal experiment	Beagle dogs N = 12	(Topical application), BIC is not significantly affected	2011
Melatonin	Calvo-Guirado et al. (2010)	animal experiment	Beagle dogs N = 12	BIC↑	2010
	Sun et al. (2020)	animal experiment	SD rats N = 30		2020
	Palin et al. (2018)	animal experiment	Wistar rat N = 18		2018
	Salomó-Coll et al. (2016b)	animal experiment	American Foxhound dogs = 5		
Glucocorticoid	Petsinis et al. (2017)	Retrospective study	Patient N = 31	Glucocorticoid intake did not affect BIC and 3-year survival of dental implants	2017
	Keller et al. (2004)	animal experiment	New Zealand rabbits N = 40	The resulting osteoporosis affects BIC	2006

Insulin	Ferreira et al. (2006)	Retrospective study	Patient N = 121	diabetes caused by abnormal insulin metabolism are more likely to cause peri-implantitis	2006
	Wang et al. (2011)	animal experiment	Wistar rat N = 30	Direct insulin infiltration improves BIC	2011
	de Molon et al. (2013)	animal experiment	Wistar rat N = 80	Insulin deficiency made BIC、torque value↓	2013
	Coelho et al. (2018)		Göttingen minipig N = 9		2018
	Rybaczek et al. (2015)	animal experiment	Wistar rat N = 40	no change in bone area around medullary implants or in bone and BIC	2015
Adiponectin	Yin et al. (2019)	animal experiment	Female SD rats N = 18	BIC↑	2019
PTH	Kuchler et al. (2011a)	Clinical Randomized Controlled Trial	Patient N = 24	NBV/TV↑	2011
	Daugaard et al. (2012)	animal experiment	American Hound dogs N = 20	osseointegration of cancellous bone↑	2012
	Gomes-Ferreira et al. (2020)	animal experiment	Wistar rat N = 24	Bone volume, mass and bone turnover↑	2020
	Park et al. (2020)	animal experiment	SD rats N = 30	Promoting bone formation around implants	2020
Vitamin D	Guido Mangano et al. (2018)	Retrospective study	Patient N = 822	Vitamin D deficiency incidence of early implantation failure is increasing	2016
	Salomó-Coll et al. (2016a)	animal experiment	Foxhound dogs N = 6	Topical application of vitamin D to dental implants can reduce alveolar bone loss, BIC↓	2016
	Dvorak et al. (2012)	animal experiment	SD rats N = 51	Vitamin D deficiency has a negative effect on bone formation around cortical implants	2012
IGF-I	Tang et al. (2015)	animal experiment	Mongrel dog N = 25	Implant bone repair after tooth extraction ↑	2000
CGRP	Yuan et al. (2020)	animal experiment	C57BL/6 or CGRP—/-	CGRP promotes macrophage polarization and enhances osseointegration	2020

Source: Yi, M., Yin, Y., Sun, J., Wang, Z., Tang, Q., & Yang, C., (2022). Hormone and implant osseointegration: Elaboration of the relationship among function, preclinical, and clinical practice. Front. Mol. Biosci., 9, 965753. doi: 10.3389/fmolb.2022.965753.

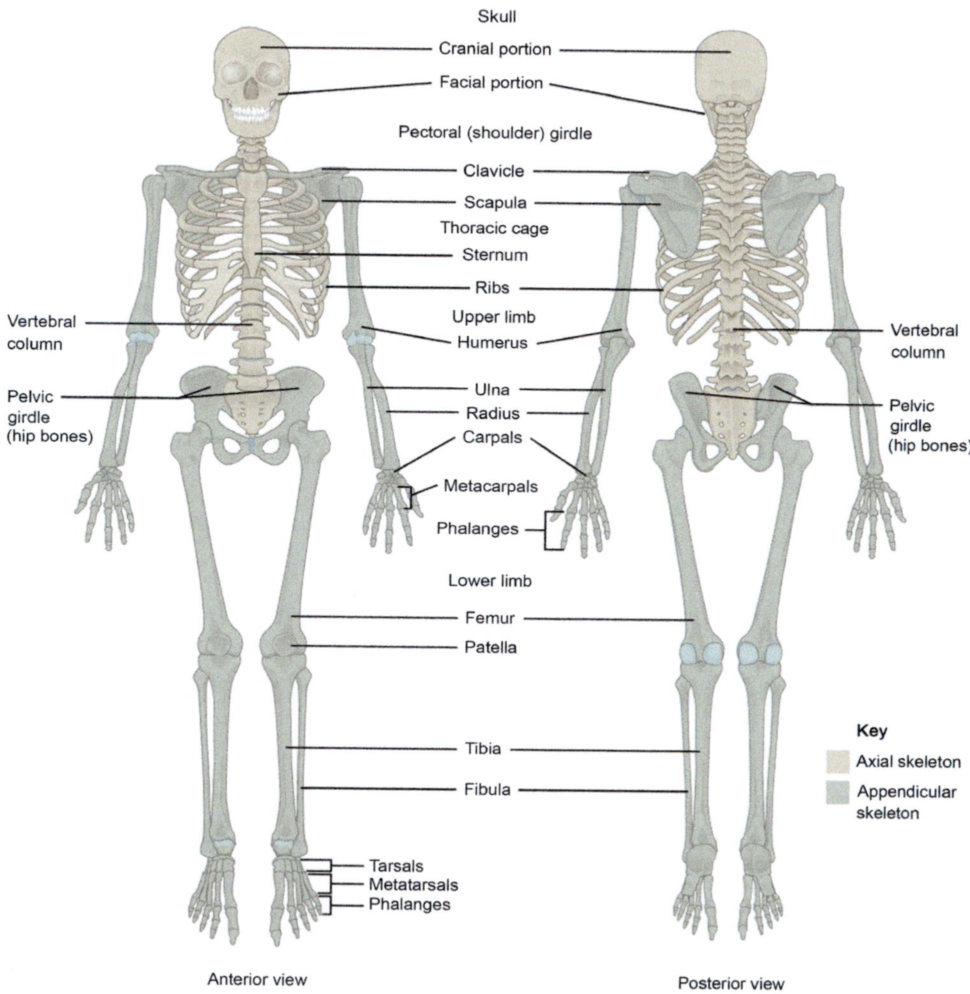

Figure 6.4. *Skeleton.*

Source: https://courses.lumenlearning.com/suny-dutchess-ap1/chapter/human-skeletal-system/.

Only the mandible, or lower jaw, which forms a condyloid joint with each temporal bone, is movable among the 14 facial bones. All other joints found between the bones of the face are sutured. The two upper jaw bones, or maxillae, constitute the anterior part of the hard palate, or roof of the mouth. The maxillae and mandible have sockets for the roots of the teeth. The frontal bone and the two nasal bones combine to form the bridge of the nose; cartilage supports the remaining portion of the nose. Each orbit contains a lacrimal bone on the medial side, which houses the lacrimal sac, a channel for tears. The maxilla, frontal bone, and temporal bone articulate with each other, and the two zygomatic bones together form the prominence of the cheek. The posterior part of the hard palate is composed of the two palatine bones. The lower portion of the nasal septum is formed by the plow-shaped vomer, which articulates with the ethmoid bone. The conchae, a group of six scroll-like bones that curl down the sides of the nasal cavities on either side of the vomer, aid in increasing the surface area of the nasal mucosa.

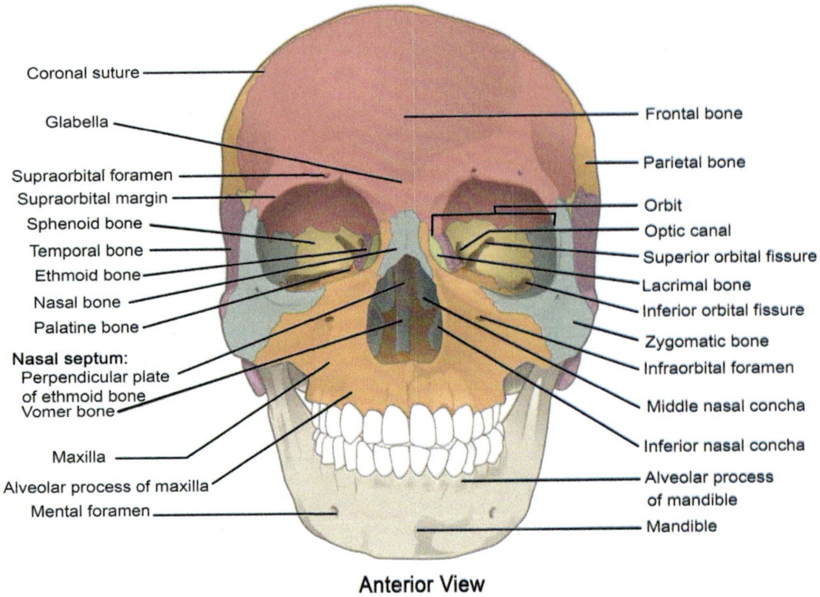

Figure 6.5. *The human skull.*

Source: https://courses.lumenlearning.com/suny-ap1/chapter/the-skull/.

The maxillae, frontal, sphenoid, and ethmoid bones contain air cavities known as paranasal sinuses (Figure 6.6). These sinuses are lined with ciliated epithelium that is continuous with the mucosa of the nasal cavity, as implied by the term "paranasal," and they open into the nasal cavities. The sinuses become noticeable when they become congested, preventing the drainage of the mucus they produce into the nasal cavities. This congestion can occur due to allergies such as hay fever or upper respiratory infections like colds. However, these sinuses serve a purpose: they contribute to voice resonance, causing more air to vibrate and raising the pitch of the voice. Additionally, they help reduce the weight of the skull since air is lighter than bone.

Each temporal bone's mastoid process contains air cavities called the mastoid sinuses, which open into the middle ear. Prior to the discovery of antibiotics, infections of these sinuses called mastoiditis were frequently brought on by middle ear infections.

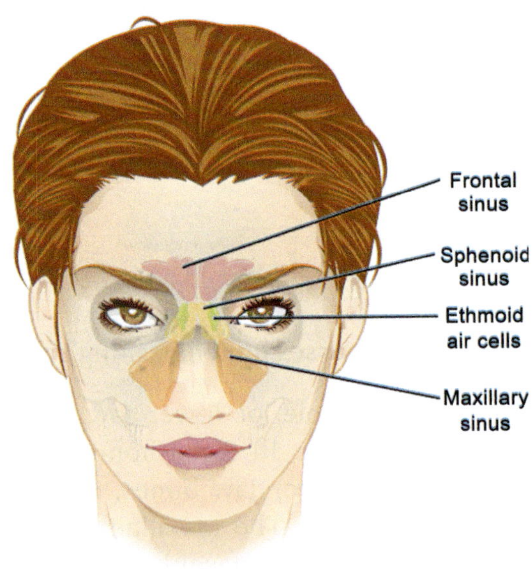

Figure 6.6. *Paranasal sinuses.*

Source: By OpenStax College – Anatomy & Physiology, Connexions Web site. http://cnx.org/content/col11496/1.6/, Jun 19, 2013., CC BY-SA 3.0, https://commons.wikimedia.org/w/index.php?curid=30850944.

The malleus, incus, and stapes are the three auditory bones located inside each middle ear cavity. These bones transfer vibrations from the eardrum to the inner ear receptors as part of the hearing process.

6.6.2. Vertebral Column

The individual bones known as vertebrae make up the vertebral column, also known as the spinal column or backbone. The names of the vertebrae identify their location within the spinal column. There are four to five small coccygeal vertebrae fused into one coccyx, seven cervical vertebrae, 12 thoracic vertebrae, five lumbar vertebrae, and five sacral vertebrae fused into one sacrum.

The seven cervical vertebrae are located in the neck. The first cervical vertebra, known as the atlas, forms a pivot joint with the odontoid process of the second cervical vertebra, known as the axis. It also articulates with the occipital bone to support the skull. This pivot joint allows us to turn our heads from side to side. The remaining five cervical vertebrae do not have individual names.

The thoracic vertebrae articulate with the ribs on the back of the trunk. The lumbar vertebrae, which are the largest and strongest bones in the spine, are located in the small of the back. The sacrum enables the sacroiliac joints, which connect the two hip bones. The coccyx, which is the skeletal remnant of the tail vertebrae, serves as an attachment point for certain muscles of the pelvic floor, or perineum (Figure 6.7).

Ligaments bind the vertebrae together, allowing them to articulate sequentially and form a flexible backbone that supports the head and trunk. In addition, they create the vertebral canal, a continuous tunnel that houses the spinal cord and provides protection against mechanical damage. The canal is lined with meninges within the bones. The spinous and transverse processes are projections for the muscles responsible for bending the vertebral column. Some vertebrae have facets, small flat surfaces that enable articulation with other bones. For instance, the facets of the thoracic vertebrae can connect with the ribs.

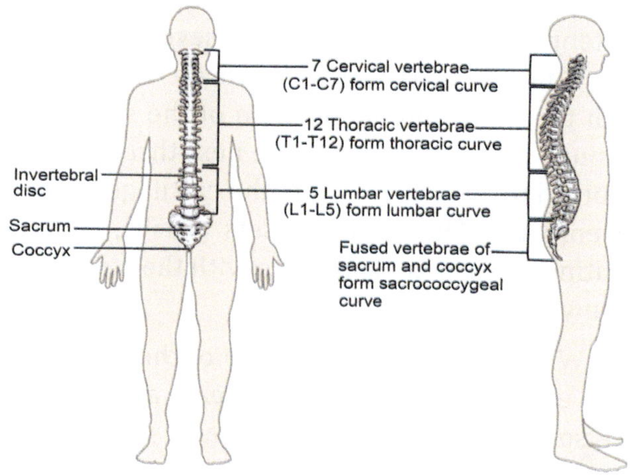

Figure 6.7. *Vertebral column.*

Source: https://courses.lumenlearning.com/suny-ap1/chapter/the-vertebral-column/.

The body of a vertebra serves as its supporting structure, with fibrous cartilage discs separating the bodies of adjacent vertebrae. These discs allow for some movement between vertebrae and act as shock absorbers and cushions (symphysis joints). The entire backbone is highly flexible due to the numerous joints it possesses.

In the normal spine's anatomic position, there are four natural curves named after the vertebrae that form them. These curves include the lumbar, sacral, thoracic, and cervical curves, which are oriented forward, backward, and forward, respectively. These curves play a crucial role in facilitating upright walking by aligning the skull with the rest of the body.

6.6.3. Rib Cage

The sternum, or breastbone, and the 12 pairs of ribs make up the rib cage. The rib cage is composed of three sections: the lower xiphoid process, the central body, and the upper manubrium.

Each rib articulates with the thoracic vertebrae posteriorly. The first seven pairs of ribs, known as true ribs, directly articulate with the body and manubrium of the sternum through costal cartilages. The next three pairs, referred to as false ribs, join the cartilage of the seventh rib. The final two sets of ribs, called floating ribs, do not articulate with the sternum in any way.

While the primary purpose of the rib cage is to enclose and protect the heart and lungs, it also shields the liver and spleen, which are located in the upper abdominal cavity. The flexibility of the rib cage is crucial for its additional function, which involves the external intercostal muscles pulling the ribs upward and outward. This action expands the chest cavity, facilitating inhalation by expanding the lungs.

6.6.4. The Shoulder and Arm

The arms are connected to the axial skeleton by the shoulder girdles. Each is composed of the clavicle (collarbone) and scapula (shoulder blade). The scapula, a large and flat bone, possesses various projections such as the coracoid process and spine, which serve as anchor points for certain muscles responsible for forearm and upper arm movement. The humerus, or upper arm bone, along with the glenoid fossa, a shallow depression, form a ball-and-socket joint.

On one side, the clavicle articulates with the scapula, while on the other side, it connects to the manubrium of the sternum. The clavicles provide support for the scapulae, preventing excessive forward movement of the shoulders. Despite its wide range of motion, the shoulder joint must maintain stability for effective movement.

The humerus, a long bone in the upper arm, is worth noting. Observe the deltoid tubercle, also known as the tuberosity, within the figure. This serves as the anchor point for the triangular-shaped deltoid muscle, which covers the shoulder joint. The scapula and humerus come together at the proximal end to form a ball-and-socket joint. At a distance, the humerus and the ulna of the forearm form a hinge joint. The elbow, being a hinge joint, allows movement solely in one plane, back and forth, without any lateral movement.

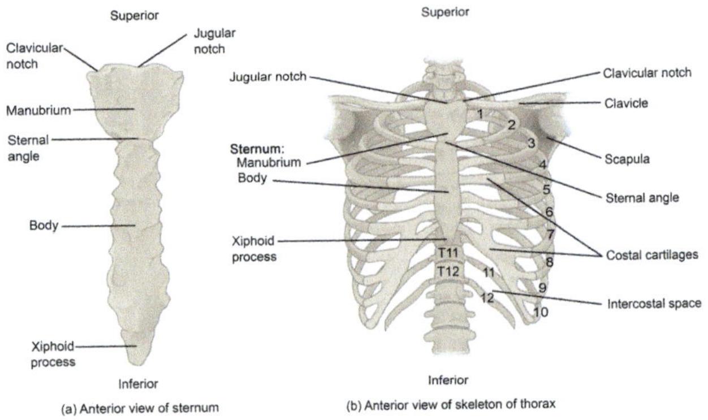

Figure 6.8. *Rib cage – anterior view.*

Source: https://courses.lumenlearning.com/suny-mcc-ap1/chapter/the-thoracic-cage/.

The ulna and radius are the two bones that make up the forearm. The ulna's semilunar notch articulates with the humerus' trochlea, forming part of the elbow's hinge joint. The proximal articulation of the radius and ulna creates a pivot joint, allowing the hand to rotate from palm up to palm down. You can personally observe this by holding your arm palm up and noticing that the radius and ulna are parallel. Additionally, you can see that your upper arm remains still as you turn your hand palm down. This is because the radius crosses over the ulna, enabling the hand to move in various ways without requiring the entire arm to move (Figure 6.8).

The eight tiny wrist bones, known as carpals, have gliding joints that allow for sliding. The proximal ends of the metacarpals, which are the five bones that make up the palm of the hand, and the distal ends of the ulna and radius also articulate with the carpals. The wrist's flexion to extension should be nearly 180° due to the flexibility of the carpal and metacarpal joints. However, the thumb's carpometacarpal joint allows for greater movement compared to the fingers. This joint, known as the saddle joint, enables the thumb to glide over the palm and facilitates grasping.

The finger bones are called phalanges. Each thumb has two phalanges, while each finger has three. Hinge joints, which allow movement in a single plane, are located between the phalanges.

6.6.5. The Hip and Leg

The two hip bones, known as the coxae or innominate bones, which articulate with the axial skeleton at the sacrum, make up the pelvic girdle, also known as the pelvic bone. The pubis, ischium, and ilium—the three main components of each hip bone—are depicted in Figure 6.12, which shows the pelvises of a man and a woman. The upper, flared part of the ilium is what creates the sacroiliac joint. The lower, posterior portion of the ischium is where one sits. The frontmost, lower portion is called the pubis. At the pubic symphysis, a disc of fibrous cartilage sits between the two pubic bones where they articulate with one another. Take note of the pelvic pubic angle for both the male and female. The larger pelvic outlet that results from the broader female angle is an adaptation to childbirth.

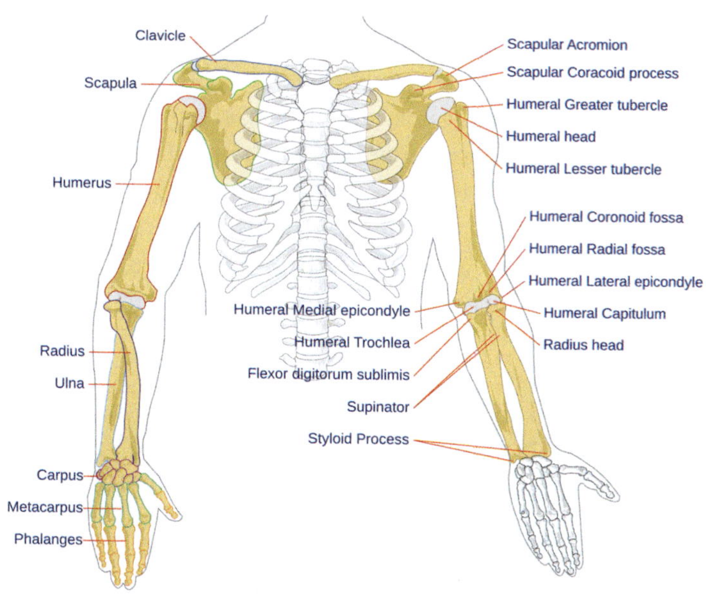

Figure 6.9. *Bones of the arm and shoulder girdle.*

Source: https://en.wikipedia.org/wiki/File:Human_arm_bones_diagram.svg.

The hip bone socket that creates a ball-and-socket joint with the femur is called the acetabulum. The socket of the acetabulum is significantly deeper than that of the glenoid fossa of the scapula.

Because the hip and shoulder are different weight-bearing joints, this is very important functionally. Even with intense joint stress from activities like running and jumping (landing), the hip joint is resistant to dislocation due to the deep acetabulum (Figure 6.9).

The femur is the long bone of the thigh, which forms a highly mobile ball-and-socket joint with the hip bone. At the proximal end, the greater and lesser trochanters serve as attachment points for muscles, while at the distal end, the femur forms a hinge joint with the tibia in the lower leg. Both bones have condyles that shape the joint. The patella, or kneecap, is situated in front of the knee joint, within the quadriceps femoris tendon.

The tibia is the weight-bearing bone of the lower leg. On the anterior side of the leg, one can feel the anterior crest, a ridge, and the tibial tuberosity, a bump. At the distal end, there is the medial malleolus, also known as the "inner ankle bone." The fibula, although not involved in weight-bearing or the knee joint, plays a crucial role. The lateral malleolus of the fibula, located directly above the foot, is referred to as the "outer ankle bone." Despite not bearing weight, the fibula serves as an attachment point for leg muscles, contributing to ankle stability. The malleoli of the tibia and fibula overlap the sides of the talus, creating a more stable configuration with two bones rather than one. Unlike the radius and ulna in the forearm, the tibia and fibula do not form a pivot joint.

In addition to providing stability to the lower leg and foot, as well as supporting the entire body, the tibia and fibula play distinct roles in the musculoskeletal system.

The seven ankle bones are called tarsals. They are larger and stronger than the carpals of the wrist, as expected, and their gliding joints provide less mobility. The talus transfers weight between the calcaneus and the tibia, with the calcaneus, or heel bone, being the largest. The five long bones in each foot are called metatarsals, and the toe bones are called phalanges. The big toe has two phalanges, while the other toes have three. The phalanges of the toes join together to form hinge joints. The big toe is not as mobile as the thumb because the foot lacks a saddle joint. Ligaments support the foot's two primary arches, which are transverse and longitudinal. These arches provide our steps with resilience and are adaptations for fully upright walking. Important components of the hip and leg bones are listed in Figures 6.10 and 6.11; Table 6.4.

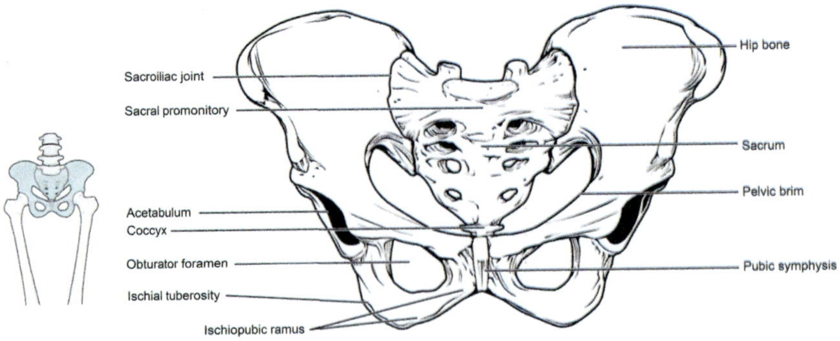

Figure 6.10. *Hip bones and sacrum.*

Source: girdle-and-pelvis/.

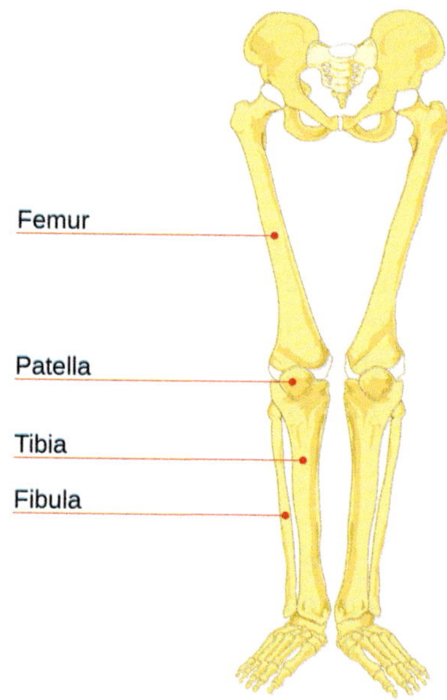

Figure 6.11. *Bones of the leg.*

Source: By The original uploader was Jecowa at English Wikipedia. – Transferred from en.wikipedia to Commons by Rocket000 using CommonsHelper., Public Domain, https://commons.wikimedia.org/w/index.php?curid=10979543.

Table 6.4. Bones of the Hip and Leg—Important Parts

Bone	Part	Description
Pelvic (2 hip bones)	• Ilium • Iliac crest • Posterior superior iliac spine • Ischium • Pubis • Pubic symphysis • Acetabulum	• Flared, upper portion • Upper edge of ilium • Posterior continuation of iliac crest • Lower, posterior portion • Anterior, medial portion • Joint between the 2 pubic bones • Deep depression that articulates with femur
Femur	• Head • Neck • Greater trochanter • Lesser trochanter • Condyles	• Round process that articulates with hip bone • Constricted portion distal to head • Large lateral process for muscle attachment • Medial process for muscle attachment • Rounded processes that articulate with tibia
Tibia	• Condyles • Tibial tuberosity • Anterior crest • Medial malleolus	• Articulate with the femur • Round process for the patellar ligament • Vertical ridge • Distal process; medial "ankle bone"
Fibula	• Head • Lateral malleolus	• Articulates with tibia • Distal process; lateral "ankle bone"
Tarsals (7)	• Calcaneus • Talus • Cuboid, navicular • Cuneiform: 1st, 2nd, 3rd	• Heel bone • Articulates with calcaneus and tibia — —

6.7. Joints – Articulations

A joint is where two bones meet, or articulate.

6.7.1. The Classification of Joints

Joints are categorized according to the range of motion they allow. An immobile joint, such as the suture connecting two cranial bones, is referred to as a synarthrosis. A slightly movable joint, like the symphysis joint between adjacent vertebrae, is known as an amphiarthrosis. A diarthrosis is a joint that exhibits free movement. This category encompasses ball-and-socket joints, pivots, hinges, and other types of joints, making it the largest category.

6.7.1.1. Synovial Joints

All diarthroses, or freely movable joints, are classified as synovial joints due to their structural similarities. Each bone's articular cartilage covers the joint surface, providing a smooth surface. The joint capsule, composed of fibrous connective tissue, acts as a protective sleeve for the joint. The synovial membrane, lining the joint capsule, secretes synovial fluid into the joint cavity. This synovial fluid, with its slick and viscous nature, reduces friction during bone movement.

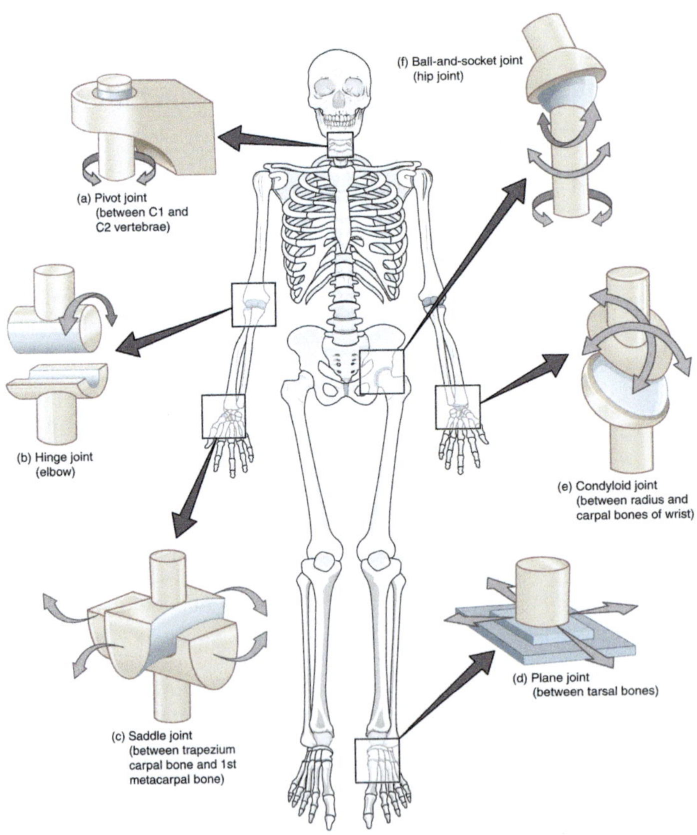

Figure 6.12. *Types of joints.*

Source: https://upload.wikimedia.org/wikipedia/commons/e/ed/909_Types_of_Synovial_Joints.jpg.

Bursae, also known as bursas, are small sacs filled with synovial fluid that are located between the joint and the tendons that pass over it in many synovial joints. Bursae facilitate smooth movement of the tendons when the bones move. Overuse of a joint can lead to inflammation and pain in the bursae, a condition known as bursitis (Figures 6.12 and 6.13).

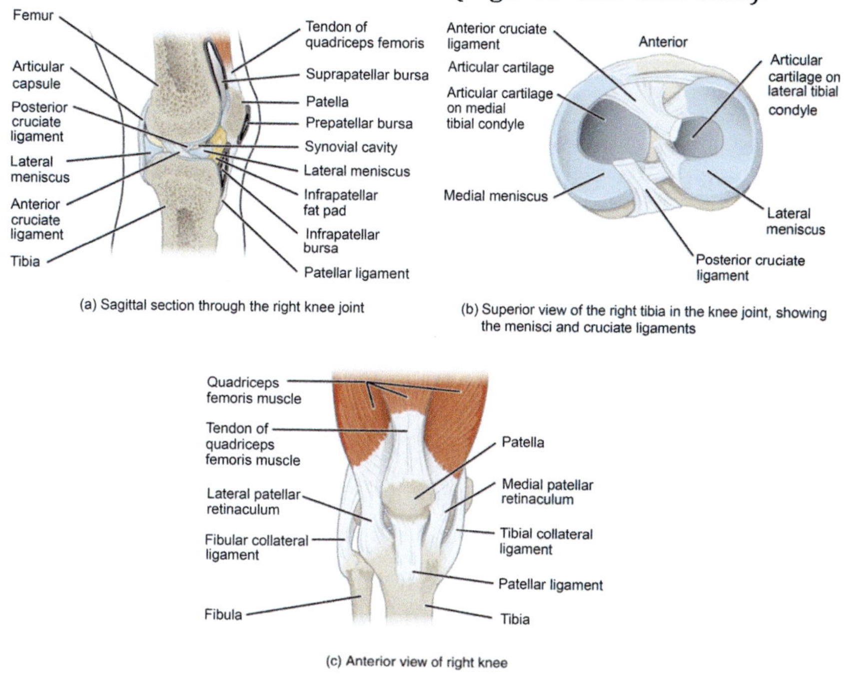

Figure 6.13. *Structure of a synovial joint.*

Source: https://courses.lumenlearning.com/suny-ap1/chapter/anatomy-of-selected-synovial-joints/.

A Closer Look

Osteoporosis

Bone is an active tissue; calcium is constantly being removed to maintain normal blood calcium levels. Usually, however, calcium is replaced in bones at a rate equal to its removal, and the bone matrix remains strong.

Osteoporosis is characterized by excessive loss of calcium from bones without sufficient replacement. Research has suggested that a certain gene for bone buildup in youth is an important factor; less buildup would mean earlier bone thinning. Contributing environmental factors include smoking, insufficient dietary intake of calcium, inactivity, and lack of sex hormones. Osteoporosis is most common among elderly women because estrogen secretion decreases sharply at menopause (in older men, testosterone is still secreted in significant amounts). Factors such as bed rest or inability to get even minimal exercise will make calcium loss even more rapid.

As bones lose calcium and become thin and brittle, fractures are much more likely to occur. Among elderly women, a fractured hip (the neck of the femur) is an all-too-common consequence of this degenerative bone disorder. Such a serious injury is not inevitable, however, and neither is the thinning of the vertebrae that bows the spines of some elderly people. After menopause, women may wish to have a bone density test to determine the strength of their bone matrix. Several medications are available that diminish the rate of bone loss. A diet high in calcium and vitamin D is essential for both men and women, as is moderate exercise. Young women and teenagers should make sure they get adequate dietary calcium to form a strong bone matrix because this will delay the serious effects of osteoporosis later in life.

Summary

- The osseous system is a component of the human body composed of osseous tissue, ligaments, cartilage, and other connective tissues that fulfill essential functions for the body.
- Cancellous bone, which exhibits visible pores or cavities, bears resemblance to a sponge. This constitutes the secondary form of osseous tissue. Although they are present, the blood vessels, extracellular matrix, and osteoblasts are not arranged in haversian systems.
- The skeleton is initially composed of cartilage and fibrous connective tissue during embryonic development, which are progressively replaced by bone.
- The axial skeleton, which forms the body's axis, and the appendicular skeleton, which supports the appendages or limbs, are the two divisions of the human skeleton.
- The articulations that connect the cranial bones are all fixed joints referred to as sutures. Although it might appear peculiar to discuss an immobile joint, any point where two bones converge is denoted as a joint or articulation.
- The individual bones recognized as vertebrae constitute the vertebral column, also acknowledged as the spinal column or backbone. The designations of the vertebrae identify their location within the spinal column.
- Ligaments bind the vertebrae together so they can articulate successively to form a flexible backbone that provides support to the head and trunk.
- Each rib articulates with the thoracic vertebrae posteriorly. The first seven pairs of ribs are known as true ribs because they directly articulate with the sternum's body and manubrium through costal cartilages.
- The femur is the thigh's elongated bone, forming a highly mobile ball-and-socket joint with the hip bone.
- Joints are categorized based on the range of motion they allow. An immobile joint, like the suture connecting two cranial bones, is referred to as a synarthrosis.

References

1. Anderson, H. C., (2003). Matrix vesicles and calcification. *Curr. Rheumatol. Rep., 5*, 222–226.
2. Blair, H. C., & Athanasou, N. A., (2004). Recent advances in osteoclast biology and pathological bone resorption. *Histol. Histopathol., 19*, 189–199.
3. Boyden, L. M., Mao, J., Belsky, J., Mitzner, L., Farhi, A., Mitnick, M. A., Wu, D., et al., (2002). High bone density due to a mutation in LDL receptor-related protein 5. *N Engl. J. Med., 346*, 1513–1521.
4. Boyle, W. J., Simonet, W. S., & Lacey, D. L., (2003). Osteoclast differentiation and activation. *Nature, 423*, 337–342.
5. Brodsky, B., & Persikov, A. V., (2005). Molecular structure of the collagen triple helix. *Adv Protein Chem., 70*, 301–339.
6. Burger, E. H., Klein-Nuland, J., & Smit, T. H., (2003). Strain-derived canalicular fluid flow regulates osteoclast activity in a remodeling osteon: A proposal. *J. Biomech., 36*, 1452–1459.

7. Burr, D. B., (2002). Targeted and nontargeted remodeling. *Bone, 30*, 2–4.

8. Cohen, M. M. Jr., (2006). The new bone biology: Pathologic, molecular, clinical correlates. *Am. J. Med. Genet. A, 140*, 2646–2706.

9. Delaisse, J. M., Andersen, T. L., Engsig, M. T., Henriksen, K., Troen, T., & Blavier, L., (2003). Matrix metalloproteinases (MMP) and cathepsin K contribute differently to osteoclast activities. *Microsc. Res. Tech., 61*, 504–513.

10. Hauge, E. M., Qvesel, D., Eriksen, E. F., Mosekilde, L., & Melsen, F., (2001). Cancellous bone remodeling occurs in specialized compartments lined by cells expressing osteoblastic markers. *J. Bone Miner. Res., 16*, 1575–1582.

11. Hock, J. M., Centrella, M., & Canalis, E., (2004). Insulin-like growth factor I (IGF-I) has independent effects on bone matrix formation and cell replication. *Endocrinology, 122*, 254–260.

12. Jorgensen, N. R., Teilmann, S. C., Henriksen, Z., Civitelli, R., Sorensen, O. H., & Steinberg, T. H., (2003). Activation of L-type calcium channels is required for gap junction-mediated intercellular calcium signaling in osteoblastic cells. *J. Biol. Chem., 278*, 4082–4086.

13. Kobayashi, S., Takahashi, H. E., Ito, A., Saito, N., Nawata, M., Horiuchi, H., Ohta, H., et al., (2003). Trabecular minimodeling in human iliac bone. *Bone, 32*, 163–169.

14. Lindsay, R., Cosman, F., Zhou, H., Bostrom, M., Shen, V., Cruz, J., Nieves, J. W., & Dempster, D. W., (2006). A novel tetracycline labeling schedule for longitudinal evaluation of the short-term effects of anabolic therapy with a single iliac crest biopsy: Early actions of teriparatide. *J. Bone Miner. Res., 21*, 366–373.

15. Little, R. D., Recker, R. R., & Johnson, M. L., (2002). High bone density due to a mutation in LDL receptor-related protein 5. *N Engl. J. Med., 347*, 943–944.

16. Logan, C. Y., & Nusse, R., (2004). The Wnt signaling pathway in development and disease. *Annu. Rev. Cell Dev. Biol., 20*, 781–810.

17. Martin, T. J., & Sims, N. A., (2005). Osteoclast-derived activity in the coupling of bone formation to resorption. *Trends Mol. Med., 11*, 76–81.

18. S Standring. Churchill Livingstone, Musculoskeletal system, (2004). In: Standring, S., (ed.), *Gray's Anatomy* (39th edn., pp. 83–135). New York, Elsevier.

19. Parfitt, A. M., (2002). Targeted and nontargeted bone remodeling: Relationship to basic multicellular unit origination and progression. *Bone, 30*, 5–7.

20. Plotkin, L. I., Aguirre, J. I., Kousteni, S., Manolagas, S. C., & Bellido, T., (2005). Bisphosphonates and estrogens inhibit osteocyte apoptosis via distinct molecular mechanisms downstream of extracellular signal-regulated kinase activation. *J. Biol. Chem., 280*, 7317–7325.

21. Plotkin, L. I., Manolagas, S. C., & Bellido, T., (2002). Transduction of cell survival signals by connexin-43 hemichannels. *J. Biol. Chem., 277*, 8648–8657.

22. Reddy, S. V., (2004). Regulatory mechanisms operative in osteoclasts. *Crit. Rev. Eukaryot. Gene. Expr., 14*, 255–270.

23. Ross, F. P., & Teitelbaum, S. L., (2005). $\alpha_v\beta_3$ and macrophage colony-stimulating factor: Partners in osteoclast biology. *Immunol. Rev., 208*, 88–105.

24. Shin, C. S., Lecanda, F., Sheikh, S., Weitzmann, L., Cheng, S. L., & Civitelli, R., (2000). Relative abundance of different cadherins defines differentiation of mesenchymal precursors into osteogenic, myogenic, or adipogenic pathways. *J. Cell Biochem., 78*, 566–577.

25. Smit, T. H., Burger, E. H., & Huyghe, J. M., (2002). A case for strain-induced fluid flow as a regulator of BMU-coupling and osteonal alignment. *J. Bone Miner. Res., 17*, 2021–2029.

26. Smit, T. H., Burger, E. H., & Huyghe, J. M., (2002). Is BMU-coupling a strain-regulated phenomenon? A finite element analysis. *J. Bone Miner. Res., 15*, 301–307.

27. Helen Thompson, *Switching Farming Made Human Bone Skeleton Joint Lighter*. (2014), Smithsonian Magazine.

28. Taichman, R. S., (2005). Blood and bone: Two tissues whose fates are intertwined to create the hematopoietic stem cell niche. *Blood, 105*, 2631–2639.

29. Teitelbaum, S. L., & Ross, F. P., (2003). Genetic regulation of osteoclast development and function. *Nat. Rev. Genet., 4*, 638–649.

30. Ubara, Y., Fushimi, T., Tagami, T., Sawa, N., Hoshino, J., Yokota, M., Kaitori, H., et al., (2003). Histomorphometric features of bone in patients with primary and secondary hyperparathyroidism. *Kidney Int., 63*, 1809–1816.

31. Ubara, Y., Tagami, T., Nakanishi, S., Sawa, N., Hoshino, J., Suwabe, T., Kaitori, H., et al., (2005). Significance of minimodeling in dialysis patients with adynamic bone disease. *Kidney Int., 68*, 833–839.

32. Vaananen, H. K., Zhao, H., Mulari, M., & Halleen, J. M., (2000). The cell biology of osteoclast function. *J. Cell Sci., 113*, 377–381.

33. Weiner, S., Sagi, I., & Addadi, L.,(2005). Structural biology: Choosing the crystallization path less traveled. *Science, 309*, 1027–1028

34. White, T. D., & Pieter, A. F., (2005). *The Human Bone Manual*. Academic Press: San Diego, CA.

35. Xing, L., & Boyce, B. F., (2005). Regulation of apoptosis in osteoclasts and osteoblastic cells. *Biochem Biophys. Res. Commun., 328*, 709–720.

Chapter

IMMUNE SYSTEM PHYSIOLOGY

7

Contents

Unit Introduction

The immune system, a sophisticated collection of defensive mechanisms present in humans and other higher vertebrates, aids in the rejection of pathogens, or organisms that cause disease. Two complementary immune systems—specific acquired immunity and nonspecific innate immunity—work together to provide immunity against disease. While specific immune responses are directed against specific types of invaders, nonspecific protective mechanisms repel all microorganisms in the same way. Together, the two systems prevent organisms from penetrating and multiplying inside the body. These immune systems also aid in the body's removal of aberrant cells that have the potential to become cancer.

Orientation and Directional Terms:

Term	Definition	Illustration
Antigen	Antigen is a substance that can bind to a specific antibody or T-cell receptor.	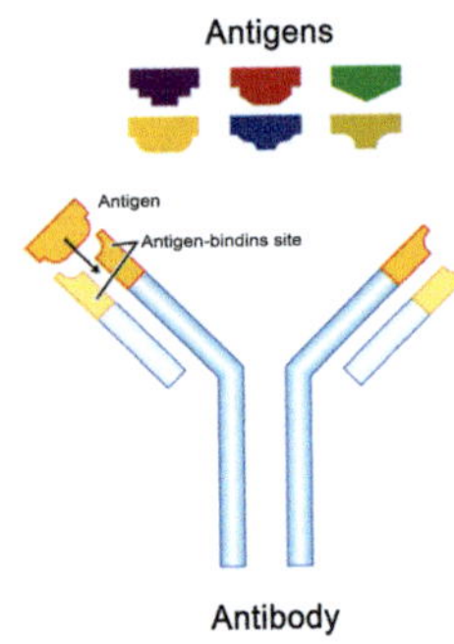
B cells	B cells, also known as B lymphocytes, are a type of white blood cell that produce antibodies. They are a key part of the adaptive immune response and are responsible for humoral immunity in mammals.	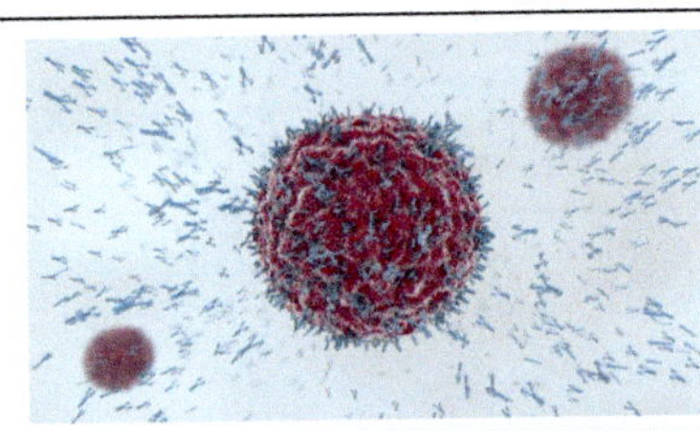
Cell-mediated immunity	Cell-mediated immunity (CMI) is a beneficial host response that involves the production of cytokines and chemokines by T-cells.	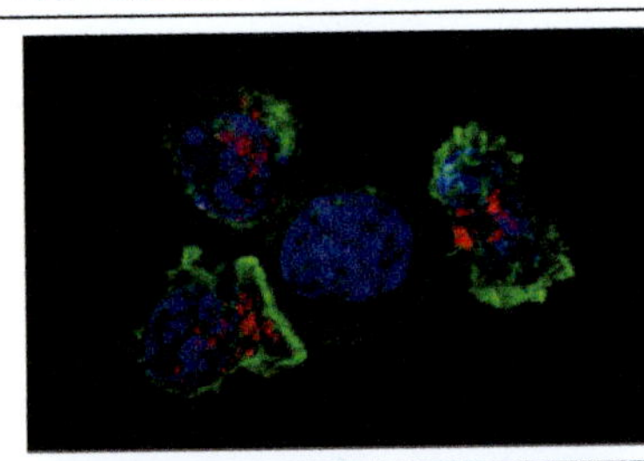
Cytokines	Cytokines are a group of small proteins that are important for cell signaling and regulating the immune system.	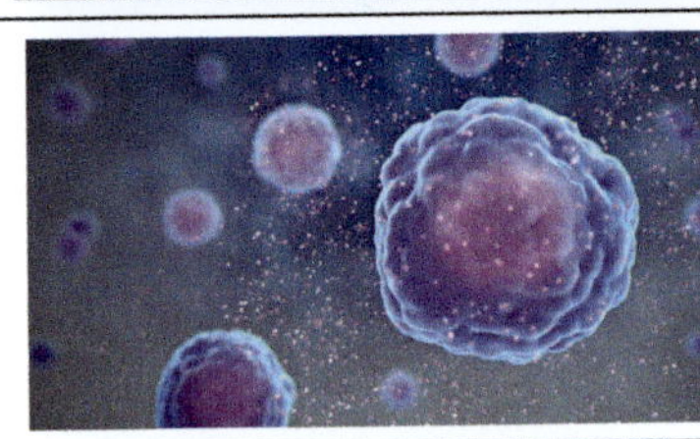
Humoral immunity	Humoral immunity is a type of adaptive immunity that protects the body's extracellular spaces.	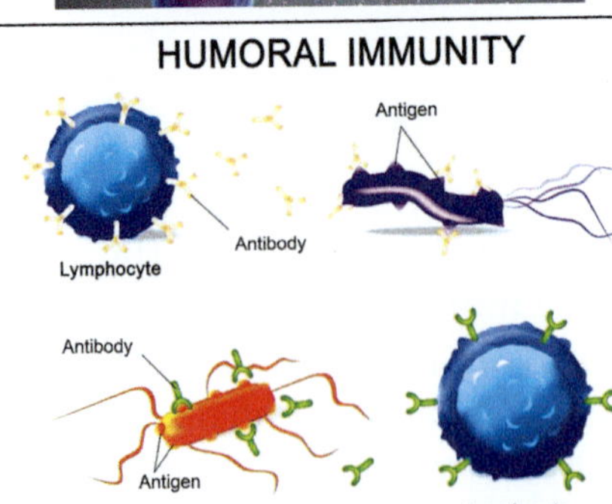

7.1. Mechanisms of the Immune System

7.1.1. Nonspecific, Innate Immunity

The majority of microorganisms encountered in day-to-day life are repelled before they can produce obvious disease signs and symptoms. Given the diversity of these potential pathogens, which include viruses, bacteria, fungi, protozoa, and worms, an organism can greatly benefit from a general defense mechanism that disperses this diverse population of microscopic invaders equally. The innate immune system offers this kind of nonspecific protection through a variety of defense mechanisms, including chemical barriers like antimicrobial proteins that injure or destroy invaders, physical barriers like the skin, and cells that attack foreign cells and body cells harboring infectious agents. The subsequent sections provide a detailed explanation of how these defense mechanisms function to keep the body safe (Figure 7.1).

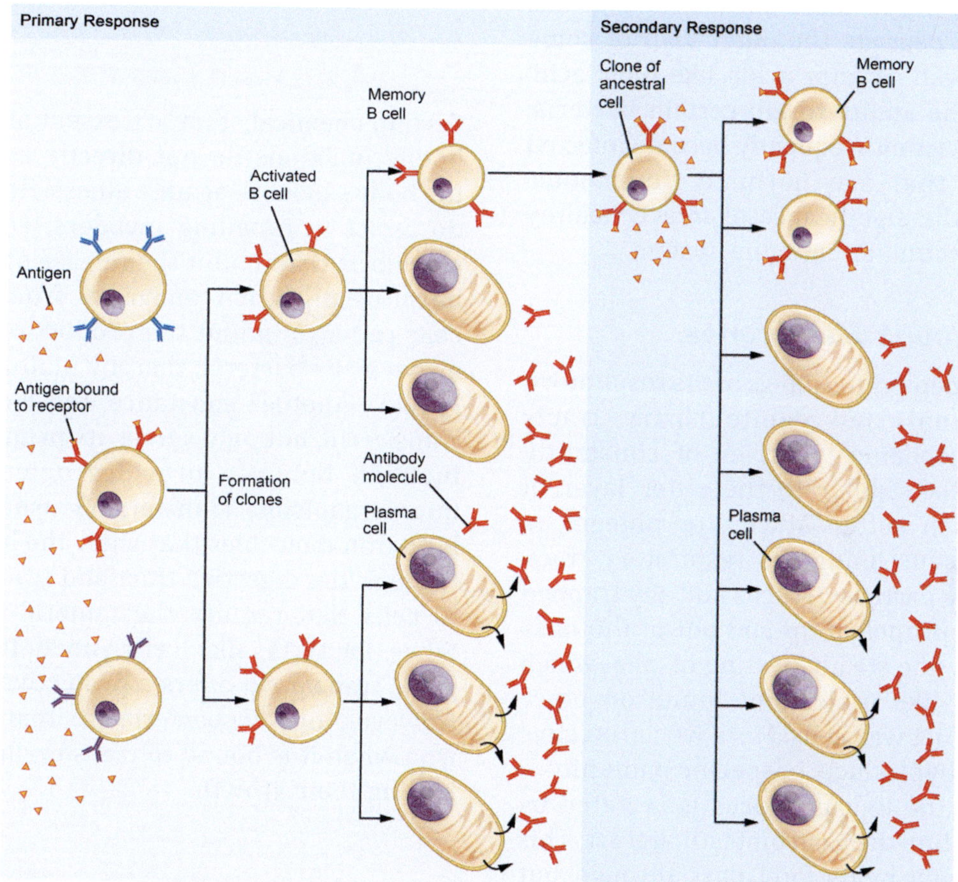

Figure 7.1. *Clonal selection of a B cell: Activated by the binding of an antigen to a specific matching receptor on its surface, a B cell proliferates into a clone. Some clonal cells differentiate into plasma cells, which are short-lived cells that secrete antibodies against the antigen. Others form memory cells, which are longer-lived and, by proliferating rapidly, help to mount an effective defense upon a second exposure to the antigen.*

Source: https://commons.wikimedia.org/wiki/File:2222_Clonal_Selection_of_B_Cells.jpg.

7.1.2. External Barriers to Infection

The first line of defense against the infiltration of bacteria or parasites is the skin, as well as the mucous membrane linings of the gastrointestinal, respiratory, and genitourinary tracts.

7.1.2.1. Skin

Keratin is produced by the hard outer layer of cells in human skin. This layer of cells acts as a mechanical barrier to infection and is continuously renewed from below. Furthermore, lipid-secreting skin glands release lysozyme, an enzyme found in tears and saliva that has the ability to degrade the outer wall of some bacteria, as well as fatty acids like oleic acid, which have the ability to kill certain bacteria. Serious burn victims frequently become infected by bacteria that are normally innocuous, highlighting the significance of intact, healthy skin for a functioning immune system.

7.1.2.2. Mucous Membranes

The mucous membrane linings of the respiratory, gastrointestinal, and genitourinary tracts provide a mechanical barrier of constantly renewing cells, similar to the outer layer of skin but much softer. Mucus, or phlegm, is secreted by cells lining the respiratory tract, capturing tiny particles. Mucus and any trapped particles are propelled up and out of the nose and throat by the steady beating of cilia, which are tiny hair-like projections found on other respiratory tract wall cells. Moreover, protective antibodies—byproducts of specific immunity—are found in the mucus. Mucus is secreted by the cells that line the gastrointestinal tract. This mucus not only helps food pass through but also has the ability to trap or deter potentially hazardous particles from adhering to the gut's lining cells. Underlying gastrointestinal lining cells secrete protective antibodies. Moreover, the lining of the stomach secretes hydrochloric acid, which is potent enough to eradicate a variety of microorganisms.

7.1.3. Chemical Barriers to Infection

Certain microbes have the ability to bypass the body's defenses and infiltrate the internal tissues. Once there, they encounter various chemicals that have the potential to hinder their growth. These substances include those produced by naturally occurring bacteria, chemicals whose primary purpose is to harm or eliminate invaders, and chemicals whose protective effects are incidental to their main purpose.

7.1.4. Chemicals with Incidental Protective Effects

Certain chemicals that are essential for normal bodily functions do not directly contribute to the body's defense against illness. However, they do assist in repelling invaders. For example, chemicals that inhibit the release of potentially harmful digestive enzymes from deceased cells can also inhibit the production of similar enzymes by bacteria, thereby limiting bacterial growth. Another substance, the blood protein transferrin, not only serves its primary cellular function but also provides defense against microorganisms. Transferrin's usual role is to bind iron molecules that enter the bloodstream through the digestive tract and transport them to cells that require the mineral for growth. Since bacteria, like cells, need free iron to grow, transferrin offers a protective advantage. However, invasive bacteria are unable to access iron when it is bound to transferrin, effectively halting their growth.

7.1.5. Antimicrobial Proteins

7.1.5.1. Complement

Many proteins directly aid in the body's non-specific defense mechanism by assisting in the destruction of invasive microbes. One subset of these proteins is known as complement because it supports the body's other defense systems in their efforts to drive out invaders. Complement can be activated by a variety of microorganisms in non-specific ways. Complement proteins, once activated, combine to lyse—that is, disintegrate—dangerous infectious organisms lacking coats of defense. While some microorganisms are able to avoid these mechanisms, they are susceptible to the actions of scavenger cells, which consume and eliminate infectious agents, as well as the mechanisms of a particular immune response. Complement works with defense systems that are both specific and nonspecific.

7.1.5.2. Interferons

Interferons, a different class of proteins that also offer defense, prevent the replication of many viruses, though not all of them. A virus's infected cells release interferon, which alerts other body cells to stop the virus from spreading. Interferon was initially thought to be a single substance when it was discovered in 1957, but since then, multiple types have been found, each produced by a distinct type of cell. Alpha interferon is produced by white blood cells other than lymphocytes, beta interferon is produced by fibroblasts, and gamma interferon is produced by natural killer cells and cytotoxic T lymphocytes (killer T cells).

By interfering with the transcription of viral nucleic acid, all interferons prevent the spread of viruses. Interferons also have additional inhibitory effects by controlling the degree to which lymphocytes and other cells express specific crucial molecules on their surface membranes.

7.1.6. Proteins From Naturally Occurring Bacteria

Naturally occurring gut-dwelling bacteria that do not cause disease can inhibit the growth of invasive bacteria in the small and large intestines. These bacteria that live in the stomach secrete a range of proteins that help them survive by preventing the invasive bacterial species from growing.

7.1.7. Cellular Defenses

An infectious agent will come into contact with cells that have the job of removing foreign substances from the body if it is not successfully repelled by the chemical and physical barriers mentioned above. These are the non-specific effector cells of the innate immune response. Among them are scavenger cells, such as natural killer cells, which target bodily cells that contain infectious organisms, and a variety of cells that directly combat infectious agents. Some of these cells use the process of phagocytosis to engulf and destroy infectious agents, while other cells employ different strategies. These cells work in concert with elements of acquired immunity to combat infection, just like other components of innate immunity.

7.1.8. Scavenger Cells

Leukocytes, or white blood cells, are the main type of scavenger cells found in all higher animals and many lower ones that eliminate infectious agents. There are two primary types of scavenger cells found in most vertebrates, which includes all birds and mammals. Greek terms for "little eaters" and "big eaters," macrophages and microphages, were given to them by Russian biologist Élie Metchnikoff in 1884, marking the first time their significance was acknowledged (Figure 7.2).

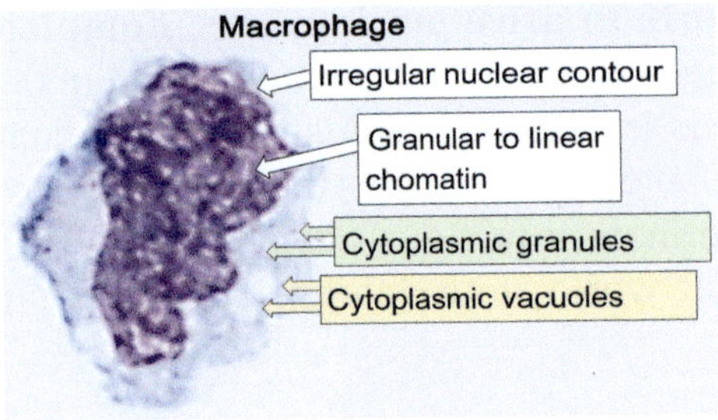

Figure 7.2. *Macrophages, the principal phagocytic (cell-engulfing) components of the immune system, ingest and destroy foreign particles such as bacteria.*

Source: By Mikael Häggström, M. D. Author info – Reusing images – Conflicts of interest: NoneMikael Häggström, M.D.Consent note: Consent from the patient or patient's relatives is regarded as redundant, because of absence of identifiable features (List of HIPAA identifiers) in the media and case information (See also HIPAA case reports guidance). – Own work, CC0, https://commons.wikimedia.org/w/index.php?curid=122541440.

7.1.8.1. Granulocytes

Due to the presence of various chemical-containing granules in their cytoplasm, microphages are now commonly referred to as either granulocytes or polymorphonuclear leukocytes, owing to the distinctive shape of their nuclei. Some granules possess the ability to break down proteins through digestion, while others contain bacteriocidal proteins that can kill bacteria. The three types of granulocytes, namely neutrophils, eosinophils, and basophils, are distinguished by the staining properties of their cytoplasmic granules and the shape of their nuclei. Variations in the chemical composition of the granules are reflected in differences in their staining properties. Neutrophils, accounting for 60-70% of white blood cells, are the most abundant type of granulocytes. They are responsible for engulfing and eliminating microbes, particularly bacteria. Eosinophils, although less common, are highly effective at breaking down the cells that make up the cuticle or body wall of larger parasites. Basophils, which release histamine, heparin (a drug that inhibits blood coagulation), and other chemicals involved in certain allergic reactions, are even less common. Mast cells, another type of tissue cell, function similarly to basophils in terms of structure and function, aiding in immune responses.

Granulocytes, with a lifespan of only a few days, are continuously produced from stem cells in the bone marrow. They enter the bloodstream, circulate for a few hours, and then cease circulation before eventually dying. Granulocytes are mobile cells that are attracted to foreign substances through chemical signals. These signals can be generated by invasive microorganisms, injured tissues, or the interaction of microbes with blood plasma proteins. Certain microbes are indigestible and do not perish upon consumption, while others produce toxins that poison granulocytes and evade phagocytosis. Therefore, granulocytes must be supported by the mechanisms of specific immunity, as they are not highly effective on their own.

7.1.8.2. Macrophages

The mature form of the monocyte, the macrophage, is the other primary type of scavenger cell. Monocytes, which circulate in the bloodstream but are produced in smaller quantities than granulocytes by bone marrow stem cells, are similar to granulocytes. However, unlike granulocytes, monocytes differentiate into macrophages, which settle in a variety of tissues, particularly lymphoid tissues (e.g., liver and lymph nodes), which act as filters to catch bacteria and other foreign objects that enter through the blood or lymph. Macrophages have a different function from granulocytes despite being more effective scavengers due to their longer lifespan. In contrast to granulocytes, macrophages exhibit comparatively slow motility. They are drawn to distinct stimuli and typically reach invasion sites after granulocytes. Although the digestive process is slower and less thorough, macrophages recognize and ingest foreign particles using mechanisms that are essentially similar to those of granulocytes. This is a crucial factor because macrophages stimulate particular immune responses, a process that granulocytes are not involved in (Figure 7.3).

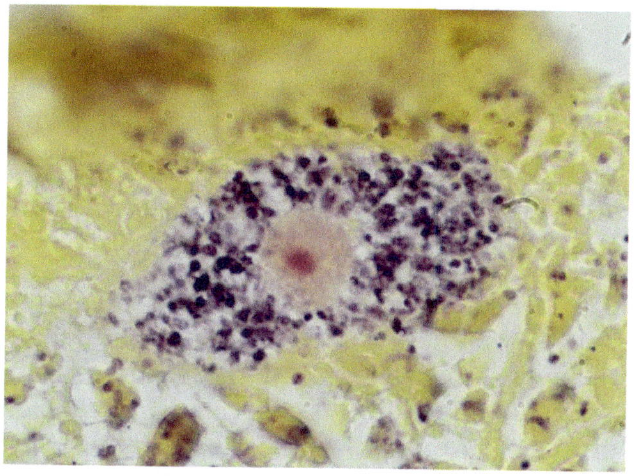

Figure 7.3. *Macrophage attacking a bacterial cell.*

Source: By Mikael Häggström, M.D. Author info – Reusing images – Conflicts of interest:NoneMikael Häggström, M.D. – Own work, CC0, https://commons.wikimedia.org/w/index.php?curid=138526356.

7.1.8.3. Natural Killer (NK) Cells

Natural killer cells eliminate the body's own cells that have either developed cancer or contracted a virus, rather than directly attacking foreign invaders. The identification of natural killer (NK) cells dates back to 1975, when investigators noticed cells in lymphoid tissues and blood that were not ordinary lymphocytes or the scavengers mentioned earlier, but still had the ability to destroy cells. NK cells resemble lymphocytes in appearance, but they are different in that they have granules that contain cytotoxic substances.

NK cells use a method independent of specific immunity to identify dividing cells. After attaching themselves to these dividing cells, they release their granules, which pass through the membrane and into the cytoplasm. The dividing cells leak and perish as a result of this.

With B and T lymphocytes being the most prevalent types of lymphocytes in the body, NK cells are the third most common type. They originate from hematopoietic stem cells and undergo maturation in the liver and bone marrow.

7.1.9. Nonspecific Responses to Infection

The body fights infection through a variety of nonspecific mechanisms known as early induced responses. These consist of the inflammatory response and the acute-phase response, which can either completely eradicate infection or contain it until certain acquired immune responses have had time to mature. Although nonspecific immune responses happen more quickly than acquired immune responses, they do not offer long-lasting protection against specific pathogens.

The effects of nonadaptive immune responses are mediated by a variety of chemical signals referred to as cytokines. These cytokines include tumor necrosis factor-alpha (TNF-α), which initiates the inflammatory response, and members of the protein family known as interleukins, which induce fever and the acute-phase response.

7.1.10. Acute-Phase Response

Macrophages release interleukin-1 (IL-1) and interleukin-6 (IL-6) to combat infections when the body is invaded by pathogens. One of their effects is to increase body temperature, which often leads to fever following an infection. The interleukins raise body temperature by influencing the hypothalamus in the brain, which regulates body temperature, as well as by influencing the energy mobilization of muscle and fat cells. Fever is believed to be beneficial in eliminating infections because most bacteria thrive in temperatures lower than the average body temperature. However, fever is merely a component of the acute-phase response, which is a broader innate defense mechanism. The interleukins not only induce an increase in body temperature, but also stimulate the liver cells to release more proteins into the bloodstream. Collectively, these proteins are known as acute-phase proteins. When these proteins bind to bacteria, they activate complement proteins that eliminate the infection. Acute-phase proteins function similarly to antibodies, but they have a broader spectrum of activity, targeting various microorganisms rather than selectively targeting specific pathogens. Another effect of interleukins is the elevation of circulating neutrophils and eosinophils, which contribute to the fight against infection.

7.1.11. Inflammatory Response

Tissue damage caused by infections often triggers an inflammatory reaction. Pain, swelling, redness, and fever are indications of inflammation that result from the release of chemicals by macrophages. These compounds increase the permeability of capillaries, promote coagulation, and enhance local blood flow. Redness is caused by increased blood flow, while swelling and pain are caused by the infiltration of cells and fluids into tissues due to capillary leakage. These effects attract more phagocytic cells to the area, aiding in the removal of pathogens. Neutrophils and eosinophils are the first cells to arrive, usually within an hour, followed by macrophages a few hours later. In addition to engulfing pathogens, macrophages contribute to the healing process by eliminating cellular debris from damaged tissue cells and neutrophils that undergo self-destruction after consuming microbes. If the infection persists, T cells and antibodies from specialized immunity arrive at the site to combat it.

7.1.12. Specific, Acquired Immunity

For centuries, it has been widely recognized that individuals who survive a particular disease generally develop immunity to it in the future. Thucydides, the Greek historian, documented during the 5th century BCE, amidst the devastating plague in Athens, that the sick and dying would have been left without any care if it were not for the dedication of those who had already recovered from the illness. It was well-established that no one ever contracted the plague twice. This principle holds true for a wide range of other diseases, such as mumps, chickenpox, smallpox, and measles, with only a few exceptions. However, having had measles does not guarantee protection against chickenpox, and vice versa. Each infection can only confer immunity specific to that particular disease due to the presence of acquired immunity, also known as adaptive immunity.

Certain infectious diseases, such as the common cold, influenza, pneumonia, and diarrheal illnesses, appear to defy the concept of specific immunity as they can be contracted repeatedly. However, the recurrence of these illnesses can be attributed to the similar symptoms caused by various infectious agents, leading to the same disease. For example, the common cold encompasses a cluster of symptoms that can be caused by over 200 different viruses. Therefore, infection with a specific agent does not provide protection against other pathogens that have not been encountered, although it does guard against reinfection by the same pathogen.

Acquired immunity relies on the crucial role of lymphocytes, specialized white blood cells. The various mechanisms by which lymphocytes function to confer specific immunity are extensively discussed. While early research on specific immunity dates back to the late 1800s, our comprehensive understanding of this topic has primarily emerged since the 1960s, and new insights continue to be discovered (Figure 7.4).

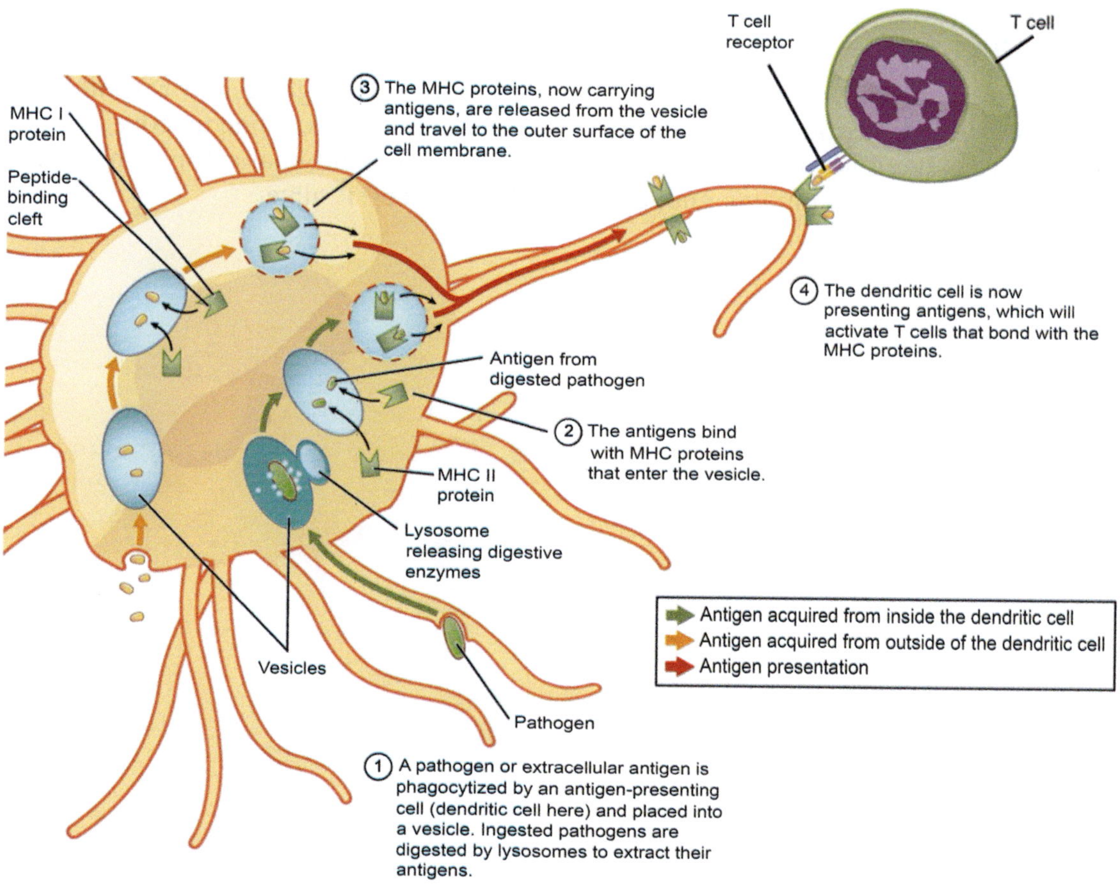

Figure 7.4. *Diagram of the activities of T- and B-cells.*

Source: https://courses.lumenlearning.com/suny-ap2/chapter/the-adaptive-immune-response-t-lymphocytes-and-their-functional-types/.

Acquired immunity depends on the activities of T and B lymphocytes (T and B cells). One part of acquired immunity, humoral immunity, involves the production of antibodies by B cells. The other part, cell-mediated immunity, involves the actions of T cells. When an antigen (such as a bacterium) enters the body, it is attacked and engulfed by macrophages, which process and display parts of it on their cell surface. A helper T cell, recognizing the antigen displayed, initiates the maturation and proliferation of other T cells. Cytotoxic (killer) T cells develop and attack foreign and infected cells. B cells stimulated by the presence of antigen are activated by helper T cells to divide and form antibody-producing cells (plasma cells). Released antibody binds to antigen, marking the cell for destruction. Helper T cells also induce the development of memory T and B cells needed to mount future immune responses on reinfection with the same pathogen.

7.2. The Nature of Lymphocytes

7.2.1. General Characteristics

7.2.1.1. Location in the Lymphatic System

Lymphocytes are the cells responsible for the body's ability to recognize and respond to a vast array of different foreign substances, including those found in microbes. When inactive, lymphocytes are small round cells filled mostly with a nucleus. Despite having minimal cytoplasm compared to other cells, each lymphocyte contains enough organelles to keep it alive.

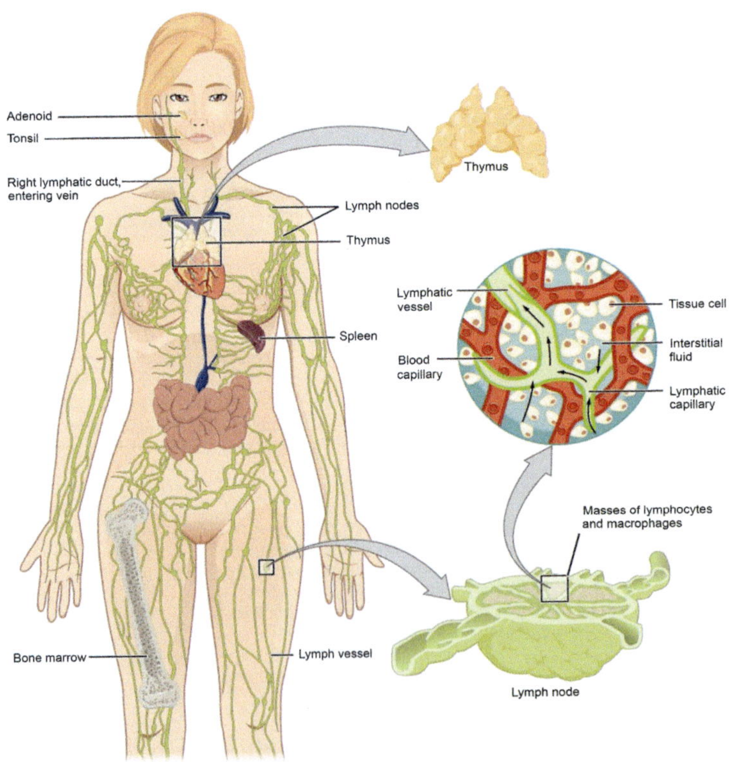

Figure 7.5. *Diagram of the human lymphatic system. The human lymphatic system, showing the lymphatic vessels and lymphoid organs.*

Source: https://courses.lumenlearning.com/suny-ap2/chapter/anatomy-of-the-lymphatic-and-immune-systems/.

While lymphocytes typically move slowly on their own, they can travel quickly through the body when carried by the blood or lymph. An adult human typically has around 2×10^{12} lymphocytes, with roughly 1% in the bloodstream and the majority concentrated in various tissues throughout the body, such as the bone marrow, spleen, thymus, lymph nodes, tonsils, and intestinal lining. These tissues make up the lymphatic system, and those containing high concentrations of lymphocytes are known as lymphoid. In lymphoid structures, lymphocytes are free to move within a network of lymph capillaries, ensuring they interact with other cells and foreign materials in an organized manner (Figure 7.5).

7.2.1.2. T- and B-Cells

Bone marrow stem cells give rise to lymphocytes. These stem cells constantly proliferate, releasing immature lymphocytes into the circulation. Certain cells proceed to the thymus, where they proliferate and undergo differentiation into T lymphocytes, also known as T cells. The 'T' in T cells stands for thymus-derived, indicating that the thymus is where these cells mature. T cells leave the thymus and travel through the bloodstream to other lymphoid organs, where they can further proliferate in response to the appropriate stimuli. T cells make up approximately half of all lymphocytes. Certain lymphocytes continue to differentiate in the bone marrow before directly moving to the lymphoid organs. They are known as B lymphocytes, or B cells. Like T cells, B cells can develop and proliferate even more in the lymphoid organs when given the appropriate stimuli. Since they are derived from bone marrow, it is appropriate to refer to them as B cells in humans and other mammals. However, the letter 'B' actually stands for the bursa of Fabricius, a lymphoid organ exclusive to birds, which is where B cells were originally discovered.

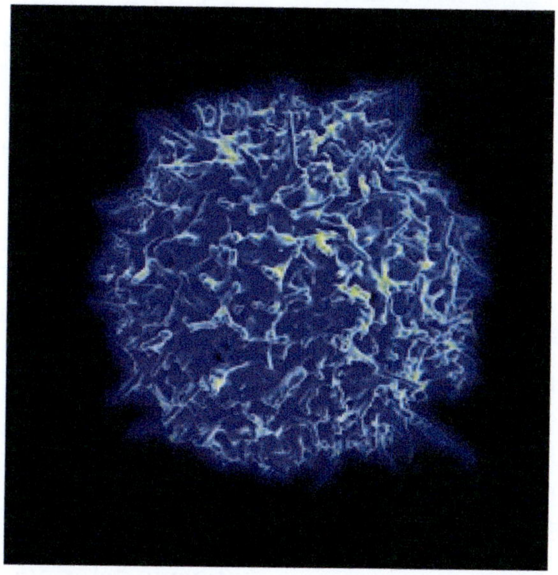

Figure 7.6. *Human T-cell; human T-lymphocyte. A scanning electron micrograph of a T-cell (T-lymphocyte) from the immune system of a healthy person.*

Source: By NIAID/NIH – NIAID Flickr's photostream, Public Domain, https://commons.wikimedia.org/w/index.php?curid=18233598.

Although they employ distinct mechanisms, B and T lymphocytes possess the ability to recognize and aid in the elimination of foreign molecules (antigens), such as those encountered in invasive organisms. Antibodies, which are proteins secreted by B cells, have the capacity to bind to antigens. Given that antibodies circulate throughout the bodily secretions known as humors, the defense provided by B cells is referred to as humoral immunity. Conversely, T cells directly target invaders instead of producing antibodies. This alternative form of acquired immunity is termed cell-mediated immunity, as it relies on the direct involvement of cells rather than antibodies. While B cells and antibodies interact with extracellular invaders, T cells exclusively identify infectious agents that have infiltrated body cells. However, it should be noted that T cells also exert a significant influence on B cell function, thereby blurring the distinction between these two forms of specific acquired immunity. An immune response often employs both humoral and cell-mediated attacks to target foreign substances. Additionally, both classes of lymphocytes can enhance or activate a variety of nonspecific immune responses (Figure 7.6).

7.2.2. Ability to Recognize Foreign Molecules

7.2.2.1. Receptor Molecules

The ability of lymphocytes to identify foreign molecules sets them apart from other types of cells. Receptor molecules aid in the process of recognition. A unique protein, known as a receptor molecule, possesses a shape that complements a specific region of an alien molecule. Due to their complementary shapes, the foreign molecule and the receptor can fit together, much like a key fitting into a lock.

Receptor molecules can be found in bodily fluids or attached to the surface of lymphocytes. Both B and T lymphocytes have receptor molecules on their cell surfaces, but only B cells produce and secrete a significant amount of antibodies, which are receptor molecules that are not attached. The structure of antibodies matches that of the receptor molecules on the surface of B cells.

7.2.2.2. Antigens

An antigen refers to any foreign substance that specifically binds to a receptor molecule produced by lymphocytes, often a complex protein. Antigens can be found on the surface of foreign substances such as dust, pollen, or transplanted tissue, as well as on invasive microorganisms like viruses, bacteria, protozoa, and fungi. When an antigen attaches to a receptor molecule, it may or may not trigger an immune response. Antigens that do cause an immune response are known as immunogens. Therefore, while all antigens are not immunogens, all immunogens are antigens. There are chemical groups, called haptens, that can bind to a lymphocyte receptor and act as antigens, but they do not affect the immune system. Haptens can become immunogenic when they are attached to a larger, more complex molecule, such as a protein. This property is useful for immune response research (Figure 7.7).

A wide range of unique three-dimensional patterns can be observed on various surfaces of antigens. Each pattern is known as an epitope, or antigenic determinant, and it can interact with different lymphocyte receptors. Complex antigens display an "antigenic mosaic" and possess the ability to elicit responses from various types of specific lymphocytes. Certain antigenic determinants provoke a more robust immune response compared to others, likely due to the presence of more responsive lymphocytes. It is possible for an epitope to be shared by two or more distinct substances. In such cases, immune components that have been activated by a single antigen can react with any other antigen that shares the same epitope. These antigens are referred to as cross-reacting antigens.

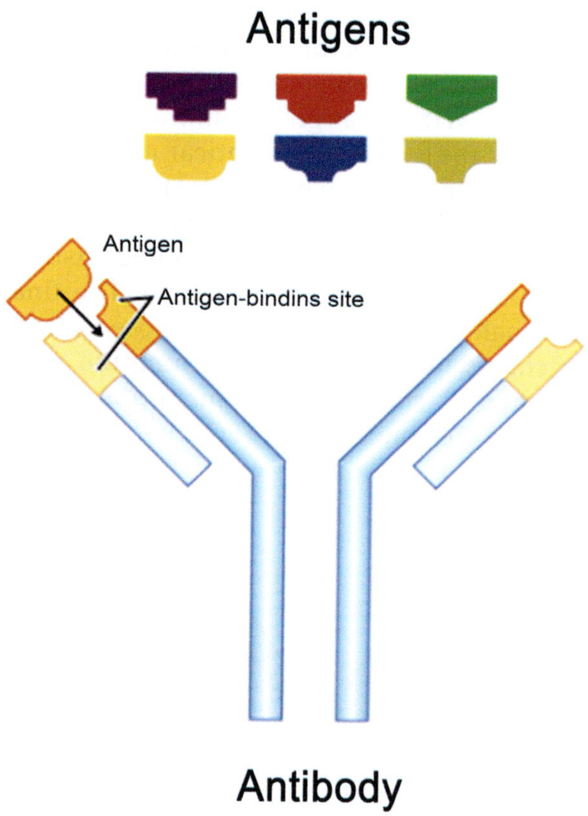

Figure 7.7. *Antigen, antibody, and lymphocyte. Phagocytic cells destroy viral and bacterial antigens by eating them, while B cells produce antibodies that bind to and inactivate antigens.*

Source: By Fvasconcellos 19:03, 6 May 2007 (UTC) – Color version of Image:Antibody.png, originally a Work of the United States Government, Public Domain, https://commons.wikimedia.org/w/index.php?curid=2067564.

T cells and B cells recognize different forms of antigens, which influences the antigens they are capable of detecting. B cells target antigens present on invaders in the bloodstream, while T cells exclusively detect invaders located inside cells. This implies that foreign materials engulfed by cells or viruses that replicate within cells cannot be targeted by antibodies but can be eliminated by T cells.

7.2.2.3. Diversity of Lymphocytes

The totality of lymphocytes within the immune system, or the specific immune system, is capable of identifying almost any complex molecule created by nature or science. The B and T lymphocytes produce trillions of distinct antigen receptors, which contribute to their extraordinary capacity. Every lymphocyte produces a unique receptor that is arranged structurally to react differently to various antigens. When a cell comes into contact with an antigen it recognizes, it is proliferated, leading to an increase in the number of lymphocytes that carry that specific receptor.

How does the body possess such a wide array of receptors that are always prepared to react to invading molecules? To comprehend this, it is helpful to have a quick review of genes and proteins. Antigen receptor molecules are proteins made up of a few polypeptide chains, comprising amino acids linked together by peptide bonds. The sequence of amino acids that forms a specific polypeptide chain is dictated by a distinct region of DNA, known as a gene. If each polypeptide region of every antigen receptor was encoded by a different gene, the human genome would require trillions of genes just to encode these immune system proteins. As the human genome consists of around 25,000 genes, individuals cannot inherit a gene for each specific antigen receptor component. Instead, there is a mechanism in place that generates a vast array of receptors from a limited number of genes.

For every kind of polypeptide chain, there exists a pool of inherited gene segments. These gene segments are then assembled into a single gene for each polypeptide, which forms an individual antigen receptor as each lymphocyte develops. This rearrangement of alternative gene segments can result in a vast array of combinations, mostly occurring at random. Through an imperfect recombination process called junctional diversification, gene segment ends can be shortened or lengthened, leading to additional diversity. To ensure that each mature lymphocyte produces only one type of receptor, a genetic rearrangement takes place when the lymphocytes derived from stem cells first become functional. Consequently, it is possible to generate an infinite variety of diverse antigen receptors from a pool of only hundreds of genes.

Additional mechanisms also contribute to receptor diversity. Somatic mutation, another process superimposed on the previously described mechanism, plays a role. Mutation refers to the natural occurrence of minute alterations in DNA during cell division. The term "somatic" is used when these alterations affect body cells, as opposed to germ-line cells such as eggs and sperm. Somatic mutation commonly occurs in the DNA that codes for antigen receptors in lymphocytes, although it can occur accidentally in any body cell. As a result, descendant cells of a stimulated lymphocyte may possess new antigen receptor variants, some of which may offer an even better fit for the antigen that triggered the initial stimulation.

7.2.2.4. B-Cell Antigen Receptors and Antibodies

B lymphocyte antigen receptors are identical to the binding sites of antibodies that these lymphocytes produce upon stimulation, except for the presence of an additional tail that penetrates the cell membrane and attaches to the cell surface. Therefore, a comprehensive explanation of the extensively studied structure and characteristics of antibodies will encompass both.

7.2.3. Basic Structure of the Immunoglobulin Molecule

Antibodies belong to the class of proteins called globulins, owing to their globular structure. Collectively, antibodies are referred to as immunoglobulins (Ig for short). The basic molecular structure of all immunoglobulins consists of four polypeptide chains that are identical. Within a given immunoglobulin molecule, there are two identical chains: two light (L) chains and two heavy (H) chains. Simply put, "heavier" and "lighter" denote larger and smaller, respectively. Genes encoding distinct chains are produced independently. The final immunoglobulin molecule is composed of the four chains joined together, forming the most fundamental configuration an antibody can assume: a flexible Y shape (Figure 7.8).

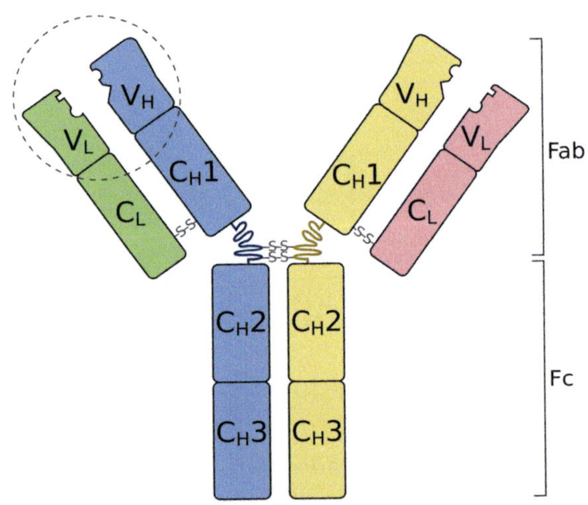

Figure 7.8. *Antibody structure.*

Source: By Tokenzero – Own work, based on File:Immunoglobulin basic unit.svg by Y_tambe, CC BY-SA 4.0, https://commons.wikimedia.org/w/index.php?curid=93798019.

The four-chain structure of an antibody, or immunoglobulin, molecule. The basic unit is composed of two identical light (L) chains and two identical heavy (H) chains, which are held together by disulfide bonds to form a flexible

Y shape. Each chain is composed of a variable (V) region and a constant (C) region. Part of the heavy and light chains come together to form the antigen-binding, or antibody-combining, site, which is located at the tip of each arm of the Y-shaped molecule. There are two or more of these identical sites on every immunoglobulin molecule. The epitope, also known as the antigenic determinant, is the portion of the antigen that the antibody can recognize thanks to its antigen-binding site. The epitope can fit into the antigen-binding site and be "recognized" by the antibody if its shape matches that of the site. The antigen is then held inside the binding site by the formation of weak chemical bonds.

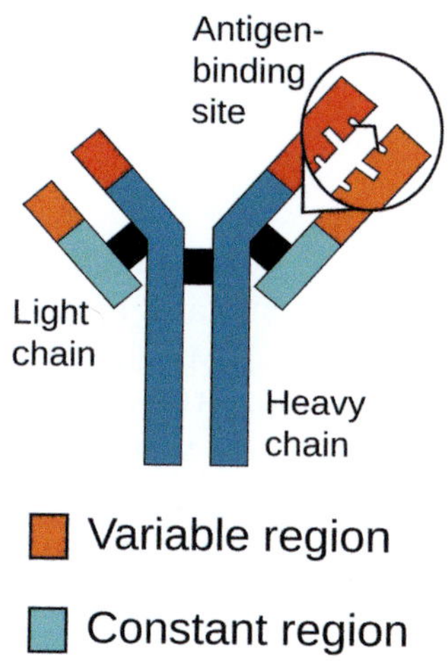

Figure 7.9. *Variable and constant domains of an antibody.*

Note: Variable (V) and constant (C) domains exist within the light (L) and heavy (H) chains of an antibody, or immunoglobulin, molecule. The folded shapes of the domains are maintained by disulfide bonds (–S–S–).

Source: https://en.m.wikipedia.org/wiki/File:Antibody_chains.svg.

Constant (C) and variable (V) are the two regions that make up each arm of the antibody, which consists of the heavy and light chains. These regions are identified based on similarity in amino acid sequences; that is, constant regions are found in all antibody molecules belonging to the same class (IgG, IgM, IgA, IgD, or IgE), whereas variable regions exhibit significant variation in amino acid sequences between antibody molecules. This makes sense since the antibody-binding site's distinct shape is determined by the variable regions. The constant regions of heavy chains make up the entire molecule's tail, which is free of antigen binding (Figure 7.9).

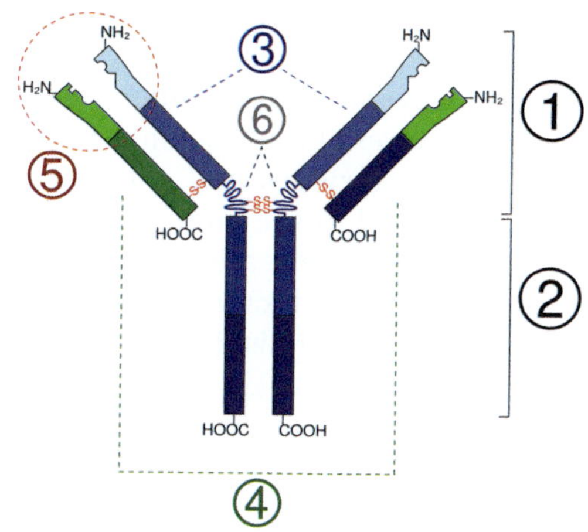

Figure 7.10. *Diagram of the hinge region of an antibody molecule.*

Source: By Y_tambe – Y_tambe's file, CC BY-SA 3.0, https://commons.wikimedia.org/w/index.php?curid=1573513.

The variable and constant regions of the light and heavy chains are structurally folded into domains, which serve as functional units. Each light chain consists of one constant domain (C_L) and one variable domain (V_L). Each heavy chain consists of one variable domain (V_H) and three or four constant domains (CH_1, CH_2, CH_3, CH_4). The unique biological characteristics of immunoglobulins are attributed to the H-chain constant domains, excluding CH_1, which form the "tail" of the Y-shaped molecule. These characteristics include the ability to bind to specific antigenic determinants. Once the antigen is bound to the antibody, its fate is determined by the antibody's tail (Figure 7.10).

7.2.4. Classes of Immunoglobulins

Given that these segments vary among immunoglobulins, the term "constant region" is a little misleading. Instead, they share many characteristics with large groups. A class of immunoglobulins is defined as having all of the same fundamental types of constant domains in their H chains. IgG, IgM, IgA, IgD, and IgE are the five primary classes; some of these contain several unique subclasses. The structural differences of the H chains determine the unique characteristics and roles of each class. To further add to the immense diversity of immunoglobulins, there are two basic types of L chains: lambda and kappa chains. Either of these chains can be linked to any of the H chain classes (Figure 7.11).

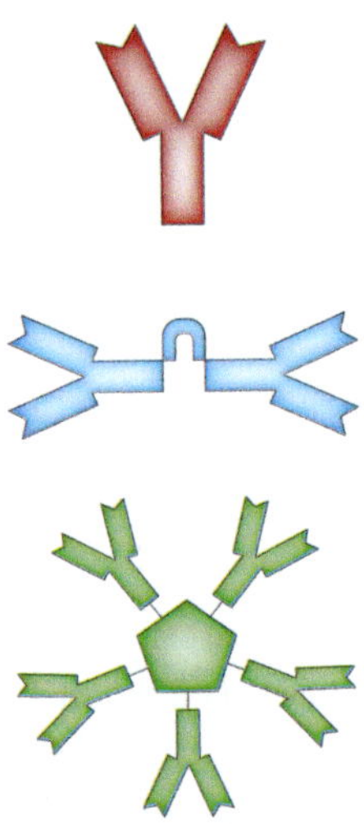

Figure 7.11. *Classes of antibodies. The five main classes of antibodies (immunoglobulins): IgG, IgA, IgD, IgE, and IgM.*

Source: By Martin Brändli (brandlee86) - Own work, CC BY-SA 2.5, https://commons.wikimedia.org/w/index.php?curid=560511.

7.2.4.1. IgG

The most prevalent type of immunoglobulin is called IgG. Blood and tissue fluids contain the highest concentrations of this substance. Every IgG molecule has two identical antigen-binding sites because it is made up of the basic four-chain immunoglobulin structure, which consists of two identical H chains and two identical L chains (either kappa or lambda). IgG is divided into four subclasses, each having unique biological characteristics but only slight variations in their H chains. Since IgG is the only type of immunoglobulin that can pass through the placenta, it offers the growing fetus some level of immune protection. These molecules are also secreted into breast milk and can enter an infant's bloodstream after ingestion, where they provide immunity.

7.2.4.2. IgM

The most prevalent form of immunoglobulin to be found on the surface of B cells as the antigen receptor is IgM, the first class of immunoglobulin produced by developing B cells. Five of the fundamental Y-shaped units come together to form a big pentamer molecule with 10 antigen-binding sites when IgM is secreted from the cells. The ability of this big antibody molecule to adhere to antigenic determinants found on the outer coats of bacteria is especially strong. Agglutination, or the clumping together of microorganisms, is the result of this IgM attachment.

7.2.4.3. IgA

The primary antibody class present in a variety of bodily secretions, such as saliva, tears, intestine and respiratory secretions, and colostrum—the first milk secreted by nursing mothers—is IgA. There is not much IgA in the serum. B cells found in the body's mucous membranes produce IgA. To enable the newly formed IgA molecule to be secreted across epithelial cells that line various ducts and organs, two IgA molecules are joined together and linked to a specific protein. Despite the fact that IgG is the most prevalent class of immunoglobulin, the body produces more IgA every day than any other class of antibody. IgA is present in smaller amounts at all times due to its less stability than IgG.

7.2.4.4. IgD

Most B cells, although not all of them, have IgD molecules on their surface during their initial development. However, only a small amount of this IgD is released into the bloodstream. The exact role of IgD is still unknown, although it may play a part in determining whether antigens activate B cells.

7.2.4.5. IgE

IgE is produced in minimal quantities by a small percentage of B cells and can be found in the blood. Similar to IgG, each IgE molecule consists of a single four-chain unit and possesses two antigen-binding sites. However, unlike IgG, each of its H chains contains an additional constant domain (CH4), which grants IgE the unique ability to bind to the surface of mast cells and basophils. When antigens attach to these bound IgE molecules, the cell is stimulated to release chemicals involved in allergic reactions, such as histamines. IgE antibodies also contribute to the defense against parasite infections.

7.2.5. Normal Production of Antibody

The blood levels of immunoglobulin, which indicate the equilibrium between the ongoing degradation of these proteins and their production, are generally fairly constant in most individuals. IgG (including its subclasses) is present in approximately four times the amount of IgA, 10–15 times that of IgM, 300 times that of IgD, and 30,000 times that of IgE. Undoubtedly, the continuous response to antigenic stimulation accounts for a portion of the normal production of immunoglobulin. However, even animals raised in environments completely devoid of microbes and their byproducts produce significant, albeit smaller, amounts of immunoglobulin. Therefore, a large portion of immunoglobulin must be the result of all B cells that are, in a sense, "ticking over," even in the absence of specific stimulation. Consequently, it should come as no surprise that traces of antibodies that react with antigenic determinants—to which an animal has never been exposed—that are recognized by cells that have receptors can be found using incredibly sensitive techniques.

Any one of the constant-region classes can be used by any B cell to create the immunoglobulin that they secrete. As mentioned above, the majority secrete IgM when first stimulated. While some continue in this manner, others eventually begin producing IgG, IgA, or IgE. Memory B cells produce IgG or IgA right away because they are specifically trained to react to repeated infections by a particular antigen. The exact factors that control the ratio of one class of antibody to another are unclear. The type and location of the antigen's deposition, for instance, can affect the production of IgE (parasites, for example), and the release of cytokines by T cells locally is evidently a mediating factor in this process.

7.2.6. T-Cell Antigen Receptors

7.2.6.1. Structure of the T-Cell Receptor

Only on the cell membrane are T-cell antigen receptors present. Due to this, isolating T-cell receptors in the laboratory was a challenging task, and their discovery did not occur until 1983. T-cell receptors are composed of two polypeptide chains. The most common type of receptor is known as alpha-beta, which consists of two distinct chains: alpha and beta. The less prevalent variety is the gamma-delta receptor, which is composed of one gamma chain and one delta chain. A single T cell can have up to 20,000 different alpha-beta or gamma-delta receptor molecules on its membrane surface (Figure 7.12).

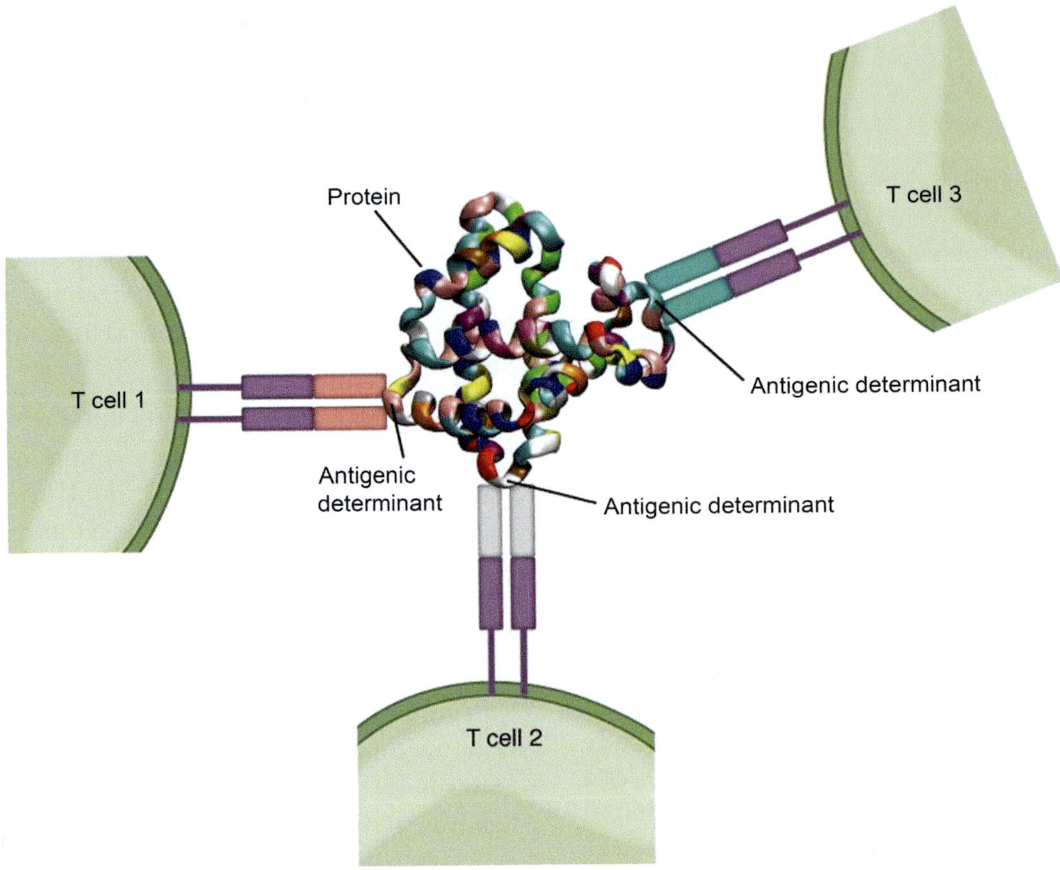

Figure 7.12. *The basic structure of a typical T-cell antigen receptor.*

Source: https://courses.lumenlearning.com/suny-ap2/chapter/the-adaptive-immune-response-t-lymphocytes-and-their-functional-types/.

A portion of the T-cell receptor molecule extends from the cell surface into the surrounding tissue, while the remainder of the molecule is embedded in the cell's membrane. Each chain has two folded domains: a constant domain and a variable domain, arranged similarly to antibody molecule chains. Additionally, the variable domains of the chains form an antigen-binding site, just as they do in the structure of antibodies. In contrast to the basic antibody molecule, which has two antigen-binding sites, the T-cell receptor only has one.

There are numerous structural parallels between T-cell receptors and antibodies. It follows that the arrangement of the genes encoding T-cell receptor chains is comparable to that of immunoglobulin genes. There are parallels between the processes that T cells employ to produce T-cell diversity and the ones that B cells use to produce antibody diversity. These similarities imply that both systems descended from an earlier, more basic recognition system.

7.2.7. Function of the T-Cell Receptor

T cell receptors and B cell receptors have different functions, despite their structural similarities. The distinct functions that B and T cells perform within the immune system are a result of these functional differences. T cells are unable to attach to free-floating antigens, but B cells can secrete antibodies to antigens found in blood and other bodily fluids. Instead, T cells attach themselves to segments of foreign proteins that are expressed on the exterior of bodily tissues. Consequently, once a virus infects a cell, it evades circulating antibodies and becomes susceptible to the defense mechanism of T cells.

However, the process by which fragments of foreign material end up on the exterior of a biological cell begins with the material's entry into the cell, which can occur through infection or phagocytosis. Subsequently, a portion of the invader is broken down by the host cell and presented on the cell's surface, where it binds to a protein on the cell surface. This cell-surface protein is one of the molecules encoded by the major histocompatibility complex (MHC) genes. MHC proteins are commonly referred to as HLA (human leukocyte antigens) because they were initially discovered on leukocytes, or white blood cells, in humans. The two main types of MHC molecules are class I molecules, found on the surfaces of almost all nucleated body cells or the majority of body cells, and class II molecules, found only on the surfaces of certain T cells, macrophages, and cells resembling macrophages, as well as the majority of B cells (Figure 7.13).

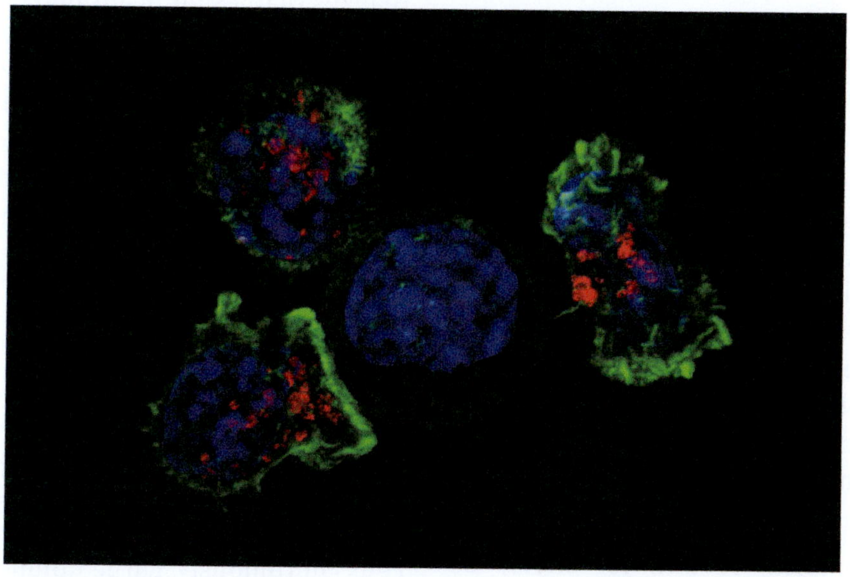

Figure 7.13. *A cytotoxic T-cell recognizes antigens on the surface of a cancer cell in the center, enabling the T-cell to bind to and kill the infected cell.*

Source: By The National Institutes of Health – https://www.flickr.com/photos/nihgov/20673870162/in/album-72157656657569008/, Public Domain, https://commons.wikimedia.org/w/index.php?curid=49182097.

Helper T cells and cytotoxic T cells are the two recognized subtypes of mature T cells. Regulatory T cells are a third subset of mature T cells that some scientists believe to exist. Class I

MHC molecules are recognized by some T cells, while class II molecules are bound by other T cells. Cytotoxic T lymphocytes eliminate bodily cells that could endanger the person, such as cancerous cells and germ-laden cells. Helper T cells assist in activating other white blood cells (lymphocytes and macrophages) by secreting a range of cytokines that mediate changes in other cells, rather than directly killing them. The operational mechanisms of regulatory T cells remain unclear. Helper T cells utilize class II MHC molecules on the surfaces of macrophages or B cells to identify foreign antigens and carry out their functions. Regulatory T cells and cytotoxic T cells typically target cells that have antigens linked to class I molecules. Cytotoxic and regulatory T cells are often grouped together due to their recognition of the same class of MHC molecule; however, populations of both cell types have been associated with class II molecules. Almost any cell in the body that has been infected by a pathogen can bind to cytotoxic T cells.

T cells possess an additional receptor on their surface known as a coreceptor, which enhances the attachment between the T cell and the target cell. Helper T cells have the CD4 coreceptor on their surface, which binds to class II MHC molecules, while the CD8 coreceptor on the surface of cytotoxic T cells recognizes class I MHC molecules. These auxiliary receptors strengthen the interaction between the T cell and the target cell.

The CD3 complex, or CD3 for short, is a collection of molecules that are linked to the T-cell receptor and are essential for T-cell activation. These molecules, known as signal transducers, facilitate the conversion of extracellular antigen-receptor binding into internal cellular signals. B-cell receptors and similar signal transducing molecules are also connected.

7.2.8. Life Cycle of T- and B-Lymphocytes

7.2.8.1. T-Cells

T-cell precursors do not yet express antigen receptors and are therefore unresponsive to stimulation from them when they depart the bone marrow in preparation for maturing in the thymus. T cells proliferate numerous times inside the thymus as they move through a network of thymus cells. They develop antigen receptors during multiplication and become helper or cytotoxic T cells. As was noted in the previous section, the function and the presence of the unique surface proteins, CD4 and CD8, allow these cell types to be identified despite having a similar appearance. When T cells proliferate in the thymus, they also tend to die there. This appears wasteful until one realizes that a significant percentage of antigen receptors produced randomly from various antigens are those that recognize self antigens, i.e., compounds found on the body's own components—and that developed lymphocytes possessing these receptors would target the body's own tissues.

The majority of these self-reactive T cells perish before leaving the thymus, allowing only the T cells with the ability to recognize foreign antigens to emerge. These are transported by the blood to the lymphoid tissues, where they can proliferate once more and engage in immune responses when given the right stimuli. In young animals, the thymus continues to produce T cells continuously. Large numbers of T cells are produced in humans prior to birth, but during adulthood, production gradually decreases and is significantly reduced in old age, by which point the thymus has shrunk and partially atrophied. However, because some of the T cells that have emerged from the thymus continue to divide and function for an extended period of time, cell-mediated immunity endures throughout life.

7.2.8.2. B-Cells

B-cell precursors are continually produced in the bone marrow throughout an individual's life. However, similar to T-cell generation, the rate at which B cells are produced decreases as a person ages. If B cells are not encouraged to mature, most of them will die. However, those that do mature can survive for a long time in lymphoid tissues, ensuring a constant supply of new B cells in the body. While B cells that can recognize self antigens are usually eliminated, they are not as effectively removed as self-reactive T cells. This means that some self-reactive B cells always remain in the B-cell population, alongside the majority that can identify foreign antigens. The reason that self-reactive B cells typically do not cause harm will be explained in the next section.

7.2.9. Activation of T- and B-Lymphocytes

A lymphocyte may encounter the antigen during its lifetime or it may not, but if it does, it can be stimulated to proliferate into a large number of identical cells, known as clones. Since every cloned cell has the same antigen receptor as the original lymphocyte, they are all antigen-specific. One of the core concepts of immunology is the process known as clonal selection.

Clonal selection leads to the production of effector cells and memory cells. The relatively short-lived activated cells, called effector cells, provide protection to the body during an immune response. Activated T cells, including cytotoxic T cells and helper T cells, execute cell-mediated responses, while effector B cells, also known as plasma cells, release antibodies.

The primary immune response is the generation of effector cells in response to an antigen for the first time. At this stage, memory cells are also generated, but they remain inactive. However, when the same antigen that initially triggered their formation is encountered again by the organism, the body initiates a second immune response, led by these long-lasting memory cells, which in turn generate a new population of effector and memory cells. Immunological memory, a secondary mechanism resulting from childhood exposure to the causative pathogen, is responsible for lifelong immunity to diseases like measles.

7.2.10. Activation of T-Cells

7.2.10.1. Helper-T-Cell Activation

Unlike cytotoxic T cells, helper T cells do not directly destroy diseased cells. Instead, they either stimulate B cells to secrete antibodies or assist in the activation of cytotoxic T cells and macrophages to attack infected cells. Interactions with antigen-presenting cells, such as macrophages, lead to the activation of helper T cells. Antigen-presenting cells engulf a microbe, partially break it down, and then release fragments of the microbe, known as antigens, on the cell surface, where they are presented alongside class II MHC molecules. Subsequently, the surface receptor of the helper T cell binds to the MHC-antigen complex. However, the helper T cell is not activated solely by this interaction. Another signal is required, which can be generated in two different ways: either through a cytokine that stimulates the cell or through a costimulatory response between the helper T cell's surface receptor protein, CD28, and the antigen-presenting cell's signaling protein, B7. The helper T cell is activated to proliferate and stimulate the relevant immune cell if it receives both the initial signal and one of the second signals. If the T cell only receives the initial signal, it may become anergic, meaning it is unable to respond to the antigen.

The fact that helper T cells are not a single type of cell but rather fall into two broad subpopulations—TH_1 and TH_2 cells—with radically different chemistry and functions complicates discussions of helper-T-cell activation. These populations can be identified by the secreted cytokines. The cytokines gamma interferon, tumor necrosis factor-beta, and interleukin-2 (IL-2) are predominantly produced by TH_1 cells, whereas TH_2 cells primarily produce IL-4, IL-5, IL-6, IL-9, IL-10, and IL-13 interleukins. While TH_2 cells mainly help to stimulate B cells to make antibodies, TH_1 cells play a major role in stimulating cell-mediated responses, which include cytotoxic T cells and macrophages.

After the initial activation steps, helper T cells produce various proteins including signaling proteins and cell-surface receptors. These signaling molecules are crucial for activating the helper T cell and determining its functional role and differentiation. For instance, the helper T cell creates IL-2 receptors on its surface and releases IL-2 molecules, which then bind to the receptors and prompt the cell to grow and multiply.

7.2.10.2. Results of Helper-T-Cell Activation

Helper T-cell activation generally results in the production of multiple T-cell cytokines and an increase in the number of helper T cells that are capable of recognizing a particular foreign antigen. Other effects of the cytokines include the activation and multiplication of regulatory or cytotoxic T cells that recognize the same antigen, which is facilitated by IL-2. In response, other cells expressing the foreign antigen in conjunction with class I MHC molecules, which are found on nearly all cells as previously mentioned, can be attacked and killed by cytotoxic T cells. Therefore, target cells that express antigens produced by viruses or bacteria that are growing within them can be attacked by cytotoxic T lymphocytes. Regulatory T cells are distinguished from cytotoxic T cells by their capacity to inhibit the activity of B cells and even helper T cells (possibly by eliminating them). Hence, regulatory T cells function to reduce the immune response and occasionally become dominant to totally suppress it.

7.2.10.3. Activation of B-Cells

When a B cell's receptor identifies and binds to an antigen, the B cell is activated. However, the majority of the time, stimulation by an activated helper T cell—the second factor mentioned above—is required for B-cell activation. An antigen can trigger the activation of a B cell that has already come into contact with the same antigen by a helper T cell. The process of activation involves a cell-to-cell interaction between the CD40 protein on the surface of B cells and the CD40 ligand, a protein that is present on the surface of activated helper T cells. Cytokines, which the helper T cell also secretes, have the ability to interact with B cells and stimulate them further. T-dependent antigens are those that elicit a response in this way, which is the standard mechanism of B-cell activation.

T-dependent antigens predominate. On the other hand, some can activate B cells without the assistance of T cells. Typically, the T-independent antigens are large polymers with repeated antigenic determinants. Bacteria's long, tail-like flagella and outer coats are frequently composed of these polymers. According to immunologists, the high concentration of identical T-independent antigens generates a stimulus that is sufficiently potent to avoid the need for additional helper T cell stimulation.

When exposed to antigens, B cells replicate into identical cells that produce antibodies. These B cells are then encouraged by cytokines to transform into plasma cells, which generate antibodies. Each plasma cell has the ability to release thousands of immunoglobulin molecules every minute and sustain this production for days. The specific antibody is then released into the bloodstream in large quantities. While the initial surge of antibody production wanes after the stimulation is gone (such as after recovering from an infection), some antibodies remain in the body for months following.

The described process occurs within circulating B lymphocytes, specifically among memory B cells in germinal centers where few T cells are found. When memory cells with highly effective receptors encounter antigens, they multiply extensively in a different activation process. These memory cells do not secrete antibodies but instead remain in tissues and circulation for extended periods. If memory B cells encounter the same antigen with the help of T cells, they quickly divide to form activated cells that produce specific antibodies and more memory cells. The initial group of memory cells "remembers" the initial antigen contact, allowing for a rapid response if reinfected. This response leads to a rapid increase in protective antibodies, preventing illness from taking hold, particularly in cases of microbial reinfection.

7.2.11. Antibody-Mediated Immune Mechanisms

7.2.11.1. Protective Attachment to Antigens

The simple attachment of antibodies can neutralize a wide range of harmful microorganisms and toxins. Certain dangerous bacteria, like those that cause tetanus and diphtheria, for instance, release toxins that damage vital body cells. Such toxins are neutralized by antibodies, particularly IgG, when they combine with them. All viruses, as well as certain bacteria and protozoa, are among the numerous infectious microorganisms that reside within human cells and are also vulnerable to simple antibody attachment. These pathogens possess unique molecules that enable them to adhere to the host cells and pierce and infiltrate them. To stop invasion, antibodies can attach themselves to these molecules. Furthermore, antibody attachment is capable of immobilizing bacteria and protozoans with whip-like flagella. In these situations, antibodies do not eradicate or kill the microorganisms; instead, they provide protection by joining forces with the repeating protein units that comprise these structures. The complement system plays a major role in the phagocytosis—the process by which granulocytes and macrophages actually destroy microbes—that takes place during this process.

7.2.11.2. Activation of the Complement System

More than 30 proteins are referred to as complements when they work together to strengthen the body's other defense systems. Both liver cells and macrophages produce complement proteins in various tissues. The majority of these proteins are found in an inactive state in the blood and other bodily fluids. They become active in a sequential manner: the first protein in the pathway activates the other complement proteins, which then activate the subsequent proteins in turn (Figure 7.14).

The main function of complement proteins is to aid in the destruction of pathogens by piercing their outer membranes (cell lysis) or by making them more attractive to phagocytic cells such as macrophages (a process known as opsonization). Some complement components also promote inflammation by stimulating cells to release histamine and by attracting phagocytic cells to the site of infection.

Recall that complement has a non-specific action. Complement proteins do not interact with antigen-binding sites and are not recognized by them. Complement proteins actually most likely evolved before antibodies. Numerous species share similar complement functions, and when corresponding components from one species are introduced into another, they can perform the same functions. The complement system is clever because it allows antibodies to react with antigens in a way that produces the same biological effects regardless of their specificity.

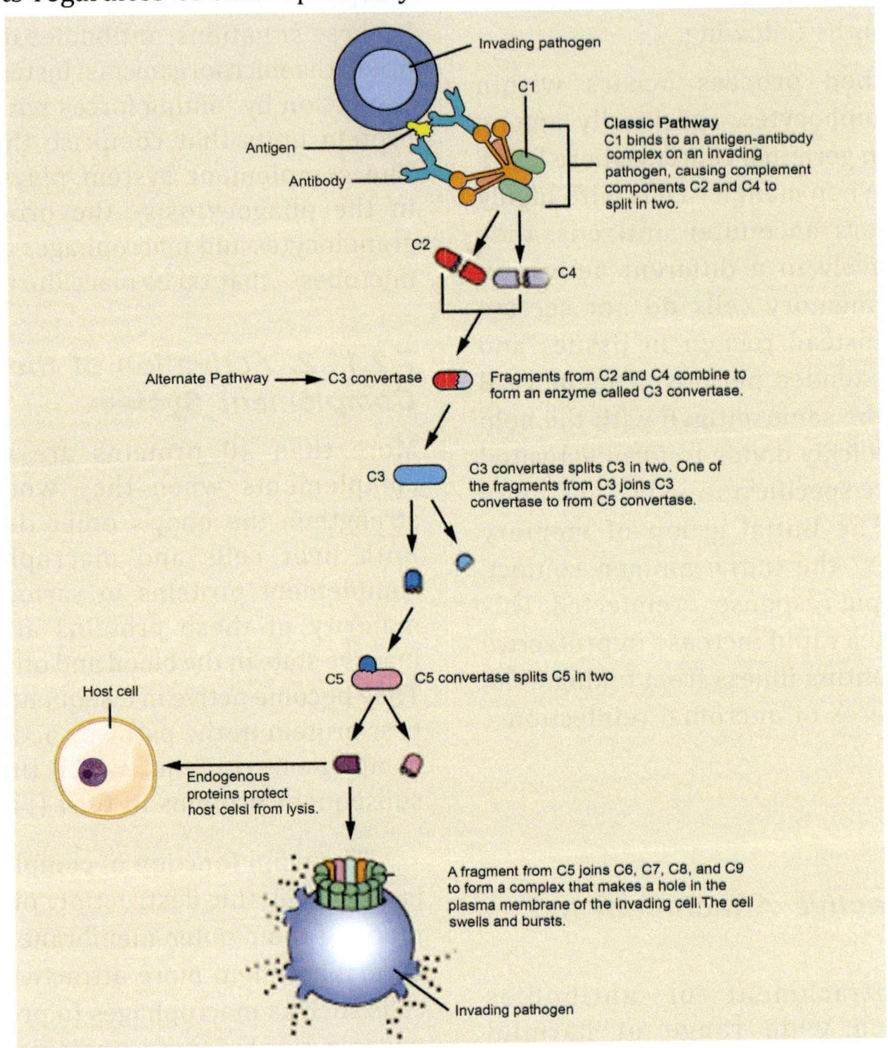

Figure 7.14. *Pathways of complement activation.*

Source: https://courses.lumenlearning.com/wm-biology2/chapter/complement-system/.

Immunologists initially believed that antigen-antibody complexes were the only substances that could activate the complement system. However, subsequent research revealed that other substances, such as a microorganism's surface components alone, could also cause complement activation. There are thus two complement activation pathways: the classical pathway, which was the first to be identified and is triggered by antigen-antibody complexes, and the alternative pathway, which can be activated by a variety of other factors such as invasive pathogens or tumor cells. (It is likely that this pathway evolved before the classical pathway, so the term "alternative" is a bit misleading. The order of discovery is reflected in the nomenclature, not the age of the evolutionary pathways.) The initial stages of the cascades of the classical and alternative pathways are made up of distinct protein components, but ultimately both pathways converge to activate the same complement components, which eradicate and destroy invasive pathogens.

The most effective immunoglobulins to activate the classical complement pathway are IgM and IgG, which are also the most abundant. However, antibodies must bind to antigens (the previously mentioned antigen-antibody complex) in order for activation to take place. Complement is not activated by free antibodies. The first complement protein in the pathway, C1, needs to interact with a bound immunoglobulin in order to initiate the cascade. C1 specifically interacts with the Y portion of the bound antibody molecule, which is its tail, i.e., the portion of the antibody that is nonspecific and does not bind to an antigen. Following its binding to the antibody, C1 is cleaved, which causes C1 to become active, split, and activate the subsequent complement component in the series. The next proteins in the pathway undergo this process again until the complement protein C3, which is the most prevalent and physiologically significant part of the complement system, is activated. This is the point at which the alternative and classical complement pathways converge: at the cleavage of the C3 molecule, resulting in the production of C3b, the large active form of C3, and C3a.

C3b carries out several functions:

1. The activation of subsequent steps in the cascade leads to the formation of a ringlike structure known as the membrane attack complex, resulting in lysis (bursting) of the target cell. This complex, composed of complement proteins C5 through C9, inserts itself into the membrane of the invading pathogen, creating a pore through which the cell contents leak out, ultimately causing cell death.
2. C3b has the ability to combine with another protein, converting more C3 protein into C3b.
3. Additionally, C3b can initiate the alternative pathway of complement activation.
4. However, the most significant outcome of C3b production is the deposition of numerous C3b molecules on the surface of the invading pathogen, a process called opsonization. This opsonization makes the microorganism more attractive to phagocytic cells such as macrophages and neutrophils. The phagocytes recognize and bind to the C3b molecule on the pathogen's surface through receptors, thereby stimulating phagocytosis. The microbe is subsequently destroyed by the digestive enzymes present in the phagocytes. If the microbes manage to evade immediate destruction and reach the bloodstream or organs such as the liver, spleen, or bone marrow, they can become coated with antibody and complement, leading to ingestion by phagocytes.

During complement activation, the release of small protein fragments serves as potent pharmacological agents that contribute to inducing an inflammatory response. These fragments attract granulocytes and monocytes, as well as trigger the release of histamine from mast cells and basophils, thereby increasing blood vessel permeability.

Thus, when a microbe enters the body, damage to its outer membrane may cause the entire complement sequence to be activated and the microbe to be killed if antibodies reactive with its surface are already present (or if the microorganism activates complement without the assistance of antibodies, through the alternative complement pathway). This mechanism is important even though it only works with certain large viruses and bacteria without protective coats. Recurrent bacterial infections can occur in individuals deficient in C3, which prevents them from completing the subsequent steps in the complement sequence.

It is evident that if the consequences of this physiologically significant series of events extended beyond the site of antigen invasion, they might cause more harm than good. Fortunately, if the active intermediates at any point in the complement sequence are unable to trigger the subsequent step, inhibitors quickly deactivate or eliminate them. This restricts the activation to the specific location within the body that requires it, with very few exceptions.

7.2.11.3. Activation of Killer Cells

Antigen-antibody complexes on certain cells are not compatible with complement because their antibody molecules are positioned widely apart on the cell surface or belong to a class of antibodies that do not readily activate the complement system (e.g., IgG and IgE, IgA, and IgD). Some cells are impermeable to activated complement because their outer membranes are extremely durable or rapidly repairable. Some are still too large for phagocytes to engulf. However, killer cells found in lymphoid tissues and blood can target these cells. The receptors on killer cells, which can be either natural killer cells or cytotoxic T cells, attach to the IgG antibody molecule's tail—the part that does not bind to antigen. Once attached, killer cells cause the target cell to swell and rupture by introducing a protein known as perforin. Killer cells help eliminate bodily cells infected by viruses and certain parasites, but they do not damage bacteria.

7.2.11.4. Other Antibody-Mediated Mechanisms

There is a slight variation in the protection provided by IgA antibodies, which are carried to the surface of passageways lined with mucous membranes. The respiratory tract and gut lining do not contain complement proteins; hence, complement activation is not involved. Here, the primary immune defense mechanism is the combination of IgA with microbes to prevent them from penetrating the lining's cells. Subsequently, the bound microbes are eliminated from the body. Additionally, it appears that IgA regulates certain forms of cell-mediated immunity.

IgE antibodies also operate through distinct mechanisms. As previously mentioned, the majority of IgE molecules bind to specific receptors on basophils and mast cells. Instead of inducing antigen ingestion, the interaction between antigens and IgE antibodies on these cells triggers the release of pharmacologically active chemical contents from granules. The chemicals released often dislodge large multicellular parasites such as hookworms, while also causing sudden increased permeability of local blood vessels, adhesion and activation of platelets (blood cell fragments that initiate clotting), release of their own active agents, contraction of smooth muscle in the gut or respiratory tubes, and secretion of fluids. Eosinophil granulocytes and IgE are particularly effective in eliminating parasites like flatworms that cause schistosomiasis. Eosinophils adhere to the IgE-bound worms and release substances from their granules that degrade the parasite's robust outer layer. Consequently, IgE antibodies appear to play a unique protective role against larger parasites, despite the potential issues they may cause when reacting with otherwise harmless antigens.

7.2.11.5. Transfer of Antibodies From Mother to Offspring

Unless, extremely rarely, a newborn animal contracts the infection while still inside its mother's womb, it does not have the opportunity to naturally develop protective antibodies. However, it is born into an environment that is identical to that of its mother, containing every possible microbiological invader to which she is exposed. The fetus has few or none of its mother's lymphocytes, despite having elements of innate immunity. In most cases, the placenta prevents the mother's lymphocytes from entering the uterus, where they would recognize the fetal tissues as foreign antigens and trigger an immune response similar to rejecting an incompatible organ transplant.

In many species, a representative sample of the mother's antibodies crosses the placenta. This occurs based on the structure of the placenta, which varies between species. During the second two-thirds of pregnancy in humans, maternal IgG antibodies cross the placenta and enter the fetal bloodstream, but not those of other immunoglobulin classes. Similar transfer occurs in many rodents, but primarily across the yolk sac.

Because the placentas of horses and cattle have more layers of cells than those of other animals, no antibodies are transferred during fetal life, and the resulting newborn lacks any components of specific immunity. However, there is another mechanism that compensates for this shortcoming. Colostrum, or early milk, is highly rich in antibodies, primarily IgA but also some IgM and IgG. In the first few days of life, the newborn mammal can absorb these intact proteins directly into the bloodstream from the digestive tract. Thus, drinking colostrum is necessary for young horses and cattle and somewhat less so for other mammals. Since foods other than milk contain proteins and other antigens that are also absorbed intact and may function as immunogens that the developing animal would become allergic to, the digestive tract's ability to absorb intact proteins must not last longer than one or two weeks. Despite its resistance to digestion, milk's IgA can continue to function in the gut after its complete absorption into the bloodstream has ceased. IgA is also abundant in human colostrum, with the highest concentration occurring right after birth. A newborn is as protected as its mother once it has received its full dose of maternal antibodies. This implies that the infant will also be unprotected if the mother has not grown immune to a specific infection. Because of this, a doctor might advise a prospective mother to get vaccinated against tetanus and other illnesses. However, because the immunizing agent can cross the placenta and cause serious fetal complications, it is necessary to avoid actively immunizing pregnant women against certain viral diseases like rubella [German measles].

The maternal antibodies that are passively transferred are highly significant, although their effects are transient. As the animal matures, the maternal antibodies in its bloodstream gradually lose their potency due to regular metabolic breakdown. In fact, it is during the early stages of growth that young mammals become more vulnerable to infection than they are immediately after birth, as the active development of acquired immunity is a slow and gradual process. At times, there can be adverse effects from the transfer of maternal antibodies while the fetus is still developing. Erythroblastosis fetalis, also known as hemolytic disease of the newborn, serves as a well-known example of this phenomenon. It is a condition in which the mother's antibodies destroy the child's red blood cells in the final stages of pregnancy and the initial few days after delivery. The most severe form of erythroblastosis fetalis is Rh hemolytic disease, which occurs when:

1. The fetus is Rh-positive, meaning its red blood cells carry an antigen known as the Rh factor.
2. The mother is Rh-negative, indicating that her red blood cells lack the Rh factor.

3. The mother's immune system has been previously activated against the Rh antigen, typically resulting from exposure to fetal cells during the birth of an earlier Rh-positive baby or a transfusion of Rh-positive blood.

Anti-Rh antibody injections can be administered to the mother shortly after the delivery of an Rh-positive infant to prevent Rh hemolytic disease. By eradicating any Rh-positive fetal cells in the mother's bloodstream, this antibody prevents activation of the mother's immune system in the event that she conceives another Rh-positive fetus.

7.2.12. Cell-Mediated Immune Mechanisms

T cells play crucial and distinct roles in defending against antigens that have evaded or circumvented antibody defenses, in addition to their cooperation with B cells that secrete specific antibodies. Immunologists have long known that antibodies do not always provide protection against viral infections, as many viruses can spread directly from one cell to another without encountering antibodies in the bloodstream. Furthermore, it is well-established that individuals with immunodeficiency are not overly susceptible to viral infections but are highly vulnerable to bacterial infections. In such cases, cell-mediated immunity offers protection by eliminating bodily cells that harbor actively growing viruses or other intracellular parasites, such as the bacteria responsible for leprosy and tuberculosis. This process deprives microorganisms of their growth medium and exposes them to antibodies.

Cell-mediated immunity operates through two mechanisms, which are discussed in the section on Activation of T and B lymphocytes. Activated helper T cells release cytokines, particularly gamma interferon, which significantly enhances the ability of macrophages to eliminate ingested microbes. This can tip the balance against microbes that would otherwise be resistant to destruction. Gamma interferon also stimulates natural killer cells. The second mechanism of cell-mediated immunity involves cytotoxic T lymphocytes. These cells bind to target cells displaying relevant antigens on their surface, especially those produced by emerging viruses, causing enough damage to infected cells to induce their death.

Multiple mechanisms exist for cytotoxic T cells to eliminate infected cells. The primary killing mechanism employed by a specific cytotoxic T cell is contingent upon several costimulatory signals. To put it briefly, cytotoxic T lymphocytes can eliminate their target cells by using pore-forming substances like perforins and different cytoplasmic granule components, or by causing the target cell to undergo a series of events that initiate a programmed cell death known as apoptosis. Granular cytotoxic T cells typically kill cells directly at the site of cell-to-cell contact by releasing the powerful contents of their cytotoxic granules. As a result, the target cell's cell membrane becomes permeable, allowing the cell to die and its contents to seep out. Nongranular cytotoxic T lymphocytes frequently cause cell death by activating the cell-surface protein Fas, which triggers apoptosis. The target cell's Fas protein is activated and sends a signal to the target cell's nucleus, starting the process of cell death, when a protein on the surface of the cytotoxic T cell interacts with it. In essence, the target cell kills itself, which also eliminates the virus inside the cell.

7.2.13. Immunity Against Cancer

Cancer cells are regular body cells that have undergone alterations to enable them to divide uncontrollably and disregard signals of restraint. Consequently, cancer cells group together to form tumors, which invade and colonize tissues before eventually impairing organ function and resulting in death. In the early 20th century, pioneering immunologist Paul Ehrlich noted that although immune mechanisms eliminate aberrant cells, the massive cell division and multiplication that occurs during fetal life must provide numerous opportunities for such cells to emerge and proliferate. In the 1950s and 1960s, a number of immunologists proposed the theory of immune surveillance. This theory suggests that T-cell-mediated immunity developed as a specific defense against cancer cells and that T cells constantly patrol the body, searching for abnormal body cells that carry antigens on their surface, which are not found on healthy body cells. Despite its compelling elements, the immunosurveillance theory remains just a theory and a contentious one at that.

There is no doubt that the immune system can occasionally differentiate between cancerous and normal cells, even though the immune system's function in preventing cancer has not been fully understood. It is clear from the study of tumor immunology that antigens carried by cancer cells differ from those on healthy cells. Tumor-associated antigens, which are expressed abnormally on both normal and cancer cells, and tumor-specific antigens, which are only present on cancer cells and not on their counterparts, are the two main categories of tumor antigens that immunologists distinguish between. These antigens are produced in excess on cancer cells and have been demonstrated to elicit an immune response in both situations, albeit one that may not be potent enough to eradicate the tumor.

Why does a tumor continue to grow if an immune response against it is induced? Through animal experiments, a number of mechanisms have been identified that allow tumors to avoid recognition and destruction by the immune system:

1. The surfaces of cancer cells may lose antigens that are recognizable by the immune system.
2. Cancer cells may lose all class I MHC molecules from their surface, which prevents cytotoxic T cells from recognizing the cells.
3. Some cancer cells produce immunosuppressive chemicals that can inhibit T cells directly or that can activate regulatory T cells.
4. Some cancer cells shed their antigens, and these antigens, which are released into the bloodstream, can bind to the receptors on cytotoxic T cells. This binding can hinder the ability of T cells to attach to cancer cells and eliminate them.
5. Certain cancer cells can evade immune responses by growing rapidly or forming dense masses that prevent immune cells from making contact with most of them.

If other dysfunctions of the immune system, such as immunological deficiency and immune suppression, are not addressed, cancer can develop and spread more rapidly. Patients with immunodeficiency disorders and transplant recipients who have been on immunosuppressive medication for a long time are at a higher risk of developing specific cancers. For example, individuals with acquired immunodeficiency syndrome (AIDS) are more susceptible to virally-related cancers like Kaposi sarcoma. As immune responses weaken with age, the incidence of cancer also increases significantly. However, since genetic mutations associated with cancer also accumulate with age, impaired immune responses may not be the primary cause of cancer development in the elderly.

Extensive research has been conducted to develop potent cancer immunotherapies. One approach focuses on immunizing patients against the specific cancer that is developing within them. This method targets antigens that are unique to tumors and are present on cancer cells. Although these antigens are considered "foreign" and could potentially be recognized by the immune system, they are often modified versions of normal self antigens. Nevertheless, researchers are striving to create vaccines that can stimulate an immune response strong enough to eliminate the cancer.

Scientists have made significant progress in understanding how T-cells are activated and how the immune system is regulated, leading to the development of human monoclonal antibodies customized for treating certain types of cancer. For example, the identification of CTLA-4 as a molecule that suppresses immune responses against tumors paved the way for the creation of ipilimumab (Yervoy), an antibody approved by the FDA in 2011 to treat advanced melanoma. Similarly, the discovery of PD-1 as a negative regulator of the immune system on T cells led to the development of effective anti-PD-1 cancer immunotherapies.

7.2.14. Prophylactic Immunization

The artificial development of specific immunity, also known as "prophylactic vaccination," is a method that has dramatically reduced the incidence of pain and mortality caused by various infectious diseases. Prophylactic immunization can be categorized into two types: passive immunization, which provides protection by transferring preformed antibodies or lymphocytes from an individual who has already developed an immune response to the relevant antigen, and active immunization, which provides protection by administering a vaccine containing inactivated or dead forms of the pathogen or harmless live forms of the pathogen that stimulate the immune system to produce lymphocytes and antibodies against the pathogen or its toxins.

7.2.14.1. Passive Immunization

Passive immunization is employed in situations where the effects of an infectious agent or toxic substance are so rapid and severe that the individual is unable to mount an immune response on their own. In such cases, the administration of preformed antibodies can help combat the pathogen or toxin, potentially saving lives. This approach is used for individuals who have been bitten by venomous snakes or exposed to botulism, as well as those with advanced infections such as gas gangrene, tetanus, or diphtheria, where bacterial toxins have entered the bloodstream. It is also utilized in cases of rabid animal bites, although active vaccination is initiated simultaneously due to the slower spread of infection to the central nervous system. Passive immunization is employed as a temporary protective measure for individuals traveling to regions where hepatitis B is prevalent. Individuals with B-cell deficiencies, who are unable to produce antibodies on their own, can receive antibodies through passive immunization. Furthermore, as previously mentioned, the administration of anti-Rh antibodies via passive immunization can prevent erythroblastosis fetalis.

Human or non-human animal blood can be used to prepare protective immunoglobulins, mostly of the IgG class. Animals (such as horses or rabbits) that have already acquired a particular immunity to the relevant antigens produce these antiserums. This is why serum therapy was originally referred to as passive immunization. Human IgG is metabolized gradually in the recipient's body, with a halving of concentration occurring approximately every three weeks. This allows for the effective maintenance of antibody levels for two to three months. Due to the higher likelihood of triggering an immune response and causing serum sickness, IgG from other species is avoided whenever possible, and human antiserum is used instead.

7.2.14.2. Active Immunization

The objective of active immunization is to ensure that the body possesses an adequate number of T and B cells or antibodies that can respond to a potential toxin or infectious agent before the manifestation of the toxin or infection. Once primed, the immune system can either prevent the pathogen from spreading or rapidly activate the various defense mechanisms mentioned earlier to halt the infection or toxin.

Living microbes are not required to be present in the vaccines used for active immunization. It is crucial that these vaccines contain the necessary antigens to stimulate a protective response. These antigens should be provided in a harmless form that is persistent and present in sufficient quantity to trigger an immune response similar to that of a natural infection. Formaldehyde treatment can neutralize bacterial toxins, including those responsible for tetanus and diphtheria, without compromising their ability to function as immunogens. Toxoids, which are modified toxins, are typically administered by adsorbing them onto an inorganic gel. This approach enhances the probability of the toxoid being retained within a macrophage. Toxoids elicit effective and long-lasting immunity against bacterial toxins. In cases where immunization against multiple antigenic determinants is desired or when the important antigenic component is unknown, the entire microbe, killed in a way that does not significantly alter it, may be used. These so-called "killed" vaccinations are used to protect against influenza, typhoid, pertussis (whooping cough), and the plague, among other things. In other instances, scientists have developed attenuated (weaker) strains of viruses or bacteria. These attenuated vaccinations induce infection but do not result in the full range of disease signs and symptoms, as the infectious agent only slightly multiplies in the body and never returns to its virulent form. Using live microbes in these vaccines offers the most effective prophylactic, as they mimic a mild form of the natural infection. Examples of live vaccinations include the oral poliomyelitis vaccine, yellow fever, measles, rubella, and tuberculosis vaccinations. It is important to note that live vaccinations can cause the entire disease in individuals with immunological deficiencies, even though they are sufficiently attenuated for healthy individuals.

Although some vaccines are administered orally, the majority are given by injection. Mucosal vaccines, which are applied to mucosal surfaces such as the lining of the gut, nasal passages, or urogenital tract, may ultimately prove to be the most effective vaccinations due to their ability to stimulate IgA responses. Thanks to recombinant DNA technology, researchers can now immunize individuals against antigens from pathogenic microorganisms using modified bacteria and viruses that are safe for humans. This involves inserting a gene from a pathogenic organism, which codes for an antigen capable of triggering a protective immune response without causing the full-blown disease, into the DNA of a harmless microorganism. The microbe then immunizes the host by producing the protective antigen of the pathogen. This approach has led to the development of an effective oral cholera vaccine.

In some cases, a disease can arise from distinct strains of the same microorganism, each characterized by a unique antigenic determinant. In such situations, immunity against infection by other strains cannot be achieved through prophylactic immunization against any single strain or natural infection. For example, there are numerous virus strains that cause the common cold, but it is not feasible to vaccinate against all of them. However, when it comes to bacterial pneumonia caused by pneumococci, there are over 60 distinct strains, with certain strains being more prevalent than others. For individuals who are particularly vulnerable, a vaccine containing antigens from up to 14 of the most prevalent strains can be beneficial (Figure 7.15).

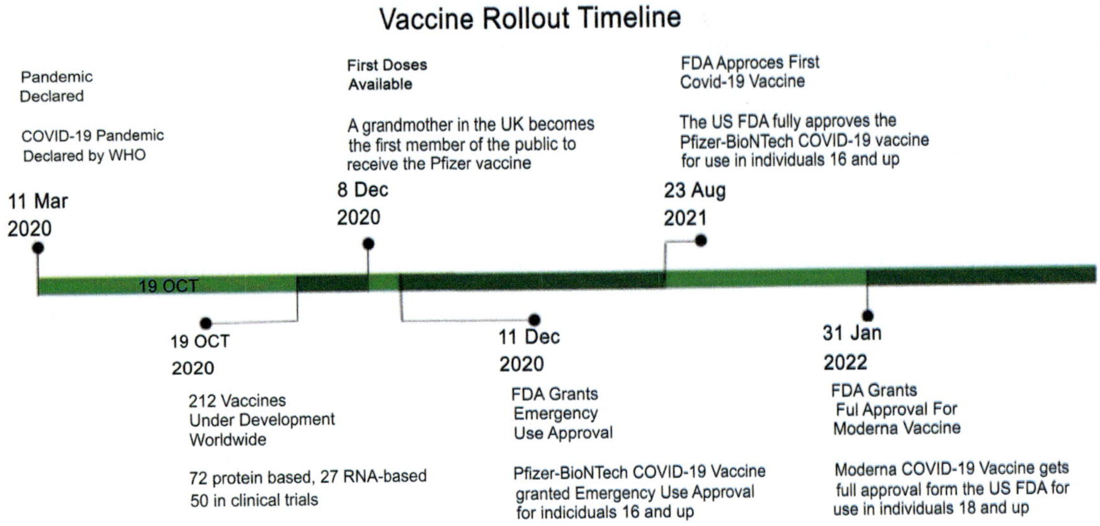

Figure 7.15. *A brief timeline of selected events related to the COVID-19 vaccine rollout.*

Source: Md Khairi, L. N. H., Fahrni, M. L., & Lazzarino, A. I., (2022). The race for global equitable access to COVID-19 vaccines. Vaccines. 10(8), 1306. https://doi.org/10.3390/vaccines10081306.

A Closer Look

Tonsil

Tonsils are small masses of lymphatic tissue located in the wall of the pharynx at the rear of the throat in humans and other mammals. In humans, the term is used to refer to three sets of tonsils, most commonly the palatine tonsils. These are a pair of oval-shaped masses protruding from each side of the oral pharynx behind the oral cavity. The exposed surface of each tonsil is marked by numerous pits that lead to deeper lymphatic tissue. Debris often gets trapped in the pits and causes inflammation, a condition known as tonsillitis.

The function of the palatine tonsils is believed to be associated with preventing infection in the respiratory and digestive tracts by producing antibodies that help eliminate infectious agents. However, the tonsils themselves frequently become infected, requiring surgical removal (tonsillectomy). Usually, children are more susceptible to tonsillitis than adults, as the tonsils tend to degenerate and decrease in size with age.

Another important pair of tonsils is the pharyngeal tonsils, commonly known as adenoids. These are diffuse masses of lymphatic tissue located on the upper wall of the nasal pharynx. Enlargement of these tonsils can obstruct nasal breathing, interfere with sinus drainage, and lead to sinus and middle ear infections. When nasal breathing is blocked, mouth breathing becomes necessary. Prolonged mouth breathing can exert pressure on the developing facial bones in children and may cause facial deformities. Surgical removal, often performed alongside a tonsillectomy, is frequently recommended for children. The adenoids tend to decrease in size during adulthood.

The third pair of tonsils are the lingual tonsils, which are aggregations of lymphatic tissue on the surface at the base of the tongue. The surface of these tonsils also has pits leading to lower lymphatic tissue, similar to the other two types of tonsils. However, these pits are effectively drained by small glands (mucous glands), and infection is rare.

Summary

- The immune system, a sophisticated collection of defensive mechanisms present in humans and other higher vertebrates, aids in the rejection of pathogens, or organisms that cause disease.
- The mucous membrane linings of the respiratory, gastrointestinal, and genitourinary tracts provide a mechanical barrier of constantly renewing cells, similar to the outer layer of skin but much softer.
- Leukocytes, or white blood cells, are the main type of scavenger cells found in all higher animals and many lower ones that eliminate infectious agents.
- The fully developed form of the monocyte, known as the macrophage, is the other primary category of scavenger cell. Monocytes, which circulate in the bloodstream but are generated in smaller quantities than granulocytes by bone marrow stem cells, bear resemblance to granulocytes.
- Natural killer cells eliminate the body's own cells that have either developed cancer or contracted a virus, rather than directly attacking foreign invaders.
- Lymphocytes are the cells responsible for the body's ability to recognize and respond to a vast array of different foreign substances, including those found in microbes.
- Bone marrow stem cells give rise to lymphocytes; these stem cells proliferate constantly, releasing immature lymphocytes into the circulation.
- The most prevalent form of immunoglobulin to be found on the surface of B cells as the antigen receptor is IgM, the first class of immunoglobulin produced by developing B cells.

References

1. Abbas, A. K., Lichtman, A. H., & Pillai, S., (2019). *Cellular and Molecular Immunology.* Elsevier.
2. Alberts, B., Johnson, A., Lewis, J., Raff, M., Roberts, K., & Walter, P., (2002). Molecular biology of the cell. *Garland Science.*
3. Arce-Sillas, A., Álvarez-Luquín, D. D., Tamaya-Domínguez, B., Gomez-Fuentes, S., Trejo-García, A., Melo-Salas, M., Cárdenas, G., et al., (2016). Regulatory T cells: Molecular actions on effector cells in immune regulation. *J. Immunol. Res., 2016,* 1720827.
4. Denson, L. A., (2013). The role of the innate and adaptive immune system in pediatric inflammatory bowel disease. *Inflamm. Bowel. Dis., 19*(9), 2011–2020.
5. Di Rosa, R., Pietrosanti, M., Luzi, G., Salemi, S., & D'Amelio, R., (2014). Polyclonal intravenous immunoglobulin: An important additional strategy in sepsis? *Eur. J. Intern. Med., 25*(6), 511–516.
6. Gack, M. U., & Diamond, M. S., (2016). Innate immune escape by Dengue and West Nile viruses. *Curr. Opin. Virol., 20*, 119–128.
7. Gu, M., (2018). Efficient differentiation of human pluripotent stem cells to endothelial cells. *Curr. Protoc. Hum. Genet., 98*(1), e64.
8. Hung, C. Y., Hsu, A. P., Holland, S. M., & Fierer, J., (2019). A review of innate and adaptive immunity to coccidioidomycosis. *Med. Mycol., 57*(Supplement_1), S85–S92.

9. Janeway, C. A., Travers, P., Walport, M., & Shlomchik, M., (2001). Immunobiology: The immune system in health and disease. *Garland Science.*

10. Lawrence, H., Mawdesley, A. E., Holland, J. P., Kirby, J. A., Deehan, D. J., & Tyson-Capper, A. J., (2016). Targeting toll-like receptor 4 prevents cobalt-mediated inflammation. *Oncotarget., 7*(7), 7578–7585.

11. Male, D., Brostoff, J., Roth, D., & Roitt, I., (2014). *Immunology* (8th edn.). Elsevier.

12. Man, K., Jiang, L. H., Foster, R., & Yang, X. B., (2017). Immunological responses to total hip arthroplasty. *J. Funct. Biomater., 8*(3).

13. McCusker, C., Upton, J., & Warrington, R., (2018). Primary immunodeficiency. *Allergy Asthma Clin. Immunol., 14*(Suppl 2), 61.

14. Murphy, K., & Weaver, C., (2016). Janeway's immunobiology. *Garland Science.*

15. Parham, P., (2014). *The Immune System* (4th edn.). Garland Science.

16. Paul, W. E., (2014). *Fundamental Immunology* (7th edn.). Lippincott Williams & Wilkins.

17. Pedraza-Sánchez, S., Méndez-León, J. I., Gonzalez, Y., Ventura-Ayala, M. L., Herrera, M. T., Lezana-Fernández, J. L., Bellanti, J. A., & Torres, M., (2018). Oral administration of human polyvalent IgG by mouthwash as an adjunctive treatment of chronic oral candidiasis. *Front Immunol., 9*, 2956.

18. Pellicciotta, M., Rigoni, R., Falcone, E. L., Holland, S. M., Villa, A., & Cassani, B., (2019). The microbiome and immunodeficiencies: Lessons from rare diseases. *J. Autoimmun., 98*, 132–148.

19. Roitt, I., Brostoff, J., & Male, D., (2014). *Immunology* (7th edn.). Wiley-Blackwell.

20. Surace, M., DaCosta, K., Huntley, A., Zhao, W., Bagnall, C., Brown, C., Wang, C., et al., (2019). Automated multiplex immunofluorescence panel for immuno-oncology studies on formalin-fixed carcinoma tissue specimens. *J. Vis. Exp.,* (143).

21. Valent, P., Akin, C., Bonadonna, P., Hartmann, K., Brockow, K., Niedoszytko, M., Nedoszytko, B., et al., (2019). Proposed diagnostic algorithm for patients with suspected mast cell activation syndrome. *J. Allergy Clin. Immunol. Pract., 7*(4), 1125–1133.e1.

22. Williamson, L. E., Flyak, A. I., Kose, N., Bombardi, R., Branchizio, A., Reddy, S., Davidson, E., et al., (2019). Early human B cell response to ebola virus in four U.S. survivors of infection. *J. Virol., 93*(8)

23. Yap, G. S., & Gause, W. C., (2018). Helminth infections induce tissue tolerance mitigating immunopathology but enhancing microbial pathogen susceptibility. *Front Immunol., 9*, 2135.

Chapter

HUMAN REPRODUCTIVE SYSTEM

8

Contents

Unit Introduction

Reproduction is the process by which organisms produce offspring, to put it simply. All living things are distinguished from nonliving things by this miracle, which unites them. However, while the reproductive system is necessary for the survival of a species, it is not necessary for the survival of an individual.

In the process of human reproduction, two types of sex cells, or gametes, are necessary. The male gamete, sperm, and the female gamete, a secondary oocyte (along with the first polar body and corona radiata), must unite in the female reproductive system to form a new individual. Both the male and female reproductive systems are essential for reproduction to take place. It is a common mistake to refer to a woman's gametic cell as an egg or ovum, as it is inaccurate. The female gamete must be fertilized by the male gamete before it can be considered an "ovum" or "egg."

The male and female reproductive systems have different shapes and structures, but they both have roles in the development, maintenance, and transportation of either oocytes or sperm. While the female's reproductive organs are fully contained within the pelvis, the male's genitals are located both inside and outside the pelvis.

Orientation and Directional Terms:

Term	Definition	Illustration
Spermatogenesis	Spermatogenesis is the process of sperm cell production. It involves the multiplication and differentiation of germ cells, leading to the production of spermatozoa in the seminiferous tubules.	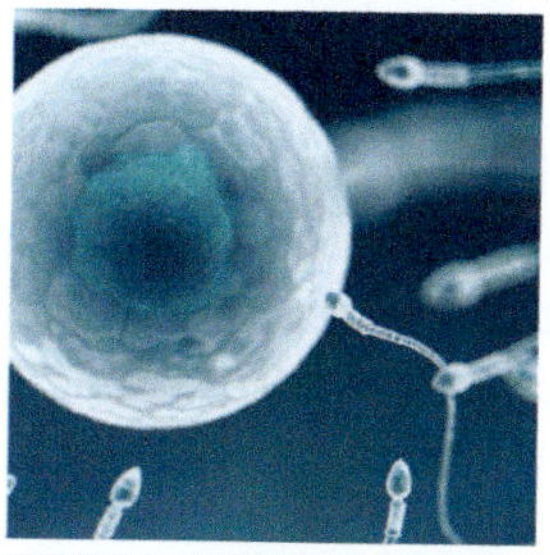
Oogenesis	Oogenesis is the type of gametogenesis through which ova, also called the female gametes, are formed. The produced female gamete is known as an ovum.	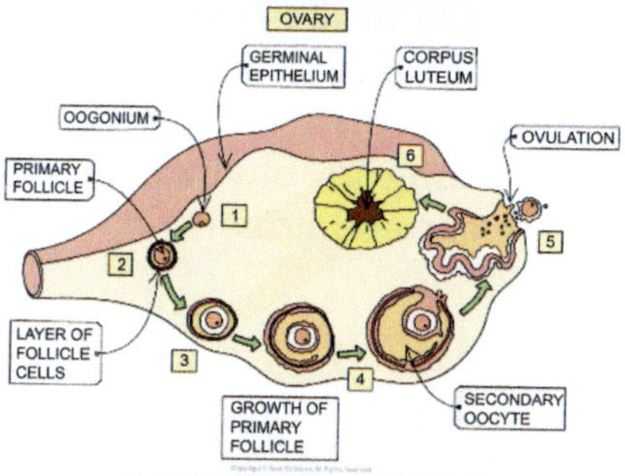
Epididymis	Epididymitis is an inflammation of the coiled tube, called the epididymis, at the back of the testicle.	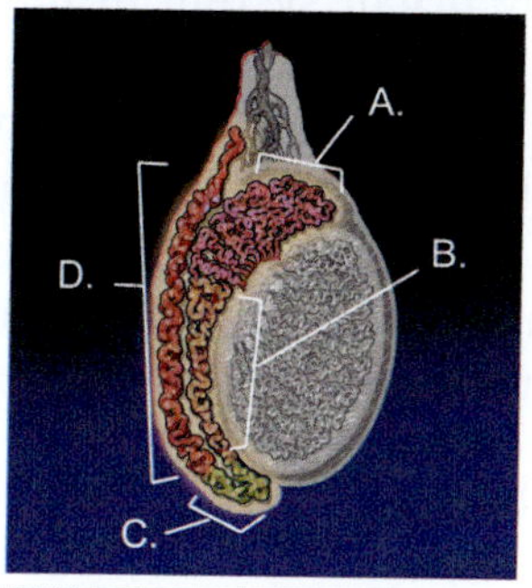
Seminal vesicles	The seminal vesicles are a pair of convoluted tubular accessory glands that lie behind the urinary bladder of male mammals.	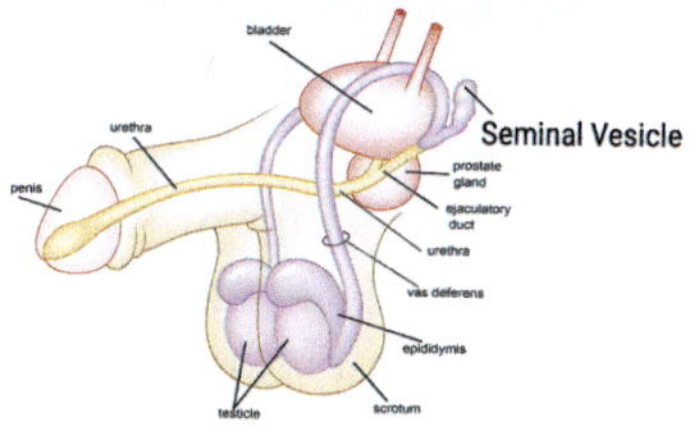
Prostate gland	The prostate gland is located just below the bladder in men and surrounds the top portion of the tube that drains urine from the bladder (urethra).	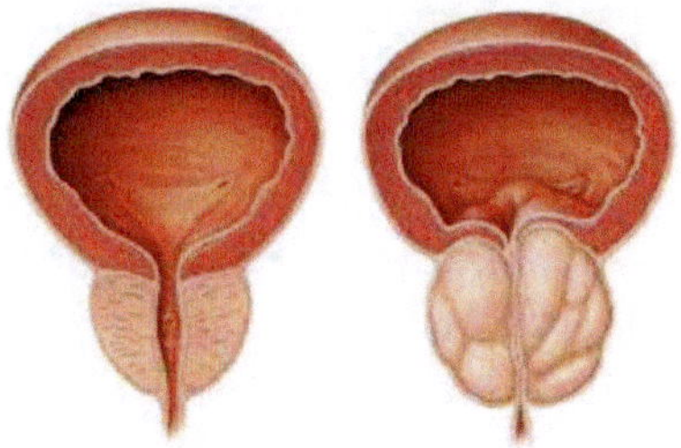

8.1. Reproductive System

The reproductive system in humans is responsible for the production and fertilization of gametes, such as sperm and eggs, as well as the development of a fetus. Both males and females have gonads that produce these gametes, which are haploid cells that combine during fertilization to form a diploid zygote. In addition to producing gametes, the gonads also produce sex hormones that regulate the development of sex organs, sexual maturation, and reproduction. Other organs in the reproductive system have various functions, including maturing gametes, transporting them to the fertilization site, and providing an environment for offspring development and growth.

8.1.1. Sex Differences in the Reproductive System

The only organ system in humans that differs noticeably between males and females is the reproductive system. Male and female embryos share the same basic structures that will give rise to the reproductive systems, but by the time they are born, the reproductive systems are distinct. How is this possible?

8.1.2. Sex Differentiation

Around the seventh week after conception in male embryos with XY chromosomes, a gene called SRY on the Y chromosome triggers the production of multiple proteins. These proteins stimulate undifferentiated gonadal tissue to become testes, which then release hormones like testosterone. These hormones induce further changes in the developing fetus, leading to the formation of a male reproductive system. In the absence of a Y chromosome, the embryo will develop ovaries that produce estrogen, resulting in the development of a female reproductive system (Figure 8.1).

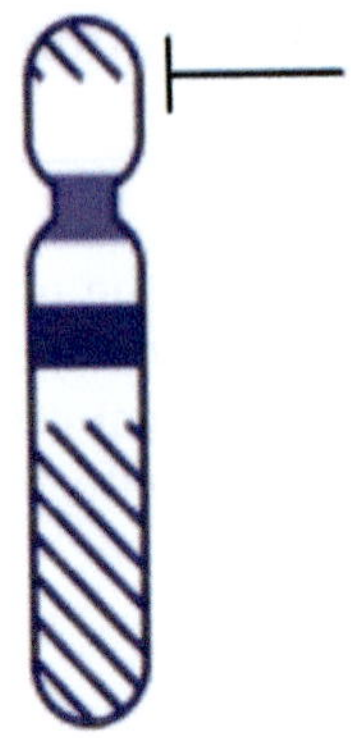

Figure 8.1. *The SRY gene on the short arm of the Y chromosome causes the undifferentiated gonads of an embryo to develop into testes. Otherwise, the gonads develop into ovaries.*

Source: https://bio.libretexts.org/@api/deki/files/16812/Screen_Shot_2019-03-29_at_9.41.42_PM.png?revision=1&size=bestfit&width=239&height=170.

8.1.3. Homologous Structures

In fetuses that are male or female, undifferentiated embryonic tissues give rise to distinct structures. Homologous structures are those that develop from the same tissues in both males and females. For instance, the embryo's undifferentiated gonads give rise to homologous structures like the testes and ovaries. Similarly, homologous structures derived from the same embryonic tissues are the penis and clitoris.

8.1.4. Sex Hormones and Maturation

The male and female reproductive systems are distinct from birth, but they are not fully developed and cannot produce gametes or sex hormones. It is during puberty that maturation of the reproductive system takes place, as hormones from the hypothalamus and pituitary gland signal the testes or ovaries to begin producing sex hormones once more. The primary sex hormones involved are testosterone and estrogen, which play a crucial role in the growth and maturation of the reproductive organs, rapid body growth, and the emergence of secondary sex characteristics like body and facial hair, as well as breast development.

8.1.5. Role of Sex Hormones in Transgender Treatment

Hormone therapy, whether feminizing or masculinizing, involves the use of external hormones to induce changes in physical appearance. It is a cost-effective and highly successful method for developing secondary sex characteristics, such as body hair or breast tissue, that align with an individual's gender identity. For many transgender individuals, hormone therapy is the initial, and sometimes sole, medical intervention pursued to attain a more masculine or feminine appearance. In certain cases, hormone therapy may be a prerequisite for undergoing surgical procedures. Transgender women typically take estrogen and anti-testosterone medications like cyproterone acetate and spironolactone, while transgender men are prescribed testosterone.

8.1.6. Male Reproductive System

Figure 8.2 illustrates the external structures comprising the male reproductive system. The scrotum, a sac of skin between the thighs, houses the two testes (singular: testis). Sperm and testosterone are both produced by the testes. The epididymis (plural: epididymes) is a coiled structure situated atop each testis. The maturation and storage of sperm occur in the epididymes. The urethra is located within the tubular organ known as the penis, which can become erect when an individual becomes sexually aroused. During sexual climax, sperm exit the body through the urethra (orgasm). This release of sperm is referred to as ejaculation.

In addition to these organs, the body also contains various internal ducts and glands. The ducts, such as the vas deferens, transport sperm from the epididymis to the urethra. Meanwhile, the glands, such as the prostate gland and seminal vesicles, produce fluids that contribute to semen. Semen is the fluid that carries sperm through the urethra and out of the body, providing substances that regulate pH levels and offer nutrients to support the sperm's energy (Table 8.1).

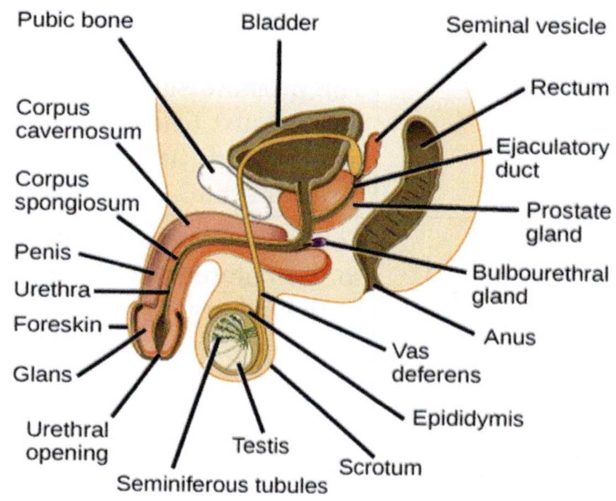

Figure 8.2. *The main organs of the male reproductive system.*

Note: Focus on the seminiferous tubules, testis, scrotum, epididymis, vas deferens, urethra, penis, and the glands that produce semen.

Source: https://courses.lumenlearning.com/wm-biology2/chapter/reproductive-system/.

Table 8.1. *The Major Components of the Male Reproductive System*

Components of the Male Reproductive System		
Structure	**Location and Description**	**Function**
Bulborethral glands (2)	Pea sized organs posterior to the prostate on either side of the urethra.	Secretion of gelatinous seminal fluid called pre-ejaculate. This fluid helps to lubricate the urethra for spermatozoa to pass through, and to help flush out any residual urine or foreign matter. (< 1% of semen).
Epididymis	Tightly coiled ducts lie just outside each testis, connecting the efferent ducts to the vas deferens.	Storage and maturation of sperm.
Penis	Three columns of erectile tissue: two corpora cavernosa and one corpus spongiosum. The urethra passes through the penis.	Male reproductive organ and also male organ of urination.
Prostate gland	The prostate surrounds the urethra just below the urinary bladder and can be felt during a rectal exam.	Stores and secretes a clear, slightly alkaline fluid constituting up to one-third of the volume of semen. Raises vaginal pH (25–30% of semen).
Seminal vesicles (2)	Convoluted structure attached to vas deferens near the base of the urinary bladder.	About 65-75% of the seminal fluid in humans originates from the seminal vesicles. It contains proteins, enzymes, fructose, mucus, vitamin C, flavins, phosphorylcholine, and prostaglandins. The high fructose concentrations provide nutrient energy for the spermatozoa as they travel through the female reproductive system.
Testes	Inside scrotum, outside of body.	Gonads that produce sperm and male sex hormones. Production of testosterone by Leydig cells in the testicles.
Urethra	Connects bladder to outside body, about 8 inches long.	A tubular structure that receives urine from the bladder and carries it to the outside of the body. It also serves as a passage for sperm.
Vas deferens	Muscular tubes connect the left and right epididymis to the ejaculatory ducts to facilitate the movement of sperm. Each tube measures approximately 30 cm in length.	During ejaculation, the smooth muscle in the vas deferens wall contracts, propelling sperm forward. Sperm is transferred from the vas deferens into the urethra, collecting fluids from accessory sex glands en route.

Source: https://courses.lumenlearning.com/wm-biology2/chapter/reproductive-system/.

8.1.7. Female Reproductive System

Figure 8.3 depicts the body structures that comprise the female reproductive system. These structures include the paired ovaries, which are small, oval organs that secrete estrogen and produce eggs. The two uterine tubes, also known as Fallopian tubes, originate near the ovaries and terminate at the uterus. Their function is to transport eggs from the ovaries to the uterus. Fertilization typically occurs as an egg travels through the Fallopian tube. The uterus, a muscular organ with a pear shape, serves as a gestational chamber for the fetus until birth. Its muscular walls have the ability to contract forcefully during labor, facilitating the expulsion of the baby through the vagina. The uterus can also expand significantly to accommodate the growing fetus. The vagina, a tubular tract, connects the uterus to the external body. Sperm are typically deposited into the vagina during ejaculation and sexual activity. Additionally, since the baby passes through the vagina during delivery, it is also referred to as the birth canal.

The term "vulva" encompasses all of the external reproductive system structures in females. Among these structures is the clitoris, which bears resemblance to the male penis. Furthermore, there are two pairs of labia (plural: labium), which encircle and protect the vaginal and urethral openings (Table 8.2).

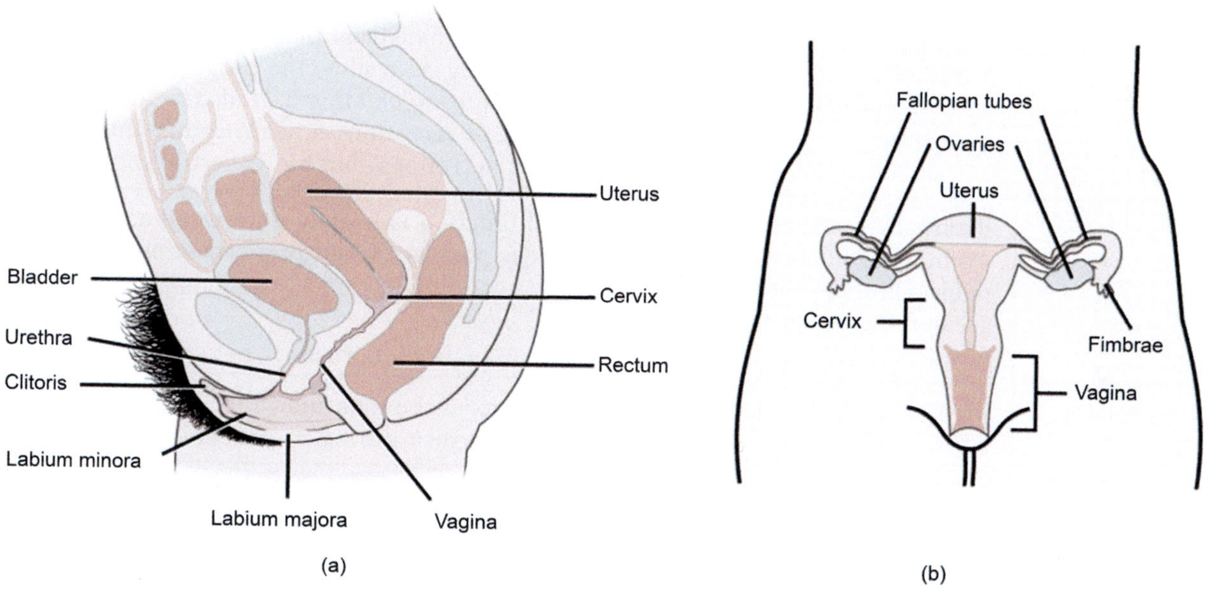

Figure 8.3. *The main organs of the female reproductive system lie within the abdominal cavity. Pay attention to ovaries, uterine tube, uterus, cervix, and vagina.*

Source: https://courses.lumenlearning.com/wm-biology2/chapter/reproductive-system/.

Table 8.2. *Components of the Female Reproductive System*

Components of the Female Reproductive System		
Structure	**Location and Description**	**Function**
Ovaries (2)	Ovoid structures on either side of the uterus in the pelvic cavity.	The primary sex organs of females are the ovaries, which contain ovarian follicles that house the oocytes. Oocytes are released during the ovulation stage of the menstrual cycle.
Fallopian tubes (2)	Extend from lateral areas of the uterus to near the ovaries.	The oocyte is transported to the uterus after fertilization, and it is in the uterus where fertilization by sperm actually occurs.
Uterus	Pear shaped structure divided into the fundus and the cervix.	Site of fetal development during gestation.
Vagina	Located between the rectum and urethra, it is a smooth muscle lined with an epithelial mucous membrane.	The reproductive system includes the pathway for menstrual blood and tissue to exit the body, as well as the passage for the fetus during childbirth. It also produces a variety of secretions for lubrication and receives secretions that aid in fertilization.
Vulva	Externally located: labia majora and minora, mons pubis, clitoris, vestibule, greater and lesser vestibular glands.	Sexual function is heavily innervated and provides pleasure when properly stimulated.
Perineum	Area between vagina and anus.	It helps form the muscular floor of the pelvis and can be torn during vaginal childbirth.
Mammary glands	Superficial to pectoral muscles.	Provide nourishment to the baby through milk secretions.

Source: https://courses.lumenlearning.com/wm-biology2/chapter/reproductive-system/.

8.1.8. Comparing Male and Female Reproductive Systems

8.1.8.1. Similarities

There are fundamental similarities between the male and female reproductive systems, as well as specific differences. They are homologous, meaning that the majority of the reproductive organs in both sexes develop from similar embryonic tissue. The gonads in both systems produce sex organs (egg and sperm or ovum). Additionally, the reproductive organs in both systems mature and start to function during puberty as a result of the gonads secreting sex hormones (Table 8.3).

Table 8.3. *Similarities and Differences between the Male and Female Reproductive Systems*

Indifferent	Male	Female
Gonad	Testis	Ovary
Müllerian duct	Appendix testis	Fallopian tubes
Müllerian duct	Prostatic utricle	Uterus, proximal vagina
Wolffian duct	Rete testis	Rete ovarii
Mesonephric tubules	Efferent ducts	Epoophoron
Wolffian duct	Epididymis	Gartner's duct
Wolffian duct	Vas deferens	–
Wolffian duct	Seminal vesicle	–
Wolffian duct	Prostate	Skene's glands
Urogenital sinus	Bladder, urethra	Bladder, urethra, distal vagina
Urogenital sinus	Bulborethral gland	Bartholin's gland
Genital swelling	Scrotum	Labia majora
Urogenital folds	Distal urethra	Labia minora
Genital tubercle	Penis	Clitoris
Prepuce	Foreskin	Clitoral hood
–	Bulb of penis	Vestibular bulbs
–	Glans penis	Clitoral glans
–	Crus of penis	Clitoral crura

Source: https://courses.lumenlearning.com/wm-biology2/chapter/reproductive-system/.

8.1.9. Differences

Based on each person's unique function within the reproductive cycle, the female and male reproductive systems differ from one another. A healthy, sexually mature male produces sperm continuously. Fetal development is the time when women's "eggs" stop developing. This indicates that she is born with a fixed number of oocytes and is unable to create more.

The ovaries have 6 to 7 million oogonia at five months gestation, which is when meiosis begins. From birth until puberty, the oogonia produce primary oocytes that are stopped in prophase I of meiosis. Following puberty, one or more oocytes resume meiosis and go through their first meiotic division during ovulation during each menstrual cycle. One polar body and a secondary oocyte are produced as a result. In metaphase II, the division of meiosis is stopped. One ovum and an extra polar body are produced when the second meiotic division is completed, which is triggered by fertilization.

A newborn baby girl's ovaries hold roughly a million oocytes. By the time puberty arrives, this number has dropped to between 400,000 and 500,000. 500–1000 oocytes ovulate on average in a woman's lifetime during reproduction. Every 28 days, a primary oocyte is released from one of the ovaries when a young woman reaches puberty, which occurs between the ages of 10 and 13. This lasts until the woman enters menopause, which typically happens around age 50. Oocytes are present from birth and develop with age in a female.

8.2. Structures of the Male Reproductive System

8.2.1. Testes and Scrotum

The two testes, or testis in singular, are the gonads that produce testosterone and sperm in male mammals, including male humans. Figure 8.4 depicts these and additional organs of the male reproductive system in humans. The scrotum, a pouch of smooth muscle and skin that hangs behind the penis, houses the testes.

8.2.1.1. Testes Structure

The testes are made up of hundreds of tiny tubes known as seminiferous tubules, which serve as the organs' functional units. The testis is divided into sections known as lobules, which contain the tightly packed, coiled seminiferous tubules. Internal walls, also known as septa, divide lobules from one another.

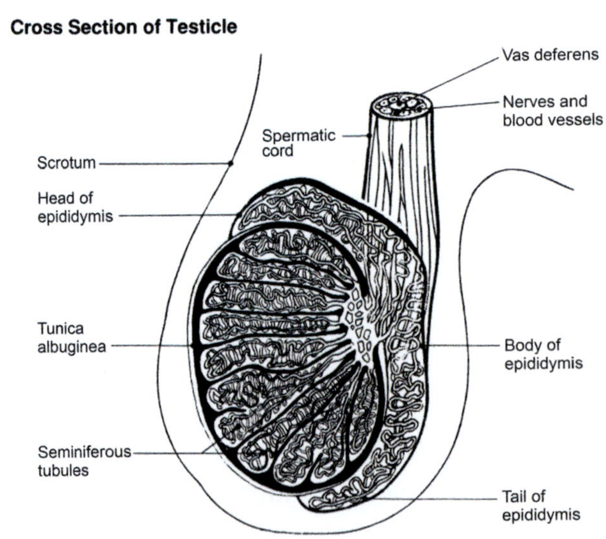

Figure 8.4. *This drawing includes a testis, epididymis, and vas (or ductus) deference.*

Source: https://bio.libretexts.org/@api/deki/files/17888/Testicle.jpg?revision=1&size=bestfit&width=395&height=342.

Each of the hundreds of lobules in the testis contains one or more tightly coiled seminiferous tubules. Approximately 30 m (90 ft) of these densely packed tubules are typically found in a single testis! The cross-sectional drawing of a seminiferous tubule in Figure 8.4 illustrates that the tubule contains sperm at multiple stages of development.

The three structures are connected to create a tract through which sperm can travel. The testes are composed of microscopic tubes called seminiferous tubules where sperm is produced. Sperm is stored in the epididymis after maturation until it is ejaculated via the vas deferens.

8.2.2. Other Scrotal Structures

In addition to the testes, the scrotum houses the epididymis and sections of the vas deferens. These organs play a vital role in sperm production and transportation.

8.2.2.1. Epididymis

The efferent ducts, which transport immature sperm to the associated epididymis, are formed when the seminiferous tubules within each testis converge. Each epididymis (plural: epididymes) is a tightly coiled tubule that measures approximately 20 feet (20 meters) in length. The epididymis is typically divided into three sections, as depicted in Figure 8.4: the head, located above the testis, the body, which extends down the side of the testis, and the tail, which connects to the vas deferens near the base of the testis. The two epididymes have the dual function of maturing sperm and storing it until ejaculation, when they transfer the sperm to the vas deferens and exit the body.

8.2.2.2. Vas Deferens

The vas deferens, also known as the sperm ducts, are a pair of slender tubes that originate from the scrotal epididymis and extend upward into the pelvic cavity. Each tube is approximately 30 centimeters (1 foot) long. They are composed of smooth muscle and ciliated epithelium. These structures assist the vas deferens in transporting sperm from the epididymes to the ejaculatory ducts, which are accessory structures of the male reproductive system.

8.2.3. Accessory Structures

There are various internal accessory structures in the male reproductive system in addition to those found within the scrotum. The prostate, bulborethral (Cowper's) glands, seminal vesicles, and ejaculatory ducts are a few of them (*refer* Figure 8.5). An explanation of the main reproductive structures shown in Figure 8.5.

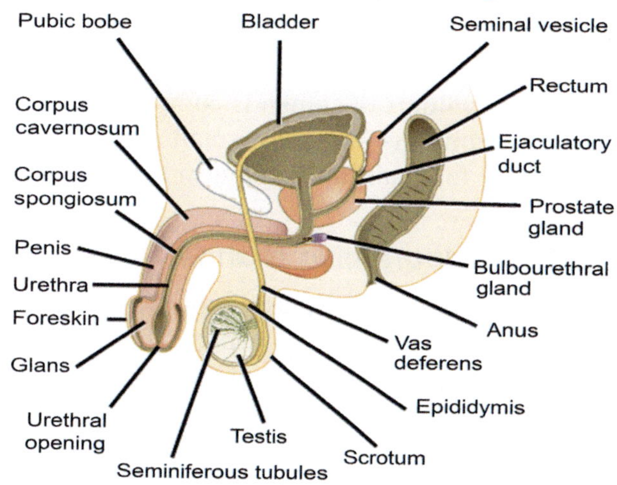

Figure 8.5. *The ejaculatory duct, seminal vesicles, and the bulbourethral gland that produce semen. The figure also shows the other major structures of the male reproductive system.*

Source: https://bio.libretexts.org/@api/deki/files/30089/male_rep_anat.png?revision=1&size=bestfit&width=757&height=328.

8.2.3.1. Seminal Vesicles

The seminal vesicles are a pair of glands, each containing a single folded and coiled tube. They measure approximately 5 cm (2 in.) in length and possess an excretory duct that connects with the vas deferens to form one of the two ejaculatory ducts. The fluid secreted by the seminal vesicles constitutes about 70% of the total volume of semen, which is the fluid containing sperm that is ejaculated from the penis. This fluid is alkaline in nature, providing semen with a basic pH that aids in supporting the longevity of sperm in the acidic environment of the female vagina. Along with proteins and fructose, the fluid from the seminal vesicles contains other substances that nourish sperm.

8.2.3.2. Ejaculatory Ducts

The junction of the seminal vesicle ducts in the prostate gland and the vas deferens is where the ejaculatory ducts form. They join the urethra and vas deferens. Sperm from the vas deferens and secretions from the prostate gland and seminal vesicles combine to form semen, which is transported by the ejaculatory ducts. Among other things, the chemicals that the glands secrete into the semen as it travels through the ejaculatory ducts regulate its pH and nourish the sperm. The liquid itself provides a medium for the sperm to swim in. "

8.2.3.3. Prostate Gland

The seminal vesicles are situated directly beneath the prostate gland. This organ, bearing resemblance to a walnut, is positioned around the urethra and its junction with the two ejaculatory ducts. About 30% of the volume of semen is composed of a slightly alkaline fluid secreted by the prostate gland. This fluid contains enzymes, small amounts of proteins, and a high concentration of zinc, which is essential for maintaining sperm motility and quality.

8.2.3.4. Bulborethral Glands

The bulborethral glands, also known as Cowper's glands, are located just below the prostate gland and are about the size of a pea. These glands secrete a protein-rich, clear, alkaline fluid. The secretions from each gland are transported into the urethra through a short duct, contributing only a small portion to the total volume of semen. The purpose of the bulborethral secretions is to lubricate the urethra and neutralize any acidic urine that may remain.

8.2.4. Penis

Delivering sperm to the female reproductive tract is the reproductive role of the penis, an external male organ. This function is referred to as intromission. Urine is expelled from the body through the penis as well.

8.2.4.1. Structure of the Penis

The structure of the penis is depicted in Figure 8.6, which also shows its position in relation to other reproductive organs. The root of the penis is the portion of the genitalia that is hidden inside the body. The portion of the penis that is external to the body is called the shaft. The term "glans penis" refers to the larger, bulbous end of the shaft.

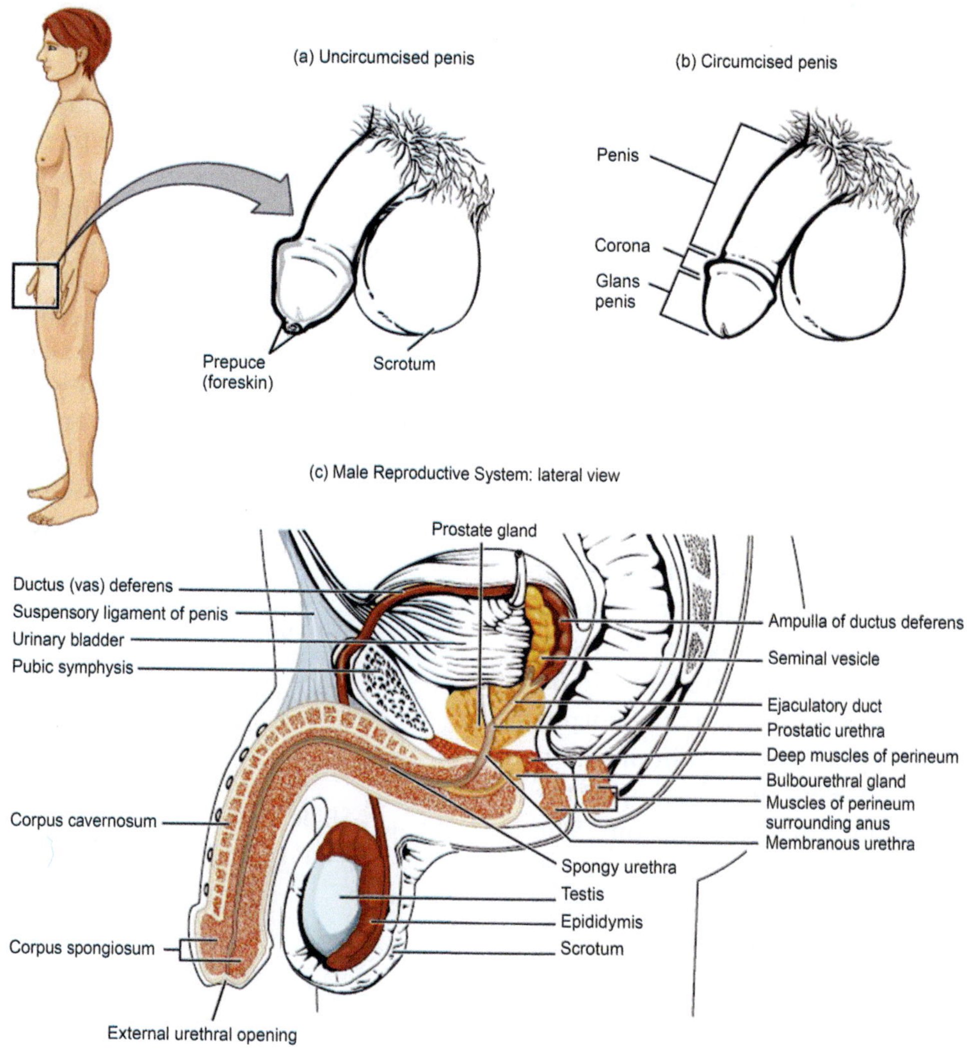

Figure 8.6. *This section shows the internal anatomy of the penis and related structures.*

Source: https://courses.lumenlearning.com/suny-ap2/chapter/anatomy-and-physiology-of-the-male-reproductive-system/.

The penis is composed of the glans penis, shaft, and root. The corpus spongiosum is a column of erectile tissue that contains the urethra, while the corpora cavernosa are the other two columns that contribute to penile erection.

8.2.4.2. Urethra

The urethra travels through the penis to transport urine from the bladder or semen from the ejaculatory ducts out of the body. It starts at the urinary bladder, passes through the prostate gland, and joins the ejaculatory ducts. The external urethral orifice, located at the tip of the glans penis, serves as the opening for the release of urine or semen.

8.2.4.3. Tissues of the Penis

The skin covering the penis is called epithelium, which is unattached and movable. In uncircumcised males, the glans penis is mostly covered by the foreskin, which is a type of epithelium. Beneath the foreskin, there is a layer of mucous membrane. The foreskin is connected to the penis by the frenulum, located on the underside of the penis.

The penis consists mostly of spongy tissues that can fill with blood, stiffening the organ. The corpus cavernosum urethrae are now called corpus spongiosum. You can see the urethra in the center of the corpus spongiosum.

The interior of the penis is composed of three columns of spongy tissue that can fill with blood and expand, allowing the penis to achieve an erect state, as depicted in Figure 8.7. This spongy tissue is known as the corpus cavernosum, or corpora cavernosa in plural. It is arranged in two columns along the top of the shaft and one column along the bottom. The bottom column of spongy tissue, also referred to as the corpus spongiosum, is where the urethra passes through. The majority of the glans penis is also made up of spongy erectile tissue. Veins and arteries running along the top of the penis enable blood to flow through the spongy tissues.

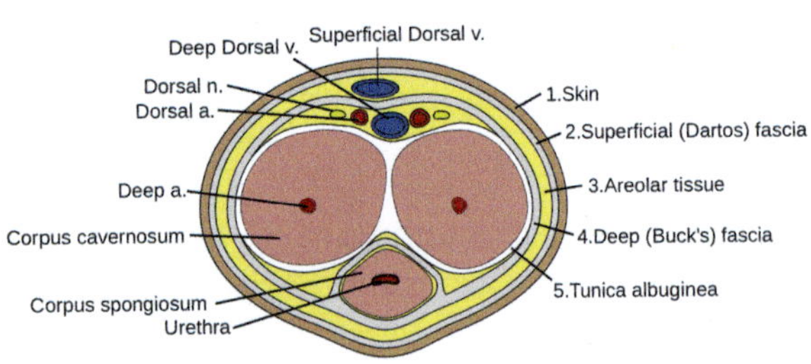

Figure 8.7. *Cross-section of the penis.*

Source: https://en.m.wikipedia.org/wiki/File:Penis_cross_section.svg.

8.2.5. Functions of the Male Reproductive System

In Figure 8.8's false-color image, real human sperm can be observed. Due to their status as the smallest human cell, they are significantly enlarged in the image. In reality, human sperm cells are tiny, even when compared to those of other animals. A normal, healthy man typically releases vast quantities of sperm during each ejaculation, despite their small size. In contrast, mouse sperm are approximately twice as long as human sperm. One teaspoon of semen may contain hundreds of millions of sperm cells. The production of sperm is one of the primary functions of the male reproductive system.

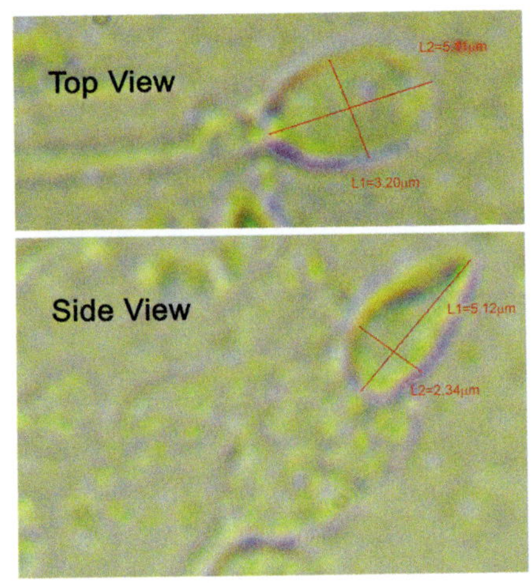

Figure 8.8. *Human spermatozoa (sperm cells).*

Source: By Ethan Kung – Own work, CC BY-SA 4.0, https://commons.wikimedia.org/w/index.php?curid=90891385.

8.2.5.1. Sperm Anatomy

The drawing of a sperm in Figure 8.9 illustrates the various structures that assist a mature sperm cell in reaching and penetrating an egg.

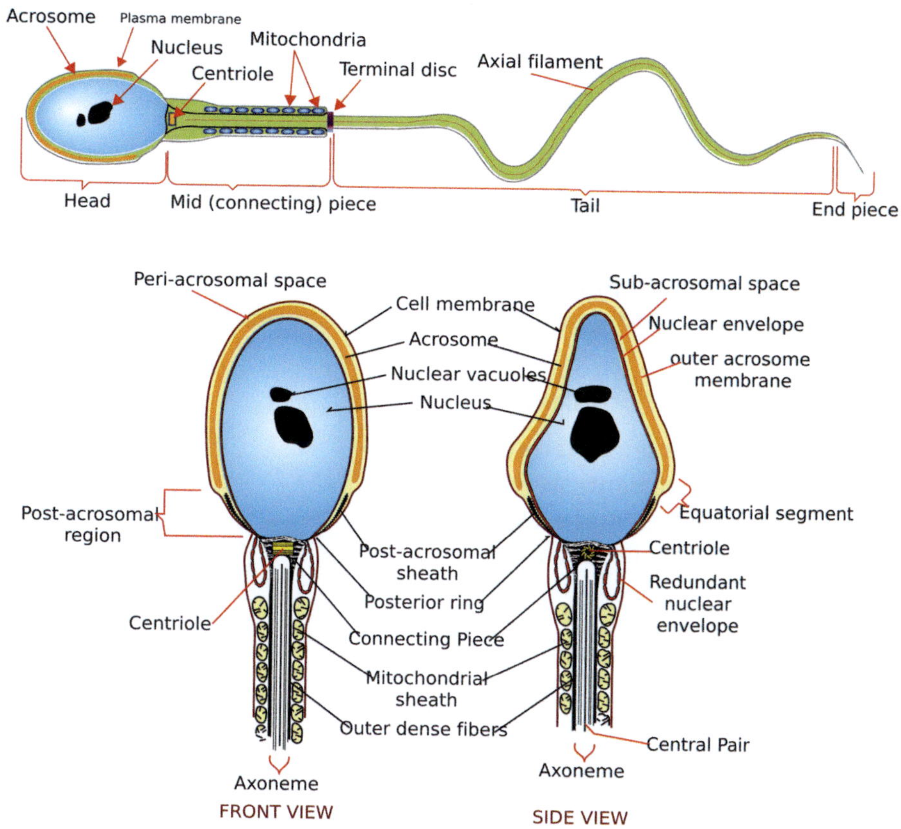

Figure 8.9. *Each normal mature sperm cell has the structures labeled in this image. The acrosome is located at the front end, just behind the nucleus. The midpiece connects the nucleus to the tail.*

Source: By Mariana Ruiz Villarreal – I did the diagram myself based on the one found on the book "Gray's anatomy" 36th edition, Williams & Warwick (1980); and a diagram found of the review "Formation and organization of the mammalian sperm head" from Kiyotaka Toshimori and Chizuro Ito. (Chiba, Japan)., Public Domain, https://commons.wikimedia.org/w/index.php?curid=699220.

- The head is the part of the sperm that contains the nucleus—and not much else. The nucleus, in turn, contains tightly coiled DNA that is the male parent's contribution to the genetic makeup of a zygote (if one forms). Each sperm is a haploid cell, containing half the chromosomal complement of a normal, diploid body cell.
- The front of the head is an area called the acrosome. The acrosome contains enzymes that help the sperm penetrate an egg (if it reaches one).
- The midpiece is the section of the sperm located between the head and the flagellum tail. Packed with mitochondria, the midpiece produces the energy required for the flagellum's movement.
- The flagellum, also known as the tail, is capable of rotating like a propeller, enabling the sperm to navigate through the female reproductive tract in search of an egg.

8.2.5.2. Spermatogenesis

Spermatogenesis is the process responsible for sperm production. While the production of sperm generally decreases with age, spermatogenesis typically begins at puberty in males and continues uninterrupted until death. In a young and healthy male, approximately half of the hundreds of millions of sperm produced daily are likely to mature into viable sperm.

8.2.5.3. Where Sperm Are Produced?

Spermatogenesis takes place in the seminiferous tubules of the testes. Adequate concentrations of testosterone are necessary for this process, which is secreted by Leydig cells located adjacent to the seminiferous tubules.

Temperature plays a significant role in sperm production within the seminiferous tubules. The testes are positioned outside the body in the scrotum precisely for this reason, making it the most crucial factor. Generally, the temperature inside the scrotum is approximately 2°C (almost 4°F) lower than the core body temperature, which is ideal for spermatogenesis. The smooth muscles lining the scrotum contract to regulate the internal temperature of the organ as needed. When the temperature drops too low, the scrotal muscles contract, drawing the scrotum closer to the warmer body. Conversely, when the temperature inside the scrotum rises too high, the opposite occurs.

8.2.5.4. Events of Spermatogenesis

Figure 8.10 provides an overview of the key cellular processes involved in spermatogenesis. A diploid stem cell known as a spermatogonium (plural: spermatogonia) is the starting point of the multi-phase process. The entire process, including the maturation of the epididymis, takes at least 10 weeks to complete.

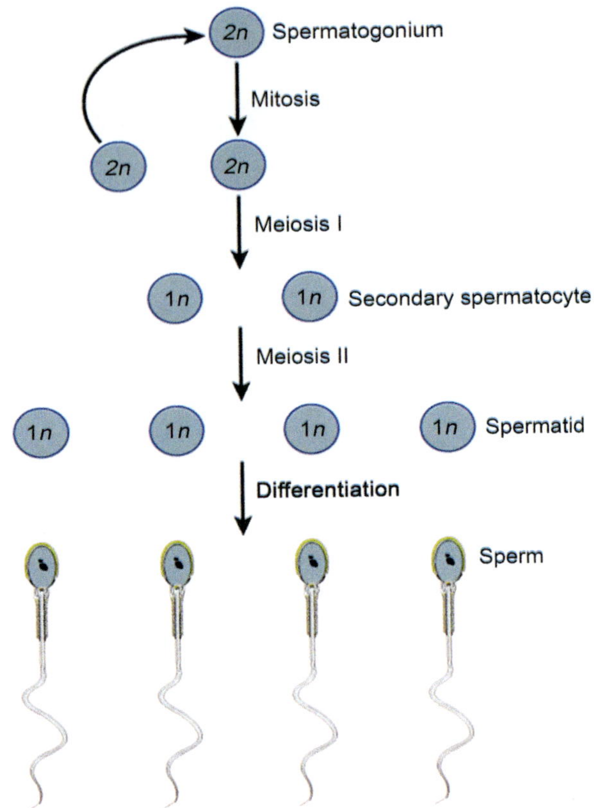

Figure 8.10. *Spermatogenesis includes one mitotic division and two meiotic divisions. Also, on the right, the cross-section of the seminiferous tubule shows the locations of the lumen, cells of spermatogenesis, Sertoli, and Leydig cells in the tube.*

Source: https://courses.lumenlearning.com/wm-biology2/chapter/gametogenesis/.

- A spermatogonium undergoes mitosis to produce two diploid cells called primary spermatocytes. One of the primary spermatocytes goes on to produce sperm. The other replenishes the reserve of spermatogonia.
- The primary spermatocyte undergoes meiosis I to produce two haploid daughter cells called secondary spermatocytes.
- The secondary spermatocytes rapidly undergo meiosis II to produce a total

of four haploid daughter cells called spermatids.

- The spermatids begin to form a tail, and their DNA becomes highly condensed. Unnecessary cytoplasm and organelles are removed from the cells, and they form a head, midpiece, and flagellum. The resulting cells are sperm (spermatozoa).

As seen in Figure 8.10, spermatogenesis events start close to the seminiferous tubule wall, which is home to spermatogonia, and proceed inward toward the tubule lumen. At every stage of spermatogenesis, Sertoli cells come into contact with developing sperm as they extend from the wall of the seminiferous tubule inward toward the lumen. In spermatogenesis, Sertoli cells have multiple functions.

- They secrete endocrine hormones that help regulate spermatogenesis.
- They secrete substances that initiate meiosis.
- They concentrate testosterone (from Leydig cells), which is needed at high levels to maintain spermatogenesis.
- They phagocytize the extra cytoplasm that is shed from developing sperm cells.
- They secrete a testicular fluid that helps carry sperm into the epididymis.
- They maintain a blood-testis barrier, so immune system cells cannot reach and attack the sperm.

8.2.5.5. Maturation in the Epididymis

The testes produce sperm, but these are not yet motile (able to "swim"), despite having tails. With the aid of peristaltic contractions, the non-motile sperm are moved to the epididymis in the testicular fluid secreted by Sertoli cells. The sperm acquire motility in the epididymis, enabling them to swim up the female genital tract and arrive at an egg. The epididymis houses the mature sperm until ejaculation takes place.

8.2.5.6. Ejaculation

The body releases sperm during ejaculation, which usually happens during an orgasm. During a normal ejaculation, hundreds of millions of mature sperm are propelled from the penis within a small amount of thick, whitish fluid called semen.

8.2.5.7. How Ejaculation Occurs?

Sperm are propelled from the epididymes, where mature sperm are stored, during ejaculation by the peristalsis of the muscle layers of the vas deferens and other auxiliary structures. Sperm are forced by the contractions of the muscles to pass through the ejaculatory ducts and vas deferens, and finally exit the penis through the urethra. The ejaculation happens in spurts because of the peristaltic action of the muscles.

8.2.5.8. The Role of Semen

During ejaculation, sperm pass through the ejaculatory ducts and combine with secretions from the prostate gland, bulborethral glands, and seminal vesicles to form semen (Figure 8.11). A little less than a teaspoonful, or roughly 3.7 mL, of semen is produced with each ejaculate on average. The vast majority of this semen volume is made up of glandular secretions; the hundreds of millions of sperm cells add relatively little to the total volume.

Semen secretions play a vital role in supporting and enhancing sperm survival and mobility. These secretions serve as a fluid in which sperm can move, containing essential nutrients like fructose that provide energy for the sperm. Semen also includes alkaline substances that counteract the acidic conditions of the female reproductive system, preserving the integrity of sperm DNA and extending the lifespan of sperm inside the female body.

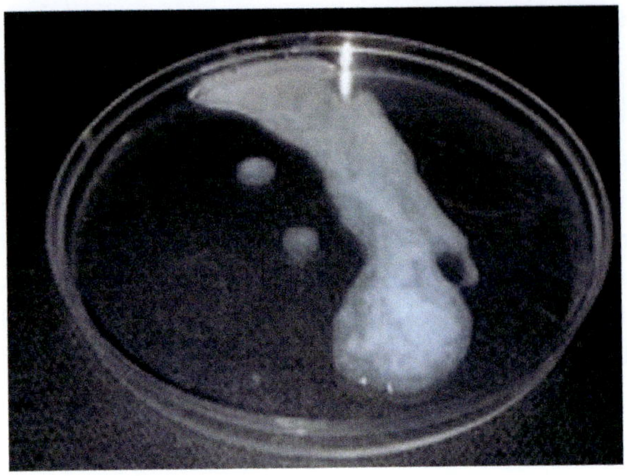

Figure 8.11. *This petri dish shows normal human semen in a typical ejaculate.*

Source: By Digitalkil – Own work, Public Domain, https://commons.wikimedia.org/w/index.php?curid=12892579.

8.2.5.9. Erection

The penis' primary function in reproduction is intromission, or the depositing of sperm in the vagina of the female reproductive tract, in addition to giving sperm a means of exiting the body. The ability of the penis to achieve an erection—a stiff, erect state—is necessary for intromission. Unlike the majority of other mammals, the human penis is devoid of the erectile bone. Rather, it depends solely on engorgement with the blood of its spongy tissue columns to achieve its erect state. The arteries supplying blood to the penis widen when a person becomes sexually aroused, allowing more blood to fill the spongy tissue. The blood-sucking veins that lead from the penis are compressed and pressed against by the now enlarged spongy tissue. As a result, until an erectile size is reached, more blood enters the penis than exits. The penis not only carries sperm but also excretes urine from the body. These two tasks cannot be completed at the same time. The brain's centers regulate the sphincters that keep urine from exiting the bladder during an erection, preventing them from relaxing and allowing urine to pass through the urethra.

8.2.5.10. Testosterone Production

The generation of the male sex hormone testosterone is the final major function of the male reproductive system. This primarily affects the testes in adult males. The production of testosterone is regulated by the pituitary gland's luteinizing hormone (LH). Testicular Leydig cells secrete testosterone in response to LH stimulation. Testosterone plays a crucial role in male sexual development during puberty. It promotes the development of secondary male sex characteristics, such as facial hair, and the maturation of the male reproductive organs. In addition, mature males require testosterone to maintain normal spermatogenesis in the testes. Spermatogenesis also relies on the pituitary gland's follicle stimulating hormone (FSH), as it helps concentrate testosterone in the Sertoli cells of the testes to sustain sperm production at adequate levels. The proper functioning of the prostate gland also depends on testosterone. Furthermore, testosterone contributes to erection by facilitating the deposition of sperm in the female reproductive system.

8.2.6. Disorders of the Male Reproductive System

8.2.6.1. Erectile Dysfunction

Erectile dysfunction (ED) is a common sexual disorder that affects approximately 40% of individuals with penises. It is characterized by the consistent inability of a sexually mature person to achieve or sustain an erection.

8.2.6.2. Causes of Erectile Dysfunction

When the corpora cavernosa and corpus spongiosum, the spongy tissue columns inside the penis shaft, swell with blood, the penis usually stiffens and becomes erect. Therefore, anything that prevents the penis's natural blood flow may hinder its ability to fill with blood and become erect. Failure of the normal nervous system to control sexual arousal or penile engorgement can also result in difficulties getting or keeping an erection.

Physiological as well as psychological factors are specific causes of ED. The use of therapeutic drugs (like antidepressants), aging, kidney failure, diseases (like diabetes or multiple sclerosis), tobacco smoking, and treatments for other disorders (like prostate cancer) are examples of physiological causes. Though less frequent, psychological factors can include mental illnesses, stress, and anxiety related to performance. Additionally, obesity, cardiovascular disease, poor eating habits, and general poor physical health may increase a person's risk of developing ED. An untreated groin hernia may also contribute to ED.

8.2.6.3. Treatments for Erectile Dysfunction

How erectile dysfunction (ED) is treated depends on its underlying causes or influencing factors. For example, quitting smoking can have a significant positive impact on ED in tobacco users. Additionally, improving overall physical health through regular exercise and weight loss can be beneficial. However, the most commonly prescribed initial treatment for ED is the use of oral medications, such as Cialis® and Viagra®, which enhance penile blood flow. Other potential treatments include injecting medication into the penis, using topical creams, or utilizing a vacuum pump to create negative pressure, which aids in drawing blood into the penis. If all other treatments prove unsuccessful, more invasive methods may be considered as a last resort. These methods typically involve surgical implantation of inflatable tubes or rigid rods into the penis. Interestingly, the venom of the Brazilian wandering spider, known as the most venomous spider in the world, may paradoxically offer a novel treatment for ED. It has been reported that the spider's venom can cause prolonged erections, known as priapism, which can potentially damage reproductive organs and lead to infertility if left untreated. Researchers are currently studying one of the components of the spider's venom in very small doses as a potential treatment for ED.

8.2.6.4. Epididymitis

The inflammation of the epididymis is called epididymitis. The epididymis is one of the paired organs in the scrotum where sperm develop and are stored. Discomfort or pain and swelling in the scrotum are the most common symptoms of epididymitis, which is relatively common, especially in young people. In the United States alone, more than half a million cases of epididymitis are diagnosed each year among individuals aged 18 to 35. Epididymitis can be categorized as acute or chronic.

8.2.6.5. Acute vs. Chronic Epididymitis

Acute and chronic epididymitis differ in their duration; acute epididymitis is short-lived, while chronic epididymitis can last for years or even a lifetime.

1. **Acute Epididymitis:** Acute epididymitis is typically caused by bacterial infections and manifests fairly quickly. Bacteria can reach the epididymis from the urethra through the reproductive and urinary systems. Sexually transmitted bacteria are the primary cause of acute epididymitis in sexually active individuals. In addition to pain and swelling, redness, warmth in the scrotum, and fever are typical signs of acute epididymitis. A urethral discharge might also be present.

2. **Chronic Epididymitis:** More than three months of epididymitis is considered chronic epididymitis. For some, the illness might persist for years. It could happen with or without a confirmed diagnosis of bacterial infection. Occasionally, it is linked to lower back pain that develops following a lower back-stressing activity, like prolonged driving or heavy lifting.

8.2.6.6. Treatment of Epididymitis

Antibiotics are typically used to treat both acute and chronic epididymitis when a bacterial infection is suspected.

Antibiotic therapy for chronic epididymitis may be recommended for a maximum of four to six weeks in order to fully eradicate any potential bacteria. Anti-inflammatory medications are frequently used in addition to other treatments to lessen tissue inflammation and painkillers to manage moderate to excruciating pain. It may also be advised to use cold compresses and physical support the scrotum in order to reduce pain and swelling.

Treatment is crucial for both acute and chronic epididymitis, regardless of symptoms, as untreated cases may result in serious complications. If acute epididymitis is left untreated, it can result in an abscess, or a buildup of pus, or it can spread to other organs. If left untreated, chronic epididymitis can result in irreversible harm to the testicles and epididymis, as well as infertility.

8.2.6.7. Male Reproductive Cancers

Why does Figure 8.12's Brazilian hospital look like that? Wear a massive blue mustache as a symbol of "Movember" on its "face." This is a global initiative to increase funds for prostate cancer research as well as awareness of the disease.

Figure 8.12. *The mustache is a symbol for "Movember," a campaign against prostate cancer.*

Source: By Movember Foundation - www.movember.com, CC BY-SA 4.0, https://commons.wikimedia.org/w/index.php?curid=77785878.

8.2.6.8. Prostate Cancer

Before reaching the penis, the urethra travels through the prostate gland after exiting the bladder. During ejaculation, the prostate secretes zinc and other chemicals into the semen. Prostate cancer is the most common cancer in the US and the second largest cause of cancer-related deaths among those who have a prostate gland. By the time they are 80 years old, about 80% of American men who have prostate cancer will have cancerous cells in their glands.

8.2.6.9. How Prostate Cancer Occurs?

Prostate cancer occurs due to the prostatic glandular cells that give rise to tumor cells. If left unchecked, the tumor eventually has the potential to invade neighboring structures like the seminal vesicles. Additionally, tumor cells have the ability to spread and reach other organs throughout the body through the lymphatic or circulatory systems. Prostate cancer metastases most frequently affect lower urinary tract organs, lymph nodes, the rectum, and bones.

8.2.6.10. Symptoms of Prostate Cancer

In the initial stages of prostate cancer, there may be no indications. When symptoms do occur, they are primarily related to urination due to the location of the prostate gland in the urethra. Typical symptoms include blood in the urine, painful urination, difficulty initiating and maintaining a steady stream of urine, and frequent urination. Prostate cancer can also cause sexual function issues such as difficulty achieving an erection or experiencing painful ejaculation.

8.2.6.11. Risk Factors for Prostate Cancer

- There are certain risk factors for prostate cancer, some of which can be modified while others cannot. Modifiable risk factors include a diet high in meat, a sedentary lifestyle, obesity, and high blood pressure.
- Non-modifiable risk factors include older age, a family history of prostate cancer, and African ancestry. Family history is a significant risk factor, indicating a clear involvement of genes. Numerous genes have been implicated in the development of prostate cancer.

8.2.6.12. Diagnosing Prostate Cancer

A biopsy is the only definitive test that can confirm a diagnosis of prostate cancer. During this procedure, a small portion of the prostate gland is surgically removed and subsequently examined under a microscope. A biopsy is performed only when there is evidence of possible prostate cancer found through less invasive testing.

If a physician discovers a prostate lump during a routine physical examination, it may prompt a blood test to check for elevated levels of prostate-specific antigen (PSA). PSA is a protein secreted by the prostate that typically circulates in the bloodstream. Elevated PSA levels can indicate prostate cancer, although there may be other explanations as well. Magnetic resonance imaging (MRI) or ultrasound procedures may also be used to obtain additional information about the cancer and images of the prostate gland.

8.2.6.13. Treatment of Prostate Cancer

Prostate cancer is typically diagnosed in men around the age of 70. Due to its slow growth, elderly patients may not require immediate treatment. Instead, a technique called active surveillance is employed to closely monitor these patients over the following years to ensure that the cancer is not spreading and posing an urgent threat. At least half of the patients who are expected to pass away from other causes before experiencing symptoms from prostate cancer are treated accordingly.

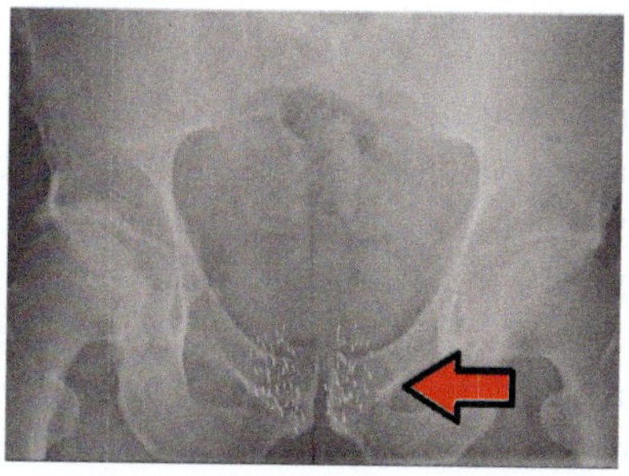

Figure 8.13. *Brachytherapy is a form of radiation therapy for prostate cancer. Radioactive "seeds" like the ones shown here are inserted into the prostate gland. The seeds emit radiation that eradicates cancer cells.*

Source: https://bio.libretexts.org/@api/deki/files/18071/Brachytherapybeads.png?revision=1&size=bestfit&width=326&height=240.

Younger patients, or those whose tumors are growing more quickly, may be treated with radiation therapy (brachytherapy – Figure 8.13), chemotherapy, and/or surgery to remove the prostate. Urinary incontinence and erectile dysfunction are two serious side effects that can occur with any of these treatment options. To choose the best course of action for their unique situation, patients should educate themselves on the advantages and disadvantages of various treatments and consult with their healthcare provider about them.

8.2.6.14. Testicular Cancer

Testicular cancer is a rare form of reproductive cancer that typically affects young individuals. The paired reproductive organs in the scrotum that produce testosterone and sperm are known as testes. Individuals of European ancestry have a significantly higher risk of testicular cancer, around four to five times higher, compared to individuals of African ancestry. The cause of this disparity is still unclear.

8.2.6.14.1. Signs and Symptoms of Testicular Cancer

A lump or swelling in one of the testes is often one of the early signs of testicular cancer. The lump may or may not be painful. If there is discomfort, it may feel dull or sharp in the scrotum or lower abdomen. Some testicular cancer patients describe a feeling of heaviness in the scrotum. Although testicular cancer rarely spreads beyond the testis, when it does, it typically metastasizes to the lungs, which can cause coughing or difficulty breathing (dyspnea).

8.2.6.14.2. Diagnosis of Testicular Cancer

The primary method of diagnosing testicular cancer is the identification of a lump in the testis. There will likely be additional diagnostic testing following this initial finding. An ultrasound examination may be performed to determine the precise location, dimensions, and features of the lump. Blood tests can be used to detect and measure tumor-marker proteins that are unique to testicular cancer. CT scans can also be conducted to determine if the cancer has spread beyond the testis. Unlike in the case of prostate cancer, a biopsy is not recommended as it increases the risk of cancer cells spreading to the scrotum.

8.2.6.14.3. Treatment of Testicular Cancer

Testicular cancer has one of the highest cure rates among all cancers. There are three main treatment options for testicular cancer: surgery, radiation therapy, and/or chemotherapy. Surgery to remove the affected testis is typically the initial treatment. With a nearly 100% five-year survival rate, surgery is often curative if the cancer is detected early. If the remaining testis is healthy, it can maintain fertility, hormone production, and other normal functions even after one testis is removed. In cases where there is no evidence of cancer spread, radiation therapy and/or chemotherapy may be used in addition to surgery to eliminate any remaining tumor cells. However, surveillance is often employed instead of further treatment after surgery.

8.3. Structures of the Female Reproductive System

This old stone carving's geometric pattern depicts the vagina, a potent fertility symbol. The Hindu symbol, known as yoni, represents the importance that Hindu culture places on the capacity for childbirth. The female reproductive system consists of multiple organs, including the vagina.

8.3.1. Female Reproductive Organs

The internal and external organs that make up the female reproductive system are responsible for secreting sex hormones like estrogen, producing haploid gametes known as eggs (or oocytes), and carrying and giving birth to a fetus. The internal reproductive organs are the vagina, uterus, Fallopian (uterine) tubes, and ovaries, as Figure 8.14 illustrates. The clitoris and labia are two of the external organs that are referred to as the vulva collectively.

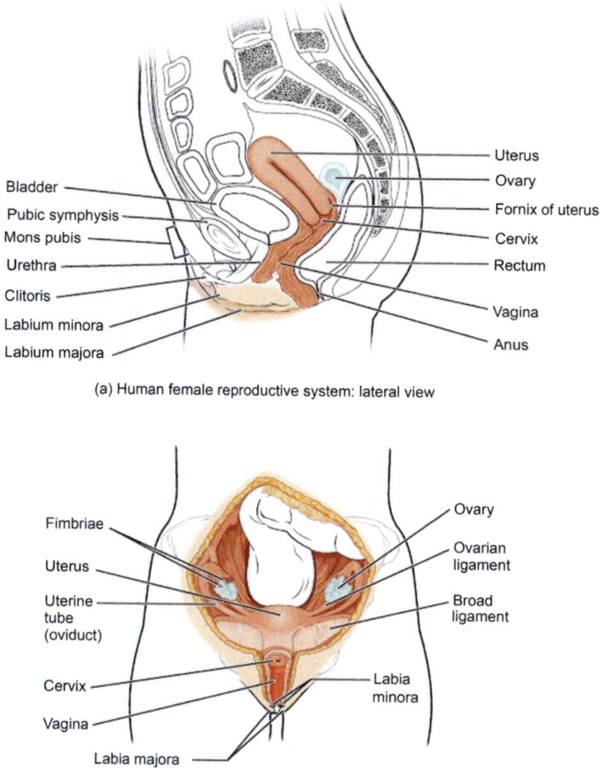

(a) Human female reproductive system: lateral view

(b) Human female reproductive system: anterior view

Figure 8.14. *Structures of the internal female reproductive organs.*

Source: https://courses.lumenlearning.com/suny-ap2/chapter/anatomy-and-physiology-of-the-female-reproductive-system/.

The vagina is a muscular and elastic canal that extends from the vulva to the cervix, which is the neck of the uterus. It measures approximately 7 to 9 centimeters in length. During sexual intercourse, sperm is typically ejaculated into the vagina, which also accommodates the penis. The term "birth canal" is used to refer to the vagina in the context of natural childbirth. Additionally, the vagina facilitates the passage of menstrual blood from the uterus.

8.3.1.1. Structure of the Vagina

In terms of structure, the vagina is a muscular canal that serves as the entrance to the reproductive tract. It is approximately 10 centimeters long and acts as the exit point for the uterus during menstruation and childbirth. The superior part of the vagina, known as the fornix, meets the protruding uterine cervix. The anterior and posterior walls of the vagina form longitudinal columns or ridges. The walls of the vagina are lined with an inner mucous membrane that has transverse folds called rugae, as well as an outer layer of smooth muscle and fibrous adventitia. The middle and inner layers work together to allow the vagina to expand during sexual activity and childbirth. The opening of the vaginal orifice may be partially surrounded by the slender, perforated hymen, which can rupture during penile-vaginal sex, childbirth, or intense physical activity. The Bartholin's glands and the lesser vestibular glands, located near the clitoris, secrete mucus to maintain moisture in the vestibular area.

A normal population of microorganisms resides in the vagina, helping to protect against infection by pathogenic bacteria, yeast, and other organisms that may enter the vagina. The majority of vaginal bacteria in a healthy individual belong to the genus Lactobacillus. This group of beneficial bacterial flora produces lactic acid, which maintains the vagina's acidic pH (below 4 points) and provides protection. These acidic conditions reduce the likelihood of potential pathogens surviving. The vagina acts as a self-cleaning organ, aided by other vaginal secretions and lactic acid. However, douching or washing out the vagina with liquid can disrupt the delicate balance of beneficial microorganisms and increase the risk of irritation and infections. In fact, the American College of Obstetricians and Gynecologists advises women to refrain from douching and allow the vagina to maintain its normal, healthy population of beneficial microbiota.

8.3.1.2. Uterus

The uterus, also known as the womb, is a pear-shaped, muscular organ measuring approximately 7.6 centimeters (3 in.) in length. It is located in the middle of the pelvis, behind the bladder and above the vagina. Ligaments and supporting tissue keep the uterus in place within the pelvis. During gestation, a fetus develops in the uterus, which provides mechanical support and protection to the growing child. During childbirth, contractions of the uterine muscle wall expel the fetus from the uterus.

8.3.1.3. Parts of the Uterus

The cervix, also known as the neck of the uterus, is formed by the lower end of the uterus, as illustrated in Figure 8.15. The cervix measures approximately 2.5 cm (1 in.) in length and extends into the vagina below. The uterine cavity and the vaginal lumen are connected by a small canal that runs the entire length of the cervix. This allows for the entry of sperm deposited in the vagina into the uterus, as well as for the passage of a baby during childbirth from the uterus to the vagina. The cervix secretes mucus from its glands, which, depending on its thickness and water content, can act as a barrier to prevent germs from entering the uterus during pregnancy or as a transport medium to assist sperm in entering the uterus around ovulation. The term "uterine body" refers to the remaining portion of the uterus above the cervix. The two Fallopian tubes are attached to the upper end of the uterus.

8.3.1.4. Tissues of the Uterus

The uterus is composed of three tissue layers known as the endometrium, myometrium, and perimetrium, as shown in Figure 8.15. The uterine endometrium is the innermost layer of tissue, consisting of mucous membranes and other epithelial tissue. During each menstrual cycle, this layer thickens and eventually sheds during the subsequent cycle if no egg is fertilized. When fertilization occurs, hormones preserve the thicker endometrium, which provides nourishment to the developing embryo. As the pregnancy progresses, the endometrium grows into the maternal part of the placenta. The placenta is a temporary organ composed of a network of fetal and maternal blood vessels that facilitate the exchange of substances between the mother's and fetus's blood.

The middle layer of the uterus is called the myometrium. It is primarily composed of a thick layer of smooth muscle. During childbirth, the uterus can contract and expel an infant due to powerful smooth muscle contractions.

The outermost layer of the uterus is known as the perimetrium. It covers the external surface of the uterus. In reality, this layer consists of two layers of epithelium that secrete fluid into the space between them. The uterus is able to move slightly within the pelvis, thanks to this fluid, which prevents it from rubbing against other organs.

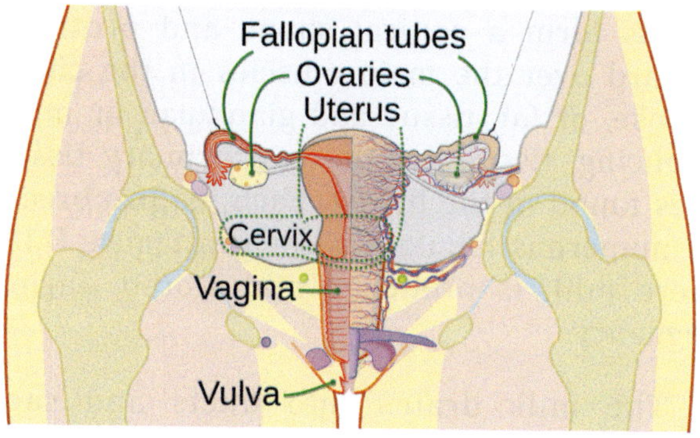

Figure 8.15. *The cervix of the uterus connects it to the vagina. The thick walls of the uterus are composed of layers of tissues known as the endometrium, myometrium, and perimetrium.*

Source: By CDC, Mysid – Vectorized in Inkscape by User:Mysid from a CDC image (https://www.cdc.gov/cancer/nbccedp/cc_basic.htm), public domain.https://web.archive.org/web/20050206211444/http://www.cdc.gov/cancer/nbccedp/cc_basic.htm, Public Domain, https://commons.wikimedia.org/w/index.php?curid=2885139.

8.3.1.5. Fallopian Tubes

The uterus and the ovaries are separated by two thin tubes called the Fallopian tubes (Figure 8.16). The broad upper ends of the Fallopian tubes, known as infundibula, are located quite close to the ovaries even though they are not attached to them. Additionally, the infundibula contain fringe-like projections known as fimbriae, which wave in response to movement and aid in directing eggs from the ovaries into the Fallopian tubes. On either side of the body, the lower ends of the Fallopian tubes are joined to the upper portion of the uterus, allowing passage for the uterus. Fertilization occurs in the fallopian tubes.

8.3.1.6. Ovaries

The ovaries are the gonads, arranged in pairs, each measuring roughly 2 to 3 centimeters in length, or the size of an almond. The pelvic cavity contains the ovaries, which are supported by numerous ligaments. The ovaries are the ovum-producing organs of the internal reproductive system. They are reproductive organs that normally grow in pairs and produce ova. Both the ovaries and the testes are gonads and endocrine glands, making them comparable. The ovaries secrete progesterone and estrogen. Estrogen is responsible for the development and maintenance of the reproductive organs in their fully developed, functional states, as well as the emergence of secondary sex traits in females during puberty. Progesterone and estrogen work together to promote changes in the endometrium during the menstrual cycle.

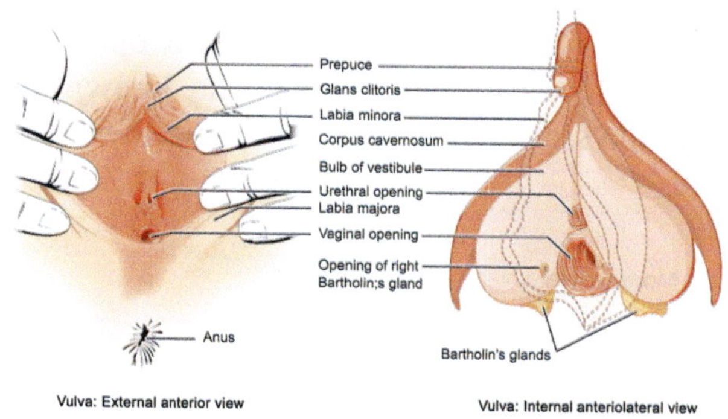

Figure 8.16. *External female genitalia (vulva).*

Source: https://courses.lumenlearning.com/suny-ap2/chapter/anatomy-and-physiology-of-the-female-reproductive-system/.

8.3.1.7. Vulva

The term "vulva" refers to all of the external reproductive structures combined (Figure 8.17). A fat pad situated above the pubic bone at the anterior region is called the mons pubis. Pubic hair grows over it after puberty. The labia majora are folds of skin covered in hair that start immediately posterior to the mons pubis (labia = "lips"; majora = "larger"). Medially, the labia majora are joined by the thinner and more pigmented labia minora (labia = "lips"; minora = "smaller"). The purpose of the labia minora, despite their inherent diversity in size and form, is to shield the urethra and the opening to the reproductive system.

The clitoris, also known as the glans clitoris, is an organ that arises from the same cells as the glans penis and has an abundance of nerves that make it important for orgasm and sexual sensation. The superior and anterior portions of the labia minora come together to encircle the clitoris. The hymen is a thin membrane that can occasionally cover part of the vaginal opening. The hymen, which is only partially formed at birth, cannot be used as a sign of "virginity" because secretions such as menstrual fluid must be able to leave the body regardless of penile-vaginal sex. The urethral and anus openings are where you can find the vaginal opening. The larger vestibular glands, also known as Bartholin's glands, have outlets on either side of it.

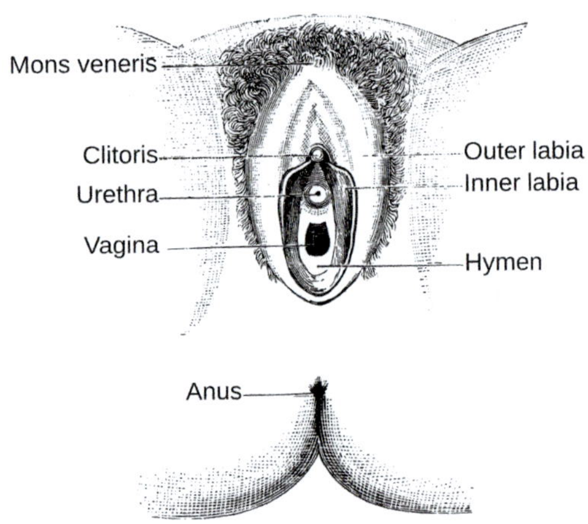

Figure 8.17. *External and internal view of a vulva.*

Source: https://en.m.wikipedia.org/wiki/File:Haultain_and_Ferguson_-_external_female_genital_organs.svg.

8.3.1.8. Breasts

Although the breasts do not directly contribute to reproduction, their mammary glands allow them to nourish a newborn after birth. The breasts form a conical shape and protrude outward over the main muscles in the chest. Adipose, or fat, tissue and glandular, or milk-producing, tissue are the two primary tissue types found in the breast. Each mature breast has numerous lobules, as seen in Figure 8.18, where milk is produced and stored during pregnancy.

The milk drains into ducts and sacs during nursing, also known as lactation, and then converges at the nipple. When an infant suckles, milk is expelled from the breast through the nipple. The areola, an area with darker pigmentation, encircles the nipple. During breastfeeding, glands in the areola secrete an oily fluid that lubricates and shields the nipple.

Two lactation induction protocols for transgender women—the Zil Goldstein and Newman-Goldfarb protocols—were mentioned by survey participants in 2018. These protocols were initially developed to assist cisgender women in breastfeeding a child born to a surrogate mother. The Newman-Goldfarb protocol recommends a dosage of 10 mg of domperidone taken four times a day, while the Zil Goldstein protocol begins with 10 mg of the medication three times per day. In both regimens, the dosage is then increased to 20 mg four times per day. Since the Food and Drug Administration (FDA) has not approved domperidone, patients obtain the medication from alternative sources. Additionally, the sex hormones progesterone and estradiol are utilized in both regimens. Therefore, it is advised to physically stimulate the nipples in order to induce milk production. There have been anecdotal reports of transgender women inducing lactation in recent years. However, none of these reports are supported by empirical data. Consequently, there is a significant lack of evidence-based medicine for this particular population.

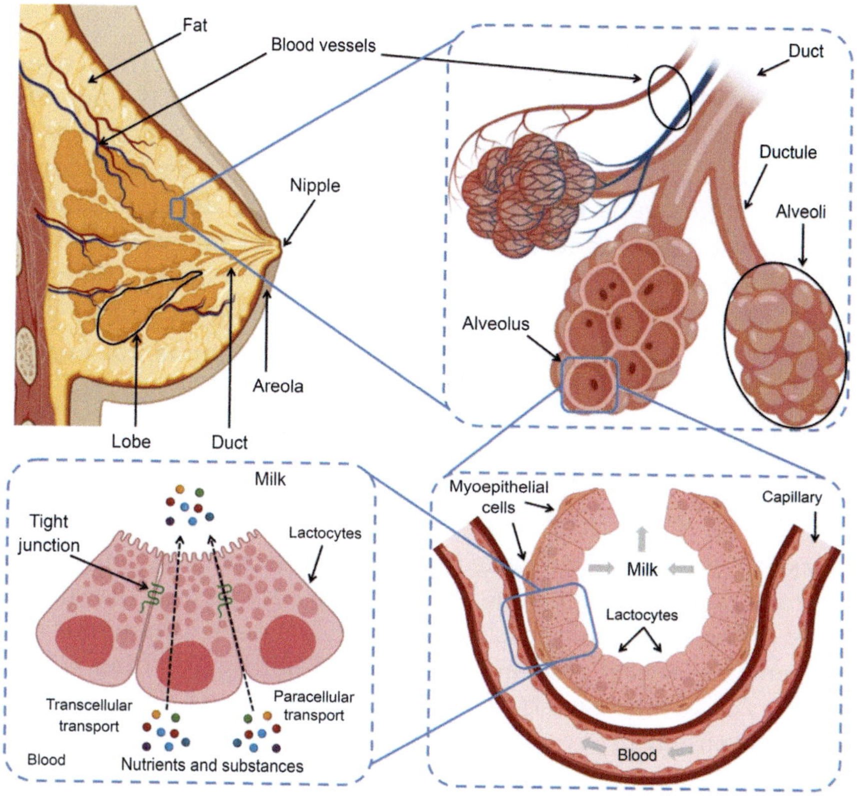

Figure 8.18. *The breasts are not really reproductive organs, but they play a reproductive role as mammary glands that can produce milk to feed an infant. Milk is produced in the glands of the lobules. Then the milk is created through ducts when the infant sucks on the nipples.*

Source: Hatmal, M. M., Al-Hatamleh, M. A. I., Olaimat, A. N., Alshaer, W., Hasan, H., Albakri, K. A., Alkhafaji, E., Issa, N. N., Al-Holy, M. A., Abderrahman, S. M., et al., (2022). Immunomodulatory properties of human breast milk: MicroRNA contents and potential epigenetic effects. Biomedicines, 10(6), 1219. https://doi.org/10.3390/biomedicines10061219.

8.3.2. Menstrual Cycle

Throughout the reproductive years, the natural changes that occur in the female reproductive system each month are referred to as the menstrual cycle. The cycle is crucial for both egg production and uterine preparation for pregnancy. It is regulated by pituitary and ovarian hormones and involves changes in the uterus and ovaries. Day 1 of the cycle marks the beginning of the menstrual cycle, during which the uterus starts to shed the built-up endometrium, resulting in bleeding. Throughout the rest of the cycle, the endometrium thickens again, only to be shed once more at the start of the next cycle if pregnancy does not occur. The ovarian menstrual cycle involves follicle development, ovulation of the secondary oocyte, and follicle degeneration in the absence of pregnancy. Although the phases differ in the two organs, uterine and ovarian changes during the menstrual cycle are typically categorized into three stages.

8.3.2.1. Menarche and Menopause

The onset and cessation of the menstrual cycle define the female reproductive years. The first menstrual period, or menarche, typically occurs when a child reaches the age of 12 or 13. There is a significant variation in the age at which menarche occurs. It can sometimes happen as late as 16 years old, but it can also occur as early as 8 years old and still be considered normal. In the developing world, the average age is typically lower than in the developed world. It is believed that nutritional differences contribute to a significant portion of this variation. Menopause is the term used to describe the end of a woman's reproductive years when her menstrual cycles cease. Menopause can occur naturally at any age between approximately 45 and 55 years old, although the average age is 52. There are numerous biological and environmental factors that influence the age at which menopause occurs. It may occur earlier as a result of specific medical conditions or therapies.

8.3.2.2. Variation in the Menstrual Cycle

The duration and phases of the menstrual cycle can vary significantly, not only between individuals but also within a single person's monthly cycle. The interval between the first day of one menstrual cycle and the first day of the subsequent cycle is typically 28 days, although it can range from 21 to 45 days. When a woman's longest and shortest cycles differ by less than eight days, her cycles are considered regular. The actual menstrual period typically lasts five days, though it can last anywhere from two to seven days.

8.3.3. Ovarian Cycle

The ovarian cycle is composed of the events of the menstrual cycle that occur in the ovaries. It consists of changes that happen in one of the follicles of the ovaries. The ovarian cycle is divided into three stages: the follicular phase, ovulation, and luteal phase. Figure 8.19 provides illustrations of these stages.

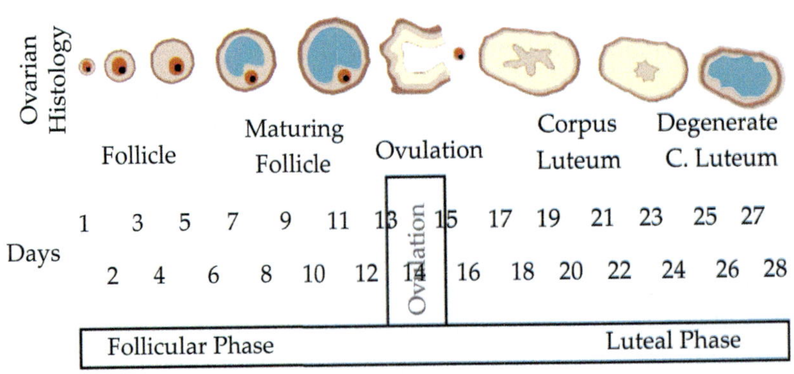

Figure 8.19. *The diagram illustrates the maturation of follicles in the ovary, ovulation, and the formation of the corpus luteum during the follicular and luteal phases of the ovaries. The diagram displays the phases and days of the ovarian cycle. It represents a cycle in which fertilization does not occur, resulting in the degeneration of the corpus luteum during the luteal phase.*

Source: https://bio.libretexts.org/@api/deki/files/16855/Screen_Shot_2019-03-30_at_3.04.15_PM.png?revision=1&size=bestfit&width=672&height=302.

8.3.3.1. Follicular Phase

The ovarian cycle begins with the follicular phase. Typically, it lasts between 12 and 14 days during a 28-day menstrual period. Many ovarian follicles are stimulated to start maturing during this phase, but typically only one, known as the Graafian follicle, fully matures and becomes ready to release an egg.

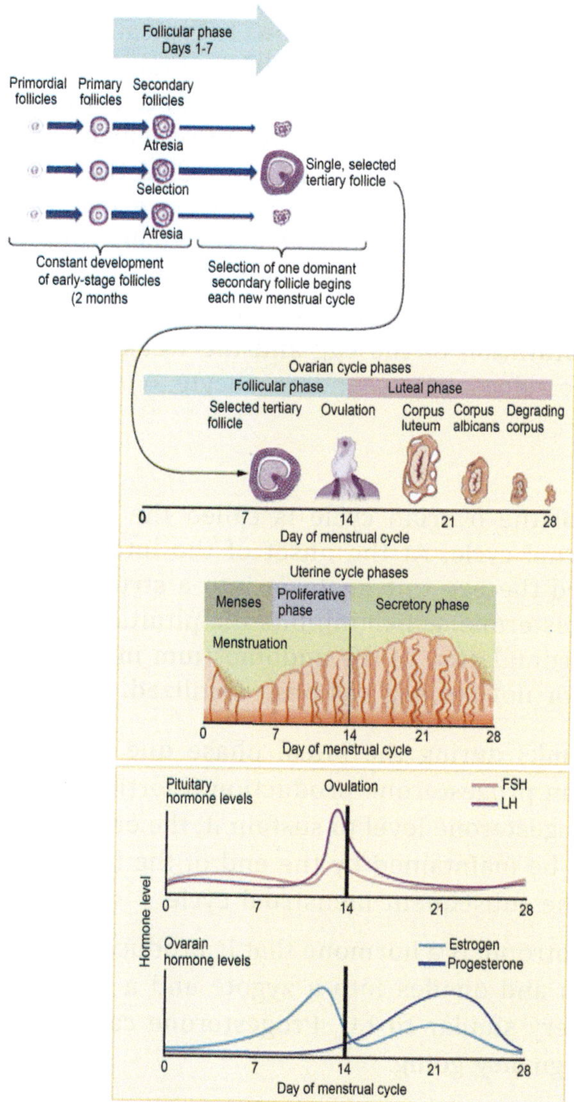

Figure 8.20. *Pituitary and ovarian hormone levels. FSH in the pituitary and estrogen in the ovaries increase during the first half of the menstrual cycle. LH in the pituitary surges shortly before ovulation occurs due to the rise in estrogen in the ovaries. After ovulation, the level of progesterone and estrogen increases in the ovaries due to the formation of the corpus luteum if pregnancy does not occur.*

Source: https://courses.lumenlearning.com/suny-ap2/chapter/anatomy-and-physiology-of-the-female-reproductive-system/.

The remaining developing follicles break apart and cease to grow. The pituitary gland secretes FSH, which raises blood levels and promotes follicular development. Estrogen is released by maturing follicles, and during the follicular phase, its level rises. The chart in Figure 8.20 shows these and other changes in hormone levels that occur during the menstrual cycle.

8.3.4. Ovulation

The second stage of the ovarian cycle is ovulation. It typically occurs on day 14 of a 28-day menstrual cycle. During this phase, the Graafian follicle ruptures and releases its egg. Ovulation is triggered by a sharp increase in the blood concentration of luteinizing hormone (LH) produced by the pituitary gland. This increase is known as the LH surge, which is depicted in the top hormone graph above. The LH surge usually takes place on day 12 of the cycle and lasts for one or two days. The spike in LH is caused by the ongoing increase in estrogen from the maturing ovarian follicle. During the follicular phase, rising estrogen levels actually suppress the pituitary's secretion of LH. However, as the follicular phase nears its end, estrogen levels rise to a point where this suppression is nullified, and estrogen triggers the release of a significant amount of LH. The rise in LH levels leads to the maturation of the egg and the weakening of the follicle wall, allowing the fully developed follicle to release its secondary oocyte.

8.3.4.1. Luteal Phase

The third and final phase of the ovarian cycle is called the luteal phase. It typically lasts for 14 days in a 28-day menstrual cycle. At the onset of the luteal phase, FSH and LH induce the Graafian follicle that released the egg to transform into a structure called a corpus luteum. The corpus luteum secretes progesterone, which inhibits the pituitary's production of FSH and LH and promotes the continuous accumulation of the endometrium in the uterus. The conclusion of this phase depends on whether or not the egg has been fertilized.

The corpus luteum shrinks during the luteal phase due to decreasing FSH and LH levels, which results in a decrease in progesterone production if fertilization has not taken place. In the absence of a high enough progesterone level to sustain it, the endometrium begins to degrade. The endometrium can no longer be maintained by the end of the luteal phase, and the endometrium sheds (menses) to initiate the subsequent menstrual cycle.

Human chorionic gonadotropin is a hormone that is produced by the outer layer of a blastocyst that forms after fertilization and divides into a zygote and a blastocyst. This hormone protects the corpus luteum and is very similar to LH. Progesterone can then be secreted by the corpus luteum to keep the new pregnancy going.

8.3.5. Uterine Cycle

The uterine cycle consists of the events of the menstrual cycle that occur inside the uterus. The endometrium, which is the layer of tissue lining the uterus, undergoes changes primarily during this cycle. The uterine cycle is divided into three phases: menstruation, the proliferative phase, and the secretory phase. Figure 8.21 provides illustrations of these stages.

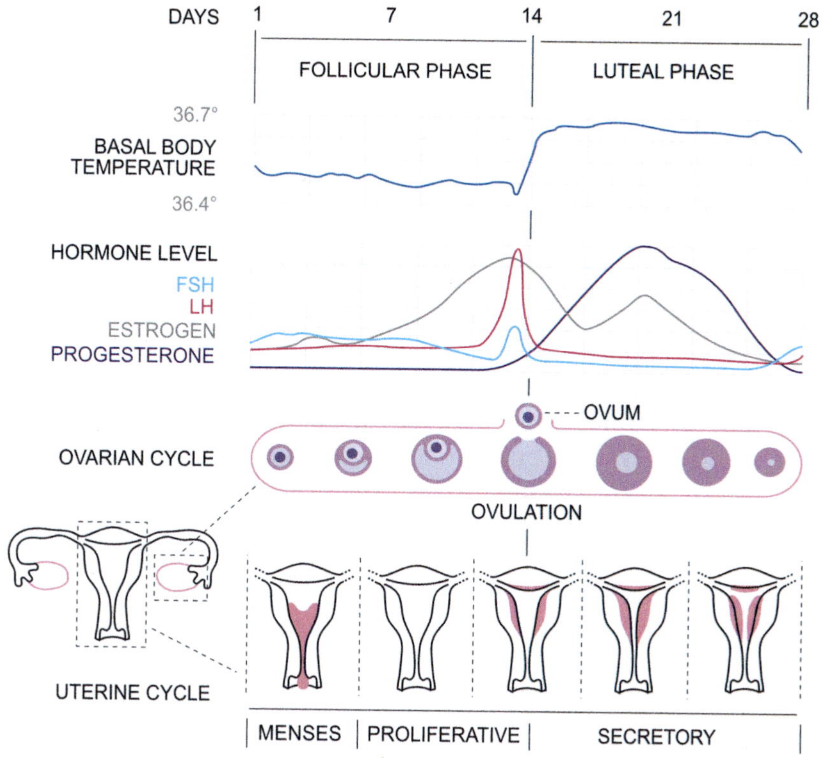

Figure 8.21. *The uterine cycle begins with menstruation, which starts on day 1 of the cycle. The proliferative phase ranges from day 7 to 14. The secretory phase lasts for the second half of the uterine cycle.*

Source: By Isometrik – Own work, CC BY-SA 3.0, https://commons.wikimedia.org/w/index.php?curid=8703107.

8.3.5.1. Menstruation

The first part of the uterine cycle is known as menstruation, sometimes referred to as the menstrual period or menses. It occurs if fertilization did not take place during the preceding menstrual cycle. The uterine endometrium, which has developed over the previous cycle, degenerates and sheds from the uterus during menstruation. On average, approximately 35 mL of blood is lost during the menstrual cycle. Uterine cramps are commonly experienced during this time and can be quite severe in certain individuals.

8.3.5.2. Proliferative Phase

The second stage of the uterine cycle is known as the proliferative phase. During this phase, the maturing cells of the ovarian follicle secrete estrogen, which stimulates the growth or proliferation of the uterine lining. Additionally, estrogen promotes the secretion of more mucus by the uterine cervix. This mucus is thinner and aids in the passage of sperm through the cervix and into the uterus, thereby increasing the chances of fertilization.

8.3.5.3. Secretory Phase

The third and final phase of the uterine cycle is known as the secretory phase. During this stage, the corpus luteum of the ovary produces progesterone, which stimulates further changes in the endometrium to facilitate the implantation of the blastocyst. Progesterone promotes uterine secretions, enhances blood flow to the uterus, and reduces the contractility of the uterine smooth muscle tissue.

8.4. Functions of the Female Reproductive System

A pregnant woman watches her belly grow and patiently awaits the growth of her fetus. The primary objective of reproduction is to create offspring, and the female reproductive system is specifically designed for this purpose. Its functions include the production of gametes, such as eggs, the secretion of sex hormones like estrogen, providing a site for fertilization, gestating a fetus in the event of fertilization, facilitating childbirth, and enabling nursing. The only missing component is sperm.

8.4.1. Egg Production

All of the eggs that will ever be produced, possibly up to a million, are present in the ovaries at birth. However, the eggs do not begin to develop until a female reaches sexual maturity and puberty. After that, an ovary normally releases one mature egg each month. This continues until menopause, which marks the end of monthly periods, usually around the age of 52. By that time, hormone levels may have dropped to the point where viable eggs are almost completely depleted, disrupting the monthly cycle. The release of an egg from either ovary during the reproductive years appears to be random. In rare cases, an egg may be released simultaneously from both ovaries, resulting in the conception of fraternal twins (dizygotic, or "two-zygote," twins) if both eggs are fertilized. Genetically, these twins are no more similar than non-twin siblings.

8.4.2. Oogenesis

Oogenesis, the process by which a fetus with XX chromosomes produces eggs in its ovaries, is illustrated in Figure 8.22. The production of eggs, which are haploid gametes, involves multiple steps and various cell types. Oogenesis is completed long before a child is born, occurring during the mitotic process of diploid germ cells known as oogonia (singular: oogonium). Each of these cell divisions produces two diploid cells. The primary oocyte, one of the oocytes, is reserved to help maintain an oogonia reserve. Meiosis I, the initial cell division of meiosis, begins in the primary oocyte but is not completed until puberty.

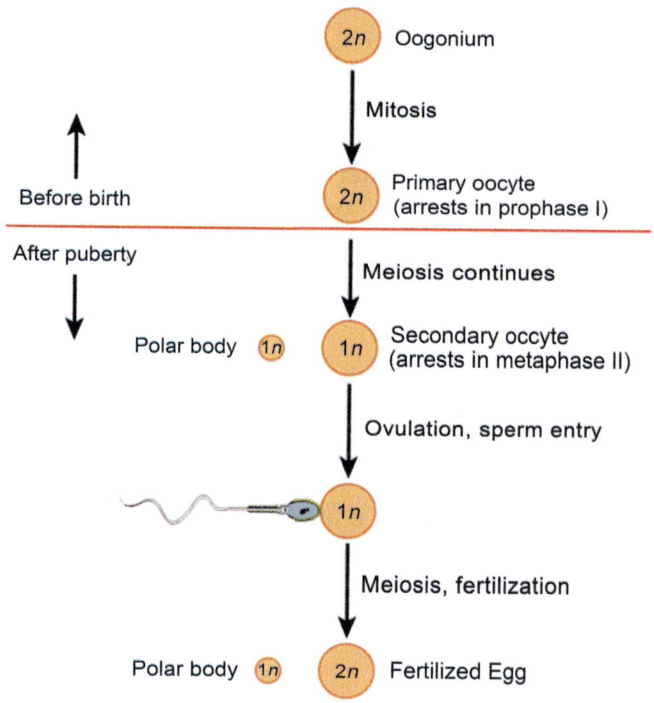

Figure 8.22. *The formation of a secondary oocyte, which has the potential to become a zygote, begins with the mitosis of an oogonium. This is followed by two meiotic cell divisions. In humans, the first polar body does not undergo the second meiotic division. The secondary oocyte completes meiosis II after the penetration of sperm.*

Source: https://courses.lumenlearning.com/wm-biology2/chapter/gametogenesis/.

8.4.2.1. Maturation of a Follicle

Approximately once a month, starting during puberty, an ovary's follicle matures and releases an egg. The follicle undergoes changes in the quantity and type of its cells as it matures. Meiosis is also resumed by the follicle's primary oocyte. It completes meiosis I, which begins long before birth, resulting in a smaller cell called the first polar body and a secondary oocyte. Both the first polar body and the secondary oocyte are haploid cells. The cytoplasm of the primary oocyte is mostly present in the larger secondary oocyte, while the first polar body quickly dissolves and disappears. Meiosis II is initiated by the secondary oocyte and can only be completed if the egg is fertilized.

8.4.2.2. Release of an Egg

The maturation of a follicle in an ovary and the formation of the secondary oocyte typically take 12 to 14 days. Subsequently, the ovary ruptures and the follicle bursts open, releasing the secondary oocyte. This process is known as ovulation. The now-empty follicle begins to develop into the corpus luteum, a structure. The finger-like fimbriae of the expelled secondary oocyte usually sweep it into the adjacent Fallopian tube.

8.4.2.3. Uterine Changes

While the follicle in the ovary matures, changes also occur to prepare the uterus for an embryo in case fertilization occurs. For example, the endometrium thickens and becomes more vascularized. The cervix undergoes changes around ovulation to facilitate the sperm's reach to the oocyte for fertilization. The cervical mucus becomes thinner and more alkaline as the cervical canal widens. These modifications facilitate the movement of sperm from the vagina into the uterus and create a more favorable environment for sperm.

8.4.2.4. Fertilization – or Not

Normally, sperm fertilize eggs in the Fallopian tubes, primarily in the section of the tube that passes above the ovary (Figure 8.23). Sperm must swim from the vagina where they are deposited, via the cervical canal to the uterus, and then via the uterus's body to one of the Fallopian tubes for fertilization to take place. Tubular fluids aid in the passage of sperm through the Fallopian tube and toward the secondary oocyte at the other end. Additionally, the secondary oocyte aids in the process of fertilization. It releases chemicals that direct the sperm and enable the egg's surface to adhere to the sperm's surface. After that, the sperm can be absorbed by the egg, enabling fertilization.

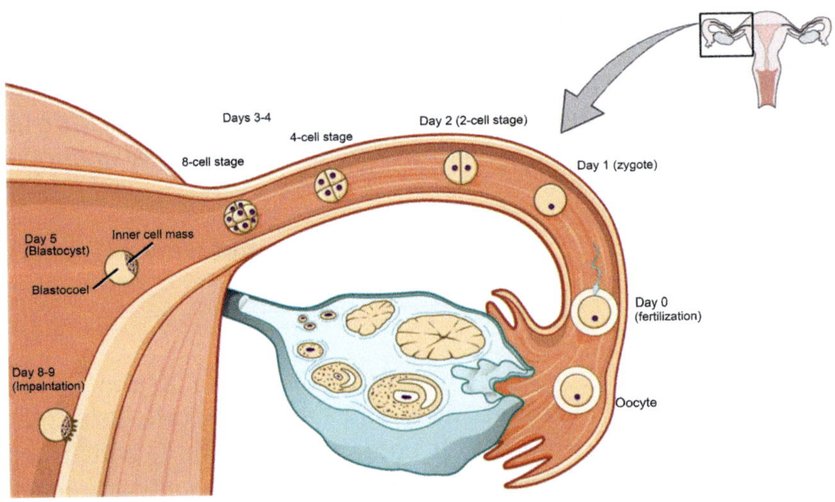

Figure 8.23. *The fimbriae of the fallopian tube sweep the egg into the fallopian tube. Sperm travels through the cervix and uterus and enters the fallopian tube, fertilizing the egg. The embryo then travels towards the uterus.*

Source: https://courses.lumenlearning.com/suny-wmopen-biology2/chapter/human-pregnancy-and-birth/.

8.4.2.5. If Fertilization Occurs

The secondary oocyte rapidly completes meiosis II, forming a diploid zygote and another polar body, if a sperm fertilizes it as it travels through the Fallopian tube. Like the first polar body, this second one usually disintegrates and vanishes. After that, the zygote travels through the fallopian tube and into the uterus, where it divides into multiple mitotic cells. Up to five days after fertilization, when it enters the uterus, it is nothing more than a ball of cells known as a blastocyst. After a day or two, the blastocyst inserts itself into the uterine lining, initiating the process of gestation.

8.4.2.6. If Fertilization Does Not Occur

The secondary oocyte travels to the uterus without ever completing meiosis II if it is not fertilized by a sperm during its passage through the Fallopian tube. If it is still in the Fallopian tube, it will probably be expelled in a few days. The woman's body will expel any leftover material during her subsequent menstrual cycle.

8.4.2.7. Pregnancy

The process of carrying one or more children from fertilization to delivery is commonly known as pregnancy. It serves as one of the primary functions of the female reproductive system. Pregnancy has a profound impact on nearly every other bodily system, including the respiratory, cardiovascular, and urinary systems, among others. The development of the offspring is heavily influenced by the mother organism, who must eliminate the waste products excreted by the offspring and provide all the necessary nutrients and materials for their normal growth and development. During pregnancy, the pregnant individual requires an increased intake of various nutrients to meet the needs of the fetus, with certain nutrients like calcium, iron, folic acid, and omega-3 fatty acids being particularly crucial. To ensure the best possible outcome, it is recommended to take prenatal vitamin supplements and maintain a nutritious diet. Furthermore, it is important for a pregnant individual to refrain from consuming substances, such as alcohol, that may harm the developing fetus, especially during the early stages of pregnancy when major organs and organ systems are still forming.

Typically, pregnancy lasts for 40 weeks when counting from the first day of the last menstrual cycle (or 38 weeks when counting from the time of fertilization). However, a pregnancy lasting between 37 and 42 weeks is still considered within the normal range. From the perspective of the mother organism, the entire duration of pregnancy is divided into three trimesters, each lasting approximately three months. By dividing the entire gestation period into sections, we can gain an overview of the common changes that occur during pregnancy. However, when viewed from the perspective of the developing offspring, the main divisions are different, focusing on the phases of the fetus and embryo. From the moment of implantation in the uterus until the first eight weeks of life, the developing organism is referred to as an embryo. From that point onward, and throughout the remainder of the pregnancy, it is referred to as a fetus.

8.4.2.7.1. First Trimester

Starting at the moment of fertilization and lasting for the following 12 weeks is the first trimester. A person may exhibit pregnancy signs and symptoms even before they become aware of their pregnancy. In addition to experiencing a tender nipple area, increased appetite, and more frequent urination, they might notice that their menstrual period has skipped. In the first trimester, nausea and vomiting are common side effects for many people. Although it can happen at any time of day, this is commonly referred to as "morning sickness" because it usually happens in the morning. Some people lose weight due to morning sickness in the first trimester.

8.4.2.7.2. Second Trimester

The weeks 13 through 28 of pregnancy are when the second trimester happens. During this trimester, a pregnant person might feel more energized. In the second trimester, symptoms such as nausea and vomiting that she had in the first trimester usually go away. Additionally, weight gain begins to occur during this trimester. The fetus is growing to the point where the mother can feel its movements by week 20 or so. In Figure 8.24, a picture of the pregnancy timeline is given. (For comparison, the same woman is depicted at the end of the third trimester on the right of Figure 8.24).

8.4.2.7.3. Third Trimester

The third trimester lasts from week 29 until the baby is born, or roughly 40 weeks. The uterus grows quickly during this trimester, taking up an increasing amount of the woman's abdomen. Moreover, weight gain happens faster. The fetus's movements intensify and increase in frequency during the third trimester, sometimes causing discomfort for the mother. Growing larger fetuses can cause symptoms in the mother such as heartburn, varicose veins, back pain, lower extremity swelling, and increased urination due to their weight and increased space. Because the fetus turns to a downward position prior to birth so that its head rests on the cervix, the woman's abdomen frequently changes shape by the end of the third trimester. This increases pressure on the rectum and pelvic floor while decreasing bladder capacity and relieving pressure on the upper abdomen.

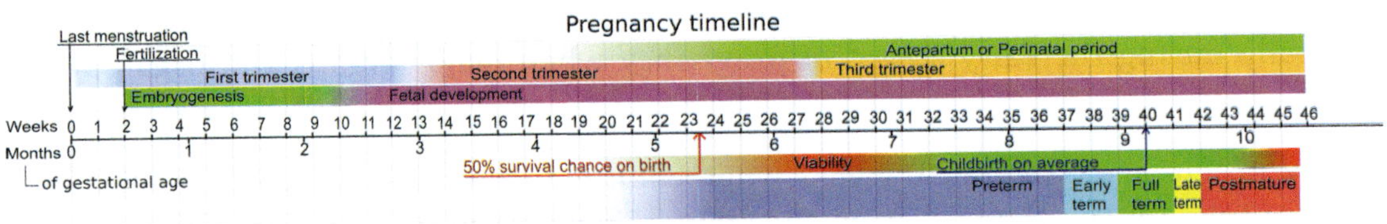

Figure 8.24. *Pregnancy: A timeline.*

Source: https://en.m.wikipedia.org/wiki/File:Pregnancy_timeline.png.

8.4.2.7.4. Childbirth

The amniotic sac, a membrane filled with fluid that surrounds the fetus inside the uterus, bursts in a torrent of fluid close to the time of birth. This is referred to as "rupture of membranes." Labor usually commences one day after this incident, although it may sometimes begin earlier. The process of childbirth, in which the fetus and placenta are expelled from the body through regular uterine contractions, is known as labor. Three distinct phases of labor can be identified, as depicted in Figure 8.25: dilation, birth, and postpartum.

Uterine contractions initiate during the dilation phase of labor and intensify in strength and frequency over time. The cervical canal widens as a result of the contractions exerting pressure on the baby's head (typically) against the cervix. This process continues until the cervical canal is dilated to approximately 10 cm (3.9 in.) in width, which may require up to 20 hours or more. This degree of cervical canal dilation is necessary for the baby's head to pass through.

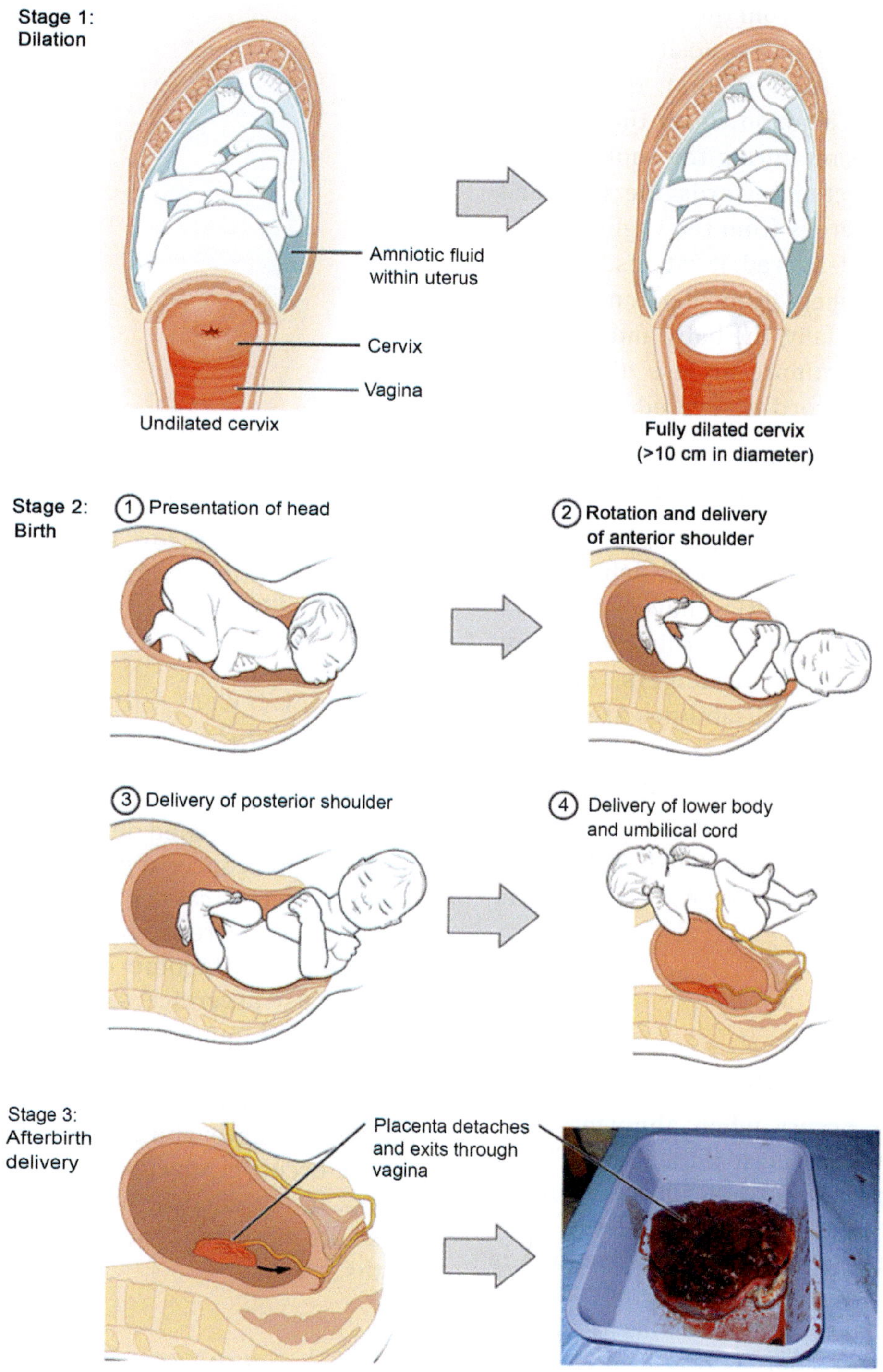

Figure 8.25. *The three stages of labor are dilation of the cervix, the birth of the baby, and the delivery of the afterbirth (placenta).*

Source: https://courses.lumenlearning.com/atd-herkimer-developmentalpsych/chapter/childbirth/.

The baby emerges from the birth canal and vagina, usually in a headfirst position, entering the outside world. At this point, the mother typically begins to bear down on the fetus to facilitate its expulsion during the contractions. With its face directed towards the mother's back, the fetus emerges from the vagina. When the shoulders are delivered, it rotates 90°. This phase can last anywhere from 20 minutes to two hours or longer. Usually, the baby and placenta separate within a minute or less of delivery when the umbilical cord is severed.

During the postpartum stage, the placenta is delivered. This stage may last from a few minutes to half an hour.

Everyone is concerned about delivery, but individuals with disabilities have additional reasons to be concerned. According to a study conducted by Lipson and Rogers, delivery options for people with disabilities are chosen randomly without taking their input into consideration. Due to the assumption that a disabled person would not be able to handle the procedure, they are compelled to undergo a cesarean section for delivery.

8.4.3. Disorders of the Female Reproductive System

8.4.3.1. Cervical Cancer

Cervical cancer occurs when abnormal cells grow in the cervix, the neck of the uterus. These cells have the potential to invade surrounding tissues or spread to other parts of the body, such as the lungs or abdomen. The location of the cervix and the appearance of normal and abnormal cervical cells under a microscope are depicted in Figure 8.26.

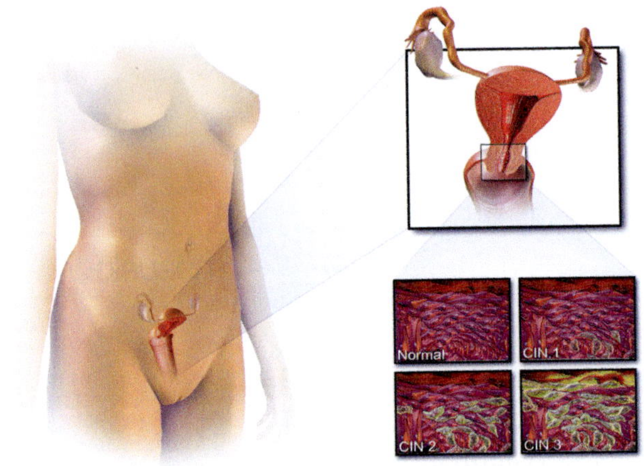

Figure 8.26. *Cancer of the cervix.*

Source: By Blausen Medical Communications, Inc. – see ticket for details, CC BY 3.0, https://commons.wikimedia.org/w/index.php?curid=27639313.

8.4.3.1.1. Cervical Cancer Prevalence and Death Rates

Cervical cancer ranks fourth in the world in terms of cancer-related deaths and is the second most common cancer type globally, after breast cancer. Cervical cancer mortality rates have significantly decreased in the United States and other high-income countries due to the extensive use of cervical cancer screening, which has identified numerous cases of precancerous cervical changes. However, routine screening for cervical cancer is less common in developing countries, where about 75% of cases of the disease occur, primarily due to cost and other factors. In low-income nations, cervical cancer is also the most frequent cause of cancer-related deaths.

8.4.3.1.2. Symptoms of Cervical Cancer

Usually, there are no symptoms when cervical cancer is first developing. Nonetheless, symptoms are likely to appear as the illness worsens. Possible symptoms include abnormal vaginal bleeding, pelvic pain, or pain during sexual activity. Unfortunately, cervical cancer is often diagnosed at an advanced stage where treatment is less likely to be effective by the time symptoms appear.

8.4.3.1.3. Cervical Cancer Causes and Risk Factors

The human papillomavirus (HPV), a sexually transmitted virus that also causes genital warts, is responsible for over 90% of cases of cervical cancer. Cervical cancer can arise from HPV infection through disruption of normal cell division. The absence of HPV prevents mutant cervical cells from proliferating, thus maintaining the health of the cervix. However, when HPV is present, mutated cervical cells may be given the opportunity to proliferate, leading to the unchecked growth of mutated cells and the development of a tumor.

Additional risk factors for cervical cancer include the use of birth control pills, smoking, having multiple sexual partners, having a compromised immune system (due to HIV infection, for example), and early initiation of sexual activity. However, these risk factors are overshadowed by HPV infection. In individuals already infected with HPV, these risk factors are more likely to increase the risk of cervical cancer. For example, current and former smokers with HPV infection have a two to three times higher incidence of cervical cancer compared to non-smokers. Although to a lesser extent, passive smoking is also associated with an increased risk of cervical cancer.

8.4.3.1.4. Diagnosis of Cervical Cancer

Typically, a Pap smear, which involves examining microscopic abnormal cervical cells scraped from the cervix, is used to diagnose cervical cancer. If cancerous cells are found or suspected in the smear, a biopsy is usually performed to confirm the results of the Pap smear. Additional tests, such as an MRI or CT scan, may also be conducted to provide more detailed information, such as the extent of cancer spread.

8.4.3.1.5. Prevention of Cervical Cancer

With the availability of a vaccine, HPV infection can now be prevented. The first HPV vaccine was approved by the U.S. in 2006, through the Food and Drug Administration. The vaccine provides protection against the HPV strains that are most likely to cause cervical cancer. It is predicted that up to 90% of cervical cancer cases can be avoided if the vaccine is widely used. Currently, the recommended age range for vaccination is between nine and 26 years old.

HPV vaccinations are recommended for all sexes due to the virus's potential to cause various other cancers, including penis cancer. The vaccine is most effective when administered before the onset of HPV infection. In addition to vaccination, using condoms during sexual activity can also help prevent HPV infection and cervical cancer, as well as pregnancy and STDs like HIV.

It is important to note that cervical cancer remains a rare risk even in individuals who have received the HPV vaccine. Therefore, it is advised that people with a cervix still undergo routine Pap smear exams.

8.4.3.1.6. Treatment of Cervical Cancer

The course of treatment for cervical cancer typically depends on the stage of the disease at diagnosis, but it usually entails a mix of radiation therapy, chemotherapy, and/or surgery. Treatment outcomes are primarily determined by how early cancer is identified and treated. Surgery is required to remove the entire tumor and ensure that, upon microscopic inspection, no cancerous cells are present at the margins of the removed tissue in order to cure cervical cancer. The five-year survival rate is nearly 100% if cancer is detected and treated very early, while it is still in the microscopic stage.

8.4.3.2. Vaginitis

Inflammation of the vagina and, occasionally, the vulva is known as vaginal vaginitis. Yellow, gray, or green discharge, itching, pain, and a burning feeling are possible symptoms. A bad vaginal odor and pain or irritation during sex are possible additional symptoms (Figure 8.27).

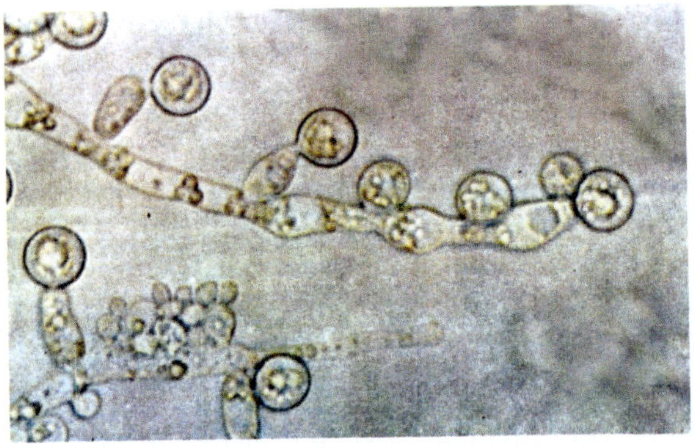

Figure 8.27. *The yeast Candida albicans—shown here growing on a culture plate—is one of the most common causes of vaginitis.*

Source: By Dr Graham Beards - Own work, CC BY-SA 3.0, https://commons.wikimedia.org/w/index.php?curid=10921762.

8.4.3.2.1. Causes of Vaginitis

Microorganism infection is the cause of about 90% of cases of vaginitis. The yeast *Candida albicans* is most frequently the cause of vaginal infections. Vaginal candidiasis is the term used to describe these infections. Bacteria, particularly *Gardnerella vaginalis*, and certain single-celled parasites, most notably the protist parasite *Trichomonas vaginalis*, which is typically spread through vaginal sex, are other potential causes of vaginal infections. Those who use birth control pills, wear tight clothing, take antibiotics for another illness, or practice poor hygiene may be more susceptible to vaginal infections. Yeast and other organisms that are typically found in the stool can contaminate the vagina due to poor hygiene. The majority of the remaining cases of vaginitis are caused by allergic reactions to different products or irritation from them. Condoms, spermicides, soaps, douches, lubricants, and even semen are examples of these irritants. Other possible causes of this kind of vaginitis include soaking in hot tubs and using tampons.

8.4.3.2.2. Diagnosis of Vaginitis

Symptoms reported by the patient are typically the initial step in diagnosing vaginitis. To determine the exact cause, a microscopic examination or culture of the vaginal discharge may follow. The causative agent can be inferred from the color, consistency, acidity, and other characteristics of the discharge. For example, a *Gardnerella vaginalis* infection may result in a high pH discharge with a fishy odor, while a *Candida albicans* infection may cause a low pH discharge resembling cottage cheese.

8.4.3.2.3. Prevention of Vaginitis

Wearing loose cotton underwear can help prevent vaginitis by maintaining dryness in the vulva. Moisture generally provides an ideal environment for yeasts and bacteria that can cause vaginitis. Additionally, it is crucial to avoid using douches, personal hygiene sprays, and perfumed soaps as they can disrupt the natural pH and bacterial balance of the vagina. When engaging in sexual activity, it is recommended to use condoms to help prevent vaginitis caused by a Trichomonas infection.

8.4.3.2.4. Treatment of Vaginitis

The appropriate treatment of vaginitis depends on the cause. In many cases of vaginitis, there is more than one cause, and all of the causes must be treated to ensure a cure.

- Yeast infections of the vagina are typically treated with topical anti-fungal medications, which are available over the counter. The medications may be in the form of tablets or creams that are inserted into the vagina. Depending on the particular medication used, treatment may involve one, three, or seven days of application.
- Bacterial infections of the vagina are usually treated with antibiotics. These may be taken orally as pills or applied topically to the vagina in creams.
- Trichomonas vaginalis infections of the vagina are generally treated with a single dose of an oral antibiotic. Sexual partners should be treated at the same time, and intercourse should be avoided for at least a week until both partners have completed treatment and been followed up by a physician.

8.4.3.3. Endometriosis

Endometriosis is a condition where tissue similar to the lining of the uterus grows outside of the uterus. This tissue can be found around the ovaries, Fallopian tubes, and uterus, and in rare cases, in other parts of the body. The areas affected by endometriosis can bleed during menstrual periods, leading to inflammation, pain, and scarring. About 6% to 10% of individuals with a uterus are estimated to have endometriosis, most commonly occurring in their 30s and forties. It is rare before puberty or after menopause (Figure 8.28).

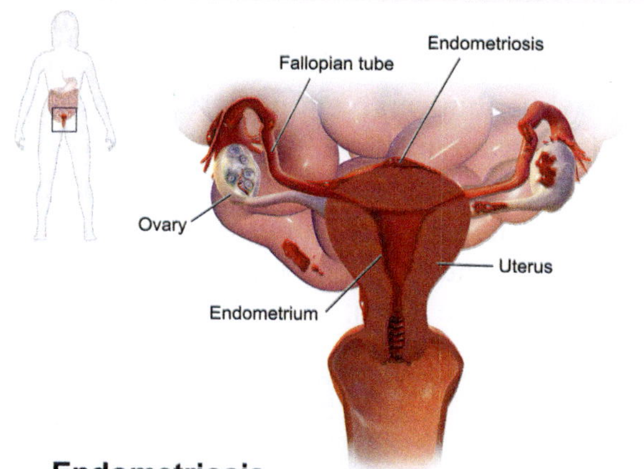

Figure 8.28. *In endometriosis, endometrial tissue may grow outside the uterus and cause health problems such as pain, bleeding, scarring, and infertility. Here, the endometrial tissue is growing in the fallopian tubes, ovaries, and on the outside of the fallopian tube and uterus.*

Source: By BruceBlaus. When using this image in external sources, it can be cited as: Blausen.com staff (2014). "Medical gallery of Blausen Medical 2014." WikiJournal of Medicine, 1(2). doi: 10.15347/wjm/2014.010. ISSN 2002-4436. – Own work, CC BY 3.0, https://commons.wikimedia.org/w/index.php?curid=29600447.

8.4.3.3.1. Signs and Symptoms of Endometriosis

Pelvic pain is the primary sign of endometriosis and can vary in intensity. The amount of endometrial tissue growing outside the uterus does not seem to be correlated with the intensity of pain. For many individuals with the condition, menstruation is the primary source of pain. However, persistent pelvic pain affects nearly half of those affected. Inflammation caused by pelvic bleeding may be the source of endometriosis pain. Internal scar tissue that connects internal organs can also cause pain.

Another issue commonly associated with endometriosis is infertility, or the inability to conceive. Infertility can affect up to half of endometriosis patients. Anatomical deformities caused by abnormal endometrial tissue or scar formation may be linked to infertility. Endometriosis can also cause chronic fatigue, headaches, nausea and vomiting, constipation or diarrhea, and heavy or irregular menstrual bleeding (Figure 8.29).

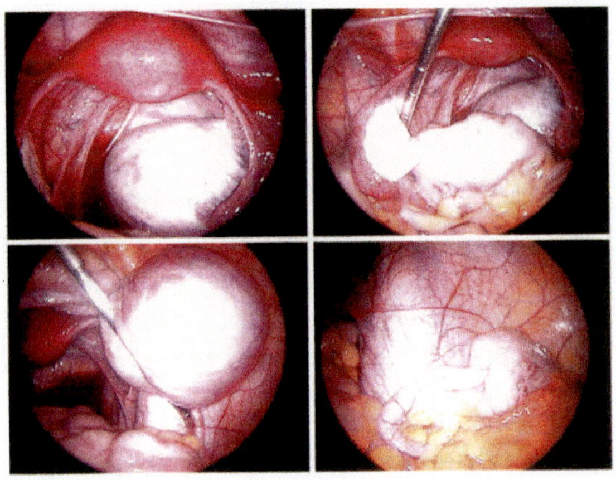

Figure 8.29. *Laparoscopy: Visually inspecting the abdomen for endometrial growth is the most reliable way to diagnose endometriosis. The camera is inserted through the abdominal wall.*

Source: By richie graham – originally posted to Flickr as jensute, CC BY 2.0, https://commons.wikimedia.org/w/index.php?curid=4178268.

8.4.3.3.2. Causes of Endometriosis

Although the exact causes of endometriosis are unknown, a number of risk factors, such as a family history of the condition, have been found. Individuals who are genetically related to someone who has endometriosis are approximately six times more likely to develop the condition themselves. There have been suggestions that endometriosis is caused by multiple gene mutations. Endometriosis is likely to be multifactorial, meaning that multiple factors interact to cause it. The most common physiological theory regarding the development of endometriosis is retrograde menstruation. This occurs when part of the endometrial debris from a menstrual flow exits the uterus through the Fallopian tubes instead of the vagina. The debris then attaches itself to the lining of the abdominal cavity or the exterior of the organs within. However, not all cases of endometriosis can be explained by retrograde menstruation, suggesting that other factors may be involved. Environmental pollutants and autoimmune reactions are two possible suggestions.

8.4.3.3.3. Diagnosis of Endometriosis

Endometriosis is typically diagnosed through patient self-reporting of symptoms and physical examination by a physician, often in conjunction with medical imaging such as ultrasound. However, a visual examination of the endometrial tissue is the only definitive method for diagnosing endometriosis. This can be achieved through a surgical technique called laparoscopy, which involves making a small incision in the abdomen to insert a tiny camera (Figure 8.29). The camera allows the doctor to visually examine the suspected endometrial tissue area.

8.4.3.3.4. Treatment of Endometriosis

The most common treatments for endometriosis are surgery to remove the abnormal tissue and the use of painkillers. Non-steroidal anti-inflammatory drugs (NSAIDs), such as naproxen, are commonly used for pain relief. In cases of severe pain, opioids may be prescribed. Both the diagnosis and surgical treatment of endometriosis can be performed using laparoscopy. To remove or cauterize the endometrial growths, a second small incision is made to insert instruments that the surgeon can manipulate externally. In younger patients who wish to preserve their reproductive organs for future parenthood, surgery is performed conservatively. However, it should be noted that 20% to 40% of endometriosis cases recur within five years following conservative surgery. In older individuals who have completed their childbearing years, a hysterectomy may be performed to remove some or all of the internal reproductive organs. This is the only treatment that has the potential to effectively treat endometriosis and prevent relapses.

8.4.4. Infertility

The inability of a sexually mature adult to naturally procreate is known as infertility. Infertility is widely recognized in the fields of science and medicine as the inability to conceive a child after engaging in consistent, unprotected sexual activity for at least one year. There are two types of infertility: primary and secondary. Primary infertility refers to the inability to conceive for individuals who have never been able to do so. On the other hand, secondary infertility is characterized by the inability to conceive again after successfully carrying a child to adulthood, despite trying for a year. Infertility is a prevalent issue, affecting approximately 61 million, or roughly 10%, of women in the United States aged 15 to 44 who struggle to become or remain pregnant.

8.4.4.1. Causes of Infertility

There are various causes of infertility. The process of pregnancy involves several steps, including the release of an egg from one of the ovaries, the passage of the egg through the Fallopian tube, fertilization of the egg by a sperm, and the implantation of the fertilized egg in the uterus. Infertility may occur if there are issues with any of these procedures.

8.4.4.2. Causes of Male Infertility

In the case of male infertility, it can be caused by an excess or lack of sperm, or by healthy, motile sperm that are unable to pass through the female reproductive system and fertilize an egg. One common cause of insufficient sperm motility or quantity is varicocele, which refers to an enlargement of the scrotal blood vessels. This condition can lead to an increase in testes' temperature, negatively impacting sperm production. In other cases, the sperm may be healthy, but the male reproductive tract is blocked, preventing the ejaculation of sperm.

A man's risk of infertility is increased by heavy drinking, drug addiction, smoking cigarettes, exposure to environmental toxins (like lead or pesticides), certain medications, serious illnesses (like kidney disease), and cancer treatment such as radiation or chemotherapy. Growing older is an additional risk factor. Male fertility typically peaks in the middle of one's 20s and begins to progressively decline after the age of 40, though it may never truly fall to zero.

8.4.4.3. Causes of Female Infertility

One of two issues typically causes female infertility: the ovaries' inability to generate viable eggs or anatomical issues with the uterus or Fallopian tubes. Ovulation disorders are the most common cause of infertility in women. There wouldn't be any eggs to fertilize without ovulation. Even regular menstrual periods can be anovulatory for a variety of reasons. Anovulatory cycles, or menstrual cycles in which ovulation does not occur, are associated with irregular or nonexistent menstrual cycles. Polycystic ovarian syndrome (PCOS), which results in hormone imbalances that can obstruct normal ovulation, is the most common cause of anovulatory cycles. Primary ovarian insufficiency is another rather common cause of anovulation. This disorder causes the ovaries to stop functioning normally and releasing viable eggs at a young age—typically before the age of 40 (Figure 8.30).

Less frequently, structural issues with the uterus or Fallopian tubes can cause infertility. Endometriosis can lead to blockage in the Fallopian tubes. Pelvic inflammatory disease, which occurs when STDs spread to the Fallopian tubes or other female reproductive organs, is another potential cause (Figure 8.30). This infection can result in blockage and scarring of the Fallopian tubes. If a woman has uterine fibroids and her Fallopian tubes are functioning properly when an egg is released, implantation in the uterus may not be possible. Uterine fibroids are non-cancerous growths of muscle and tissue that develop on the uterine walls.

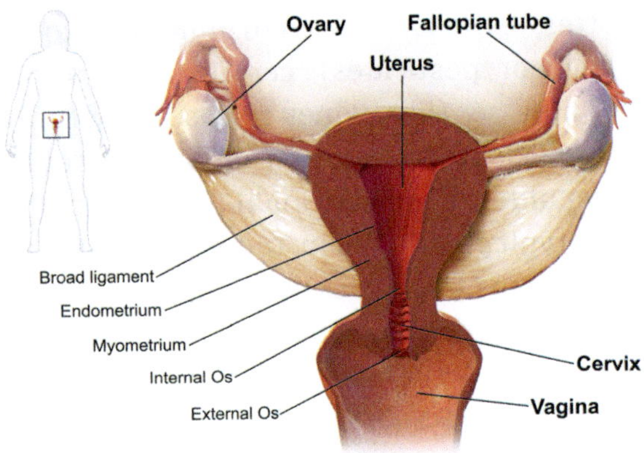

Figure 8.30. *An infection of the Fallopian tubes may cause scarring and blockage of the tubes, preventing sperm from reaching eggs for fertilization.*

Source: By BruceBlaus – Own work, CC BY 3.0, https://commons.wikimedia.org/w/index.php?curid=30462650.

Smoking tobacco, excessive alcohol consumption, stress, poor diet, intense physical activity, and being overweight or underweight increase a woman's risk of infertility. For women, older age presents greater challenges compared to men. Typically, a woman's fertility peaks in her mid-20s and gradually declines until menopause, which occurs around age 52 and causes the ovaries to stop producing eggs. Infertility issues affect approximately one-third of couples where the woman is over 35. Anovulatory cycles are more common in older women, and the quality of the eggs may be lower.

8.4.4.4. Diagnosing Causes of Infertility

Testing both partners for potential issues is frequently necessary in order to diagnose the cause(s) of infertility in a couple. It is likely that the quantity, form, and motility of sperm in the semen will be assessed. If sperm issues are discovered, further research will likely be conducted, including imaging tests to check for structural issues with the testes or ducts.

Determining if ovulation is occurring is typically the initial step for individuals with ovaries and uteruses. This can be achieved at home using a home ovulation test kit, which is available over-the-counter at most drugstores, or by closely monitoring body temperature, which slightly increases around the time of ovulation. Blood tests and ultrasound imaging of the ovaries can also be utilized to determine whether ovulation is taking place. If ovulation is occurring normally, an X-ray of the uterus and Fallopian tubes may be performed to check for blockages or other structural issues. Laparoscopy is an additional method of examining the reproductive tract for potential issues. During this surgical procedure, a tiny camera is inserted into the abdomen through a small incision, allowing the physician to closely examine the reproductive organs.

8.4.4.5. Treating Infertility

Infertility can often be successfully treated. The type of treatment depends on the cause of infertility.

1. **Treating Male Infertility:** Treatments for medical conditions that affect sperm production may involve medications or other interventions that can help restore normal sperm production. In cases where an infection is hindering sperm production, antibiotics may be beneficial. If there is an obstruction

preventing sperm ejaculation, surgery may be performed to remove it. Alternatively, sperm extraction and artificial insemination can be considered as an option. During this process, the sperm is injected into the uterus.

2. **Treating Female Infertility:** When it comes to treating female infertility, surgery can be utilized to address uterine fibroids or blocked Fallopian tubes. On the other hand, hormonal treatments that target the ovaries or the pituitary gland are commonly employed to address ovulation issues.

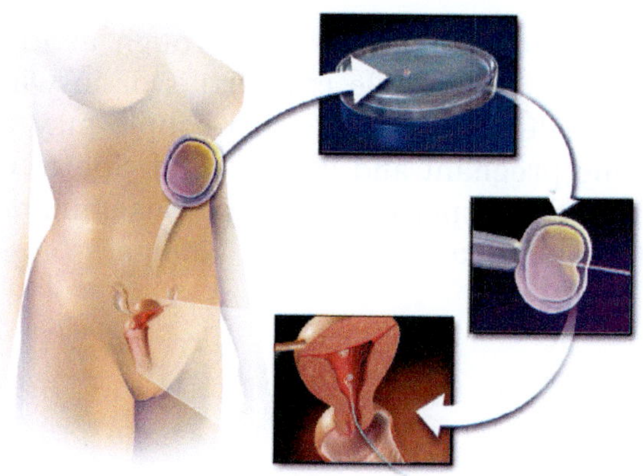

Figure 8.31. *One way ART procedures may be used to treat infertility. An egg is removed from the female reproductive tract, injected with sperm from her partner, and allowed to develop into an embryo in the lab. Then, the embryo is placed inside the woman's uterus for implantation and development during the remainder of gestation.*

Source: By BruceBlaus. When utilizing this image in external sources, it may be referenced as follows: Blausen.com personnel (2014). "Medical gallery of Blausen Medical 2014." WikiJournal of Medicine, 1(2). doi: 10.15347/wjm/2014.010.ISSN 2002-4436. - Own work, CC BY 3.0, https://commons.wikimedia.org/w/index.php?curid=29600441.

The use of hormonal treatments that stimulate ovulation can increase the chances of conceiving twins, triplets, or even more multiple births, as it often leads to the release of multiple eggs simultaneously. However, it is important to consider that multiple fetuses have a higher risk of premature birth, health and developmental issues, as well as pregnancy-related complications for the mother. Therefore, the possibility of multiple fetuses should be carefully considered when opting for this type of infertility treatment (Figure 8.31)

8.4.4.6. Assisted Reproductive Technology

Assistance with reproduction through technology is utilized to treat certain cases of infertility, known as Assisted Reproductive Technology (ART). This category of medical treatments involves the retrieval of eggs and sperm for manipulation in order to optimize the chances of fertilization. In order to facilitate in vivo fertilization, the eggs and sperm can be injected into one of the Fallopian tubes within the body. However, it is more common for the eggs and sperm to be combined externally, resulting in in vitro fertilization taking place in a laboratory test tube or dish. Figure 8.30 provides an illustration of this latter approach. The fertilized eggs may be allowed to develop into embryos through in vitro fertilization before being implanted into the woman's uterus.

The success rate of Assisted Reproductive Technology (ART) is approximately 40% for women under 35, but decreases to 20% for those over 35. Some studies suggest a slightly higher risk of birth defects in children conceived through ART, although this may be attributed to the age of the parents rather than the technology itself. Additionally, same-sex couples often utilize ART to expand their families.

8.4.4.7. Other Approaches

Other approaches for addressing infertility and assisting same-sex couples include the use of a surrogate mother, a gestational carrier, or sperm donation.

- A surrogate mother is a woman who agrees to become pregnant using the male partner's sperm and her own egg. The child, who will be biologically related to the surrogate and the male partner, is then given up for adoption by the couple. Surrogacy may be chosen by women with no eggs or unhealthy eggs. Furthermore, a woman who carries a mutant gene for a serious genetic disorder might opt for this option to prevent the transmission of the defective gene to the offspring.
- A gestational carrier is a woman who agrees to receive a transplanted embryo from a couple and carry it to term. The child, who will be the biological offspring of the couple, is given to the parents at birth. A gestational carrier might be used by women who have normal ovulation but no uterus, or who cannot safely carry a fetus to term because of a serious health problem (such as kidney disease or cancer). This method is commonly used by gay couples.
- Sperm donation is the use of sperm from a fertile man (generally through artificial insemination) for cases in which the male partner in a couple is infertile, or in which a woman seeks to become pregnant without a male partner. A lesbian couple may use donated sperm to enable one of them to become pregnant and have a child. Sperm can be obtained from a sperm bank, which buys and stores sperm for artificial insemination, or a male friend or another individual may donate sperm to a specific woman.

A Closer Look

Spermatogenesis

Spermatogenesis is the process of origin and development of sperm cells within the male reproductive organs, specifically the testes. The testes consist of tightly coiled tubules called seminiferous tubules, where the sperm cells are produced. Within these tubules, there are scattered cells known as Sertoli cells, which provide support and nourishment to the immature sperm cells by supplying them with nutrients and blood products. As the germ cells mature, the Sertoli cells assist in transporting them from the outer surface of the seminiferous tubule to the central channel.

Sperm cells are continuously produced by the testes, although not all areas of the seminiferous tubules produce sperm cells simultaneously. It takes approximately 74 days for an immature germ cell to reach full maturation, and during this growth process, there are intermittent resting phases.

The immature cells, called spermatogonia, are derived from stem cells located in the outer wall of the seminiferous tubules. These stem cells primarily consist of nuclear material, with the nucleus containing the chromosomes. The stem cells undergo mitosis, a process of cell duplication, to multiply. Half of the new cells from this initial division become future sperm cells, while the other half remain as stem cells, ensuring a constant supply of germ cells. Spermatogonia that are destined to develop into mature sperm cells are referred to as primary sperm cells. They migrate from the outer portion of the seminiferous tubule to a more central location and attach themselves to the Sertoli cells. The primary sperm cells then develop by increasing the amount of cytoplasm and organelles within the cytoplasm. After a resting phase, the primary cells divide into secondary sperm cells, with a splitting of the nuclear material. The nucleus of the primary sperm cells contains 46 chromosomes, while each secondary sperm cell and the egg contain only 23 chromosomes. When the egg and sperm combine, their chromosomes unite, blending the characteristics of both individuals and initiating the growth of the new organism.

The secondary sperm cell still needs to mature before it can fertilize an egg. Maturation involves changes in the shape and form of the sperm cell. The nuclear material becomes more condensed and oval, forming the head of the sperm. The head is partially covered by a cap called the acrosome, which aids in the sperm's entry into the egg. Attached to the opposite end of the head is the tailpiece, derived from the secondary sperm cell's cytoplasm. The mature sperm consists of a long, slender bundle of filaments that propel the sperm through undulating movement. Once matured, the sperm is transported through the long seminiferous tubules and stored in the epididymis of the testes until it is ready to leave the male body.

Summary

- Reproduction is the process by which organisms generate offspring, to put it simply. All living things are distinguished from nonliving things by this phenomenon, which unites them.
- The reproductive system in humans is responsible for the production and fertilization of gametes, such as sperm and eggs, as well as the development of a fetus.
- In fetuses, both male and female, undifferentiated embryonic tissues give rise to different structures. Homologous structures are those that arise from the same tissues in both males and females.
- The male and female reproductive systems are distinct from birth, but they are not fully developed and cannot produce gametes or sex hormones.
- The testes are made up of hundreds of tiny tubes called STs, which serve as the organs' functional units.
- The vas deferens, sometimes referred to as the SDs, are a pair of slender tubes that start at the scrotal epididymis and extend upward into the pelvic cavity.
- The seminal vesicles are directly below the prostate gland. This organ, resembling a walnut, is located around the urethra and where it connects to the two EDs.
- Delivering sperm to the female reproductive tract is the reproductive role of the penis, an external male organ.
- The urethra travels through the penis to transport urine from the bladder or semen from the ejaculatory ducts out of the body.
- Erectile dysfunction (ED) is a common sexual disorder that affects approximately 40% of individuals with penises.
- The internal and external organs that make up the female reproductive system are responsible for secreting sex hormones like estrogen, producing haploid gametes known as eggs (or oocytes), and carrying and giving birth to a fetus.

References

1. Al-Agha, O. M., & Axiotis, C. A., (2007). An in-depth look at Leydig cell tumor of the testis. *Arch. Pathol. Lab. Med., 131*(2), 311–317.
2. Albulescu, D., Constantin, C., & Constantin, C., (2014). Uterine artery emerging variants – angiographic aspects. *Curr. Health Sci. J., 40*(3), 214–216.
3. Ambedkar, V., Singh, A., Bain, J., & Singh, L. M., (2015). A rare case of femoral herniation of female internal genitalia. *J. Nat. Sci. Biol. Med., 6*(2), 454–456.
4. Anderson, D., (2014). Pudendal nerve block for vaginal birth. *J. Midwifery Womens Health., 59*(6), 651–659.
5. Ashton-Miller, J. A., & DeLancey, J. O., (2007). Functional anatomy of the female pelvic floor. *Ann. N Y Acad. Sci., 1101*, 266–296.
6. Basaria, S., (2014). Male hypogonadism. *Lancet, 383*(9924), 1250–1263.
7. Bonomi, M., Rochira, V., Pasquali, D., Balercia, G., Jannini, E. A., & Ferlin, A., (2017).

Klinefelter Italian Group (KING). Klinefelter syndrome (KS): Genetics, clinical phenotype and hypogonadism. *J. Endocrinol. Invest., 40*(2), 123–134.

8. Boyd, C. A., & Riall, T. S., (2012). Unexpected gynecologic findings during abdominal surgery. *Curr. Probl. Surg., 49*(4), 195–251.
9. Briceag, I., Costache, A., Purcarea, V. L., Cergan, R., Dumitru, M., Briceag, I., Sajin, M., & Ispas, A. T., (2015). Fallopian tubes--literature review of anatomy and etiology in female infertility. *J. Med. Life., 8*(2), 129–131.
10. Cagnacci, A., Grandi, G., Cannoletta, M., Xholli, A., Piacenti, I., & Volpe, A., (2014). Intensity of menstrual pain and estimated angle of uterine flexion. *Acta Obstet. Gynecol. Scand., 93*(1), 58–63.
11. Catenaccio, E., Mu, W., & Lipton, M. L., (2016). Estrogen- and progesterone-mediated structural neuroplasticity in women: Evidence from neuroimaging. *Brain Struct. Funct., 221*(8), 3845–3867.
12. Chen, C., Lee, S. M., Kim, J. W., & Shin, J. H., (2018). Recent update of embolization of postpartum hemorrhage. *Korean J. Radiol., 19*(4), 585–596.
13. Chung, S. H., & Kim, W. B., (2018). Various approaches and treatments for pelvic organ prolapse in women. *J. Menopausal Med., 24*(3), 155–162.
14. Ciebiera, M., Słabuszewska-Jóźwiak, A., Ledowicz, W., & Jakiel, G., (2015). Vaginal foreign body mimicking cervical cancer in postmenopausal woman – case study. *Prz Menopauzalny., 14*(3), 208–210.
15. Coy, P., García-Vázquez, F. A., Visconti, P. E., & Avilés, M., (2012). Roles of the oviduct in mammalian fertilization. *Reproduction, 144*(6), 649–660.
16. Coyle, D., Kavanagh, N., Mahmoud, A., Lowery, A. J., Khan, W., & Barry, K., (2011). Incarcerated femoral hernia containing ovary and fallopian tube in a 54-year-old. *BMJ Case Rep., 2011.*
17. Dabrowiecki, A., Newsome, J., Bercu, Z. L., & Martin, J. G., (2019). Postpartum haemorrhage requiring embolization of a hypertrophied round ligament artery. *BMJ Case Rep., 12*(8)
18. De Tayrac, R., Panel, L., Masson, G., & Mares, P., (2006). Episiotomy and prevention of perineal and pelvic floor injuries. *J. Gynecol. Obstet. Biol. Reprod. (Paris)., 35*(1 Suppl), 1S24–1S31.
19. DeMayo, F. J., Zhao, B., Takamoto, N., & Tsai, S. Y., (2002). Mechanisms of action of estrogen and progesterone. *Ann. N Y Acad. Sci., 955*, 48–59; discussion 86–88, 396–406.
20. Dimitriadis, F., Tsiampali, C., Chaliasos, N., Tsounapi, P., Takenaka, A., & Sofikitis, N., (2015). The Sertoli cell as the orchestra conductor of spermatogenesis: Spermatogenic cells dance to the tune of testosterone. *Hormones (Athens)., 14*(4), 479–503.
21. Ernest, A., Emmanuel, M., & Gregory, K., (2014). Post-coital posterior fornix perforation with vaginal evisceration. *BMC Womens Health., 14*, 141.
22. Esteves, S. C., (2014). Clinical relevance of routine semen analysis and controversies surrounding the 2010. World Health Organization criteria for semen examination. *Int. Braz. J. Urol., 40*(4), 443–453.
23. Garcia-Ortiz, J. E., Pelosi, E., Omari, S., Nedorezov, T., Piao, Y., Karmazin, J., Uda, M., et al., (2009). Foxl2 functions in sex determination and histogenesis throughout mouse ovary development. *BMC Dev. Biol., 9*, 36.

24. Garge, S., Paliwal, G., Mittal, S., & Kakani, N., (2020). Mesonephric remnant (paroophoron) presenting as a congenital lumbar sinus in a child. *J. Indian Assoc. Pediatr. Surg., 25*(1), 58–59.

25. Giarenis, I., & Robinson, D., (2014). Prevention and management of pelvic organ prolapse. *F1000Prime Rep., 6,* 77.

26. Hasanzadeh, M., Jafarian, A. H., & Mousavi, S. L., (2019). Primary clear cell carcinoma with no diethylstilbestrol exposure; case series. *Iran J. Med. Sci., 44*(2), 163–167.

27. Heindel, J. J., & Treinen, K. A., (1989). Physiology of the male reproductive system: Endocrine, paracrine, and autocrine regulation. *Toxicol. Pathol., 17*(2), 411–445.

28. Kalis, V., Chaloupka, P., Turek, J., & Rokyta, Z., (2005). The perineal body length and injury at delivery. *Ceska Gynekol., 70*(5), 355–361.

29. Khan, Y. S., Fakoya, A. O., & Sajjad, H., (2023). *StatPearls* [Internet]. StatPearls Publishing; Treasure Island (FL). Anatomy, Thorax, Mammary Gland.

30. Kleppe, M., Kraima, A. C., Kruitwagen, R. F., Van, G. T., Smit, N. N., Van, M. J. C., & DeRuiter, M. C., (2015). Understanding lymphatic drainage pathways of the ovaries to predict sites for sentinel nodes in ovarian cancer. *Int. J. Gynecol. Cancer., 25*(8), 1405–1414.

31. Lee, I. O., Lee, J. Y., Kim, S., Kim, S. W., Kim, Y. T., & Nam, E. J., (2017). Sentinel lymph node mapping with indocyanine green in vaginal cancer. *J. Gynecol. Oncol., 28*(4), e29.

32. Lee, O. D., & Tillman, K., (2016). An overview of testosterone therapy. *Am. J. Mens Health., 10*(1), 68–72.

33. Lindquist, J. D., & Vogelzang, R. L., (2018). Pelvic artery embolization for treatment of postpartum hemorrhage. *Semin. Intervent. Radiol., 35*(1), 41–47.

34. Mawhinney, M., & Mariotti, A., (2012). Physiology, pathology, and pharmacology of the male reproductive system. *Periodontol., 61*(1), 232–251.

35. Migda, M. S., Migda, M., Słapa, R., Mlosek, R. K., & Migda, B., (2019). The use of high-frequency ultrasonography in the assessment of selected female reproductive structures: The vulva, vagina, and cervix. *J. Ultrason., 19*(79), 261–268.

36. Mihu, D., & Mihu, C. M., (2011). Ultrasonography of the uterus and ovaries. *Med. Ultrason., 13*(3), 249–252.

37. Nassar, G. N., & Leslie, S. W., (2023). *StatPearls* [Internet]. StatPearls Publishing; Treasure Island (FL). Physiology, Testosterone.

38. Nizić, D., Pervan, M., & Kos, I., (2014). Šimunović Marko [Flexion and version of the uterus on pelvic ultrasound examination]. *Acta Med. Croatica., 68*(3), 311–315.

39. Park, H. J., Kim, Y. S., Yoon, T. K., & Lee, W. S., (2016). Chronic endometritis and infertility. *Clin. Exp. Reprod. Med., 43*(4), 185–192.

40. Patil, M., (2009). Assessing tubal damage. *J. Hum. Reprod. Sci., 2*(1), 2–11.

41. Peters, A., Stuparich, M. A., Mansuria, S. M., & Lee, T. T., (2016). Anatomic vascular considerations in uterine artery ligation at its origin during laparoscopic hysterectomies. *Am. J. Obstet. Gynecol., 215*(3), 393.e1–3.

42. Plant, T. M., & Marshall, G. R., (2001). The functional significance of FSH in spermatogenesis and the control of its secretion in male primates. *Endocr. Rev., 22*(6), 764–786.

43. Roach, M. K., & Andreotti, R. F., (2017). The normal female pelvis. *Clin. Obstet. Gynecol., 60*(1), 3–10.

44. Robinson, J. G., Hodges, E. A., & Davison, J., (2014). Prostate-specific antigen screening: A critical review of current research and guidelines. *J. Am. Assoc. Nurse Pract., 26*(10), 574–581.

45. Ross, A., & Bhasin, S., (2016). Hypogonadism: Its prevalence and diagnosis. *Urol. Clin. North Am., 43*(2), 163–176.

46. Sabbagh, R., Mandron, E., Piussan, J., Brychaert, P. E., & Tu Le, M., (2010). Long-term anatomical and functional results of laparoscopic promontofixation for pelvic organ prolapse. *BJU Int., 106*(6), 861–866.

47. Sanders, R. C., & Parsons, A. K., (2014). Anteverted retroflexed uterus: A common consequence of cesarean delivery. *AJR Am. J. Roentgenol., 203*(1), W117–124.

48. Soeta, N., Saito, T., Nemoto, T., Oshibe, I., & Gotoh, M., (2016). Laparoscopic repair of irreducible femoral hernia containing the fallopian tube alone: A case report. *Surg. Case Rep., 2*(1), 57.

49. Tiwana, M. S., & Leslie, S. W., (2023). *StatPearls* [Internet]. StatPearls Publishing; Treasure Island (FL). Anatomy, Abdomen and Pelvis: Testes.

50. Trevisan, C. M., Montagna, E., De Oliveira, R., Christofolini, D. M., Barbosa, C. P., Crandall, K. A., & Bianco, B., (2018). Kisspeptin/GPR54 system: What do we know about its role in human reproduction? *Cell Physiol. Biochem., 49*(4), 1259–1276.

51. Vervoort, A. J., Uittenbogaard, L. B., Hehenkamp, W. J., Brölmann, H. A., Mol, B. W., & Huirne, J. A., (2015). Why do niches develop in caesarean uterine scars? Hypotheses on the aetiology of niche development. *Hum. Reprod., 30*(12), 2695–2702.

52. Weekes, A. R., Atlay, R. D., Brown, V. A., Jordan, E. C., & Murray, S. M., (1976). The retroverted gravid uterus and its effect on the outcome of pregnancy. *Br. Med. J., 1*(6010), 622–624.

53. Yao, H. H., (2005). The pathway to femaleness: Current knowledge on embryonic development of the ovary. *Mol. Cell Endocrinol., 230*(1, 2), 87–93.

Chapter

HUMAN MUSCULATURE SYSTEM

9

Contents

Unit Introduction

Muscle fibers are specialized cells that comprise the muscular system. Their primary characteristic is the ability to contract. Muscles attached to bones, internal organs, and blood vessels are responsible for movement. Muscle contraction serves as the foundation for nearly all bodily movements. However, there are exceptions to this rule, such as the function of cilia, the flagellum on sperm cells, and the amoeboid movement of certain white blood cells.

Even simple movements like walking and running are the result of coordinated actions between joints, bones, and skeletal muscles. Additionally, more subtle movements performed by skeletal muscles contribute to various eye movements, facial expressions, and sweating.

Muscle contraction also performs several other crucial functions for the body, including maintaining posture, joint stability, and heat production. Muscle contraction is responsible for sustaining posture, whether sitting or standing, as skeletal muscles continuously make minute adjustments. Many tendons surround joints, providing support and maintaining joint stability. This is particularly noticeable in the knee and shoulder joints. Furthermore, muscle metabolism generates heat, which helps regulate the body's temperature. Muscle contraction alone accounts for approximately 85% of the body's heat production.

The human muscle system is composed of voluntary muscles that regulate movement, posture, and balance, as well as the muscles responsible for operating the skeletal system. Generally, human muscle can be categorized as smooth muscle, cardiac muscle, and striated muscle, which is also the term used for the muscles of all vertebrates. Smooth muscle, found in the walls of blood vessels and organs such as the stomach, intestines, and urinary bladder, is controlled involuntarily. The heart consists of cardiac muscle, which is also controlled involuntarily and is responsible for the organ's regular contractions. The arrangement of the human heart and smooth muscle is nearly identical to that of other vertebrate animals, with very few exceptions (Figure 9.1).

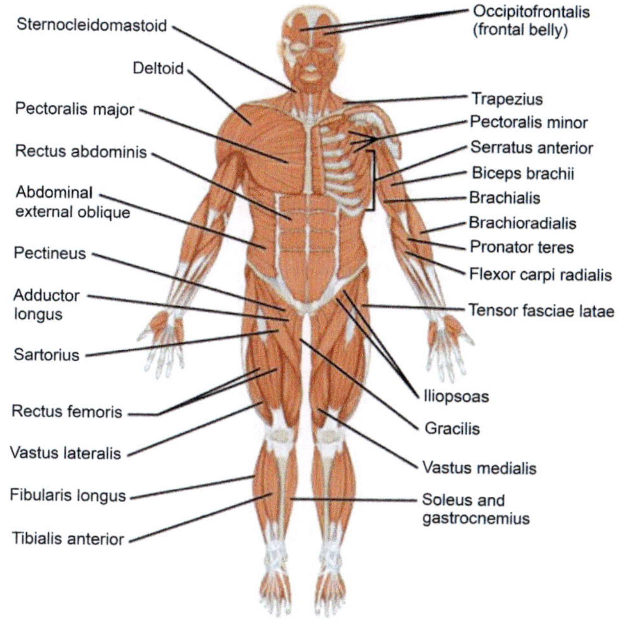

Major muscles of the body.
Right side: superficial; left side:
deep (anterior view)

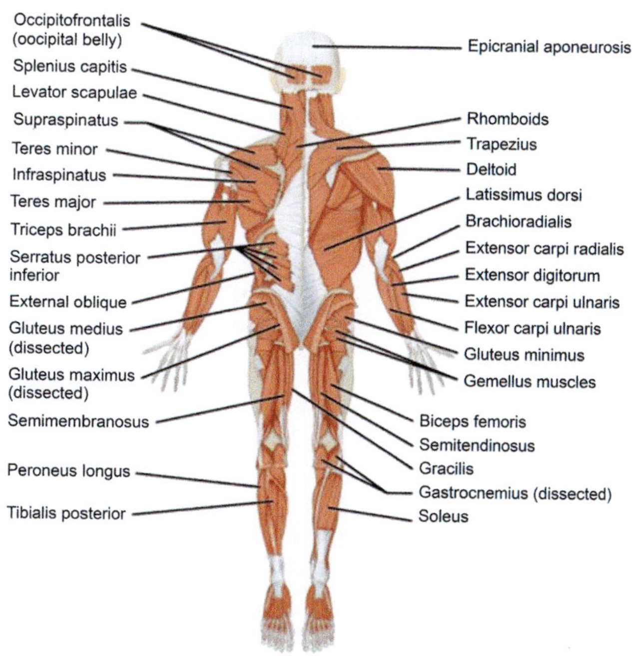

Major muscles of the body.
Right side: superficial; left side;
deep (posterior view)

Figure 9.1. *Human muscular system.*

Source: https://courses.lumenlearning.com/suny-hccc-fitness-2/chapter/naming-skeletal-muscles/.

Orientation and Directional Terms:

Term	Definition	Illustration
Muscle fiber	Muscle fibers are large, single muscle cells that control the body's physical forces. They are usually 20–100 micrometers in diameter and can be many centimeters long, with the longest fibers being about 12 centimeters.	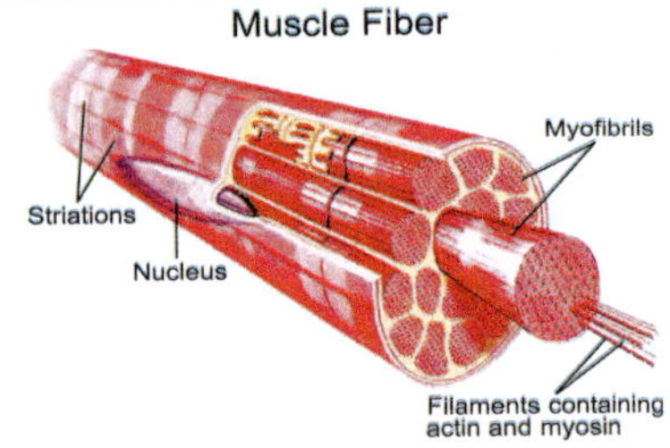
Myosin	Myosin is a protein that converts chemical energy into mechanical energy, generating force and movement.	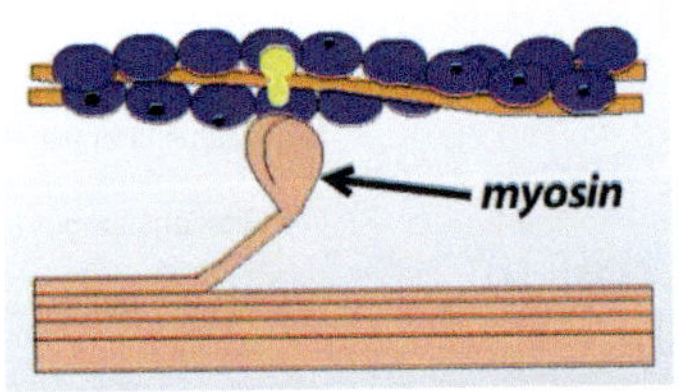
Sarcomeres	Sarcomeres are the smallest functional unit of muscle contraction. They are composed of a pattern of repeating contractile and regulatory proteins organized into thin and thick filaments.	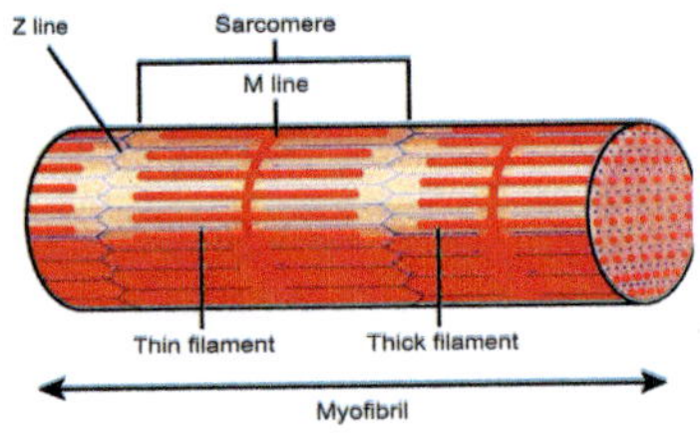
Muscle contraction	Muscle contraction occurs when muscles tighten, shorten, or lengthen during an activity. It can happen when you hold something, stretch, or exercise with weights.	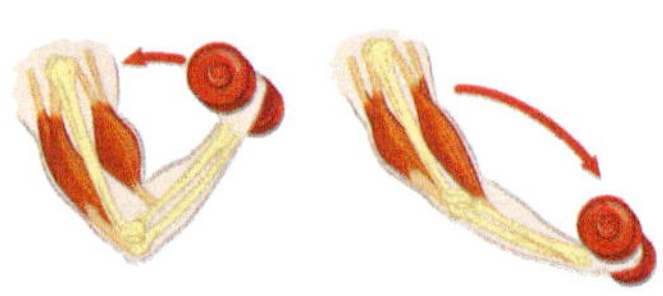
Spine	Spine is made up of small bones, called vertebrae, which are stacked on top of one another and create the natural curves of your back.	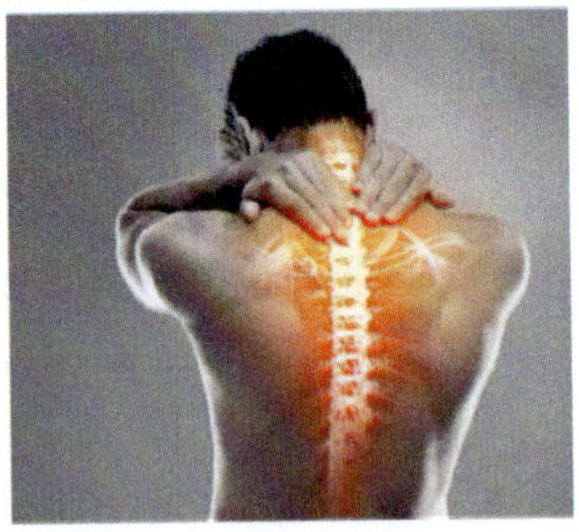

9.1. The Muscle Groups and Their Actions

A basic understanding of the gross human muscular anatomy is given in the following sections, which also include descriptions of the major muscle groups and their functions. The human body's movements are controlled by the coordinated actions of its different muscle groups.

9.1.1. The Neck

The terms rotation, flexion, extension, and side bending are used to characterize the motion of the neck (i.e., the gesture that connects the ear to the shoulder). Actions can be carried out in either an ipsilateral (moving toward the side of the contracting muscle) or contralateral (moving away from the side of the contracting muscle) direction (Figure 9.2).

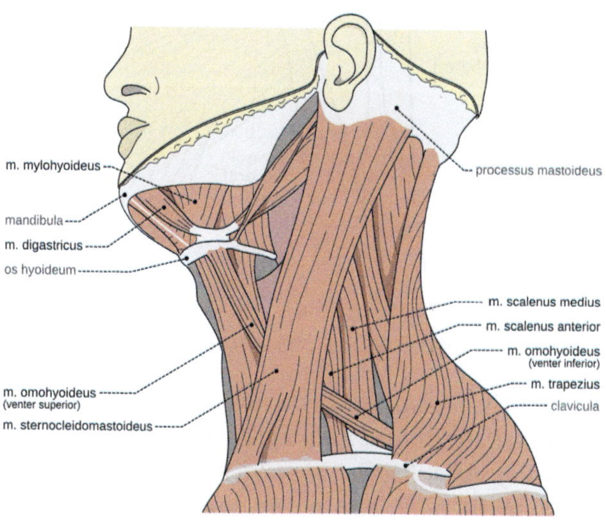

Figure 9.2. *Muscles of the neck.*

Source: By Olek Remesz (wiki-pl: Orem, commons: Orem) – Own work, based on this picture from Gray's Anatomy., CC BY-SA 2.5, https://commons.wikimedia.org/w/index.php?curid=2339732.

One of the most crucial functions of the cervical (neck) spine is rotation. The sternocleidomastoid muscle, which bends the neck to the ipsilateral side and rotates it contralaterally, is primarily responsible for rotation. To assist in forced inhalation, the sternocleidomastoid muscles on both sides of the neck work together to flex the neck and raise the sternum. The anterior and middle scalene muscles, located on the sides of the neck, elevate the first rib and rotate the neck ipsilaterally. The splenius capitis and splenius cervicis, muscles located in the back of the neck, are responsible for rotating the head.

Another crucial function of the cervical spine is side bending. Cervical side bending involves the sternocleidomastoid muscles. The neck is bent ipsilaterally to the side, and the posterior scalene muscles, located on the lower sides of the neck, raise the second rib. Neck side bending is also facilitated by the splenius capitis and splenius cervicis. The erector spinae muscles, which include the iliocostalis, longissimus, and spinalis, are large, deep muscles that run along the length of the back. All three muscles work together to bend the neck ipsilaterally to the side.

The action of touching the chin to the chest is known as neck flexion. The longus colli and longus capitis muscles in the front of the neck assist the sternocleidomastoid muscles in their primary function. The muscles involved in other neck movements, such as the splenius cervicis, splenius capitis, iliocostalis, longissimus, and spinalis, are also involved in neck extension, which is the opposite of neck flexion.

9.1.2. The Back

Many of the muscles involved in the movement of the neck and shoulders originate in the back. Furthermore, the spinal cord, which supplies almost all of the body's muscles with nerve endings, is shielded by the axial skeleton that passes vertically through the back (Figure 9.3).

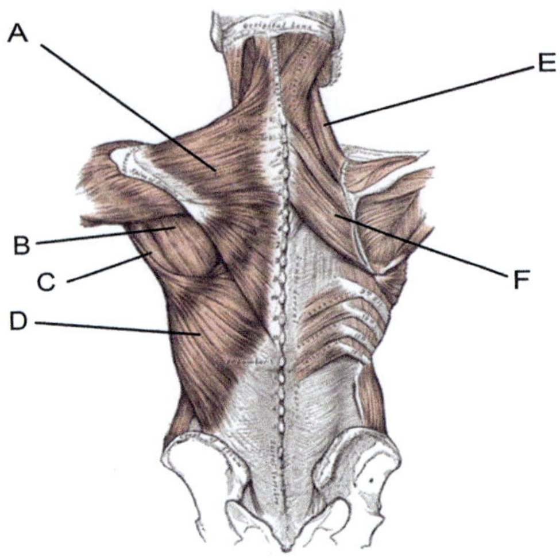

Figure 9.3. *Muscles of the back. (A) Trapezius; (B) teres major; (C) teres minor; (D) latissimus macron; (E) Levator Marcon; and (F) rhomboid hangar.*

Source: https://en.m.wikipedia.org/wiki/File:Back_Muscles.jpg.

Several back muscles are specifically used in back movements. For example, the erector spinae muscles extend (bend) the back, and they also side bend it. The back is also extended by the semispinalis dorsi and semispinalis capitis muscles. The multifidi and rotators, two tiny muscles of the vertebrae, aid in side bending, extension, and rotation of the back. By stabilizing the lumbar spine at its insertion at the 12th rib (the last of the floating ribs), the quadratus lumborum muscle in the lower back helps with inspiration of air. The rhomboid major and minor muscles in the upper back, the levator scapulae muscle that runs along the side and back of the neck, and the trapezius muscle that extends from the back of the neck to the middle of the back all work together to elevate the scapula, or shoulder blade.

9.1.3. The Shoulder

The humerus head, the clavicle (collarbone), and the scapula make up the complex ball-and-socket joint that is the shoulder. The primary movements of the shoulder include flexion, extension, internal and external rotation, abduction, and adduction (Figure 9.4).

Shoulder flexion is demonstrated when one reaches forward to pick up an object. The coracobrachialis muscle, located on the inside of the upper arm, the biceps brachii muscle on the anterior side of the upper arm, the pectoralis major muscle in the chest, and the deltoid muscle in the uppermost portion of the arm work synergistically to primarily accomplish this action.

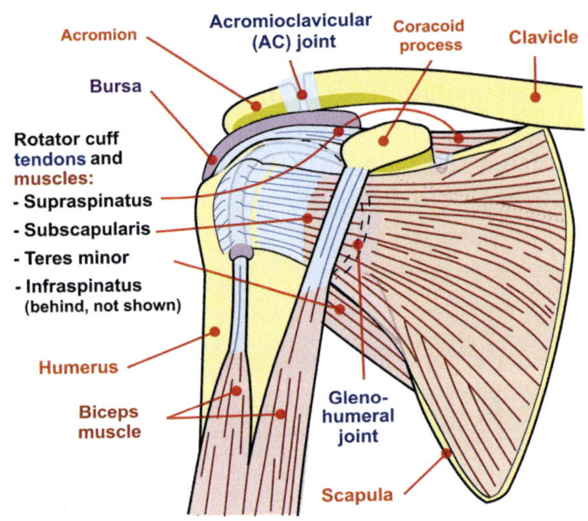

Figure 9.4. *Muscles of the shoulder.*

Source: By National Institute of Arthritis and Musculoskeletal and Skin Diseases (NIAMS); SVG version by Angelito7 – Shoulderjoint.PNG, Public Domain, https://commons.wikimedia.org/w/index.php?curid=29907860.

Shoulder flexion is the opposite of shoulder extension. When an arm is extended directly behind the body, as in a relay race, it is referred to as pure shoulder extension. The deltoid muscle, the latissimus dorsi muscle in the posterior region, the teres major muscle in the axillary region, and the triceps muscle in the posterior side of the upper arm work together to accomplish this movement. As the name implies, the triceps consist of three heads that originate from separate locations but converge at the olecranon process of the ulna, a bone in the forearm. Collectively, the three heads extend the elbow.

Arms are raised and lowered in relation to the body through shoulder adduction and abduction, respectively. You can visualize this by imagining an individual performing jumping jacks. The pectoralis major, latissimus dorsi, teres major, triceps, and coracobrachialis are the main muscles involved in adduction. The two primary shoulder abductors are the deltoid and the supraspinatus, a muscle that runs along the posterior side of the scapula.

An instance of external rotation of the shoulder can be observed in the backhand stroke of tennis. The deltoid, the teres minor in the armpit, and the infraspinatus muscle, which is located over the scapula, are the main muscles involved in external rotation. The opposite of external rotation in the shoulder is internal rotation. The motion of the shoulder when reaching into a back pocket serves as an illustration. The pectoralis major, latissimus dorsi, deltoid, teres major, and subscapularis muscles work in unison to accomplish that movement. On the anterior, or front-facing, surface of the scapula, there is a deep muscle called the subscapularis.

The rotator cuff, which is made up of the teres minor, subscapularis, supraspinatus, and infraspinatus muscles, stabilizes the humeral head, or ball part of the ball-and-socket shoulder joint. Adults frequently sustain injuries to their rotator cuff muscles, especially if they frequently perform overhead motions (e.g., hitting a ball or applying paint to a ceiling). Tendons from a number of the rotator cuff muscles pass beneath the acromion, a bony protrusion at the distal end of the scapula. (The term "proximal," which describes a relative position close to the body's center, is frequently contrasted with the term "distal," which describes a relative position far from the body's center.) Shoulder impingement syndrome is a condition that can arise from the positioning of the tendons and the subacromial bursae, which are fluid-filled sacs situated beneath the acromion, making them susceptible to compression and pinching.

9.1.4. The Arm

An instance of external rotation of the shoulder can be observed in the backhand stroke of tennis. The deltoid, the teres minor in the armpit, and the infraspinatus muscle, which is located over the scapula, are the main muscles involved in external rotation. The opposite of external rotation in the shoulder is internal rotation. The motion of the shoulder when reaching into a back pocket serves as an illustration. The pectoralis major, latissimus dorsi, deltoid, teres major, and subscapularis muscles work in unison to accomplish that movement. On the anterior, or front-facing, surface of the scapula, there is a deep muscle called the subscapularis.

The rotator cuff, which is made up of the teres minor, subscapularis, supraspinatus, and infraspinatus muscles, stabilizes the humeral head, or ball part of the ball-and-socket shoulder joint. Adults frequently sustain injuries to their rotator cuff muscles, especially if they frequently perform overhead motions (e.g., hitting a ball or applying paint to a ceiling). Tendons from a number of the rotator cuff muscles pass beneath the acromion, a bony protrusion at the distal end of the scapula. (The term "proximal," which describes a relative position close to the body's center, is frequently contrasted with the term "distal," which describes a relative position far from the body's center.) Shoulder impingement syndrome is a condition that can arise from the positioning of the tendons and the subacromial bursae, which are fluid-filled sacs situated beneath the acromion, making them susceptible to compression and pinching (Figure 9.5).

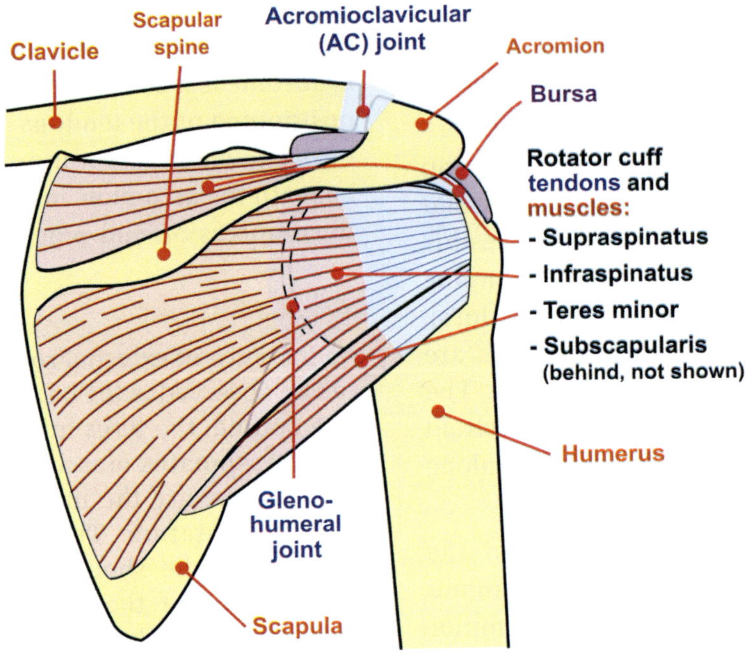

Figure 9.5. *Muscles of the upper arm.*

Source: By Jmarchn – Own work, CC BY-SA 3.0, https://commons.wikimedia.org/w/index.php?curid=67117834.

The hand moves away from the shoulder when the forearm is extended, increasing the angle at the elbow. The triceps brachii are primarily responsible for this action. The extensor muscles of the posterior compartment of the forearm, also known as the extensor compartment, which include the extensor carpi radialis longus, extensor carpi radialis brevis, extensor digitorum, extensor carpi ulnaris, and the anconeus, are additional muscles that slightly contribute to forearm extension (Figure 9.6).

Striated muscle tissue, such as the tissue of the human biceps muscle, consists of long, fine fibers, each of which is essentially a bundle of finer myofibrils. Within each myofibril, there are filaments of the proteins myosin and actin. These filaments slide past one another as the muscle contracts and expands. On each myofibril, there are regularly occurring dark bands called Z lines, where actin and myosin filaments overlap. The region between two Z lines is called a sarcomere, which can be considered the primary structural and functional unit of muscle tissue.

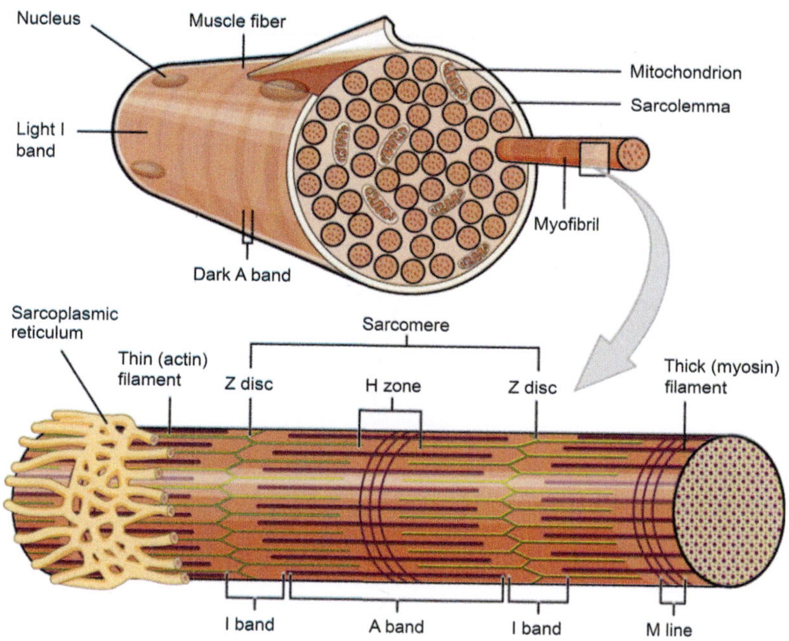

Figure 9.6. *The structure of striated, or skeletal, muscle.*

Source: https://courses.lumenlearning.com/suny-hccc-fitness-2/chapter/skeletal-muscle/.

9.1.5. The Wrist

Wrist flexion is defined as a wrist motion that pulls the hand's palm downward. The flexor pollicis longus, flexor digitorum superficialis, flexor digitorum profundus, flexor carpi radialis, and flexor carpi ulnaris perform that action.

In contrast, the angle at the back of the wrist shortens during wrist extension. The extensor carpi radialis longus and extensor carpi radialis brevis, which also abduct the hand at the wrist (moving the hand in the direction of the thumb, or first digit), the extensor digitorum, which also extends the index to little finger (the second to fifth digits), the extensor digiti minimi, which also extends the little finger and adducts the hand (moving the hand in the direction of the little finger), and the extensor carpi ulnaris, which also adducts the hand, are the muscles that cause that action. Wrist extension may also be slightly increased by other tiny muscles that cross the wrist joint.

The wrist rotation known as wrist supination causes the palm to face upward. The supinator muscle in the posterior compartment is responsible for supinating the forearm. Additionally, the biceps brachii contribute to increasing supination. The opposite movement is called pronation, which involves rotating the wrist so that the palm faces downward. The pronator teres and the pronator quadratus, muscles in the deep anterior compartment, work together to pronate the forearm (Figure 9.7).

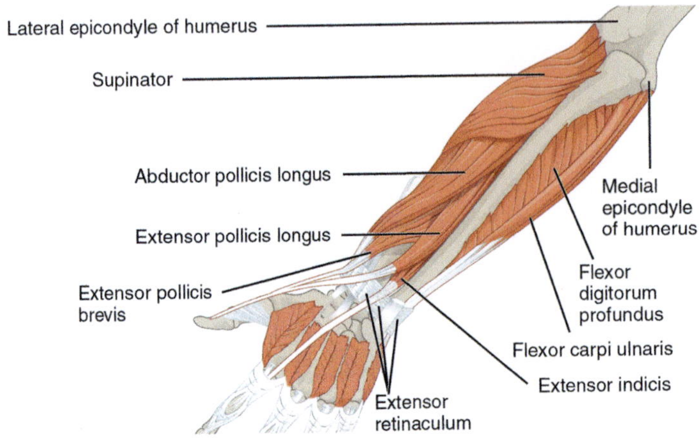

Figure 9.7. *Muscles of the forearm (posterior view).*

Source: https://commons.wikimedia.org/wiki/File:1120_Muscles_that_Move_the_Forearm_Antebrach._Prof._Ext._Sin.png.

9.1.6. The Hand

The hand is a complex structure utilized for intricate tasks and the coordination of fine motor skills. Generally, its muscles are small and possess well-developed innervation. The hand muscles are responsible for executing precise movements required even for basic activities such as keyboard typing. Given the intricacy involved, the subsequent passages exclusively focus on the primary function of each hand muscle.

Numerous muscles originating from the radius, the other bone in the forearm, or the posterior surface of the ulna exert their influence on the hand. These include the extensor pollicis brevis, responsible for extending the metacarpophalangeal (MCP) joint of the thumb; the abductor pollicis longus, which abducts and extends the thumb; the extensor pollicis, responsible for extending the distal phalanx (finger bone) of the thumb; and the extensor indicis, which extends the index finger of the thumb at the MCP joint. (MCP joints are located between the phalanges, the small bones of the fingers, and the metacarpal bones within the hand.)

While several hand muscles originate from the forearm, many of the hand's smaller muscles have both their origin and insertion within the hand itself. These muscles are referred to as the hand's intrinsic muscles. The palmar interossei adduct the fingers towards the middle finger (the third digit); the dorsal interossei abduct the fingers away from the middle finger; and the umbricals flex the MCP joints and extend the interphalangeal joints (IPs, the joints between the phalanges) of the fingers. The palmaris brevis assists in grip. All the interossei muscles flex the MCP joints and extend the IP joints.

The abductor pollicis brevis, flexor pollicis brevis, and opponens pollicis are the three muscles that comprise the thenar eminence, located on the palmar side of the base of the thumb. All of these muscles are innervated by the median nerve. The abductor pollicis brevis abducts the thumb, the flexor pollicis brevis flexes the thumb's MCP joint, and the opponens pollicis opposes the thumb to the other fingers. Thumb adduction is achieved by the adductor pollicis, which is distinct from the thenar eminence. Beneath the little finger on the palmar side of the hand lies the hypothenar eminence. It consists of three muscles that receive innervation from the deep branch of the ulnar nerve. The abductor digiti minimi abducts the little finger, the flexor digiti minimi flexes the little finger, and the opponens digiti minimi opposes the little finger using the thumb.

9.1.7. The Abdomen

The abdominal wall comprises three layers of musculature, along with a fourth layer situated in the anterior midregion. The rectus abdominis, possessing vertically oriented muscle fibers that facilitate trunk flexion and pelvic stabilization, constitutes the fourth layer of the midregion. The remaining trio of abdominal muscle layers are positioned on either side of the rectus abdominis. The transversus abdominis, the deepest among these layers, functions to compress and provide support to the abdomen, thereby furnishing static core stabilization. Its fibers run perpendicular to those of the rectus abdominis. The external oblique layers, which constitute the outermost musculature of the abdomen, descend in a downward and forward direction, while the internal oblique layers extend in an upward and forward manner from the abdominal sides. When the internal oblique layers collaborate with the external oblique on the opposite side of the body, the trunk flexes and rotates toward the side of the contracting internal oblique (also referred to as the "same-side rotator") (Figure 9.8).

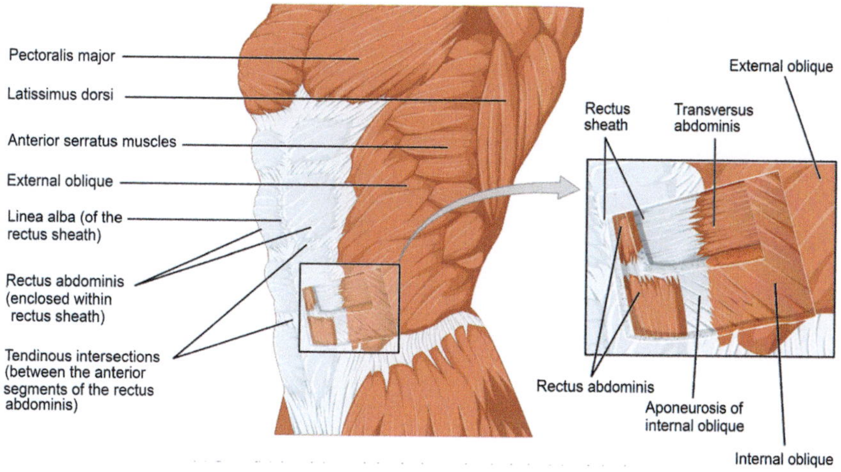

Figure 9.8. *Muscles of the abdominal wall.*

Source: By OpenStax College – https://cnx.org/contents/FPtK1zmh@8.108:y9_gDy74@5, CC BY 3.0, https://commons.wikimedia.org/w/index.php?curid=64291130.

9.1.8. The Hip

The hip joint is a complex ball-and-socket joint that is capable of supporting a substantial amount of weight. The joint's deep socket provides stability, albeit at the expense of some range of motion. This section covers several movements associated with the hip joint, including flexion, extension, abduction, and adduction. Hip flexion refers to the movement that brings the knee towards the chest. The iliopsoas, consisting of the psoas major, psoas minor, and iliacus muscles, plays a significant role in hip flexion. These muscles primarily flex the hip, while also providing support for hip stabilization and abdominal flexion. Other hip flexors include the sartorius, rectus femoris, pectineus, and gracilis. The rectus femoris also contributes to knee extension, while the sartorius aids in external hip rotation, abduction, and knee extension. The pectineus is involved in internal rotation and hip adduction. Hip extension is mainly facilitated by the muscles of the posterior thigh and buttocks. When these muscles contract, the thigh moves from a flexed position towards the midline of the body, or the trunk is bent and brought closer to an upright posture. The gluteus maximus, biceps femoris (long and short heads), semitendinosus, and semimembranosus are the primary muscles responsible for hip extension. The adductor magnus and other smaller pelvic muscles also contribute to a lesser extent.

The term "adduction movement" refers to the direction of motion of a limb that moves it from a lateral to a more axial alignment. For example, during a jumping-jack exercise, the leg undergoes abduction as it moves away from the midline and adduction as it moves back toward the midline. The primary abductors of the hip are the tensor fascia lata, gluteus medius, and gluteus minimus. These muscles are also responsible for the external and internal rotation of the thigh in both flexed and extended positions. The piriformis plays a minor additional role. On the other hand, the primary hip adductors are the adductor magnus, adductor brevis, and adductor longus. The gracilis and pectineus muscles have a minor role in hip adduction (Figure 9.9).

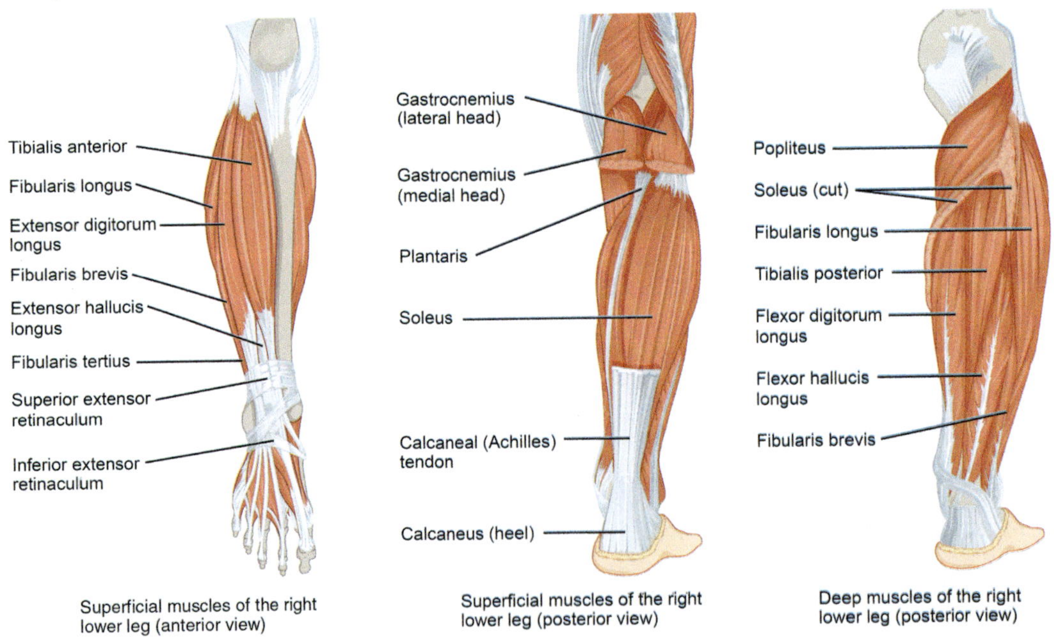

Figure 9.9. *Anterior view of the muscles of the human leg.*

Source: https://commons.wikimedia.org/wiki/File:1123_Muscles_of_the_Leg_that_Move_the_Foot_and_Toes.jpg.

9.1.9. The Upper Leg and Knee

A group of muscles collectively known as the quadriceps femoris is responsible for extending the knee, increasing the angle of the knee, and straightening the lower leg. During the forward swing phase of the gait, knee extension is utilized and is crucial for actions such as kicking. The quadriceps femoris group consists of the vastus medius, vastus lateralis, vastus intermedius, and rectus femoris muscles. The sartorius muscle plays a minor role in knee extension.

Bending the knee from its straight position is referred to as knee flexion. These muscles, commonly known as the hamstring muscles, work in opposition to the knee extension muscles. The hamstrings, which are located in the rear of the thigh, consist of the biceps femoris, semitendinosus, and semimembranosus muscles. The gastrocnemius muscle in the rear of the calf, along with a few other small muscles that cross the knee joint posteriorly, also contribute slightly to knee flexion.

9.1.10. The Lower Leg and Foot

The foot and lower leg muscles are intricate and function on multiple planes. Their actions are dependent upon both the foot's position and whether the person is bearing weight. An overview of the movements of the lower leg and foot muscles is given in the paragraphs that follow (Figure 9.10).

Ankle flexion towards the dorsum, or anterior surface of the foot, is known as dorsiflexion (when viewed from above). Several muscles, including the tibialis anterior, are involved in dorsiflexion. This muscle also contributes to foot inversion (tilting the foot towards the midline), provides stability to the foot upon ground contact, and locks the ankle during kicking. In addition to its role in dorsiflexion, the extensor digitorum longus (EDL) extends the last four toes. The peroneus tertius (fibularis tertius), which is present in some individuals in addition to the EDL, has a limited role in dorsiflexion and foot eversion (tilting the foot away from the midline).

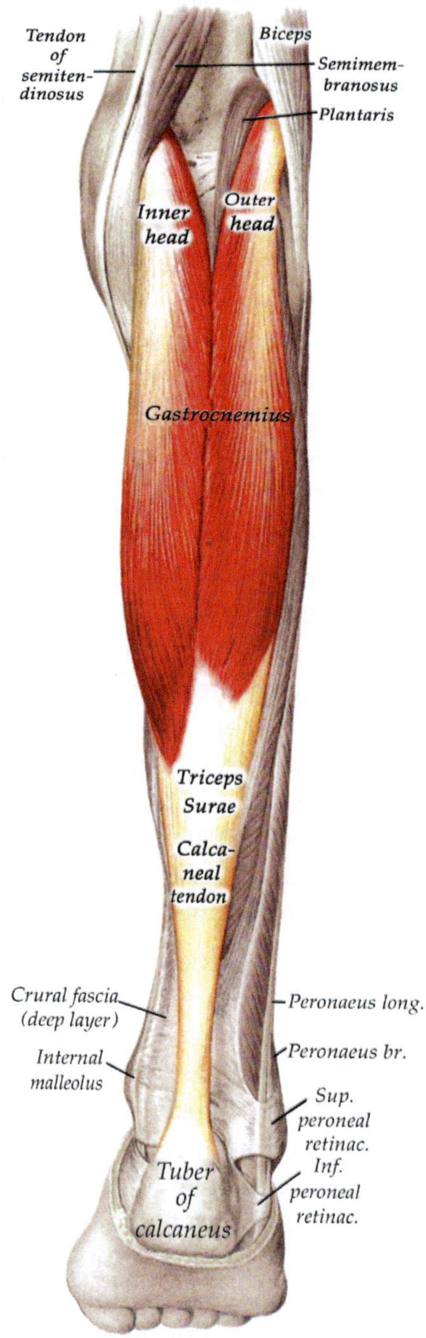

Figure 9.10. *Details of the foot.*

Source: By Dr. Johannes Sobotta – Sobotta's Atlas and Textbook of Human Anatomy 1909, Public Domain, https://commons.wikimedia.org/w/index.php?curid=89101644.

The extensor hallucis longus primarily facilitates dorsiflexion of the big toe (hallux), but it can also weakly dorsiflex and invert the ankle.

The term "plantarflexion" describes flexion of the ankle towards the sole of the foot. The easiest way to illustrate this is to have someone stand on their toes. The large calf muscles, such as the gastrocnemius and the soleus (located directly behind the gastrocnemius), are primarily responsible for plantarflexion of the ankle. While the gastrocnemius and soleus are sometimes mistaken for two separate muscles, it is generally agreed that they are indeed two separate muscles.

Additional muscles of the lower leg and foot include the plantaris (which runs obliquely between the gastrocnemius and soleus), the flexor hallucis longus (which primarily functions in flexing the big toe but also contributes to ankle flexion), the flexor digitorum longus (which flexes the second to fifth toes), the peroneus longus (which flexes the ankle and everts the foot), and the peroneus brevis (which performs plantarflexion and foot eversion).

The intrinsic muscles of the foot originate there and do not pass over the ankle joint, limiting their movement to the foot itself. These muscles include the lumbricals, which flex the metatarsophalangeal (MTP) joints and extend the distal IP and proximal IP joints of the toes, the flexor hallucis brevis, which flexes the big toe, the adductor hallucis, which flexes and contracts the big toe, and the quadratus plantae, which aids in toe flexion. The adductor hallucis has two heads, the oblique head and the transverse head, which share a common insertion point on the outside of the proximal phalanx of the big toe. The transverse head originates from the ligaments of the MTP joints of the third to fifth toes, while the oblique head originates from the base of the second to fourth metatarsal bones. The flexor digiti minimi brevis extends and adducts the fifth toe, while the dorsal interossei abduct the toes and the plantar interossei adduct them.

9.2. Evolutionary Context Human Muscle System

Modern humans have striated muscle arranged according to the basic plan shared by all pronograde quadrupedal vertebrates and mammals, or any other animals that adopt a horizontal, four-legged stance. Although the primitive quadrupedal stance and locomotion were passed down to the primates (the order of mammals to which humans belong), several groups have modified their locomotor system to focus on using the arms for propulsion through the trees since their appearance approximately 65 million years ago during the Late Cretaceous Period. The modern gibbon family represents the most extreme manifestation of that skeletal adaptation in living primates. They walk primarily on their hind limbs (bipedally) during the brief moments they spend on the ground, have comparatively long forelimbs, and maintain an erect trunk (Figure 9.11).

Modern humans are most closely related to the chimpanzee, gorilla, and orangutan. The orangutan, the most distant relative of humans in this group, possesses a locomotor system adapted for traversing the vertical tree trunks of the Asian rainforests. It adeptly grasps the trunks with both its fore and hind limbs, hence it was once referred to as "quadrumanal" or "four-handed."

Despite sharing anatomical similarities and a common ancestor with the great apes, humans (Homo sapiens) stand apart due to their highly developed brains, which endow them with the ability to reason abstractly and produce articulate speech.

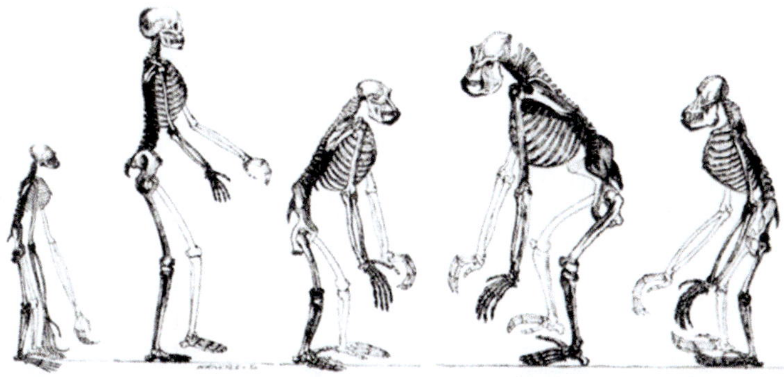

Figure 9.11. *Homo sapiens within the primate order.*

Source: https://courses.lumenlearning.com/suny-hccc-worldcivilization/chapter/the-evolution-of-humans/.

Inferences regarding the habitat and mode of mobility of the common ancestor of modern humans, chimpanzees, and gorillas must be deduced, as there is limited direct fossil evidence pertaining to this species. It is likely that the ancestor was a relatively generalized creature that resided in trees and possessed the capability to both climb and walk on all fours along branches. It appears that two locomotor trends emerged from such an ancestor. One of these trends resulted in the elongation of the forelimbs, which explains why chimpanzees and gorillas, among other contemporary animals, support their trunks by resting the knuckles of their extended forelimbs on the ground when descending. The second trend involved the relocation of the shoulder blades to the front of the trunk and, most notably, the gradual emphasis on an upright posture and hindlimb support. In other words, this trend witnessed the development of an orthograde, or upright, bipedal stance as opposed to a pronograde, or quadrupedal, one. The shape of the limb bones and the preserved footprints of early hominins discovered from that era suggest that the upright posture was likely well established around 3 million to 3.5 million years ago.

9.2.1. Changes in the Muscles of the Lower Limb

On the left is the skeletal structure of a human being, and on the right is the skeletal structure of a gorilla. The differences in the structures allow humans to walk erect on two legs with a striding gait, whereas gorillas move in a knuckle-walking fashion. These differences include shorter ischia, a broader sacrum, and broader, curved-in ilia with a lower iliac crest in the pelvis. In the legs, the femurs (thighbones) of humans are relatively long and set farther apart at the hips than they are at the knees.

Lower limb muscular alterations are the primary changes that are directly linked to the transition to bipedal locomotion. The length of the hind limb, the development of the heel, and the modification of the knee joint's shape to a flat rather than uniformly rounded surface are the three most noticeable skeletal changes. When compared to the proportions of modern humans, apes' hind limbs are comparatively short given their body size. Although they are not entirely caused by the change in locomotion, the alterations in the pelvic bones did result from it. The ability to walk on two feet allowed for the development of manual dexterity, which in turn allowed for the creation and use of tools. This has been connected to the evolution of language and other intellectual abilities in our ancestors. The end effect is a significantly larger brain. It is evident that large brains have an impact on the shape of the skull and, consequently, the head and neck muscles. Because giving birth to relatively large-brained offspring requires a wide pelvic inlet and outlet, a larger brain also directly affects the pelvis. The hip joints must be spaced farther apart in cases where the pelvic cavity is larger. Because this is the case when walking and running require bearing weight on one leg, the hip joints are put under a lot of strain (Figure 9.12).

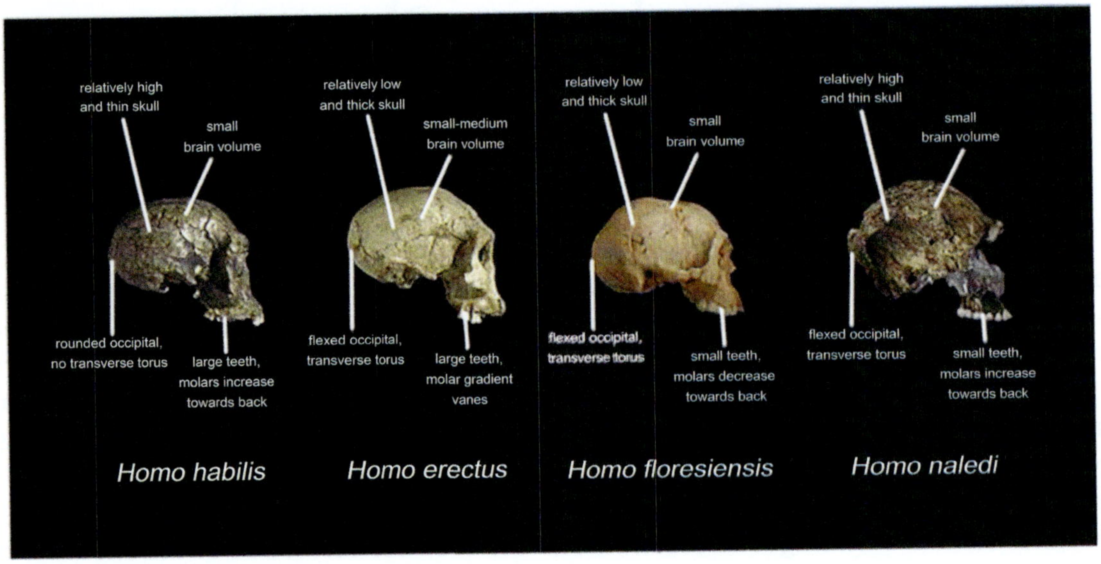

Figure 9.12. *Human beings (Homo sapiens) are anatomically similar and related to the great apes, but they are distinguished by a more highly developed brain and a resultant capacity for articulate speech and abstract reasoning.*

Source: https://courses.lumenlearning.com/suny-hccc-worldcivilization/chapter/the-evolution-of-humans/.

In order to counteract that, the gluteus minimus and gluteus medius of modern humans, which chimpanzees use as hip extensors to push their legs back, have evolved to function as abductors to balance the trunk on the weight-bearing leg during walking. The gluteus maximus, a portion of the third climbing muscle, aids in both abduction and preserving the knee's extension while bearing weight. The gluteal muscles are also primarily responsible for the hip rotation that occurs during walking. The hip joint on the same side externally rotates when the right leg is swung forward and the right foot touches the ground, while the hip joint on the opposing side internally rotates to a similar degree. The muscles that cross the hip are rearranged to enable both of these movements.

Modern humans have arranged their lower limb and trunk bones in a manner that allows for standing upright with minimal muscular effort. The extensors of the knee and the calf muscles have been realigned and rearranged, but certain muscles are still necessary for balance.

It is a common misconception that the foot is inferior to the hand. The flexor muscles of the big toe are designed to provide the final push-off in the walking cycle, even though modern humans' toes are typically incapable of useful independent movement. The muscles in the three compartments of the modern human lower leg work together to provide a stable platform that can be adjusted for walking on uneven and sloping terrain (Figure 9.13).

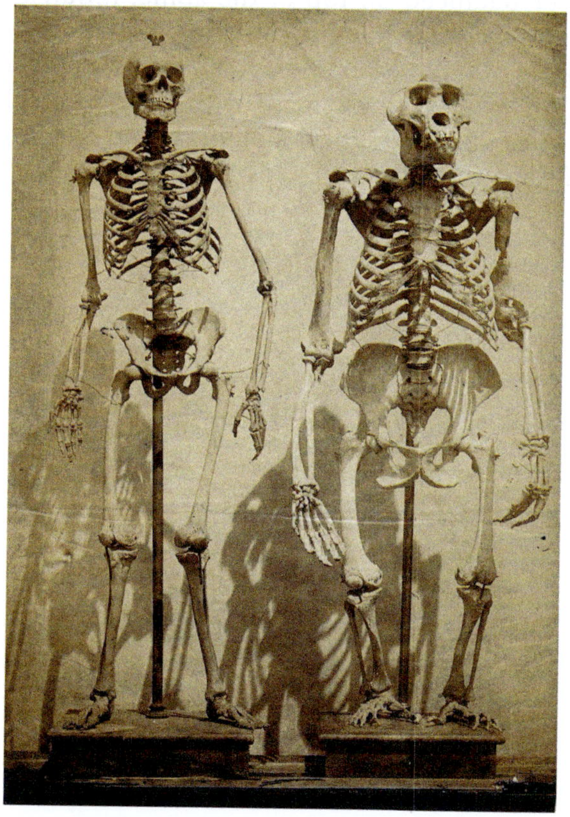

Figure 9.13. *The skeletal structure of a human being (left) and of a gorilla (right). Several differences allow the human to walk erect on two legs with a striding gait rather than move in a knuckle-walking fashion like the gorilla. In the pelvis, these differences include shorter ischia, a broader sacrum, and broader, curved-in ilia with a lower iliac crest. In the legs, the femurs (thighbones) are relatively long and are set farther apart at the hips than they are at the knees.*

Source: https://commons.wikimedia.org/wiki/File:Skeleton_of_a_human_and_a_gorilla_Wellcome_V0029412.jpg.

9.2.2. Changes in the Muscles of the Upper Limb

The generalized structure of the human upper limb has been preserved, but specific modifications have been made to accommodate an upright lifestyle. Primitive features that still exist include the ability to twist the radius bone around the ulna in a process known as pronation and supination, as well as the presence of five digits in the hand.

Unlike humans, other animals do not possess the unique ability to rotate the forearm 180°, allowing the palm to rotate. This ability is dependent on the presence of a small disk in the wrist joint and the configuration of muscles. Great apes possess both the disk and the muscle arrangement.

In quadrupedal animals, the serratus anterior muscle forms a muscular hammock that suspends the thorax, or chest, between the shoulder blades. However, in humans, the shoulder girdle is suspended from the trunk when sitting or standing upright. The arrangement of muscles such as the trapezius, rhomboid, and levator scapulae, along with the support against gravity they provide, allows the scapula, or shoulder blade, to float over the thoracic surface. Pushing forward against an object at shoulder level with the arms is similar to the support provided in quadrupedal animals.

The relationship between the muscles in the shoulder region was altered by the change in the shape of the chest to emphasize breadth rather than depth, with the pectoralis major and latissimus dorsi muscles growing in size. The human pectoralis minor muscle no longer glides over the humerus, the long bone of the upper arm, but instead clings to the coracoid process, a projection from the scapula, presumably for stability.

Although chimpanzees have very dexterous hands, modern humans have hands that are much more manipulative due to factors such as the proportions of our fingers, muscle supplementation, and rearrangement. The thumb is where most of those modifications are concentrated. For instance, only extant humans possess a distinct long thumb flexor, and humans have a particularly well-developed short thumb muscle that swings the thumb toward the palm. This aids in the oppositional movement that is necessary for the so-called precision grip, i.e., the joining of the thumb and forefinger tips together (Figure 9.14).

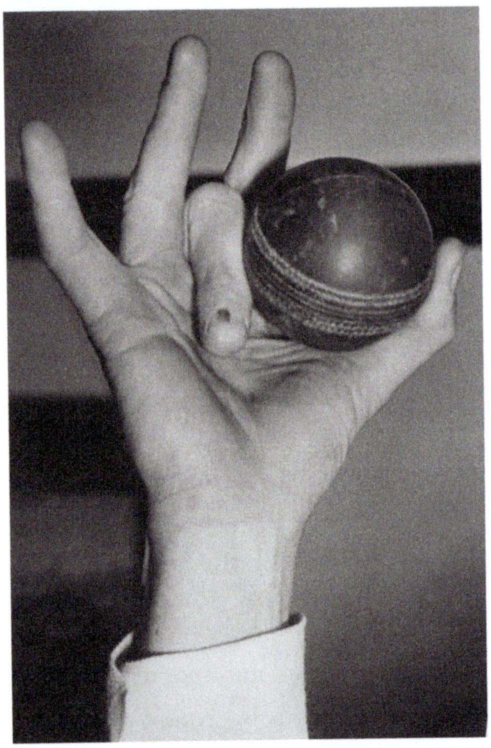

Figure 9.14. *A fully opposable thumb gives the human hand its unique power grip.*

Source: By Unknown author – [1], Public Domain, https://commons.wikimedia.org/w/index.php?curid=68856887.

9.2.3. Changes in the Muscles of the Head and Neck

The shift to an upright posture has a direct impact on the muscle group of the head and neck, which includes the muscles in the back and sides of the neck. This change is not solely due to posture, but also to the decrease in jaw size in modern humans. The reduction in bulk of nuchal muscles is a common result of these differences. With upright posture, the head is better balanced on top of the spine, requiring less muscle force compared to animals with larger jaws. However, the human head's balance still presents challenges, with certain neck muscles like the sternocleidomastoid playing different roles than in apes (Figure 9.15).

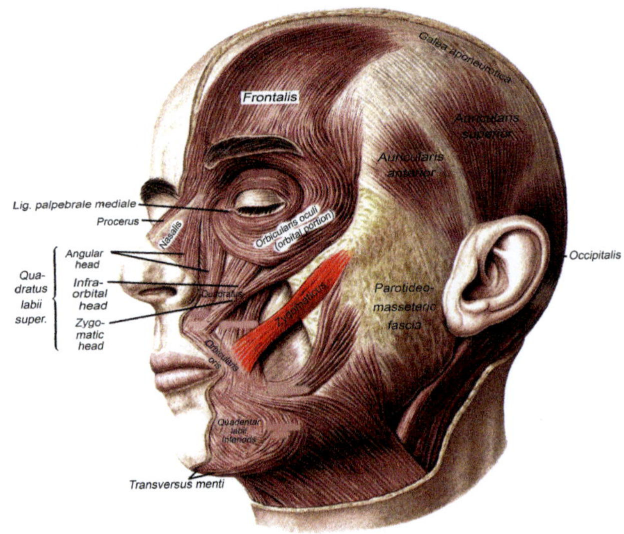

Figure 9.15. *Muscles of the face.*

Source: By Sobotta, color changed by was_a_bee. – File:Sobo_1909_260.png, Public Domain, https://commons.wikimedia.org/w/index.php?curid=30438326.

9.2.4. Changes in the Muscles of the Trunk

Maintaining an upright posture has significant effects on the support of the thoracic and abdominal viscera, but it also modifies very few trunk muscles. In animals that are pronograde, the ventral abdominal wall supports the abdominal viscera, whereas in an orthograde posture, the pelvis provides the majority of the support. This unavoidably puts more strain on the descending testicle's path through the anterior abdominal wall's muscles, known as the intestinal canal. Herniation may be the result of canal weakness.

The muscles that support the pelvic floor and regulate feces passage, known as the levator ani, also exhibit differences. All apes have lost their tails, which has caused a significant reorganization of that muscle. In comparison to apes, modern humans have more overlap and fusion between the various levator ani parts, and humans have a more substantial puborectalis muscular sling (Figure 9.16).

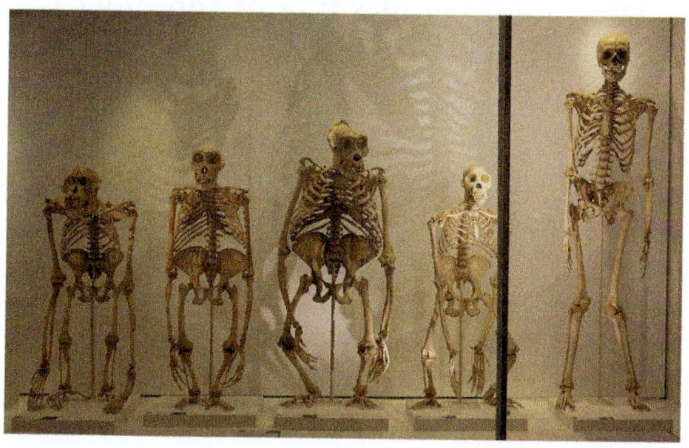

Figure 9.16. *Human and gorilla legs compared. Skeletal and muscular structures of a human leg (left) and a gorilla leg (right).*

Source: By DeFacto – Own work, CC BY-SA 4.0, https://commons.wikimedia.org/w/index.php?curid=74687030.

9.3. Muscles in the Human Body

Skeletal, smooth, and cardiac muscles are the three types of muscles in the human body. Skeletal muscle alone contains more than 650 different types of muscles. It is believed that the body has over 650 named skeletal muscles. Smooth muscle, like other muscle tissue, develops at the cellular level, allowing for billions of smooth muscle cells in the body.

The muscles in the body have important functions, including enabling movement, aiding in digestion, and assisting the heart in circulating blood.

9.3.1. Types of Muscles

Your body has three different types of muscles. They include:

1. **Skeletal Muscle:** Tendons connect your skeletal muscles to your bones. Numerous bundles of thousands of muscle fibers make up each muscle.

   These fibers are arranged in an orderly manner to create a striped pattern. As a result, skeletal muscle is sometimes referred to as striated muscle.

   The majority of skeletal muscle is used in motion. One of these muscles can contract to enable movement in a particular part of the body.

   The muscles in your skeleton are voluntary, which implies that you have control over their movement. This ability is limited to a specific category of muscle.

2. **Smooth Muscle:** It can be found in various organ systems throughout your body, including, but not limited to:

   - Digestive system;
   - Respiratory system;
   - Cardiovascular system;
   - Renal system;
   - Reproductive system.

   The center of smooth muscle cells is frequently rounded, and the sides taper off. In contrast to skeletal muscle, they lack striations. This type of muscle tissue has a more uniform appearance, commonly referred to as "smooth muscle." Smooth muscle does not contract voluntarily, meaning that you have no conscious control over its movement. Each cell contains chains of filaments that can connect to neighboring cells, forming a network resembling a mesh. This arrangement enables coordinated contraction of the cells.

3. **Cardiac Muscle:** This found exclusively in the heart, is responsible for its rhythmic contractions. It is also known as the myocardium.

   The myocardium is one of the three tissue layers in the heart, situated between the pericardium (the sac surrounding the heart) and the endocardium (the inner lining of the heart). Similar to skeletal muscle, cardiac muscle is striated and organized into fibers. The strong connections between individual cardiac muscle cells contribute to the synchronized beating of the heart.

   Like smooth muscle, cardiac muscle is involuntary. It contracts in response to electrical impulses generated by specialized heart cells.

9.3.2. Diagrams of Skeletal Muscles

There are skeletal muscles in every part of your body. The functions of some of the most well-known and frequently used skeletal muscles are shown in the following diagram.

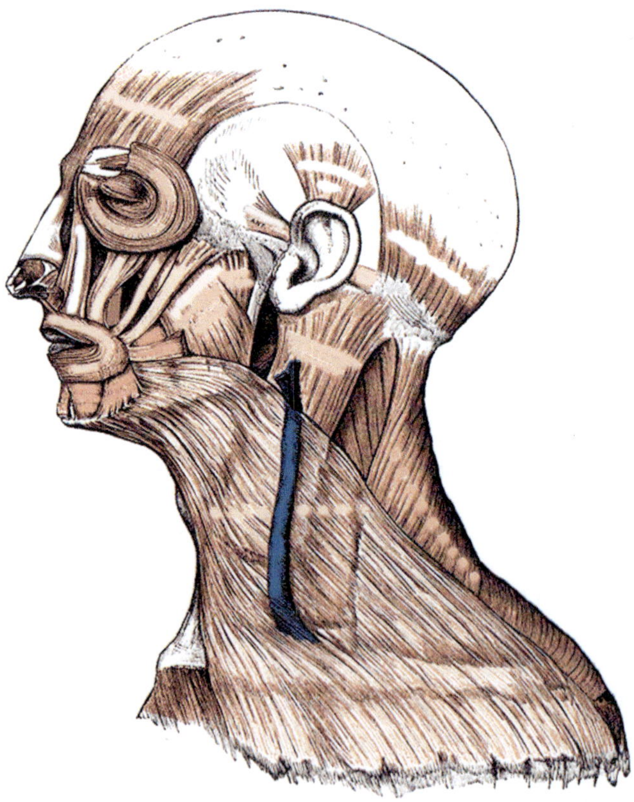

Figure 9.17. *Muscles of the head and neck.*

Source: By Henry Vandyke Carter – Henry Gray (1918) Anatomy of the Human Body (See "Book" section below). Bartleby.com: Gray's Anatomy, Plate 378, Public Domain, https://commons.wikimedia.org/w/index.php?curid=158468.

1. **Skeletal Muscle:** The functions of your skeletal muscles include:

- Enabling movement of the body;
- Providing structural support;
- Maintaining posture;
- Generating heat, which helps maintain body temperature;
- Acting as a source of nutrients such as amino acids;
- Serving as an energy source during starvation.

You may also see skeletal muscles divided according to which area of the body they serve, such as in Figure 9.17. The muscles in this area control movement of the face, head, and neck. Examples include:

- **Zygomaticus:** This muscle is involved in facial expression and lifts the corners of your mouth, such as when you smile.
- **Masseter:** The masseter is found in the jaw and is used to close your mouth and to chew food.
- **Eye (Extraocular) muscles:** This is a group of muscles that controls the movements of your eyes as well as the opening and closing of your eyelids.
- **Muscles of the Tongue:** This group of muscles help to elevate and lower the tongue as well as help it move in and out.
- **Sternocleidomastoid**: This is the major muscle that is involved when you rotate or tilt your head to the side. It is also involved in tilting your head forward.

9.3.2.1. Muscles of the Trunk

These muscles are located in the area of your torso and abdomen. Some examples include (Figure 9.18):

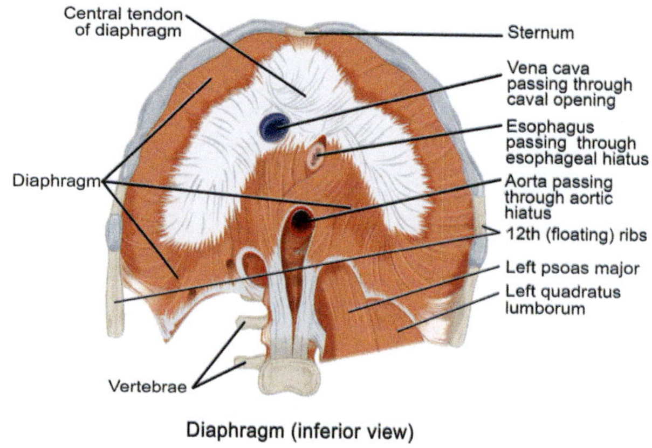

Figure 9.18. *Muscles of the diaphragm.*

Source: https://courses.lumenlearning.com/suny-ap1/chapter/axial-muscles-of-the-abdominal-wall-and-thorax/.

- **Erector Spinae:** These muscles support your spine and enable movements such as bending, arching, and twisting of the spine.
- **Oblique Muscles:** This group of muscles, including the external and internal obliques, helps you bend to the side or twist your body at the waist.
- **Intercostal Muscles**: The intercostal muscles are located around your ribs and assist in inhaling and exhaling.
- **Diaphragm:** The diaphragm separates your torso from your abdomen. It is also involved in breathing, contracting when you inhale, and relaxing when you exhale.
- **Levator Ani:** This muscle group supports the organs and tissues around your pelvis. It is also important for urination and bowel movements.

9.3.2.2. Muscles of the Upper Extremities

This includes the muscles that move your shoulders, arms, wrists, and hands. Examples of important muscles in this area include (Figure 9.19):

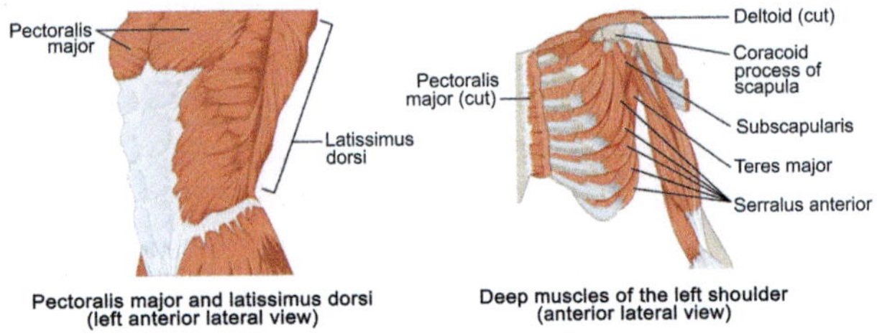

Figure 9.19. *Muscles of the upper extremities.*

Source: Illustration by Diego Sabogal. https://www.healthline.com/health/how-many-muscles-are-in-the-human-body#diagrams-of-skeletal-muscles.

- **Trapezius:** This muscle is used for several movements, including tilting your head back, raising your shoulders, and moving your shoulder blades together.
- **Pectoralis Major:** The pectoralis major is located in your upper chest and is utilized for rotational, vertical, and lateral movements of your arm.
    - **Deltoid:** The deltoid works to lift or rotate your arm at the shoulder.
    - **Biceps Brachii:** The biceps brachii flexes the forearm. When this happens, your elbow bends.
    - **Triceps Brachii**: The triceps brachii extends the forearm, straightening the elbow.

9.3.2.3. Muscles of the Lower Extremities

This area involves the muscles that move your legs and feet. Some examples that you may be familiar with are (Figure 9.20):

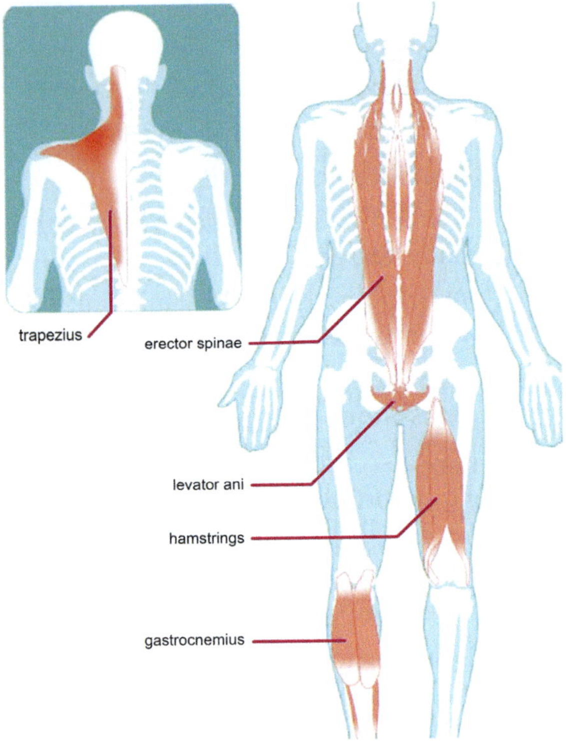

Figure 9.20. *Muscles of the lower extremities.*

Source: https://courses.lumenlearning.com/suny-ap1/chapter/muscles-of-the-pectoral-girdle-and-upper-limbs/.

1. **Gluteus Maximus:** This muscle is used for movement of your hips and thighs. It is important for maintaining posture, standing up from a sitting position, or going up stairs.
2. **Quadriceps:** This is actually a group of muscles that are located at the front of your thigh and work together to straighten your leg at the knee.
3. **Hamstrings:** Your hamstrings are located in the back part of your leg. This muscle group helps to extend your thigh and to bend your leg at the knee.
4. **Tibialis Anterior:** You use this muscle when you raise the sole of your foot from the ground.
5. **Soleus:** The soleus works to lower the

sole of your foot to the ground. It is important for maintaining your posture while you are walking.

9.3.3. Smooth Muscle

The function of smooth muscle can vary depending on its location in the body. Let's examine the functions of smooth muscle in different systems:

1. **Digestive System:** Smooth muscle contractions aid in propelling food through the digestive tract.
2. **Respiratory System:** Smooth muscle tissue can widen or narrow the airways.
3. **Cardiovascular System:** Smooth muscle in the blood vessel walls facilitates blood flow and helps regulate blood pressure.
4. **Renal System:** Smooth muscle assists in regulating urine flow from the bladder.
5. **Reproductive System:** In the female reproductive system, smooth muscle is involved in contractions during pregnancy. In the male reproductive system, it aids in propelling sperm.

Smooth muscle also plays a role in certain sensory processes. For instance, it is responsible for the expansion or contraction of the pupils.

9.3.4. Cardiac Muscle

Your heart beats because of your cardiac muscle. An electrical impulse causes a heartbeat to occur. A unique kind of cell known as a pacemaker cell initiates this electrical signal, which causes the cardiac muscle to contract (Figure 9.21).

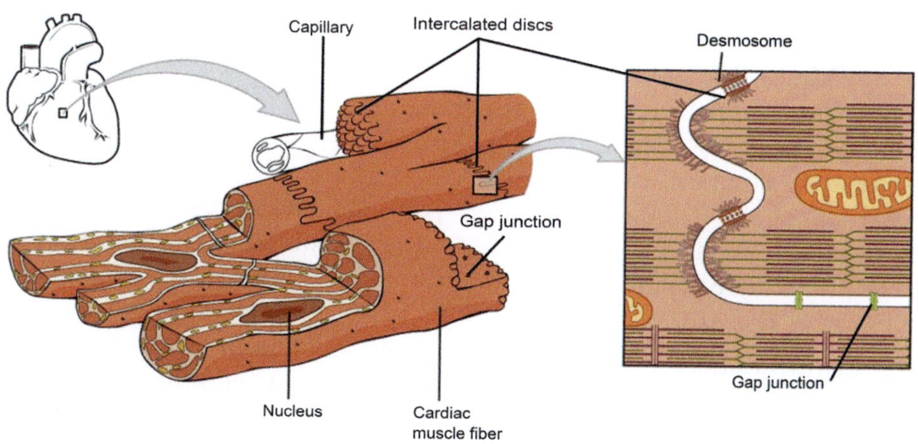

Figure 9.21. *Cardiac muscle.*

Source: https://courses.lumenlearning.com/suny-ap1/chapter/cardiac-muscle-tissue/.

The heart's electrical signal moves from the upper to lower chamber. The heartbeat is generated by the synchronized wave-like contraction of cardiac muscle cells, which are closely interconnected.

9.3.5. Muscular System Conditions

1. **Muscle Pain:** Muscle soreness refers to the discomfort caused by overworked muscles. Myofascial discomfort, caused by trigger points in the muscles, is commonly experienced in the primary upper back muscles. Muscular irritation and upper back pain are the result of weak muscles and repetitive motions.
2. **Sprains:** Ankle ligament ruptures are typically the result of a sudden motion of the foot. Future discomfort and swelling could be avoided with the use of rehabilitation treatments.
3. **Strain:** A pulled bicep is the result of overstretching and tearing the tendons and/or muscle fibers in the biceps. Pain and edema are possible complications.
4. **Bruise:** A bruise is the medical term for a cut or rupture in the muscular tissue. Symptoms include swelling and an increase in pressure around the injured muscle.
5. **Cancer of the Muscle:** This disorder, which can affect the calf muscle, is extremely rare. Cancer of the calf muscles is referred to as sarcoma in the medical community. Another potential cause of this condition is metastatic carcinoma, which originates in another part of the body and spreads to the calf.
6. **Muscle Cramps:** Calf cramps are among the most excruciating pains one may experience. Any number of medical conditions, such as pregnancy or dehydration, might be the root cause of these pains.
7. **Parkinson's Disease:** Mobility and coordination issues develop as a result of the disease, which is characterized by the slow degeneration of nerve cells in a substantial area of the brain. One of the earliest symptoms of Parkinson's disease is trembling in the hands.
8. **Multiple Sclerosis:** Degenerative changes in the myelin sheath of the exons lead to fatal redistribution of the neuronal pathways and variable neuronal degeneration in this progressive disease of the brain, spinal cord, and peripheral nervous system.

9.3.6. Muscular System Test

1. **Magnetic Resonance Imaging (MRI):** It is the most common abbreviation used to describe this diagnostic technique. The objective of this test is to obtain a comprehensive understanding of the calf muscles and other soft tissues in the body. By utilizing a powerful magnet and a computer, this technique can visualize the intricate architecture of a patient's soft tissues.
2. **Computed Tomography (CT):** This scan, also known as a CT scan, is the preferred term for this diagnostic test. It employs X-ray waves and a computer to obtain detailed images of the calf muscles and any other muscles connected to or near the calf muscles.
3. **Ultrasound:** Ultrasonography, which utilizes high-frequency sound waves, is employed for diagnostic evaluation of the calf muscle. These sound waves can penetrate the calf muscle, ligaments, and tendons, providing doctors with an accurate digital representation of the muscle's structure.
4. **Phlebography:** This procedure is also referred to as venography. It involves injecting a specific dye into the patient's veins or bone marrow, followed by a venogram to visualize the blood vessels.

5. **Biceps Ultrasound:** By directing high-frequency sound waves onto the components of the biceps, a device placed on the skin produces images. These impulses are then converted into pictures displayed on a television screen, allowing medical experts to visualize internal body structures. An ultrasonography of the biceps can help identify issues with the tendon.
6. **Serum Calcium Test:** A calcium blood test indicates the concentration of the mineral in your blood. Bone disease, thyroid disease, parathyroid abnormalities, renal disease, and other medical conditions can all be signs of high or low blood calcium levels.
7. **Serum Urea and Creatinine:** Serum Urea and creatinine aid in the identification of nitrogenous compounds generated as a metabolic byproduct. Urea is produced primarily as a result of the breakdown of dietary and cellular protein. When calcium deposits as crystals in the bone, its density decreases.

9.3.7. Muscular System Treatment

1. **Open Reduction and Internal Fixation:** When the distal third of the humerus is fractured, the bone is displaced from its position, requiring open reduction and internal fixation of the bone as well as nerve exploration to prevent damage.
2. **Closed Reduction and Slab:** In the event of a humerus fracture, the initial course of treatment involves realigning the fractured segment to its original position and applying a slab to restrict further movement until the injury has healed.
3. **RICE Therapy:** Rest, Icing, Compression (with an athletic bandage or similar), and Elevation (RICE) constitute a comprehensive injury-treatment program. Like most injuries, a palm laceration responds well to the RICE treatment protocol of rest, ice, compression, and elevation.
4. **Palm Immobilization:** The majority of palm fractures necessitate casting to limit additional movement. Immobilization is recommended by certain medical authorities as a therapeutic measure for conditions such as palm sprains.
5. **Physiotherapy for Myositis:** Contraction and release inflammation of the biceps muscles can be addressed through physical therapy. When administered by a skilled physiotherapist, this modality enhances the prognosis even for patients with chronic injuries.

A Closer Look

Splenius Capitis

The splenius capitis is a complex muscle located in the posterior (back) region of the neck and upper back. It is part of the deeper layer of muscles in the cervical spine and plays a significant role in various movements and postures of the head and neck. Understanding the anatomy, function, innervation, and clinical significance of the splenius capitis is crucial for healthcare professionals, especially those involved in diagnosing and treating neck pain and musculoskeletal disorders.

The splenius capitis muscle is broad and strap-like, extending from the lower half of the nuchal ligament, spinous processes of the seventh cervical (C7) vertebra, and the upper thoracic vertebrae (T1-T4). From these origins, it ascends diagonally upwards and laterally to insert into the mastoid process of the temporal bone and the superior nuchal line of the occipital bone. The muscle fibers are arranged in an oblique direction, crossing multiple vertebral levels.

The splenius capitis muscle primarily functions to extend, laterally flex, and rotate the head and neck. Its bilateral contraction results in head and neck extension, assisting in maintaining an upright posture. Unilateral contraction of the splenius capitis causes ipsilateral (same side) lateral flexion and contralateral (opposite side) rotation of the head and neck. For example, the right splenius capitis contracts to laterally flex the head to the right and rotate it to the left. This muscle works synergistically with other neck muscles, including the sternocleidomastoid, trapezius, and deeper cervical spine muscles, to facilitate various movements and stabilize the cervical spine.

The splenius capitis muscle receives its nerve supply from the dorsal rami of cervical spinal nerves, primarily C3 and C4. These nerves innervate the muscle fibers, providing motor signals for contraction and proprioceptive feedback. The innervation of the splenius capitis is essential for coordinating its actions with other muscles and maintaining proper head and neck alignment during movements and postural adjustments.

The splenius capitis muscle can be implicated in various clinical conditions related to neck pain and musculoskeletal dysfunction. Dysfunction or injury to the splenius capitis may result from trauma, repetitive strain, poor posture, or underlying musculoskeletal disorders. Common symptoms associated with splenius capitis dysfunction include localized neck pain, stiffness, reduced range of motion, and referred pain patterns. For example, trigger points within the muscle can cause referred pain patterns that radiate to the head, neck, shoulders, and upper back regions.

Understanding the role of the splenius capitis in contributing to neck pain and musculoskeletal dysfunction is crucial for healthcare professionals involved in the assessment, diagnosis, and management of these conditions. Manual therapy techniques, such as massage, stretching, and trigger point therapy, can be used to alleviate muscle tension and improve mobility. Additionally, strengthening exercises targeting the cervical spine and upper back muscles may help improve muscle balance and stability, reducing the risk of recurrent symptoms.

In summary, the splenius capitis muscle is an important structure in the posterior neck region, contributing to various movements and postures of the head and neck. Its anatomy, function, innervation, and clinical significance are essential considerations for healthcare professionals involved in managing neck pain and musculoskeletal disorders. A comprehensive understanding of the splenius capitis can guide assessment, diagnosis, and treatment strategies, ultimately improving patient outcomes and quality of life.

Summary

- Muscular fibers are specialized cells that constitute the musculoskeletal system. Their capacity to contract is their primary characteristic. The muscles that are attached to bones, internal organs, and blood vessels are responsible for movement.
- The muscular system of the human body consists of the voluntary muscles that govern movement, posture, and equilibrium, in addition to the muscles responsible for operating the skeletal system.
- The movements of the neck, which is the region connecting the ear to the shoulder, are described using terms such as rotation, flexion, extension, and side bending.
- Many of the muscles involved in the movement of the neck and shoulders originate in the posterior region.
- The humeral head, the clavicle (collarbone), and the scapula constitute the intricate ball-and-socket joint that is the shoulder.
- The muscles in the upper arm not only facilitate movement of the shoulder but also generate various movements of the forearm.
- Wrist flexion is defined as a wrist motion that pulls the hand's palm downward. The flexor pollicis longus, flexor digitorum superficialis, flexor digitorum profundus, flexor carpi radialis, and flexor carpi ulnaris execute that action.
- The abdominal wall comprises three layers of musculature, along with a fourth layer situated in the anterior midregion. The rectus abdominis, which possesses vertically oriented muscle fibers responsible for trunk flexion and pelvic stabilization, constitutes the fourth layer of the midregion.
- The muscles of the foot and lower leg are intricate and operate on multiple planes. Their actions are contingent upon both the position of the foot and whether the individual is bearing weight.
- The overall structure of the human upper limb has been conserved, albeit with modifications to accommodate an upright lifestyle.
- Tendons link your skeletal muscles to your bones. Numerous bundles of thousands of muscle fibers constitute each muscle.

References

1. Apple, F. S., Sandoval, Y., Jaffe, A. S., & Ordonez-Llanos, J., (2017). IFCC task force on clinical applications of cardiac bio-markers. Cardiac troponin assays: Guide to understanding analytical characteristics and their impact on clinical care. *Clin Chem., 63*(1), 73–81.
2. Bordoni, B., Jozsa, F., & Varacallo, M., (2023). *StatPearls* [Internet]. StatPearls Publishing; Treasure Island (FL). Anatomy, Head and Neck, Sternocleidomastoid Muscle.
3. Bordoni, B., Sugumar, K., & Varacallo, M., (2023). *StatPearls* [Internet]. StatPearls Publishing; Treasure Island (FL). Muscle Cramps.
4. Conable, K. M., & Rosner, A. L., (2011). A narrative review of manual muscle testing and implications for muscle testing research. *J. Chiropr. Med., 10*(3), 157–165.
5. Enoka, R. M., (2015). *Neuromechanics of Human Movement*. Human Kinetics.

6. Ferreira, C. H., Barbosa, P. B., De Oliveira, S. F., Antônio, F. I., Franco, M. M., & Bø, K., (2011). Inter-rater reliability study of the modified oxford grading scale and the peritron manometer. *Physiotherapy, 97*(2), 132–138.
7. Frontera, W. R., & Ochala, J., (2015). Skeletal muscle: A brief review of structure and function. *Calcif. Tissue Int., 96*(3), 183–195.
8. Giuriato, G., Pedrinolla, A., Schena, F., & Venturelli, M., (2018). Muscle cramps: A comparison of the two-leading hypothesis. *J. Electromyogr Kinesiol., 41*, 89–95.
9. Gordon, A. M., Homsher, E., & Regnier, M., (2000). Regulation of contraction in striated muscle. *Physiol. Rev., 80*(2), 853–924.
10. Guyton, A. C., & Hall, J. E., (2015). *Textbook of Medical Physiology.* Elsevier Health Sciences.
11. Hernandez, O. M., Housmans, P. R., & Potter, J. D., (2001). Invited review: Pathophysiology of cardiac muscle contraction and relaxation as a result of alterations in thin filament regulation. *J. Appl. Physiol. (1985), 90*(3), 1125–1136.
12. Kuo, I. Y., & Ehrlich, B. E., (2015). Signaling in muscle contraction. *Cold Spring Harb Perspect Biol., 7*(2), a006023.
13. Lieberman, D. E., (2013). *The Story of the Human Body: Evolution, Health, and Disease.* Vintage.
14. Lowey, S., Waller, G. S., & Trybus, K. M., (1993). Function of skeletal muscle myosin heavy and light chain isoforms by an in vitro motility assay. *J. Biol. Chem., 268*(27), 20414–20418.
15. Ludwig, P. E., Reddy, V., & Varacallo, M., (2022). *StatPearls* [Internet]. StatPearls Publishing; Treasure Island (FL). Neuroanatomy, Central Nervous System (CNS).
16. Mador, M. J., & Acevedo, F. A., (2015). *Exercise Physiology: A Thematic Approach.* Routledge.
17. Mills, K. R., (2005). The basics of electromyography. *J. Neurol. Neurosurg. Psychiatry., 76*(Suppl 2), ii32–35.
18. Moore, K. L., & Agur, A. M. R., (2013). *Essential Clinical Anatomy*. Lippincott Williams & Wilkins.
19. Satish V Khadilkar, Rakhil S Yadav, Bhagyadhan A Patel, *Neuromuscular Disorders: A Comprehensive Review with Illustrative Cases*, (2019). Oxford University Press.
20. Rassier, D. E., (2017). Sarcomere mechanics in striated muscles: From molecules to sarcomeres to cells. *Am. J. Physiol. Cell Physiol., 313*(2), C134–C145.
21. Roig, M., O'Brien, K., Kirk, G., Murray, R., McKinnon, P., Shadgan, B., & Reid, W. D., (2009). The effects of eccentric versus concentric resistance training on muscle strength and mass in healthy adults: A systematic review with meta-analysis. *Br. J. Sports Med., 43*(8), 556–568.
22. Rosenblueth, A., Alanis, J., & Rubio, R., (1958). A comparative study of the isometric and isotonic contractions of striated muscles. *Arch Int. Physiol. Biochim., 66*(3), 330–353.
23. Saladin, K. S., (2018). *Anatomy & Physiology: The Unity of Form and Function*. McGraw-Hill Education.
24. Squire, J., (2019). Special issue: The actin-myosin interaction in muscle: Background and overview. *Int. J. Mol. Sci., 20*(22).
25. Standring, S., (2016). *Gray's Anatomy: The Anatomical Basis of Clinical Practice.* Elsevier.
26. Sweeney, H. L., & Hammers, D. W., (2018). Muscle contraction. *Cold Spring Harb. Perspect. Biol., 10*(2).

27. Tortora, G. J., & Derrickson, B. H., (2017). *Principles of Anatomy and Physiology.* John Wiley & Sons.

28. Visone, R., Gilardi, M., Marsano, A., Rasponi, M., Bersini, S., & Moretti, M., (2016). Cardiac meets skeletal: What's new in microfluidic models for muscle tissue engineering. *Molecules, 21*(9).

29. Webb, R. C., (2003). Smooth muscle contraction and relaxation. *Adv. Physiol. Educ., 27*(1–4), 201–206.

30. Wick, C. L., & Winkelmann, Z. K., (2020). *Netter's Essential Physiology*. Elsevier.

31. Zile, M. R., Richardson, K., Cowles, M. K., Buckley, J. M., Koide, M., Cowles, B. A., Gharpuray, V., & Cooper, G., (1998). Constitutive properties of adult mammalian cardiac muscle cells. *Circulation, 98*(6), 567–579.

Chapter

10

RENAL SYSTEM

Contents

Unit Introduction

The human kidneys, which produce urine, as well as the bladder, ureters, and urethra for the passage, storage, and evacuation of urine, make up the renal system.

While the human excretory, or urinary, system shares many traits with other mammalian species, it also has some distinct structural and functional traits of its own. The system's elimination function is emphasized by the terms excretory and urinary. On the other hand, the kidneys actively retain some substances in the body and secrete others that are just as vital to survival as those that are removed.

The kidneys in the system are two thin muscular tubes called ureters that carry urine from the kidneys to the bladder. The ureters also filter out waste products that have dissolved in the blood as well as excess amounts of other substances. The kidneys regulate the electrolyte composition of the blood. Urine is stored in the bladder until it is expelled through the urethra.

Orientation and Directional Terms

Term	Definition	Illustration
Glomerulus	The glomerulus is a network of small blood vessels that filters plasma volume in the kidney. It is located between two resistance vessels and is contained within the Bowman's capsule.	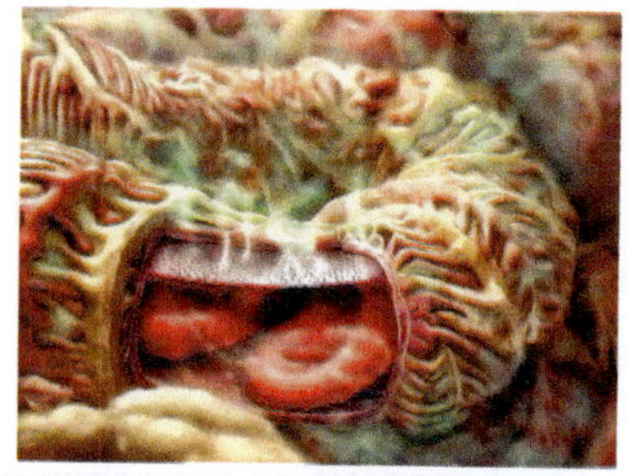
Juxtaglomerular apparatus	The juxtaglomerular apparatus is an anatomical unit located at the hilus of the glomerulus and is believed to be involved in the feedback control of renal blood flow and glomerular filtration rate.	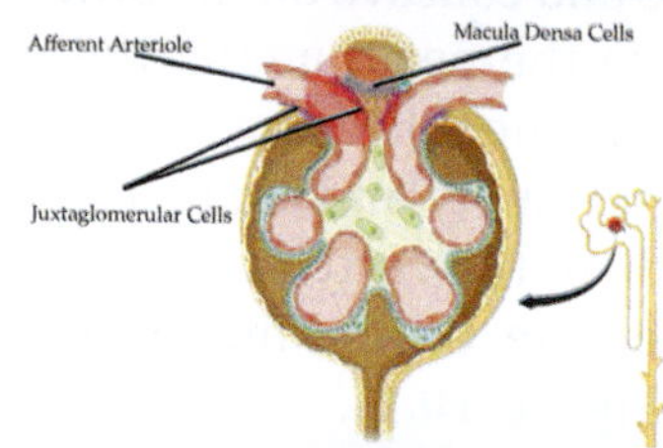
Micturition	Micturition, also known as urination, is the process of removing waste products and metabolics from the body. It's a vital function that helps maintain fluid balance, assess kidney function, and excrete medications.	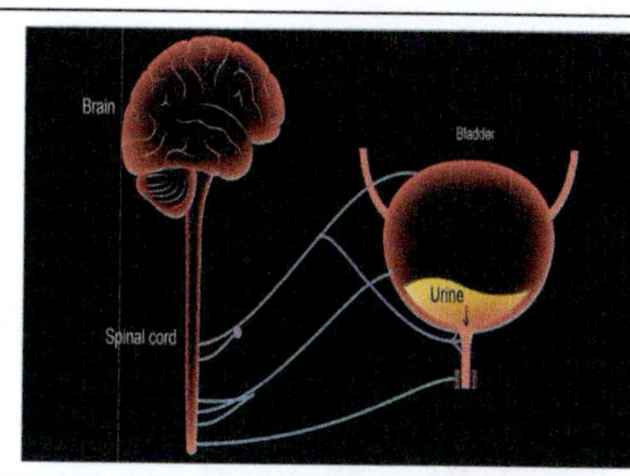
Renal corpuscle	The renal corpuscle is a structural unit of the kidney that filters blood. It is also known as the Malpighian body.	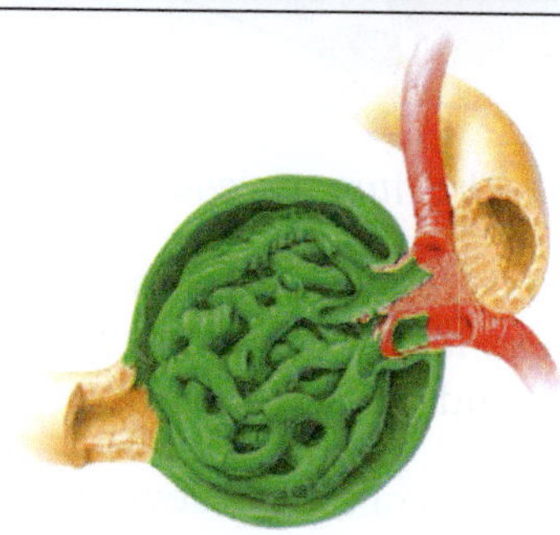
Renal tubule	A renal tubule is a small tube in the kidneys that transports nutrients, fluids, and other substances back into the bloodstream.	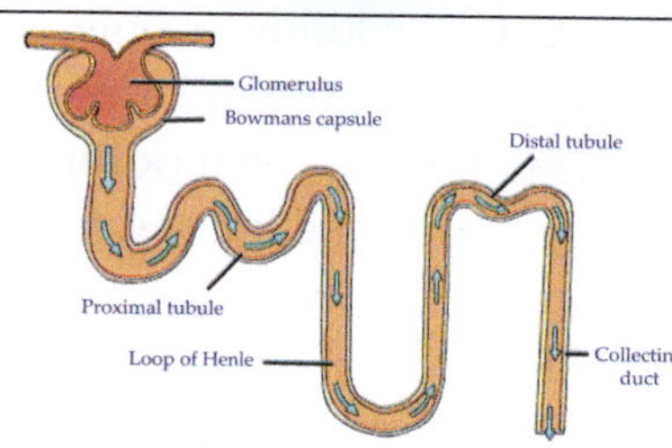

10.1. Human Excretory Organs

10.1.1. The Kidneys

10.1.1.1. General Description and Location

Bean-shaped and reddish-brown in color, the kidneys are paired organs that are convex on one long side and concave on the other. Normally found outside the peritoneum, the membrane lining the abdomen, they are situated high in the abdominal cavity and against its back wall, on either side of the vertebral column between the levels of the third lumbar and thoracic vertebrae (Figure 10.1).

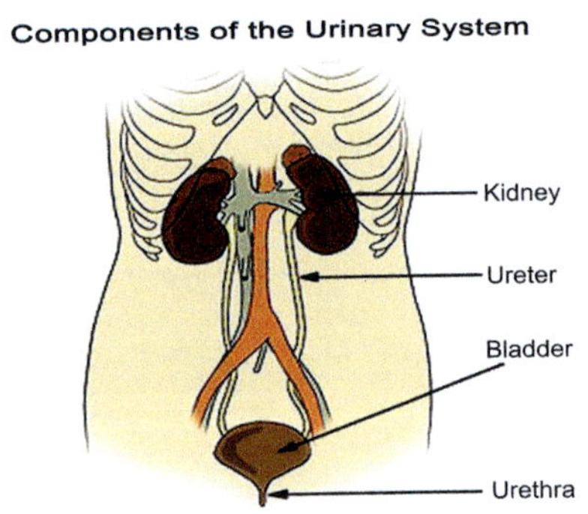

Figure 10.1. *The human renal system.*

Source: https://courses.lumenlearning.com/suny-dutchess-ap1/chapter/urinary-system-main-organs-and-their-functions/.

The long axes of the kidneys are parallel to the body's axis, but each kidney's pole, or upper end, tilts slightly inward toward the vertebral column, the backbone. The renal (kidney) sinus, which is a cavity within the kidney, is accessed through the hilus, a deep vertical cleft located in the center of the medial concave border. The hilus is the point where the lymphatic vessels, nerves, enlarged upper extension of the ureters, and renal arteries and veins enter and exit the body (Figure 10.2).

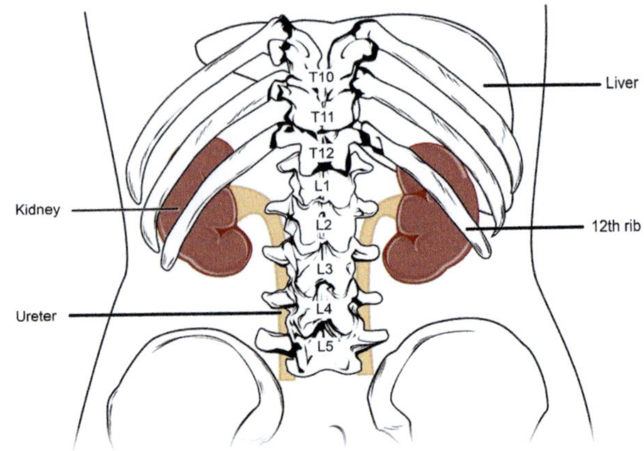

Figure 10.2. *The protection of the human renal system.*

Source: https://courses.lumenlearning.com/suny-dutchess-ap1/chapter/urinary-system-main-organs-and-their-functions/.

10.1.2. Renal Vessels and Nerves

The abdominal aorta gives rise to the renal arteries, one on each side, at a location across from the upper border of the second lumbar vertebra. Each artery near the renal hilus splits into anterior and posterior divisions after branching off into the adrenal gland and ureter. The large veins that supply the kidneys with blood typically lie in front of the corresponding arteries and almost perfectly angle into the inferior vena cava. Because the inferior vena cava is located closer to the right kidney, the left vein is longer than the right vein.

The sympathetic and parasympathetic nerves of the autonomic nervous system supply the kidneys, and the afferent and efferent fibers of the renal nerves carry nerve impulses to and from the central nervous system, respectively.

10.1.3. Internal Configuration

The renal sinus and two layers of kidney tissue that can be distinguished by texture and color are visible in a cross section of a kidney. The comparatively dark cones, known as renal pyramids, with bases pointing outward and apexes projecting singly or in groups into the renal sinus, are formed by the innermost tissue, known as the renal medulla. A renal papilla is a projection of one or more pyramid apexes into the sinus. These pyramids have uneven bases with thin striations that extend to the outermost part of the kidney. The cortex is the paler, more granular tissue located outside the medulla. It bridges the spaces between the pyramids and arches over their bases. A renal lobe is composed of the section of cortex that arches over each group of pyramids that projects into a papilla.

The renal pelvis, a funnel-shaped expansion of the upper end of the ureter, and two or three major calyxes—expansions of the cavity that extend into the kidney substance—are all parts of the renal sinus. The renal papillae project into the 4 to 12 smaller cup-shaped cavities known as minor calyxes, which are formed by successive divisions of the major calyxes. Urine enters the sinus through the urinary collecting tubules, which are tiny tubes that open into the sinus at the papillae, and is initially stored in the renal pelvis.

10.1.4. Minute Structure

Nephrons, each kidney containing approximately 1 million, are the structural components responsible for urine production in the kidneys. Each nephron is a lengthy and slender tube known as a tubule, which is intricately folded, expanded, and closed at one end to form a structure resembling a double-walled cup. Enclosed by a structure called the renal corpuscular capsule, also known as Bowman's capsule, is a collection of capillaries known as the glomerulus. Together, the glomerulus and capsule constitute a renal corpuscle, also referred to as a malpighian body. Small arteries called arterioles enter and exit the glomerulus through the open end of the capsule, facilitating the flow of blood into and out of the structure. This aperture is known as the corpuscle's vascular pole.

The length of nephron tubules ranges from 30 to 55 millimeters (1-2 inches). Within the renal cortex, the corpuscle and the proximal convoluted tubule, which is the initial segment of each tubule, are located. The tubule enters a renal pyramid, takes a U-shaped turn, and returns to the cortex near its point of entry into the medulla. The nephronic loop, also known as the loop of Henle, consists of two parallel lengths and a bend in between. After reentering the cortex, the tubule returns to the vascular pole of its own nephron, which is the aperture in the cup-shaped structure of the capsule. The final segment of the tubule, known as the distal convoluted tubule, travels from the vascular pole of the corpuscle to a collecting tubule through a brief junctional tubule. Several collecting tubules join together to form a somewhat wider tubule that carries urine to the renal pelvis and a renal papilla.

While the general disposition of all kidney nephrons is the same, there are regional variations, most notably in the length of the loops of Henle. While more superficial cortical glomeruli have much shorter loops, juxtamedullary glomeruli, which are glomeruli located deep within the renal cortex close to the medulla, have long Henle loops that extend deeply into the medulla. The length of the loops varies greatly between animal species and influences the species' capacity to concentrate urine above the osmotic concentration of plasma.

The nephron tubule's successive sections differ in size and shape, and these variations, along with variations in the cells lining the sections, are linked to particular roles in the urine-producing process (Figure 10.3).

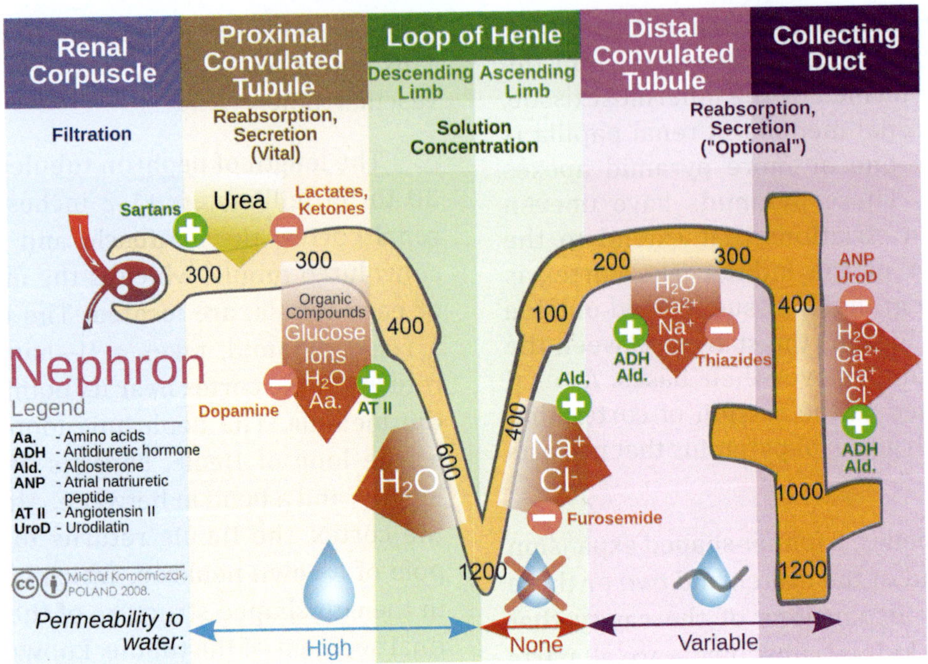

Figure 10.3. *Human kidney; nephron. Each kidney has approximately 1 million nephrons, which filter water and other substances out of the blood to produce urine.*

*Source: By Nephron-urine.svg: M. Komorniczak, polish wikipedist. Kidney nephron molar transport diagram.png: *Nephron-urine.svg: M. Komorniczak, polish wikipedist.derivative work: Juvo415derivative work: Mcstrother – Nephron-urine.svgKidney nephron molar transport diagram.png, CC BY-SA 3.0, https://commons.wikimedia.org/w/index.php?curid=12880243.*

10.1.5. Intrarenal Network of Blood Vessels

The blood-processing machinery includes the intrarenal blood vessel network.

1. **Arteries and Arterioles:** Each of the previously mentioned anterior and posterior divisions of a renal artery divides into lobar arteries, which all enter the kidney substance through or near a renal papilla. The interlobar arteries, which radiate outward between neighboring renal pyramids, are the two or three branches that each lobar artery generates. When these reach the border between the medulla and cortex, they almost immediately bifurcate into branches known as arcuate arteries, which run parallel to the kidney's surface between the medulla and cortex. Numerous arteries, referred to as interlobular arteries, branch off from the arcuate arteries and extend through the cortex, eventually terminating in capillary networks in the area immediately inside the capsule. They generate brief branches along the way known as afferent arterioles, which transport blood to the glomeruli and divide into four to eight capillary loops in each glomerulus (Figure 10.4).

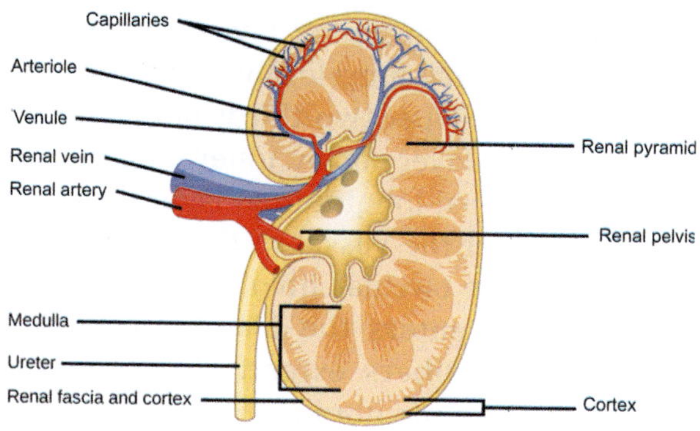

Figure 10.4. *Cross section of the right kidney showing the major parts.*

Source: https://courses.lumenlearning.com/suny-dutchess-ap1/chapter/urinary-system-main-organs-and-their-functions/.

The lining layer of the glomerulus enlarges and becomes filled with secretory granules just before and near the point where the afferent arteriole enters the structure. The process of renin secretion is believed to be facilitated by this composite structure known as the juxtaglomerular apparatus (JGA). Subsequently, they are reconstituted near the point of entry of the afferent arteriole to form the efferent arterioles that carry blood away from the glomeruli. Despite having nearly identical channel sizes, afferent arterioles have almost twice the thickness of efferent arterioles due to their thicker muscular coats.

The efferent arterioles divide into a second set of capillaries that extend across the majority of the cortex, supplying blood to the proximal and distal renal tubules. The efferent glomerular arterioles of the juxtaglomerular glomeruli split into vessels that enter the bases of the renal pyramids and vessels that supply the adjacent tubules. These vessels, known as vasa recta, run closely with the Henle loops towards the apexes of the pyramids. They then retrace their path, forming hairpin-like bends, and empty into arcuate veins that run parallel to the arcuate arteries, similar to the tubules. Normally, the cortex receives a greater blood supply than the medulla, accounting for more than 90% of the total volume. However, under certain circumstances such as severe trauma or blood loss, the cortical vessels may constrict while the juxtamedullary circulation remains intact. This can result in reduced urine flow and, in severe cases, complete cessation, as the cortical glomeruli and tubules are deprived of blood.

2. **Veins and Venules:** Names for the small veins that accompany the arterioles and arteries are similar: the renal venules. Because of their radial arrangement, the venules directly beneath the renal capsule are referred to as stellarate venules. These venules drain into interlobular venules. These then come together to form the lobar, arcuate, and interlobar veins' branches. The venae rectae, which connect the arcuate veins, receive blood from the renal pyramids. The lobar veins join together in the renal sinus to create veins that match the major renal artery divisions. Normally, these veins unite to form a single renal vein in or close to the renal hilus.
3. **Lymphatic Network:** A shallower network of lymphatic capillaries forms between and around the renal blood vessels, while a deeper network forms just inside the renal capsule. The glomeruli lack lymphatics, and the few lymphatic capillaries that are present in the renal substance are clearly connected to the connective tissue framework. The interlobular and arcuate blood vessels are accompanied

by lymphatic channels that receive drainage from the lymphatic networks within the capsule and surrounding the renal blood vessels. The major lymph channels terminate in lymph nodes next to the aorta and close to the locations where the renal arteries originate. They run parallel to the major renal arteries and veins.

10.2. The Ureters

10.2.1. General Characteristics

The ureters are small, thick-walled ducts that transport urine from the kidneys to the bladder. They have a length of approximately 25–30 centimeters (9–11–8 inches) and a diameter of 4–5 millimeters (0–16–0–2 inches). As they move along, they are connected to the peritoneum, which is the lining of the abdomen and pelvis, by connective tissue.

In both males and females, the ureters enter the bladder wall about five centimeters apart. However, this distance increases when the bladder is filled with urine. After passing obliquely through the muscular wall of the bladder for nearly two centimeters, the ureters enter the bladder cavity through small openings. This oblique course functions as a valve-like mechanism, exerting pressure on the section of each ureter located in the muscular wall of the bladder when the bladder expands. This helps prevent urine from flowing back from the bladder into the ureters.

10.2.2. Structure of the Ureteric Wall

The wall of the ureter is composed of three layers: the mucous membrane-based lining, the intermediate muscular layer, and the adventitia, or outer layer. The adventitia is made up of fibroelastic connective tissue that blends with the connective tissue behind the peritoneum. The muscular layer consists of smooth, involuntary muscle fibers arranged in two layers in the upper two-thirds of the ureter: an outer circular layer and an inner longitudinal layer. An additional longitudinal layer develops on the outside of the vessel in the lower third of the ureter. The circular fibers of each ureter disappear as it enters the bladder wall, but the longitudinal fibers extend almost to the bladder's mucous membrane.

The thickness of the mucous membrane lining increases from the renal pelvis downwards. Consequently, the lining is two to three cells deep in the pelvis and kidney calyxes, four to five cells thick in the ureter, and six to eight cells thick in the bladder. The mucous membrane of the ureters is longitudinally folded, allowing the channel to expand significantly. Neither the ureter's nor the renal pelvis' mucous membranes contain actual glands. The primary driving force behind the flow of urine from the kidney into the bladder is generated by the peristaltic (wave-like) contractions of the ureter muscles.

10.3. The Urinary Bladder

10.3.1. General Description

The primary urinary reservoir is the hollow, muscular organ known as the bladder. It lies beneath the peritoneum, behind the symphysis pubis, and on the anterior portion of the pelvic floor (see below). The hip joint in the front midline of the body is called the symphysis pubis. The amount of urine that the bladder holds determines the bladder's size and shape. It is tetrahedral and resides in the pelvis when empty; when it is distended, it expands into the lower abdomen and becomes ovoid. It has a body, which includes two inferolateral (below and to the side) and two superior (upper) surfaces, a neck, an apex, and a fundus, or base. These features are not very visible unless the bladder is empty or only slightly enlarged.

The lowest and most fixed part of the bladder is its neck, which is the region directly surrounding the urethral opening. It is securely fastened to the base of the prostate in men, a gland that surrounds the urethra.

The peritoneum covers the triangular superior surface of the bladder. The levator ani muscles, which make up the majority of the pelvic cavity floor, support the bladder. The visceral layer of the pelvic fascia covers and partially supports the bladder. The fascial layer is a layer of connective tissue that envelops the pelvic cavity's organs, blood vessels, and nerves. The pubovesical ligaments, which the fascia forms in front and to the side, function as a sort of hammock beneath the inferolateral surfaces and bladder neck.

10.3.2. Blood and Nerve Supplies

The superior, middle, and inferior vesical (bladder) arteries provide the blood supply to the bladder. The dome of the bladder is supplied by the superior vesical artery, which also supplies the ductus deferens, a portion of the male sperm passageway, through one of its branches. The base of the bladder is supplied by the middle vesical artery. The base of the bladder, the lower end of the ureter, and other nearby structures are supplied by the inferior vesical artery, which also contributes to the blood supply of the inferolateral surfaces of the bladder.

The autonomic nervous system is divided into the sympathetic and parasympathetic branches, which include the nerves that innervate the bladder. The sympathetic nerve fibers originate from the hypogastric plexus of nerves located in front of the fifth lumbar vertebra. Sympathetic nerves are believed to be involved in the relaxation of the muscular layer of the bladder wall and the contraction of the sphincter mechanism that closes the opening into the urethra. They also transmit the sensations associated with bladder distention to the central nervous system. The parasympathetic nerves, along with the pelvic splanchnic nerves, travel to the bladder from the second to the fifth sacral spinal segment. The parasympathetic nervous system regulates the contraction of the muscular walls of the bladder and the relaxation of its sphincter. Consequently, they actively participate in the process of urination and are sometimes referred to as the detrusor, or emptying, nerves.

10.3.3. Structure of the Bladder Wall

The upper surface of the bladder wall is covered in a serous coat. This covering, which extends the peritoneum lining the abdominal cavity, is known as serous because it secretes a small amount of serum, a lubricating fluid. The layers of the bladder wall that are not visible are the mucous, submucous, muscular, and fascial layers.

The fascial coat is a layer of connective tissue that covers muscles. The muscular coat is composed of bundles of smooth muscle fibers arranged in three layers. The outer and inner layers have fibers that run lengthwise, while the intermediate layer has fibers that run circularly. There is a significant intermingling of fibers between the layers. The smooth muscle coat includes the detrusor muscle, which is responsible for emptying the bladder.

The circular or intermediate muscular stratum of the vesical wall is thicker than the other layers. Despite generally flowing in a circular pattern, its fibers do interlace. The layer of fibers that makes up the internal muscular stratum is extensive and primarily oriented longitudinally. The submucous coat consists of numerous elastic fibers embedded in loose connective tissue. However, it is absent in the trigone, a triangular region with angles at the two ureter openings and the single internal urethral opening. It is believed that the thin bands of muscle that stretch between each ureteric opening and the internal urethral orifice help to keep the ureters pointing in an oblique direction when the bladder contracts. Another bundle of muscle fibers creates a slightly downward-curving fold of mucous membrane between the two ureteric openings.

The bladder's innermost lining, known as the mucous coat, is an elastic layer that is impervious to urine. Regardless of whether the bladder is enlarged or contracted, it always remains smooth and pink and securely clings to the muscular coat over the trigone. In other places, the mucous coat appears red and velvety with numerous folds when the bladder is contracted. The folds vanish when the bladder swells, but the color difference between the other parts of the mucous membrane and the paler trigonal area endures. The mucous membrane runs parallel to those of the ureters and urethra.

10.4. The Urethra

10.4.1. General Description

Urine is transported from the bladder to the outside through the urethra. In men, the urethra is approximately 20 centimeters long and carries secretions from the prostate, bulborethral, and urethral glands, as well as urine and semen. During ejaculation and urination, the urethra opens up, changing its diameter from 0 to 8 centimeters along its length. At other times, its walls come into contact and its lining forms longitudinal folds. The male urethra consists of three distinct sections: the prostatic, membranous, and spongy portions. These names are based on the structures they pass through rather than inherent qualities.

Starting at the internal urethral orifice, the prostatic section of the male urethra descends almost vertically through the prostate, forming a slight curve with its concavity forward from the base of the gland to the apex. It has a spindle shape and measures between 2.5 and 3 centimeters in length. The middle section of the urethra is the widest and most dilatable. The membranous portion of the male urethra is located between the two layers of the urogenital diaphragm membrane. Here, the urethra is surrounded by the sphincter urethrae muscle and is narrower than any other part except for its external opening. The two bulborethral glands are located on either side. The membranous urethra is not firmly encased by the layers of the urogenital diaphragm. The section of the male urethra that passes through the penis is known as the spongy part. It traverses the corpus spongiosum of the penis. Approximately 2.5 centimeters below the lower layer of the urogenital membrane, the spongy urethra receives the ducts of the bulborethral glands. Numerous mucous glands open into it, except at its outer end.

The female urethra, which only transports urine and mucous gland secretions, is significantly shorter (3 to 4 μm) and more extensible than the male counterpart. It starts at the internal opening of the urethra into the bladder and proceeds through the urogenital diaphragm, gently bending forward and downward before being encircled by the sphincter urethrae, just like in men. It is located below and behind the pubic symphysis. The urethra is incorporated into the anterior wall of the vagina, with the exception of its uppermost portion. The external urethral orifice is situated between the labia minora, the inner folds at the outer opening of the vagina, and directly in front of the vaginal opening. It is approximately 2.5 centimeters behind the clitoris.

10.4.2. Structure of Urethral Wall

The male urethra is a mucous membrane tube supported by an incomplete muscular coat and a submucous layer. When the tube is empty, the membrane folds longitudinally, with more noticeable folds in the membranous and spongy sections. The mucous membrane contains numerous glands, primarily located in the posterior wall of the spongy portion. The submucous layer, composed of fibroelastic connective tissue, contains a large number of tiny blood vessels, predominantly venules. The thin muscular coat consists of smooth (involuntary) and striated (voluntary) muscle fibers. The smooth muscular layer is longitudinally arranged and continues from the bladder's detrusor muscle, extending distally to the membranous urethra, where the external sphincter's striated muscle partially surrounds and replaces it. The external sphincter is supplied by the efferent and afferent parts of the pudendal nerve, originating from the second, third, and fourth sacral segments of the spinal cord. The female urethra also consists of muscular, submucous, and mucous coats. Similar to the male urethra, the lining of the empty channel forms longitudinal folds and contains mucous glands. The submucous coat in females is comparable to that in males, but the venules are even more prominent. This layer appears to consist of various erectile tissue in both sexes, with a higher prevalence in females. The muscular coat extends from the bladder's musculature above and runs the entire length of the female urethra. It consists of an inner longitudinal layer and an outer circular layer. The fibers from the outer layer blend with those in the anterior wall of the vagina, where the urethra is located.

10.5. Human Excretion

10.5.1. General Function of the Kidney

The kidney has developed to allow humans to live on land, where it is necessary to preserve water and salts, eliminate waste products in concentrated form, and maintain stringent volume, chemical composition, and osmotic pressure regulations for both blood and tissue fluids. Most of the water and substances that are necessary for the body are reabsorbed into the blood after being filtered out of the blood by the glomerulus's capillaries and into the lumen of the nephron, which is the passageway, under the force of arterial pressure. Urine makes up the remaining filtrate that is drained off. As a result, despite a variety of changes in the external environment, the kidneys assist in maintaining a constant internal environment.

10.5.2. Regulatory Functions

In order to maintain electrolyte and water equilibrium, which refers to the balance between water and various chemicals such as calcium, potassium, sodium, phosphorus, and sulfate in solution, the kidneys regulate three crucial and interrelated properties of the tissues: water content, acid-base balance, and osmotic pressure. Failure to keep the concentrations of waste products like urea, crystalloids like glucose, and mineral ions like sodium within strict normal limits can quickly lead to physiological dysfunction, ultimately resulting in illness or death.

If treatment is not received, the removal of both kidneys leads to uremia, which is the accumulation of urine constituents in the blood. This condition can cause death within 14–21 days. It is important to note that the term "uremia" does not imply that urea is a poisonous substance that causes disease or death. The kidneys eliminate any abnormal constituents in solution or excesses of normal constituents, such as salts and water, from the blood until the normal composition is restored. The waste products remaining after protein metabolism can only be removed by the kidneys. These waste products are not altered by the kidneys;

instead, they are transported to the urine in the same state as they are produced in other parts of the body. The kidneys have the ability to produce ammonia, which sets them apart. Additionally, the kidneys eliminate toxins and drugs. As a result, the kidneys minimize the loss of important compounds like glucose while eliminating undesirable metabolic byproducts like urea. The kidneys also remove excess hydrogen ions from the typically acid-forming diet and produce ammonia to eliminate these ions in the urine as ammonium salts, thereby maintaining the acid-base equilibrium.

The kidney is equipped with a comparatively large blood supply to support its operations. The volume of blood processed by the kidneys is approximately 1,200 milliliters per minute, or 1,800 liters (roughly 475 gallons) per day. This represents 400 times the total volume of blood and approximately one-fourth of the volume that the heart pumps out daily. Approximately 168,05 liters of water with dissolved salts are reabsorbed by the cells lining the tubules and returned to the bloodstream every 24 hours, out of the 170 liters (45 gallons) of water that are filtered from the bloodstream into the renal tubules. In a 24-hour period, the total glomerular filtrate must equal or exceed 50–60 times the volume of blood plasma, which is the blood minus its cells, in the body. An average man excretes only 1.5 liters of water (containing metabolic waste products) in a 24-hour period; however, the actual volume varies depending on fluid intake, occupational demands, and environmental factors. It can drop to 500 milliliters (roughly a pint) per day with heavy sweating; it can rise to three liters, or six times, per day with a large water intake. The kidney can adjust how much water it reabsorbs to make up for variations in plasma volume brought on by dehydration or excess water.

10.5.3. Nonexcretory Functions

In addition, the kidneys perform several nonexcretory functions. They release substances into the bloodstream. These substances can be categorized into three types: erythropoietin, which is vital for the production of hemoglobin and red blood cells, especially in response to anemia or insufficient oxygen supply to body tissues; renin, which indirectly participates in the regulation of blood pressure and electrolyte balance; and 1,25-dihydroxycholecalciferol, the metabolically active form of vitamin D. Furthermore, despite being under both neural and humoral (hormonal) control, the kidneys possess a significant level of autonomy. This means that an organ disconnected from the nervous system but sustained by circulating fluid can still function. In fact, kidney transplantation would not be feasible if this were not the case.

10.6. Renal Blood Circulation

10.6.1. Intrarenal Blood Pressures

Because the renal arteries are small and originate directly from the abdominal aorta, arterial blood can reach the kidneys at the highest possible pressure. Renal perfusion is established by the renal arterial blood pressure and the vascular resistance to blood flow, similar to other vascular beds. There is evidence to suggest that the glomerular arterioles in the kidneys contain the majority of the total resistance. Abundant sympathetic vasoconstrictor fibers are present in the muscular coats of the arterioles. Additionally, a small parasympathetic supply originating from the vagus and splanchnic nerves causes the blood vessels to dilate. Sympathetic stimulation results in vasoconstriction and decreased urine production. The walls of the vessels are also responsive to circulating hormones such as angiotensin, a constrictor closely related to renin, as well as adrenaline and norepinephrine. Prostaglandins may also play a role.

10.6.2. Factors That Affect Renal Flow

Regardless of the systemic blood pressure, the kidney can control its internal circulation as long as it is not abnormally high or low. For the kidneys to continue monitoring the blood's water and electrolyte composition without interruption, the forces that keep the blood flowing through them must not change. This regulation, known as autoregulation, is maintained even in the kidney that has been cut off from the nervous system and, to a lesser extent, in an organ that has been removed from the body but is still alive because salt solutions at physiologically appropriate concentrations are circulated through it.

There are a few theories as to how the kidney controls its own circulation, but the precise mechanism is unknown. (1) Smooth muscle cells in the arterioles may have an intrinsic basal tone, or normal degree of contraction, when they are not stimulated by humoral (hormonal) or nervous stimuli. When the perfusion pressure drops, the tone reacts to the change by reducing the degree of contraction, lowering preglomerular resistance, and maintaining blood flow. On the other hand, as perfusion pressure increases, blood flow stays constant while the degree of contraction increases. (2) The fluid in the distal tubules contains more sodium when the renal blood flow rises because the filtration rate rises. An increase in sodium levels causes the JGA to secrete renin, which in turn causes the formation of angiotensin, narrowing the arterioles and decreasing blood flow. (3) Because of the increased blood viscosity, renal blood flow does not change in response to an increase in systemic blood pressure. The interlobular arteries typically have an outer layer of plasma covering an axial (central) stream of red blood cells, allowing the afferent arterioles to remove more plasma than cells. The more tightly packed axial flow of cells in the vessels provides increasing resistance to the pressure, which must overcome this increased viscosity if the arteriolar blood pressure rises. This increases the skimming effect. Thus, there is minimal change in the total renal blood flow. Up to a certain extent, the consequences of decreased systemic pressure are subject to the same considerations in reverse. (4) Variations in arterial pressure alter the force that the kidney's interstitial fluid (tissue) exerts on veins and capillaries, causing resistance to blood flow to decrease with decreasing pressure and increased resistance to rise.

The flow of blood to the kidneys is higher when one is lying down than when one is standing, and it is also decreased by prolonged, intense physical activity, pain, anxiety, and other emotions that narrow the arterioles and cause blood to be diverted to other organs. Additionally, it is decreased by asphyxia, bleeding, and severe salt and water depletion in shock, including operative shock. Significant reductions in systemic blood pressure, such as those following a major bleeding episode, can impair renal blood flow to the point where no urine is produced for a while, potentially leading to glomerular function suppression and death. Vasoconstriction and decreased urine production result from simple fainting. When back pressure hits a critical point, obstruction of the ureter also stops urinary secretion.

10.6.3. Glomerular Pressure

These various vascular factors are of significance due to the primary function of the glomerulus, which involves filtration. This filtration process is facilitated by the blood pressure within the capillaries that line the walls of the glomerulus. The tone, whether constricted or dilated, of the afferent and efferent arterioles plays a crucial role in determining the glomerular pressure. These arterioles can open or close autonomously or in response to nervous or hormonal control.

The glomerular pressure is directly influenced by the systemic pressure.

The normal glomerular pressure is estimated to be around 45 millimeters of mercury (mmHg), which is higher compared to the pressure in other capillaries throughout the body. The glomerular filtration rate is regulated within a range where autoregulation of blood flow occurs, similar to renal blood flow. However, significant deviations from this range can occur. Severe constriction of the afferent vessel leads to a decrease in glomerular pressure, filtration rate, and blood flow. On the other hand, severe constriction of the efferent vessel results in a decrease in glomerular pressure and filtration, but an increase in blood flow.

10.6.4. Formation and Composition of Urine

The composition of the urine that exits the kidney and the plasma that enters it differs significantly (Table 10.1). These variations must be taken into consideration when studying renal function, such as the urine's low levels of sodium and calcium but its high levels of ammonia and creatinine, the pH difference between urine and plasma, the absence of protein and glucose, and the urine's high levels of these minerals.

Table 10.1. *Typical Design Values for the Concentrations of Constituents in Fresh Urine, Based on Data in Sweden and Switzerland [6]:12[7]*

Parameter	Value
pH	6.2
Total nitrogen	8830 mg/L
Ammonium/ammonia-N	460 mg/L
Nitrate and nitrite	0.06 mg/L
Chemical oxygen demand	6000 mg/L
Total phosphorus	800–2000 mg/L
Potassium	2740 mg/L
Sulphate	1500 mg/L
Sodium	3450 mg/L
Magnesium	120 mg/L
Chloride	4970 mg/L
Calcium	230 mg/L

Source: https://en.wikipedia.org/wiki/Urine.

A significant amount of ultrafiltrate, which is a fluid that has been filtered to remove blood proteins and cells, is created by the glomerulus and placed inside the capsule. As the ultrafiltrate passes through the proximal convoluted tubule, most of the liquid's water and salts are reabsorbed. Some solutes are reabsorbed entirely, while others are reabsorbed partially, depending on whether they need to be kept apart from those that should be rejected. The concentration of urine is the primary concern of the collecting ducts, distal convoluted tubule, and loop of Henle, as they provide precise control over the balance of water and electrolytes.

10.6.5. Glomerular Filtration

A substantial quantity of blood plasma is ultrafiltered from the glomerular capillaries into the capsular space, where proteins and other colloids are retained while crystalloids (substances in true solution) pass through to generate urine. Human capillaries typically possess a diameter of 5 to 10 micrometers (0.001 millimeters). Each capillary loop comprises three layers within its wall. The blood can directly come into contact with the second layer, a basement membrane, through the numerous pores, or fenestrae, formed by the flat nucleated endothelial cells arranged to constitute the inner layer. A nanometer is equivalent to 0.000001 millimeters. The basement membrane of the capillaries is a continuous layer of hydrated collagen and glycopeptides, akin to the lining of numerous other structures and organs. Previously thought to be uniform, it now appears to consist of three layers with varying quantities of polyanionic glycopeptides. Due to the relatively high concentration of sialic and aspartic acids in the membrane, it bears a negative charge, or is anionic. Glycosaminoglycans, such as heparin sulfate, are also present. The large epithelial cells, known as podocytes, constitute the third, outer layer. These cells employ minuscule cytoplasmic projections referred to as pedicels, or foot processes, to establish contact with the outer surface of the basement membrane. These processes are separated from one another by slit-like gaps that measure between 20 and 30 nanometers in width, and they are slightly enlarged at the point of contact with the basement membrane. The slit-like spaces in proximity to the basement membrane are sealed by a thin membrane known as the slit diaphragm.

Bulk flow and simple diffusion are the two physical mechanisms through which glomerular filtrate can traverse the glomerular wall barrier. Bulk flow occurs when water containing solutes passes through basement membrane pores in the glomerular filtrate. In any case, the hydrated gel structure of the basement membrane appears to be the primary barrier preventing the passage of filtrate. Larger protein molecules are restricted solely by their size, while negatively charged anionic macromolecules such as albumin (with a molecular weight of 69,000) are further hindered by the negative electrostatic charge of the membrane. Conversely, proteins with smaller molecular sizes, such as neutral gelatin (35,000), flow through without any hindrance. It is plausible that the diaphragm and slit pores have a similar effect to the endothelial cell layer in preventing the entry of blood cells and very large molecules into the body.

The integrity of the glomerulus, which relies on proper nutrition and oxygenation, is crucial for the normal process of glomerular filtration. Damage to the glomeruli caused by illness or oxygen deprivation increases their permeability, allowing plasma proteins to enter the urine. Mesangial cells are unique cells that may play a role in the development and maintenance of the basement membrane of the glomerular walls. They form a stalk or scaffolding for the capillary network and are located between the glomerular capillary loops. They may be responsible for the formation of the glomerular capillary basement membrane because they themselves are embedded in a glycosaminoglycan matrix similar to that of the membrane. Additionally, the mesangial cells are responsible for clearing the basement membrane of any large foreign molecules that may be retained there during certain medical conditions. In immunologically induced glomerular diseases, these cells proliferate and the mesangial matrix expands.

10.6.6. Tubule Function

Comparing the concentrations of different substances in the filtrate and urine can help determine the role of the tubules (Table 10.2).

It is evident that the filtrate needs to be altered in the tubules to take into consideration the variations in the filtrate and final urine—e.g., to account for the latter's complete lack of glucose, the urine's significantly lower volume than the filtrate, or the urine's acidity relative to the filtrate's neutrality.

Most of the filtrate's water and salts are reabsorbed into the blood of the capillaries that surround the tubules as it travels along the proximal tubule. Because this section of the nephron separates substances that are meant for excretion in the urine from those that must be retained in the body, some substances are reabsorbed entirely and others only partially. The proximal tubule's primary role is to reabsorb filtrate in compliance with equilibrium requirements for homeostasis, while the collecting duct and distal portion of the nephron are primarily responsible for the precise regulation of hydrogen-ion, electrolyte, and water balance. Hormonal regulation affects every single one of these chemically and physically occurring processes in the tubules. Urine and filtrate normally differ significantly, but in experimental settings, if tubule function is gradually decreased due to cooling or poisoning, the urine will start to resemble the filtrate more and more. Additionally, there is less time for the urine to change as it passes through the tubules the faster filtration happens.

Table 10.2. *Substances Filtered and Reabsorbed by the Kidney per 24 Hours*

Substances Filtered and Reabsorbed by the Kidney per 24 Hours			
Substance	**Amount Filtered (grams)**	**Amount Reabsorbed (grams)**	**Amount in Urine (grams)**
Water	180 L	179 L	1 L
Proteins	10–20	10–20	0
Chlorine	630	625	5
Sodium	540	537	3
Bicarbonate	300	299.7	0.3
Glucose	180	180	0
Urea	53	28	25
Potassium	28	24	4
Uric acid	8.5	7.7	0.8
Creatinine	1.4	0	1.4

Source: https://courses.lumenlearning.com/suny-ap2/chapter/tubular-reabsorption-no-content/#:~:text=It%20induces%20the%20production%20of,is%20lost%20in%20the%20urine.

10.6.7. Reabsorption From the Proximal Tubule

All of the filtrate's glucose, up to 70% of its water and sodium (the remaining portion is absorbed in the distal tubule), the majority of its potassium and chloride ions, some of its uric acid, 40% of its urea, and little to none of its sulfate are all impacted by reabsorption. In the proximal tubule, 75% of the total solids are reabsorbed. Amino acids, glucose, lactate, phosphate, and calcium are absorbed by the tubule's initial section; sodium, potassium, calcium, and chloride are absorbed by the entire convolution, which also slightly acidifies the fluid by eliminating bicarbonate.

There is a limited amount of reabsorption capacity in the tubule. As a result, all of the glucose that enters the filtrate is normally absorbed. However, diabetes results when plasma glucose levels are raised to a point where glucose reaches the tubule cells more quickly than it can be absorbed. Put another way, each material in the filtrate has a maximum reabsorptive capacity, and the critical rate of delivery is based on the plasma concentration and filtration rate. For any given substance, the upper maximum value of the tubular reabsorption rate is constant. As a result, all excess of the substance will be eliminated in the urine if the plasma level rises sufficiently. This also applies to glucose, which is completely reabsorbed in healthy circumstances. However, the upper limit value for phosphate is significantly lower, meaning that urine typically contains some phosphate at all times. The phosphate content of the filtrate and parathyroid hormone both have an impact on the proximal tubular reabsorption of phosphate. Phosphate is in competition with glucose for reabsorption; parathyroid hormone and vitamin D both inhibit phosphate reabsorption, while a high dietary phosphate intake increases it, at least temporarily. The amino acids also have maximum tubular reabsorption values of their own, but these are high enough to guarantee complete reabsorption under normal circumstances; in some uncommon hereditary disorders, such as cystinuria, where there is excessive cystine excretion, reabsorption is decreased.

Since approximately 70% of the sodium ions in the filtrate are reabsorbed, it is necessary to have a comparable amount of water present in the filtrate to serve as a carrier for the ions and prevent an increase in the osmotic gradient. This prevents the concentration of the sodium solution inside and outside the tubule from rising. About 80% of the oxygen utilized by the kidneys is consumed in the energy required for the reabsorption of sodium into the blood, which is equivalent to one-eighth of an individual's oxygen consumption at rest. The significant amount of water reabsorption occurs passively in response to the movement of sodium, and there is no evidence of active water transport. The overall outcome is to maintain the fluid in the tubular lumen, although its volume is greatly reduced, and it remains approximately isosmotic with the original glomerular filtrate due to sodium being the major osmotically active solute.

When sodium, a positively charged ion, is actively reabsorbed into the blood, the fluid in the proximal tubule remains electronegative compared to the peritubular fluids. This provides a driving force for the reabsorptive transport of negatively charged ions such as chloride, bicarbonate, and organic solutes. Active sodium transport is also responsible for the reabsorption of neutral molecules like urea into the blood. However, the passive movement of water out of the tubular lumen leads to an increasing luminal concentration of urea, as the tubular epithelium is less permeable to urea and creatinine compared to water or chloride. Consequently, the concentration of urea or creatinine in the tubular fluid becomes higher than that in the initial filtrate containing plasma. As a result, a significant amount of urea or creatinine is excreted in the urine because less filtered urea or creatinine is reabsorbed into the blood compared to sodium or water.

10.6.8. Reabsorption From the Loop of Henle

A third of the volume of the glomerular filtrate passes through the descending limb of the loop of Henle. This fluid, when combined with plasma, is isosmotic. The reabsorptive properties of the bend of the loop and the descending thin limb differ significantly from those of the ascending thick limb. The thin epithelium that lines the thin limb lacks the ability to actively transport substances and is permeable to water. As a result, the fluid entering the limb and the bend of the loop absorbs the concentration of the interstitial peritubular fluid surrounding it. On the other hand, the thick ascending limb, which is lined by taller cells, actively transports sodium and chloride into the peritubular fluid surrounding both limbs but has low permeability to urea and water. Due to the accumulation of sodium and chloride, the fluid in the medullary and deep cortical regions of the kidney becomes highly concentrated, sometimes reaching concentrations four times that of plasma (1,200 mosmoles per liter). We will provide more detailed information about this solute buildup, which is necessary for the production of concentrated urine, below.

10.6.9. Reabsorption From the Distal Convoluted Tubule

Plasma is more concentrated in the fluid entering the distal convoluted tubule than in the ascending limb due to the active transportation of sodium out of it. Throughout the entirety of the distal tubule, including the early portion of the collecting duct, active sodium reabsorption is ongoing. A significant concentration gradient of sodium and chloride between the luminal fluid and the plasma is maintained, with the concentration of sodium in the tubule being kept well below that of the plasma, because this portion of the nephron is comparatively impermeable to water. Also notably electronegative to the surrounding tissues is the luminal fluid in this instance. The secretion of potassium and hydrogen ions into the tubule from the blood appears to be directly linked to the mechanism of sodium reabsorption. The hormone aldosterone, which is secreted by the adrenal gland when the body lacks sodium, has a significant impact on this process.

10.6.10. The Concentration of Urine

As previously mentioned, the kidney's capacity to concentrate urine depends on the loop of Henle. The mechanism known as countercurrent exchange multiplication is thought to be responsible for the high salt concentration in the medullary fluid within the loop. The physical principle underlying this process is the same as the one used to warm and preserve heat when hot exhaust gases pass over cold incoming gas. Although the exchange is passive, the kidney's countercurrent multiplier system uses energy to "pump" sodium and chloride into the medullary fluid from the loop's ascending limb. It then diffuses into the filtrate, which is isotonic with plasma and enters the descending limb from the proximal tubule, increasing its concentration slightly above that of plasma. More sodium is then pumped out into the surrounding fluid or blood, if needed, and transported (by diffusion) back into the descending limb as this luminal fluid reaches the distal tubule and then the ascending limb. This concentrating process continues until the fluid's osmotic pressure is high enough to balance the resorptive power of the collecting ducts in the medulla, through which all of the final urine must pass. Antidiuretic hormone (ADH), which is produced by the hypothalamus and stored in the posterior pituitary gland at the base of the brain, controls the ducts' ability to absorb substances. The medullary collecting ducts open up to free solute and water passage when ADH is present. As a result, the fluid entering the ducts (on its way to the renal pelvis and later elimination) picks up the medulla's interstitial fluid concentration; i.e., the urine gets more concentrated. However, in the absence of ADH, the collecting ducts remain impermeable to both solute and water, resulting in a less concentrated fluid than plasma in the lumen from which some solute has been removed; i.e., the urine has been diluted.

ADH is secreted by the hypothalamus and released by the posterior pituitary as part of a feedback system that reacts to the plasma's tonicity. At the base of the brain, certain and sensitive receptors mediate this relationship between plasma osmotic pressure and ADH output. These receptors are particularly susceptible to sodium and chloride ions. Both steady receptor discharge and steady ADH secretion occur at normal blood tonicity. When the plasma becomes hypertonic (i.e., has a higher than normal osmotic pressure), which can be caused by dehydration or the consumption of crystalloids like common salt, receptor discharge and ADH output increase. This leads to more water being absorbed into the blood through the collecting ducts. Conversely, if the plasma's osmotic pressure drops, consuming water dilutes bodily fluids and decreases or stops the secretion of ADH. This causes the urine to become hypotonic and excrete the excess water. The situation is intricate due to the fact that, in the event of a propensity towards excessive blood volume, receptors that are sensitive to alterations in blood volume also reflexively inhibit ADH output. Urinary flow decreases and ADH output increases with exercise. Emotional disturbance, syncope, pain, injury, or the utilization of certain medications like nicotine or morphine may all lead to the same outcome. Diuresis is the term for the augmented flow of urine that occurs when the body absorbs more fluids than usual, when hormones are not active, or when certain medications are taken that prevent the tubules from reabsorbing water and salt. Water diuresis occurs when ADH secretion is inhibited by illness, excessive water consumption, or a tumor affecting the base of the brain. At the glomeruli, urine formation approaches a rate of 16 milliliters per minute. In some pituitary disorders where ADH secretion is either absent or very low—e.g., diabetes insipidus—a significant volume of diluted urine may be produced in a fixed and irreversible manner.

10.6.11. Tubular Secretion

The distinction between secretory and reabsorptive tubular mechanisms lies solely in the direction of transport. Secretory mechanisms involve the addition of chemicals from the plasma in the peritubular capillaries to the filtrate. However, apart from potassium and uric acid secretion, the occurrence of secretion is minimal and primarily takes place in the proximal tubule. Notable exceptions include the production of ammonia and the secretion of hydrogen ions, which are discussed further in the section on regulation of acid-base balance. Similar to reabsorption, secretion is driven by an electrochemical gradient and can occur passively or actively. Many medications undergo active secretion, and some of them appear to follow a common pathway, leading to potential competition for limited energy supply. Exploiting the role of tubular secretion in the elimination of penicillin can be advantageous in therapy. Concurrent administration of probenecid, a medication that competes with penicillin at its secretory site, can increase the concentration of penicillin in the blood, which is beneficial for treating specific infections. Prostaglandins, bile salts, and hippurate are among the endogenous substances secreted by the body. Uric acid, derived from nucleoproteins, can easily cross the glomerular barrier and is primarily reabsorbed in the proximal tubule, although occasional secretion by different segments of the tubule can also occur.

One of the most significant processes in the kidney is the secretion of potassium by the distal tubule, which plays a crucial role in maintaining overall potassium balance. Regardless of the amount filtered, the proximal tubule and the ascending limb of the loop of Henle reabsorb more than 75% of the filtered potassium. This percentage remains relatively constant. The distal convoluted tubule regulates the amount of potassium expelled in the urine, which is ultimately determined by the individual's food intake. In individuals with a normal diet, approximately half of the urinary potassium is secreted by the distal tubules into the urine; this secretion can be adjusted based on the body's needs. One of the many factors that influence potassium secretion is the hormone aldosterone, which is produced by the cortex of the adrenal gland. In the absence of aldosterone and other mineralocorticoids, which are adrenocortical steroids that affect electrolyte and fluid balance, potassium secretion is compromised. This can lead to potentially dangerous levels of potassium accumulation in the blood. Excessive aldosterone aids in the excretion of potassium.

10.6.12. Regulation of Acid-Base Balance

The body's cells obtain energy through oxidative processes that result in the production of acidic waste products. Acids are compounds that ionize to produce hydrogen ions, or free protons. Urine removes hydrogen ions that come from nonvolatile acids, including phosphoric, sulfuric, pyruvic, and lactic acids. When necessary, the kidney's transport mechanisms can reduce the concentration of hydrogen ions in the urine to one-quarter that of the plasma or raise it to 2,500 times that of the plasma.

Urine could theoretically become acidic due to the secretion of hydrogen ions into the tubular fluid or the selective absorption of a buffer base, which is a substance that can accept hydrogen ions (e.g., filtered baking soda). According to available data, hydrogen ion excretion requires both secretion and filtration, and both proximal and distal convoluted tubules are involved.

The proximal tubule is where the majority of the bicarbonate filtered at the glomerulus is reabsorbed before returning to the peritubular capillaries. The normal plasma bicarbonate concentration is intended to remain constant at roughly 25 millimoles per liter thanks to this mechanism. All filtered bicarbonate is reabsorbed into the blood when the plasma concentration drops below this threshold, preventing any bicarbonate from being expelled. This is commonly known as the bicarbonate threshold. Urine starts to contain more and more bicarbonate when the plasma bicarbonate level rises above 27 millimoles per liter.

Carbonic anhydrase is abundant in the brush borders of the proximal tubule cells. This enzyme assists in the conversion of CO_2 and H_2O into carbonic acid (H_2CO_3), which subsequently ionizes to produce bicarbonate ions (HCO_3-) and hydrogen ions (H+). The active secretion of hydrogen ions into the tubular fluid is most likely the initial step in the process of bicarbonate reabsorption. Under the influence of carbonic anhydrase, these ions may form from CO_2 released from the oxidation of cell nutrients and pre-existing H_2O in the cells. Bicarbonate, the filtered base, combines with hydrogen ions to form carbonic acid, which is unstable and breaks down into CO_2 and H_2O. Due to the high diffusibility of CO_2, it easily moves from the tubular fluid into the tubular cells and the blood, causing the partial pressure of CO_2 in the filtrate to increase. The water is either eliminated or treated similarly. The HCO_3^- formed inside the cells from the CO_2 generated by the hydrogen ions in the luminal fluid balances the filtered sodium that the proximal tubular cells are actively reabsorbing in the meantime. As a result, the bicarbonate that is actually reabsorbed differs from the original filtrate, but the overall outcome remains the same.

The hydrogen ions secreted into the distal tubules may be buffered by bases other than HCO_3-; in addition, the ions may mix with ammonia that the tubules also secrete. Dibasic phosphate (Na_2HPO_4), which accepts hydrogen ions to form monobasic phosphate (NaH_2PO_4), is the most significant non-bicarbonate base found in the filtrate. The amount of hydrogen ions in the urine that are buffered by bases like phosphate and bicarbonate is measured by titrating the urine with a strong base until the pH of the plasma (7.4) is reached. This is known as the urine's titratable acidity and typically ranges from 20 to 40 millimoles of H+ per day.

Under typical conditions, ammonium salts (e.g., Na^+) make up roughly two-thirds of the hydrogen ions that are secreted in the urine, such as ammoniacal chloride. Instead of being found in plasma or filtrate, ammonia (NH_3) is produced in the distal tubular cells and enters the lumen most likely by passive diffusion along a concentration gradient. Ammonium ions (NH_4^+) are created in the lumen when NH_3 combines with hydrogen ions secreted into the tubule. These ions become trapped in the lumen due to the tubular cells' lipid walls' significantly lower permeability to charged molecules than to uncharged ones.

It is now understood that the enzyme glutaminase hydrolyzes the amino acid glutamine to produce ammonia and glutamic acid. Glutamic acid is deaminated to produce glutaric acid, which is metabolized to produce another molecule of ammonia. The amount of ammonium ions in urine increases with acidity; the addition of hydrogen ions (e.g., from the food) encourages the tubular cells to produce ammonium. Ammonium salts of excess anions (negative ions) like phosphate, sulfate, and chloride are eliminated through the urine, sparing other cations (positive ions) like potassium and sodium for retention.

To sum up, there are three stages to hydrogen ion secretion. The first takes place in the proximal tubule, where filtered bicarbonate is ultimately reabsorbed into the tubule. The distal tubule is where the second and third phases occur, where ammonium and monobasic phosphate salts are produced. Therefore, the total amount of hydrogen ions secreted by tubular cells is equal to the sum of their titratable acidity, ammonium ion excretion, and bicarbonate ion reabsorption. The last can be evaluated by figuring out how much bicarbonate was filtered (i.e., bicarbonate plasma concentration divided by the glomerular filtration rate, and any bicarbonate excreted in the urine subtracted. Total hydrogen ion secretion typically ranges from 50 to 100 millimoles per day, but conditions like diabetes that are linked to excessive acid production can cause this to rise significantly.

10.6.13. Volume and Composition

Even in individuals who are in good health, the volume and composition of normal urine can vary significantly from day to day due to various factors such as food and fluid intake, as well as fluid loss through other channels influenced by external factors and physical activity. The daily volume ranges from 1–2 liters, with an average of 1–2 liters; however, after excessive perspiration, it can decrease as low as 500 milliliters, and after consuming an excessive amount of fluid, it can increase to three liters or more. Within the span of a day, there is also fluctuation. Excretion is at its lowest in the early hours and reaches its peak in the early stages of exertion and after meals. It reaches its highest point in the first few hours after waking up. Between morning and evening, two to four times as much urine is produced as during the night. Chronic renal disease (polyuria), or the excessive production of urine, usually occurs at night.

The volume of urine is regulated to maintain a constant plasma osmotic concentration, manage the overall water content of the tissues, and serve as a means for the daily excretion of about 50 grams of solids, primarily sodium chloride and urea, to the outside. Urine will contain 30 grams of urea and 10 grams of salt in a man who consumes 100 grams of protein and 10 grams of salt every day; there are many other potential constituents, but they total less than 10 grams (Table 10.3).

Table 10.3. *Some Urine Constituents (g/24 hours)*

Characteristic	Normal Values
Color	Pale yellow to deep amber
Odor	Odorless
Volume	750–2000 mL/24 hour
pH	4.5–8.0
Specific gravity	1.003–1.032

Osmolarity	40–1350 mOsmol/kg
Urobilinogen	0.2–1.0 mg/100 mL
White blood cells	0–2 HPF (per high-power field of microscope)
Leukocyte esterase	None
Protein	None or trace
Bilirubin	<0.3 mg/100 mL
Ketones	None
Nitrites	None
Blood	None
Glucose	None

Source: https://courses.lumenlearning.com/suny-ap2/chapter/physical-characteristics-of-urine/.

Normally, urine is transparent. However, it may appear murky due to the presence of calcium phosphate. Adding acetic acid can help clarify it. Occasionally, there may be microscopic deposits resembling the lining of renal tubules, known as casts. Babies' diapers often have an ammoniacal odor, caused by bacteria breaking down urea into ammonia. Certain medications and foods can also cause unusual smells. The color of urine is influenced by its concentration, typically appearing as a vivid yellow due to the pigment urochrome, a byproduct of protein metabolism. Traces of uroerythrin and urobilin pigments are also present. Beetroot, food coloring, vitamins, and specific medications can affect the color as well.

The specific gravity of urine usually ranges from 1.01 to 1.025, although it can vary. A consistently low specific gravity may indicate chronic renal disease, but some variation is normal. A healthy kidney will produce urine with a specific gravity of at least 1.025 if fluid intake is stopped for a full day. The kidney's ability to concentrate substances is limited, so urine is rarely more than four times as concentrated as plasma. The kidneys require a minimum water output of 850 milliliters to excrete their normal solute load, known as the minimum obligatory volume of urine. Dehydration occurs when the body needs to remove water from tissues if it cannot be obtained through intake. However, normal fluid intake is typically well above the minimum amount, and urine is rarely at its highest concentration. The pH of urine typically ranges from 4 to 8, with an acidic reaction (lemon juice has a pH of 2.3), while a pH of 8 is slightly alkaline, similar to a 1% sodium bicarbonate solution.

While foreign proteins in plasma are retained within the body, those with a molecular weight of less than 68,000 are excreted through the urine. Conversely, if the kidneys are compromised by illness or toxins, the glomeruli may allow a portion of normal serum albumin and globulin to pass through, resulting in urine coagulation upon warming. Typically, urine contains less than 50 milligrams of protein per 24 hours. However, protein levels in the urine can increase after physical activity, during pregnancy, and in certain individuals when standing (a condition known as orthostatic albuminuria). Certain chronic renal diseases can cause a significant increase in protein loss, with nephrotic syndrome even leading to 50 grams of protein loss in a 24-hour period. In diseases involving the proliferation of immunoglobulin-producing cells, specific and easily identifiable proteins can be detected in the urine.

Individuals with diabetes mellitus may have glucose in their urine. However, low tubular reabsorption thresholds can also result in abnormally high urine glucose levels in some healthy individuals without affecting glucose metabolism. Nursing mothers may experience lactosuria, which is an excessive amount of lactose in the urine. Normal urine contains trace amounts of ketone bodies (acetone, acetoacetic acid), but severe untreated diabetes and carbohydrate starvation, whether relative or actual, can lead to higher levels of these molecules, such as in individuals following a high-fat diet.

Hemolysis, the release of hemoglobin from red blood cells, incompatible blood transfusions, and malignant malaria (blackwater fever) can all cause the presence of hemoglobin or its derivatives in the urine. Urinary tract bleeding can result in the presence of fresh blood. In cases of jaundice, particularly the obstructive type, bile salts and pigments are elevated. In certain conditions like liver cirrhosis, urobilin levels are significantly increased.

Porphyrins are often found in trace amounts, but they can be elevated in congenital porphyria, a condition characterized by a sensitivity to sunlight or mental instability. Porphyrins may also become more prevalent following the consumption of sulfonamides and certain other medications.

The typically trace amounts of amino acids in the urine can be significantly elevated in cases of advanced liver disease, renal reabsorption failure, and certain diseases resulting from genetic errors related to protein metabolism. When the enzyme phenylalanine hydroxylase is absent, phenylalanine is converted to phenylpyruvic acid instead of tyrosine, which is why phenylketonuria, a disease marked by the presence of phenylpyruvic acid in the urine, occurs. If the urine of every newborn baby is tested, it may be easily found that this acid, which causes mental retardation, is present in the blood and tissues. In such circumstances, a phenylalanine-restricted diet might be advantageous.

The absence of the enzyme that catalyzes the oxidation of homogentisic acid results in alkaptonuria, a disease characterized by the presence of the acid in the urine. Acid deposits in the tissues can lead to spinal disorders or chronic arthritis. Other conditions include maple syrup disease, which also involves abnormally high levels of amino acids in the blood plasma and urine, and cystinuria, which is the presence of the amino acid cystine in the urine when the bladder may contain cystine stones.

10.6.14. Urine Collection and Emission

Urine exits the nephrons and passes through the last 15 or 20 collecting tubules, which open onto each renal medulla papilla and extend into a minor calyx. These then divide into two or three major calyxes, which further divide into the renal pelvis, ultimately connecting to the upper expanded segment of the ureter.

Every 10–15 seconds, a series of peristaltic waves of contraction originate in the muscle fibers of the minor calyx, propagate to the major calyxes, and eventually travel along the ureter, propelling urine down the renal pelvis and ureteral channel. If a dye is injected into the bloodstream, each wave can be observed through a cystoscope as it intermittently expels urine into the bladder through the ureteric orifice. This downward flow is facilitated by gravity and occurs more rapidly when in an upright position. Although the overall evidence suggests the presence of a pacemaker—a cluster of specialized cells capable of rhythmic contraction—near the pelviureteric junction, this has yet to be definitively demonstrated in tissue. The smooth muscle layer of the ureter is robust, and the pressure above an obstructed ureter can reach as high as 50 millimeters of mercury. Normally, the pressure in the renal pelvis is low. The ureters receive dual innervation from the hypogastric network below and the splanchnic nerves above.

10.6.15. The Bladder

The bladder is a variable-capacity hollow organ with two muscular sphincters that keep the exit closed at all other times and a strong intermediate muscle coat that empties the organ during contractions. This tough layer of muscle makes up the strong detrusor muscle. The two ureteric orifices and the internal opening of the urethra determine the region of the bladder neck, or trigone, at the base of the bladder. The involuntary internal sphincter is formed by muscle fibers looping around the urethral opening. Two layers of striated muscles under voluntary control make up the external sphincter.

The bladder's mucous membrane can stretch; when the organ is empty, it becomes ridged and smooths out. The bladder's longitudinal muscle shortens during micturition, allowing urine to pass through the urethra and widen the bladder neck. The urethra's walls are normally blocked by muscular tone, so urine only enters during micturition. Even in the event of an internal sphincter malfunction, the external sphincter can preserve continence.

The urethra and bladder possess intricate and significant innervation. There are essentially three types of nerves: (1) The parasympathetic nerves serve as the primary motor supply to the detrusor, contracting the muscle, increasing bladder pressure, relaxing the internal sphincter, and resulting in emptying. Stretch receptors in the bladder wall transmit impulses to higher centers via afferent parasympathetic channels, enabling awareness of the organ's distension and intensifying the urge to micturate. (2) The sympathetic nervous system acts as an inhibitory force on the detrusor, stimulating the closure of the ureteric and internal urethral orifices, as well as the contraction of the internal sphincter. Consequently, bladder outflow is prevented. Thus, until the point at which evacuation can no longer be postponed, the sympathetic nervous system regulates the distended bladder. Sensations from the bladder and urethral mucosa, including pain, overdistension, and temperature, are transmitted to the sympathetic nervous system via afferent pathways. (3) The somatic nerves are responsible for the contraction of the external sphincter, with their sensory fibers conveying the degree of distension in the posterior urethra.

The parasympathetic and pudendal nerves of the external sphincter transmit signals to the second, third, and fourth sacral segments of the spinal cord, which serve as reflex centers governing bladder function. This center utilizes ascending and descending spinal cord fibers to communicate with higher centers in the brain.

10.6.15.1. Bladder Function in Micturition

A number of reflexes collaborate to maintain both normal progressive micturition with complete emptying and a stable holding state for urine. The bladder contracts when its internal pressure increases and when urine passes through the urethra.

Typically, one or both bladder sphincters remain closed. As the organ fills with urine, internal pressure rises due to the contractile response of the muscle wall. The organ then actively adjusts through relaxation to retain its contents at a lower pressure. This stepwise increase and decrease in pressure occur as the bladder fills with urine, with the final pressure always gradually rising.

Initially, the small, repetitive contraction waves are not consciously felt; later, stimuli that reach the brain result in pain and a sudden increase in blood pressure. One can choose to voluntarily resist these subsequent major contractions. When the bladder content reaches 600-800 milliliters, the bladder can experience pressures of up to 100 millimeters of water. The urge to urinate begins at around 400 milliliters. However, it can be voluntarily overridden until that point. The sphincters remain contracted until this point to prevent the urethral exit from opening, but eventually, the urge to urinate becomes overwhelming and urgent. Until then, urine leakage has been prevented by voluntary detrusor inhibition and perineal muscle contraction, which have maintained the internal pressure as low as possible. Training affects the amount of bladder retention, and the threshold increases when filling occurs slowly. The threshold somewhat depends on the filling rate. Young children have less control over the situation, and even small amounts of urine can trigger reflex evacuation. Emotions have a significant impact. Under stress, small amounts of urine may involuntarily pass through the bladder because anxiety prevents the bladder from relaxing after filling.

10.6.15.2. Micturition

Micturition is a complex process that is partially controlled by the higher brain centers and partially reflexive and unconscious, mediated by the lower spinal cord centers. To initiate voluntary micturition, the brain sends signals to the bladder through the motor fibers of the pelvic nerves, which cause the detrusor to contract while also actively relaxing the two urethral sphincters. However, the previously mentioned reflexes ensure that the detrusor will continue to contract and the sphincters will remain relaxed until the evacuation is complete and the bladder is empty once the process has begun and urine has entered the urethra. The voluntary contraction of various auxiliary muscles facilitates evacuation. As the diaphragm descends and the breath is held, the abdominal wall muscles contract to exert external pressure on the bladder, while the perineal floor muscles relax simultaneously. Thus, the active process of stimulating parasympathetic sacral nerve outflow and removing the typical inhibition imposed by higher centers on the spinal cord's reflex centers are responsible for the voluntary initiation and control of micturition. When micturition begins, lower and higher brain regions work together to see it through to completion; the sensory signals from the urine-distended urethra also contribute. Therefore, the reflex process that takes over once initiated can be started by voluntarily contracting the abdominal wall to empty the bladder, even if it is not very distended or reflex emptying is not urgent.

10.7. Tests of Renal Function

10.7.1. Quantitative Tests

Renal blood flow, renal clearance, and glomerular filtration rate are three crucial quantitative tests of renal function. Additionally, tests are conducted to estimate tubular mass, tubular function, and maximal tubular activity. A renal biopsy is helpful in identifying pathological changes that impact the kidneys, and other noninvasive diagnostic techniques like radiological and other imaging methods are also beneficial. The glomerular filtration rate (GFR) is one of the most basic indicators of renal function in both clinical and experimental investigations. Measuring the specific clearance of a material thought to be eliminated by glomerular filtration alone from the body yields the GFR. The volume of plasma that contains the quantity of a substance that the kidney removes in a unit of time is known as the renal clearance of that substance (e.g., within a minute). Since no actual portion of the plasma is ever cleared in this way, the concept of clearance, or the volume of cleared plasma, is artificial.

However, it was quickly discovered that the clearance of a substance would equal the GFR if it could be found that was freely filtered by the glomeruli and was not metabolized, secreted, or reabsorbed by the renal tubules. In these particular circumstances, this is true because the amount of said substance excreted in the urine in a minute would be equal to the amount filtered at the glomeruli in the same amount of time. The clearance volume must equal the glomerular filtrate volume if the substance's concentration in the plasma, which is the same as that in the filtrate, is known.

The polysaccharide inulin, which is extracted from dahlia roots and has a molecular weight of roughly 5,000, was the first material to be found to be eliminated in this manner. Despite not occurring naturally in human plasma, inulin is safe to inject or ingest into the bloodstream. Its concentration is also easily and precisely measurable. The GFR for an adult male's body surface area is 125 milliliters per minute per 1,073 square meters. The values for the same standard area of body surface in the adult female are approximately 85% of those. The currently accepted standard for estimating GFR is inulin clearance.

The excretion rate and clearance value are not the same. Raising the plasma concentration of inulin and some other compounds does not change the amount of urine that is cleared of the agent completely. However, the total amount expelled per milliliter of filtrate per minute is the equivalent of the excretion rate, and this value is directly correlated with the plasma concentration of the filtrate.

The renal tubules must reabsorb substances, such as urea, whose clearance is less than the GFR, and they must secrete substances whose clearance is greater than the GFR. Researchers have discovered a few other drugs that are excreted by the kidney and have comparable clearance values since the discovery of inulin. Among them are sodium ferrocyanide and vitamin B12, both of which are freely circulating in plasma and unbound to protein. Before the discovery of inulin, the clearance of creatinine was used to assess renal function. As a result, creatinine clearance is still commonly used as a rough indicator of GFR. Inulin is a naturally occurring substance in plasma. Since the body produces creatinine at a nearly constant rate and its blood concentration fluctuates minimally, creatinine clearance is typically measured over a 24-hour period. There is evidence that renal tubules in humans also secrete creatinine into the urine, but this secretion is small, consistent, and has little impact on GFR measurement.

The clearance concept can be used to measure renal blood flow. When para-aminohippuric acid (PAH) is added to the bloodstream and maintained at relatively low plasma concentrations, it is rapidly eliminated into the urine through tubular secretion and glomerular filtration. According to a renal vein blood sample, 90% of PAH is removed after one circulation through the kidneys. The kidney's high degree of extraction of PAH from a single circulation suggests that PAH clearance is roughly equivalent to renal plasma flow (RPF). Around 10% of the PAH that is still present in renal venous blood is carried by blood that perfuses tubules that do not secrete PAH or nonsecretory tissue like fat or fibrous tissue. In actuality, this tiny percentage is typically disregarded, and the term "effective renal plasma flow" refers to the PAH clearance. True renal plasma flow in humans is approximately 700 milliliters per minute, based on PAH clearance of approximately 600 milliliters per minute.

Calculating the estimated GFR and RPF enables one to determine the percentage of available plasma that is filtered by the glomerulus during kidney perfusion. This is known as the filtration fraction, and in healthy people, it is typically 125/600, or roughly 20%. Approximately one-fifth of the plasma thus enters as filtrate into the glomeruli, with the remaining four-fifths proceeding into the efferent glomerular arterioles. This fraction varies in several clinical conditions, most notably high blood pressure.

It has previously been mentioned that the renal tubules have a restricted ability to carry out specific tasks. This is demonstrated, for instance, by their capacity to both dilute and concentrate urine as well as produce a gradient of hydrogen ions between the two. A synthetic analog of ADH can be injected into each nostril to test concentration power more easily than depriving the subject of water for up to 24 hours. The ability to produce ADH and the renal concentrating mechanism's sensitivity to circulating ADH are evaluated by the water deprivation test. When an analog of ADH is used, only the renal tubules' sensitivity to the hormone is evaluated.

The limitations of the kidney's capacity to eliminate acid and create a gradient in the concentration of hydrogen ions between plasma and urine were previously discussed. Urine pH can be measured after ammonium chloride is administered in divided doses over a period of two or three days to determine the best estimate of the urine's acidification power. The person's capacity to store sodium, potassium, and magnesium is one of the other particular functions that is examined. Generally speaking, these tests involve giving out diets lacking in these electrolytes and then calculating the lowest rate of excretion after a few days.

10.7.2. Radiological and Other Imaging Investigations

Imaging methods are employed to ascertain the location, structure, and degree of function of the kidneys, pelvis, and ureters. Any other, more involved examination is almost always preceded by a simple X-ray in order to determine the dimensions, shape, and location of the two kidneys as well as whether or not calcium-containing renal stones or calcification zones are present. One of the simplest ways to define these features more precisely is with excretion urography; however, noninvasive imaging techniques like magnetic resonance imaging (MRI) and ultrasonography are replacing this radiological method. Information about the composition and operation of the renal system can be obtained through excretion urography. An intravenous injection of a radiopaque compound, which is primarily excreted by glomerular filtration within an hour of the injection, is used in this test to observe the kidneys in X-rays. The first appearance of the contrast material is then indicated by a series of X-ray images called nephrograms, which also show the increasing radiographic density of the renal tissue. The X-rays also give an approximative comparison of the two kidneys' functions and show the location, size, and presence of tumors or scarring in the organs. Ultimately, the bladder is where the dye gathers, exposing any tumor or rupture there.

Distension of the calyceal system above the obstruction site may also indicate obstruction of urine flow. Urography, which employs a small catheter inserted either directly into the kidney's pelvis or into the ureteral orifice observed during a cystoscopy, provides a more distinct image of this condition. A micturating cystogram, also known as a voiding cystourethrogram (VCUG), is an essential diagnostic tool for urinary tract infections in children. It involves injecting a contrast material into the bladder. During micturition, it could indicate the reflux of urine from the bladder upward into the ureters or kidneys. Only a select group of patients should undergo this test due to the potential radiation risk to the gonads.

To perform a radioactive renogram, concentrated radioactive substances that the kidneys eliminate are injected. By placing gamma scintillation counters externally over the kidneys in the back, radiation can be detected. The counts, when recorded on moving graph paper, produce distinctive time curves for both normal and abnormal function. By introducing a radiopaque material into the renal arteries through a catheter tube inserted through a more peripheral artery in the groin region, it is possible to obtain an image of the renal circulation. The renal vascular tree is visible on a renal angiogram produced by the contrast agent. This method is particularly useful for demonstrating the presence of localized dilatations (aneurysms) or narrowing or obstructions in the circulation. Cysts, which have poor blood supply, can be distinguished from tumors, which tend to be well vascularized. With balloon-tipped catheters, bleeding can be immediately stopped. Alternatively, a supportive stent can be inserted and left inside the artery to stabilize a weakening vessel or maintain its opening.

Due to their noninvasive nature, MRIs and ultrasounds offer several advantages as they pose minimal risk to the patient. They are effective in identifying kidney or surrounding structure tumors and distinguishing them from cysts. Unique contrast agents, such as gadolinium, can be administered prior to an MRI scan to assess the metabolic properties of tissues and facilitate the examination of blood flow to a tumor. This can aid in distinguishing between benign and malignant tumors. Ultrasound techniques, being relatively user-friendly, have replaced other methods for initial kidney screening and the detection of polycystic kidneys.

10.7.3. Renal Biopsy

Renal biopsies, involving the examination of a kidney tissue sample under a microscope, are the only investigative technique that can provide precise histological information about renal anatomy. The procedure typically involves extracting a tissue sample by passing a thin needle through the back skin into the kidney substance. It usually takes only a few minutes and does not require general anesthesia. Renal biopsy has proven valuable in understanding the prognosis and natural course of various renal disorders, particularly those affecting the glomeruli. The main, albeit rare, potentially dangerous side effect of a biopsy is excessive bleeding. However, the procedure is not recommended for patients with only one kidney, a bleeding disorder, or uncontrolled extremely high blood pressure.

10.8. The Role of Hormones in Renal Function

Renal function and certain hormones and hormone-like substances are closely linked. Certain chemicals, such as vasopressin or ADH, are produced outside the kidney and enter the kidney through the bloodstream as chemical messengers. Others appear to have a localized effect and are produced within the kidney. We have already discussed how ADH regulates diuresis. By increasing the permeability of the collecting ducts to salt and water and by facilitating the movement of ions and water in a direction determined by the osmotic gradient, ADH controls water excretion. A part of the feedback mechanism that (1) concentrates urine by stimulating ADH secretion when the osmotic concentration of extracellular fluid (ECF) is high, and (2) dilutes urine by reducing ADH secretion when the osmotic concentration of ECF and plasma decreases, consists of receptors located at the base of the brain (Figure 10.5).

Adrenal cortex hormones have a significant impact on renal function, either directly or indirectly. Adrenocorticotropin (ACTH), a secretion of the pituitary gland, stimulates the adrenals, increasing the production of hydrocortisone and other corticosteroids in stressful situations, such as following an injury or surgery. The lack of hydrocortisone reduces the kidney's ability to handle normal water loads. Hydrocortisone increases protein breakdown, leading to an increase in the amount of nitrogen in the urine and affecting water metabolism. Additionally, the hormone promotes the loss of hydrogen and potassium ions by the kidney while retaining sodium. By promoting sodium ion reabsorption at the distal tubules, aldosterone affects electrolyte metabolism while simultaneously reducing the excretion of hydrogen and potassium. Aldosterone is the most crucial adrenal hormone for tubular function; its action has been compared to priming the sodium reabsorption pump. The level of aldosterone production also significantly impacts the bowel's capacity to absorb sodium, which in turn affects the overall sodium balance. A persistent loss of sodium in the urine due to aldosterone deficiency lowers blood pressure and increases the risk of fainting.

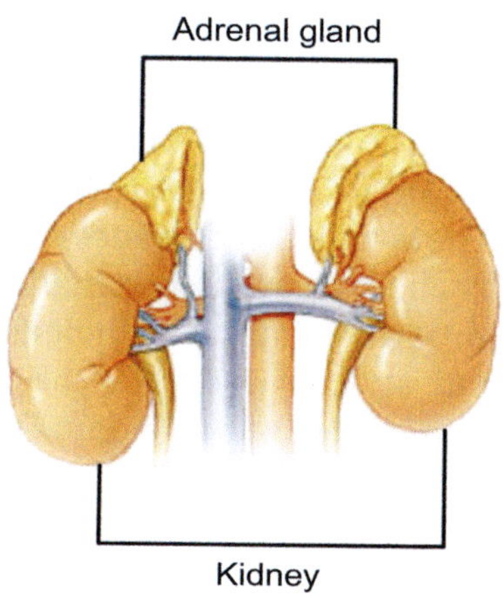

Figure 10.5. *Human adrenal gland.*

Source: https://courses.lumenlearning.com/wm-biology2/chapter/adrenal-glands/.

The function of the parathyroid glands is to mobilize calcium from the bones and other sources to raise blood calcium levels. If this hormone is released in excess, as in the case of glandular tumors, there is a significant increase in calcium loss through urine and the formation of calcium stones in the bladder and kidneys. Additionally, parathyroid hormone promotes the kidney's ability to excrete phosphate and accelerates the process by which the kidney converts hydroxylated vitamin D to its dehydroxylated form. Pituitary growth hormone reduces nitrogen loss through urine and facilitates protein synthesis. The effects of the sex hormones progesterone and estrogen on salt and water metabolism remain unclear.

Renin is found in the granules of the cells that make up the asymmetrical cuff of large granular cells in the wall of the afferent arteriole close to its entry into the nephron capsule. This structure is known as the juxtapostaglomerular apparatus (JGA). Renin is a genuine kidney internal secretion. Once it enters the plasma, it functions as an enzyme that converts one of the plasma globulins into the inactive form of angiotensin I, which subsequently leads to the production of angiotensin II, the most potent vasoconstrictor and blood pressure-elevating agent. A decrease in blood pressure stimulates the JGA to produce renin, while an increase inhibits its production. Angiotensin II production raises blood pressure in response to a drop in blood pressure and triggers the release of aldosterone from the adrenal cortex. This process serves as another example of a feedback mechanism similar to the one regulating ADH secretion.

The prostaglandins produced in the kidney tissues appear to have a local impact on various aspects of renal function. Prostaglandins are a class of fatty acids that resemble hormones and are synthesized throughout the body. Unlike true hormones, prostaglandins are not transported by the blood from their site of origin. PGE2, a distinct prostaglandin, is produced by the interstitial and collecting duct cells of the kidney, while PGI2, or prostacyclin, is produced by the renal cortex. Renal prostaglandins have multiple interactions with the renin-angiotensin system. The increased release of renin in response to reductions in renal blood flow is mediated by the prostaglandin PGI2 in the renal cortex. After its formation in the plasma, angiotensin stimulates the production of prostaglandin (PGF2) in the duct cells and interstitium, which in turn prevents angiotensin-induced vasoconstriction. As a result, prostaglandin in the renal cortex is believed to be a crucial vasodilator that preserves renal blood flow in situations where it is compromised, such as after blood loss. Prostaglandins may also directly inhibit renal tubular sodium reabsorption and the action of ADH on the distal tubule and collecting ducts; however, the significance of each of these distinct actions in a healthy human is unknown. Prostaglandins may also directly inhibit renal tubular sodium reabsorption through their interstitial and duct cell forms.

Renal blood flow may be influenced by the enzyme kallikrein, which acts as a vasodilator. Kallikrein is secreted by the renal tubules and incorporated into the urine by the distal tubules. It initiates the conversion of kininogen into bradykinin, a potent vasodilator. However, bradykinin is deactivated by an enzyme called kininase, which also converts angiotensin I into angiotensin II, a vasoconstrictor. This suggests a finely balanced internal control system where the same enzyme that deactivates the vasodilator also synthesizes the vasoconstrictor.

One potential adrenal hormone that may affect salt balance is dopamine. It is believed that tubular salt reabsorption is not influenced by sympathetic nerves that reach the kidney and release catecholamines like norepinephrine. Renal nerves are not essential for normal kidney function, as transplanted human kidneys can function properly even without a nerve supply. However, it is assumed that the kidney produces some dopamine enzymatically from its precursor, L-dopa, which is readily available in the blood. Dopamine, another catecholamine released at sympathetic nerve endings, is found in the urine in higher quantities than what could be filtered from the blood. The exact role of dopamine in blood pressure regulation, renal function, and salt balance is still unknown.

Specialized "stretch receptor" cells in the heart's atria secrete the hormone that has been most recently linked to renal function. This hormone is released in response to an increase in atrial pressure, which occurs during heart failure. Known as atrial natriuretic peptide (ANP), this hormone decreases tubular reabsorption of sodium and has a vasodilator effect on the kidney. Both actions aim to return atrial pressure to normal and increase the excretion of salt and water in the urine. It is highly likely that this hormone plays a significant role in regulating extracellular fluid volume.

10.8.1. Biological Considerations

The glomerular filtration rate (GFR) increases by up to 50% during the majority of pregnancy, corresponding to a 25% increase in renal blood flow during the middle three months of pregnancy. The frequent occurrence of glycosuria is caused by increased glucose loading of the filtrate. Additional symptoms include sodium retention and an increased risk of abnormal serous fluid accumulation (edema), as well as the presence of protein in the urine. The gravid uterus partially obstructs the ureters, resulting in enlargement and dilatation of the pelvis and ureters, along with other anatomical changes. These alterations may contribute to the heightened vulnerability to urinary tract infections during pregnancy.

The urea and uric acid content of the amniotic fluid, in which the fetus is growing steadily, increases prior to birth. This suggests that the kidneys of the fetus are functioning well before birth, as the fetus likely swallows fluid and excretes it as urine. However, even at birth, the placental circulation and the mother's kidneys still contribute to about half of the excretion work, which is then suddenly reduced.

The kidney function of the newborn infant is far from developed, with a glomerular filtration rate of only about 30 milliliters per minute per square meter of body surface, compared to 75 in adults. Tubular function does not reach adult performance until the end of the first year. The infant produces only about 20 milliliters of urine in a 24-hour period, which is diluted and frequently contains protein. The output of water and the renal clearance of sodium, potassium, and phosphate are low. Due to the kidney's inadequate ability to eliminate solids, vomiting and diarrhea can cause dehydration in the infant, which can quickly lead to renal failure.

When muscle exercise first begins, urine production increases due to the general stimulation of circulation. However, this later increases due to fatigue and perspiration from intense, prolonged exertion. It has been mentioned that urine output follows a 24-hour cycle. The modest output in the early morning hours is a useful convenience to avoid disrupting sleep. If you work the night shift, for example, your electrolyte and water output will follow suit, reversing the natural sleep cycle. When you wake up in the morning, your urine is less acidic and more alkaline. Maximum output occurs in the early hours of the day and increases after meals. Due to the wide range of water and solute output, specimens collected over a 24-hour period are required for every analytical study involving urine components.

10.9. Urinary Tract Infection

Urinary tract infections (UTIs) are among the most common and severe health problems that millions of people face globally. Nurses, being on the front lines of patient care, play a crucial role in UTI detection, management, and prevention. Gaining a comprehensive understanding of this prevalent condition is essential to provide effective, evidence-based care and improve patient outcomes. The urinary system is responsible for providing the route for drainage of urine formed by the kidneys, and it is crucial for it to be fully functional as any damage can easily affect other body systems.

- Urinary tract infections (UTIs) are caused by pathogenic microorganisms in the urinary tract.
- It is important to note that the normal urinary tract is sterile above the urethra.
- UTIs can involve the upper or lower urinary tract and can be uncomplicated or complicated depending on other patient-related conditions.

10.9.1. Classification

UTIs are classified by location and further categorized based on other factors and conditions:

- **Lower UTIs:** Lower UTIs encompass bacterial cystitis, prostatitis, and urethritis.
- **Upper UTIs:** Upper UTIs are less common and include acute and chronic pyelonephritis, interstitial nephritis, and renal nephritis.
- **Uncomplicated Lower or Upper UTIs**: Most uncomplicated UTIs are community-acquired and commonly occur in young women, but they are not usually recurrent.
- **Complicated Lower or Upper UTIs**: Complicated UTIs typically occur in individuals with urologic abnormalities or recent catheterization, and they are often acquired during hospitalization.

10.9.2. Pathophysiology

For infection to occur, bacteria must gain access to the system:

- **Access:** Infection occurs first as the

bacteria gain access into the urinary tract.

- **Attachment:** The bacteria attach to the epithelium of the urinary tract and colonize it to avoid being washed out with voiding.
- **Evasion:** The defense mechanisms are then evaded by the host.
- **Inflammation:** As the defense mechanisms react to the bacteria, inflammation starts to set in as well as other signs of infection.

10.9.3. Statistics and Epidemiology

- Urinary tract infection cases are widespread around the world and affect both the young and the old. UTI is the second most common infection in the body.
- Most cases of UTI occur among women; one out of five women in the United States will develop UTI during their lifetime.
- The urinary tract is the most common site of infection, accounting for more than 40% of the total number reported by hospitals.
- UTI affects about 600,000 patients each year.
- More than 250,000 cases of acute pyelonephritis occur in the United States each year, with 100,000 requiring hospitalization.
- Approximately 11.3 million women are diagnosed with UTIs in the United States annually.
- The expenditure in direct healthcare costs amounts to $1.6 billion.

10.9.4. Causes

UTIs are primarily caused by bacteria that have invaded the urinary tract:

- **Inability or Failure to Empty the Bladder Completely:** Stasis of urine inside the urinary bladder, which in turn attracts bacteria into entering the tract.
- **Instrumentation of the Urinary Tract:** Catheterization or cystoscopy procedures, could introduce bacteria into the urinary tract.
- **Obstructed Urinary Flow:** Abnormalities in the structure of the urinary tract, can obstruct the flow of urine and lead to an inability to empty the bladder completely.
- **Decreased Natural Host Defenses:** Immunosuppression, can predispose the patient to UTI.

10.9.5. Clinical Manifestations

A variety of signs and symptoms are associated with UTI:

- **Burning During Urination:** The patient may experience pain while urinating and describe it as a burning sensation.
- **Frequency:** The patient urinates more frequently than usual, every 3 hours.
- **Nocturia:** Waking up at night to urinate is also a sign of UTI.
- **Suprapubic or Pelvic Pain:** The patient may report pain in the suprapubic area or in the pelvic region.
- **Urgency:** There is also a sense of urgency, where the patient feels unable to hold the urge any longer and rushes to urinate.

10.9.6. Prevention

Luckily, UTI is a preventable disease that primarily focuses on the hygienic practices of the individual:

- **Avoid Bath Tubs:** It is advisable to avoid bath tubs and instead opt for showering, as bacteria in bath water may enter the urethra.
- **Perineal Hygiene:** Maintaining perineal hygiene is crucial; after each bowel movement, it is recommended to clean the perineum and urethral meatus from front to back in order to reduce concentrations of pathogens at the urethral opening.
- **Increase Fluid Intake:** Increasing fluid intake is also important, as drinking liberal amounts of fluids daily helps flush out bacteria.
- **Avoid Urinary Tract Irritants:** It is advisable to avoid urinary tract irritants such as coffee, tea, colas, alcohol, and others, as they can contribute to UTI.
- **Voiding Habit:** Developing a regular voiding habit is essential; it is recommended to void at least every 2 to 3 hours during the day and ensure the bladder is completely emptied.
- **Medications:** Lastly, it is important to take medications exactly as prescribed.

10.9.7. Complications

Early recognition of UTI and prompt treatment are essential to prevent recurrent infection and the possibility of complications.

- **Renal Failure:** UTIs that are not treated promptly could spread throughout the entire urinary system and become the cause of renal failure.
- **Urosepsis:** Additionally, the bacteria may invade the urinary system and result in urosepsis.

10.10. Urinary Catheterization Nursing Procedure and Management

Urinary catheterization is the process of inserting a catheter into the bladder to remove urine by passing it through the urethra.

10.10.1. Purposes

- To relieve urinary retention;
- To obtain a sterile urine specimen from a woman;
- To measure the amount of residual urine in the bladder;
- To obtain a urine specimen when a specimen cannot be secured satisfactorily by other means;
- To empty the bladder before and during surgery and before certain diagnostic examinations.

10.10.2. Necessary Equipment for Catheterization

- Catheters are graded on the French scale according to the size of the lumen.
- For the female adult, No. 14 and No. 16 French catheters are usually used. Small catheters are generally not necessary, and the size of the lumen is also so small that it increases the length of time necessary for emptying the bladder.
- Larger catheters distend the urethra and tend to increase the discomfort of the procedure.
- For adult males, No. 18 and No. 20 French catheters are usually used, but if these sizes appear to be too large, a smaller catheter should be used.
- No. 8 and No. 10 French catheters are commonly used for children.

10.10.3. Preparation of the Patient

1. **Adequate Exploration:** Preparation of the patient should include adequate exploration. In some instances, catheterization should be the last resort, and other techniques should be used first to draw out the urine before proceeding to catheterization.
2. **Position:** The position for female patients should be dorsal recumbent, while male patients should be in a supine position using a firm mattress or treatment table. An alternate position for female patients can be Sim's or lateral position.
3. **Provision for Privacy:**

A catheter is used to remain in place for the following purposes:

- The gradual decompression of an over-distended bladder;
- Intermittent bladder drainage;
- Continuous bladder drainage.

An indwelling catheter is equipped with a balloon that is inflated after the catheter is inserted into the bladder. Due to the inflated balloon being larger than the opening to the urethra, the catheter is retained in the bladder (Figure 10.6).

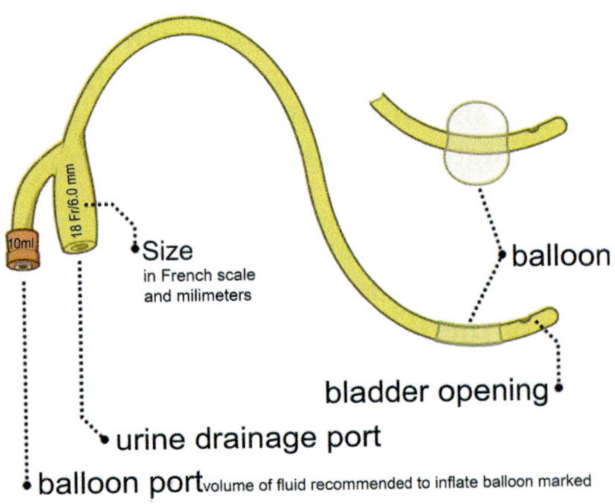

Figure 10.6. *Retention or indwelling catheter (foley).*

10.10.4. Procedure for Insertion

1. Inflate the balloon with the prefilled syringe before inserting the catheter to check for balloon patency. Aspirate the fluid back into the syringe when it is determined that the balloon is patent.
2. Hold the catheter with one hand and inflate the balloon according to the manufacturer's instructions, as soon as the catheter is in the bladder and urine has begun to drain from the bladder. Usually, 5 ml to 10 ml of sterile water is used.
3. If the patient complains of pain after the balloon is inflated, allow it to empty and replace the catheter with another one. The balloon is probably located in the urethra and is causing discomfort owing to distention of the urethra.
4. Exert slight tension on the catheter after the balloon is inflated to ensure its proper placement in the bladder.
5. Connect the catheter to the drainage tubing and drainage bag if not already connected.
6. Tape the catheter along the anterior aspect of the thigh for a female patient. Be sure there is no tension on the catheter when it is taped to the patient.
7. Hang the drainage bag on the frame of the bed below the level of the bladder.

10.10.5. Caring for the Patient with an Indwelling Catheter

1. Be sure to wash your hands before and after caring for a patient with an indwelling catheter.
2. Clean the perineal area thoroughly, especially around the meatus, twice a day and after each bowel movement.

This will help prevent organisms from entering the bladder.

3. Use soap or detergent and water to clean the perineal area and rinse it well.
4. Make sure that the patient maintains a generous fluid intake. This will help prevent infection and naturally irrigate the catheter by increasing urinary output.
5. Encourage the patient to be up and about as ordered.
6. Record the patient's intake and output.
7. Note the volume and character of urine and carefully record observations.
8. Teach the patient the importance of personal hygiene, particularly emphasizing the significance of thorough cleaning after bowel movements and frequent handwashing.
9. Promptly report any signs of infection, such as a burning sensation and irritation at the meatus, cloudy urine, a strong odor in the urine, an elevated temperature, and chills.
10. Plan to change indwelling catheters only when necessary, as the recommended interval between changes can range from 5 days to 2 weeks. The less frequently a catheter is changed, the lower the likelihood of developing an infection.

10.10.6. Removing the Indwelling Catheter and Aftercare of the Patient

1. When removing the indwelling catheter, ensure that the balloon is deflated beforehand. This can be accomplished by inserting a syringe into the balloon valve or by cutting the balloon valve.
2. Encourage the patient to take several deep breaths to promote relaxation while gently removing the catheter.
3. Wrap the catheter in a towel or disposable, waterproof drape. After catheter removal, thoroughly clean the meatus area with antiseptic swabs.
4. Monitor the patient's fluid intake, ensuring it is generous, and document the patient's intake and output. Instruct the patient to use a bedpan or urinal for voiding.
5. Carefully observe the urine for any signs of abnormality.
6. Record and report any unusual signs, such as discomfort, a burning sensation during voiding, bleeding, and changes in vital signs, particularly the patient's temperature. Remain vigilant for any signs of infection and promptly report them.

A Closer Look

Renal Failure and Hemodialysis

Renal failure, which refers to the inability of the kidneys to function properly, can be attributed to three main causes: prerenal, intrinsic renal, and postrenal.

The term "prerenal" indicates that the issue lies "before" the kidneys, specifically in the blood flow to the kidneys. Any condition that reduces blood flow to the kidneys can lead to renal damage and failure. Examples include severe hemorrhage or significantly low blood pressure following a myocardial infarction (MI).

On the other hand, "intrinsic renal" signifies that the problem originates within the kidneys themselves. Diabetes and hypertension can damage the blood vessels of the kidneys, accounting for 70% of all cases of end-stage renal failure. Bacterial infections or exposure to certain chemicals, such as certain antibiotics, can also cause damage to the nephrons. Polycystic kidney disease, a genetic disorder characterized by the dilation and dysfunction of kidney tubules, may not exhibit severe damage until middle age (40 to 60 years), but can progress to renal failure.

Lastly, "postrenal" refers to issues that occur "after" the kidneys, within the rest of the urinary tract. Obstruction of urine flow can be caused by kidney stones, a twisted ureter, or prostatic hypertrophy.

The treatment of renal failure involves addressing the specific cause, if possible. In cases where the cause cannot be resolved and kidney damage is permanent, the individual is diagnosed with chronic renal failure. Hemodialysis, which utilizes an artificial kidney machine to perform the functions that the patient's nephrons can no longer carry out, is employed. The patient's blood is circulated through small tubes surrounded by a fluid called dialysate, which has the same chemical composition as plasma. Waste products and excess minerals diffuse from the patient's blood into the fluid within the machine.

While hemodialysis does prolong the lives of individuals with chronic renal failure, it does not fully replace the functionality of healthy kidneys. However, the increasing success rate of kidney transplants offers the possibility of a normal life for those with chronic renal failure.

Summary

- The human kidneys, which generate urine, as well as the bladder, ureters, and urethra for the passage, storage, and evacuation of urine, constitute the renal system.
- The abdominal aorta gives rise to the renal arteries, one on each side, at a location opposite the upper border of the second lumbar vertebra.
- The renal sinus and two layers of kidney tissue that can be distinguished by texture and color are observable in a cross-section of a kidney.
- Nephron tubules vary in length from 30 to 55 millimeters (1–2 inches). The renal cortex contains the corpuscle and the proximal convoluted tubule, which represents the initial segment of each tubule.
- The lining layer of the glomerulus enlarges and becomes filled with secretory granules just before and close to the point where the afferent arteriole enters the structure.
- The efferent glomerular arterioles of the juxtaglomerular glomeruli split into vessels that enter the bases of the renal pyramids and vessels that supply the adjacent tubules.
- The ureters enter the bladder wall approximately five centimeters apart in both sexes, though this distance increases when the bladder is enlarged with urine.
- The main urinary reservoir is the hollow, muscular organ referred to as the bladder. It is situated beneath the peritoneum, behind the symphysis pubis, and on the anterior portion of the pelvic floor.
- The bladder's innermost lining, known as the mucous coat, is an elastic layer that is impermeable to urine.

References

1. Agnoli, G. C., & Garutti, C., (1976). Renal water-electrolyte excretion and its control mechanisms. Current status of knowledge. *Minerva Med., 67*(56), 3673–3702.
2. Araki, I., & De Groat, W. C., (1997). Developmental synaptic depression underlying reorganization of visceral reflex pathways in the spinal cord. *J. Neurosci., 17*(21), 8402–8407.
3. Asplin, J. R., & Coe, F. L., (2007). Hyperoxaluria in kidney stone formers treated with modern bariatric surgery. *J. Urol., 177*(2), 565–569.
4. Bhaskar, A., & Oommen, V., (2018). A simple model for demonstrating the factors affecting glomerular filtration rate. *Adv. Physiol. Educ., 42*(2), 380–382.
5. Buckley, B. S., & Lapitan, M. C., (2010). Epidemiology Committee of the Fourth International Consultation on Incontinence, Paris, 2008. Prevalence of urinary incontinence in men, women, and children--current evidence: Findings of the Fourth International Consultation on Incontinence. *Urology, 76*(2), 265–270.
6. von Münch, Elisabeth; Winker, Martina (May 2011). Technology review of urine diversion components (PDF). Deutsche Gesellschaft fürInternationale Zusammenarbeit (GIZ) GmbH. p. 12. Archived (PDF) from the original on 2020-10-28. Retrieved 2020-11-28.
7. Udert, K.M.; Larsen, T.A.; Gujer, W. (2006-12-01). "Fate of major compounds in source-separated urine". *Water Science and Technology*. **54** (11–12): 413–420. doi:10.2166/

wst.2006.921. ISSN 0273-1223. PMID 17302346. Archived from the original on 2022-03-08. Retrieved 2021-08-02.

8. Centers for Disease Control and Prevention (CDC), (2007). Prevalence of chronic kidney disease and associated risk factors–United States, 1999–2004. *MMWR Morb. Mortal Wkly Rep., 56*(8), 161–165.
9. Chen, M. T., Huang, C. N., Chou, Y. H., Huang, C. H., Chiang, C. P., & Liu, G. C., (1997). Percutaneous drainage in the treatment of emphysematous pyelonephritis: 10-year experience. *J. Urol., 157*(5), 1569–1573.
10. Comiter, C. V., (2002). The male sling for stress urinary incontinence: A prospective study. *J. Urol., 167*(2 Pt 1), 597–601.
11. Costantini, F., & Kopan, R., (2010). Patterning a complex organ: Branching morphogenesis and nephron segmentation in kidney development. *Dev. Cell, 18*(5), 698–712.
12. Cupples, W. A., (2007). Interactions contributing to kidney blood flow autoregulation. *Curr. Opin. Nephrol. Hypertens., 16*(1), 39–45.
13. Ferraro, P. M., Curhan, G. C., D'Addessi, A., & Gambaro, G., (2017). Risk of recurrence of idiopathic calcium kidney stones: Analysis of data from the literature. *J. Nephrol., 30*(2), 227–233.
14. Fowler, C. J., Griffiths, D., & De Groat, W. C., (2008). The neural control of micturition. *Nat. Rev. Neurosci., 9*(6), 453–466.
15. Ghossein, C., Serrano, A., Rammohan, M., & Batlle, D., (2002). The role of comprehensive renal clinic in chronic kidney disease stabilization and management: The Northwestern experience. *Semin. Nephrol., 22*(6), 526–532.
16. Glowacki, L. S., Beecroft, M. L., Cook, R. J., Pahl, D., & Churchill, D. N., (1992). The natural history of asymptomatic urolithiasis. *J. Urol., 147*(2), 319–321.
17. Gomes, C. M., Broderick, G. A., Sánchez-Ortiz, R. F., Preate, D., Rovner, E. S., & Wein, A. J., (2000). Artificial urinary sphincter for post-prostatectomy incontinence: Impact of prior collagen injection on cost and clinical outcome. *J. Urol., 163*(1), 87–90.
18. Gosling, J. A., & Dixon, J. S., (1974). Species variation in the location of upper urinary tract pacemaker cells. *Invest. Urol., 11*(5), 418–423.
19. Hannestad, Y. S., Rortveit, G., Sandvik, H., Hunskaar, S., Norwegian EPINCONT Study, & Epidemiology of Incontinence in the County of Nord-Trøndelag, (2000). A community-based epidemiological survey of female urinary incontinence: The Norwegian EPINCONT study. Epidemiology of incontinence in the County of Nord-Trøndelag. *J. Clin. Epidemiol., 53*(11), 1150–1157.
20. Hickling, D. R., Sun, T. T., & Wu, X. R., (2015). Anatomy and physiology of the urinary tract: Relation to host defense and microbial infection. *Microbiol Spectr., 3*(4)
21. Holstein-Rathlou, N. H., Sosnovtseva, O. V., Pavlov, A. N., Cupples, W. A., Sorensen, C. M., & Marsh, D. J., (2011). Nephron blood flow dynamics measured by laser speckle contrast imaging. *Am. J. Physiol. Renal. Physiol., 300*(2), F319–329.
22. Huang, J. J., & Tseng, C. C., (2000). Emphysematous pyelonephritis: Clinicoradiological classification, management, prognosis, and pathogenesis. *Arch. Intern. Med., 160*(6), 797–805.

23. Johnson, J. R., Ireton, R. C., & Lipsky, B. A., (1986). Emphysematous pyelonephritis caused by *Candida albicans*. *J. Urol., 136*(1), 80–82.

24. Jones, E. E., (1991). Ectopic pregnancy: Common and some uncommon misdiagnoses. *Obstet. Gynecol. Clin. North Am., 18*(1), 55–72.

25. Kaplan, S. A., Roehrborn, C. G., Rovner, E. S., Carlsson, M., Bavendam, T., & Guan, Z., (2006). Tolterodine and tamsulosin for treatment of men with lower urinary tract symptoms and overactive bladder: A randomized controlled trial. *JAMA, 296*(19), 2319–2328.

26. Kohler, T. S., Yadven, M., Manvar, A., Liu, N., & Monga, M., (2008). The length of the male urethra. *Int. Braz. J. Urol., 34*(4), 451–454; discussion 455–456.

27. Komlosi, P., Bell, P. D., & Zhang, Z. R., (2009). Tubuloglomerular feedback mechanisms in nephron segments beyond the macula densa. *Curr. Opin. Nephrol. Hypertens., 18*(1), 57–62.

28. Kötsche, W., (1994). The development of veterinary boards and veterinary institutes in Germany in the 18th and 19th centuries. *Berl. Munch Tierarztl Wochenschr., 107*(2), 55–57.

29. Kreidberg, J. A., (2003). Podocyte differentiation and glomerulogenesis. *J. Am. Soc. Nephrol., 14*(3), 806–814.

30. Lieske, J. C., Rule, A. D., Krambeck, A. E., Williams, J. C., Bergstralh, E. J., Mehta, R. A., & Moyer, T. P., (2014). Stone composition as a function of age and sex. *Clin. J. Am. Soc. Nephrol., 9*(12), 2141–2146.

31. Lukacz, E. S., Sampselle, C., Gray, M., Macdiarmid, S., Rosenberg, M., Ellsworth, P., & Palmer, M. H., (2011). A healthy bladder: A consensus statement. *Int. J. Clin. Pract., 65*(10), 1026–1036.

32. Mendu, M. L., Lundquist, A., Aizer, A. A., Leaf, D. E., Robinson, E., Steele, D. J., & Waikar, S. S., (2016). Clinical predictors of diagnostic testing utility in the initial evaluation of chronic kidney disease. *Nephrology (Carlton), 21*(10), 851–859.

33. Minassian, V. A., Yan, X., Lichtenfeld, M. J., Sun, H., & Stewart, W. F., (2012). The iceberg of health care utilization in women with urinary incontinence. *Int. Urogynecol. J., 23*(8), 1087–1093.

34. Mount, D. B., (2014). Thick ascending limb of the loop of Henle. *Clin. J. Am. Soc. Nephrol., 9*(11), 1974–1986.

35. Platt, J. F., Rubin, J. M., Bowerman, R. A., & Marn, C. S., (1988). The inability to detect kidney disease on the basis of echogenicity. *AJR Am. J. Roentgenol., 151*(2), 317–319.

36. Rieken, M., Ebinger, M. N., Bonkat, G., Wyler, S., & Bachmann, A., (2010). Complications of laser prostatectomy: A review of recent data. *World J. Urol., 28*(1), 53–62.

37. Roy, A., Al-bataineh, M. M., & Pastor-Soler, N. M., (2015). Collecting duct intercalated cell function and regulation. *Clin. J. Am. Soc. Nephrol., 10*(2), 305–324.

38. Schierlitz, L., Dwyer, P. L., Rosamilia, A., Murray, C., Thomas, E., De Souza, A., Lim, Y. N., & Hiscock, R., (2008). Effectiveness of tension-free vaginal tape compared with transobturator tape in women with stress urinary incontinence and intrinsic sphincter deficiency: A randomized controlled trial. *Obstet. Gynecol., 112*(6), 1253–1261.

39. Shamliyan, T. A., Wyman, J. F., Ping, R., Wilt, T. J., & Kane, R. L., (2009). Male urinary incontinence: Prevalence, risk factors, and preventive interventions. *Rev. Urol., 11*(3), 145–165.

40. Singh, P., Enders, F. T., Vaughan, L. E., Bergstralh, E. J., Knoedler, J. J., Krambeck, A. E., Lieske,

J. C., & Rule, A. D., (2015). Stone composition among first-time symptomatic kidney stone formers in the community. *Mayo Clin. Proc., 90*(10), 1356–1365.

41. Smith, P. P., (2010). Aging and the underactive detrusor: A failure of activity or activation? *Neurourol. Urodyn., 29*(3), 408–412.
42. Suchy-Dicey, A. M., Laha, T., Hoofnagle, A., Newitt, R., Sirich, T. L., Meyer, T. W., Thummel, K. E., et al., (2016). Tubular secretion in CKD. *J. Am. Soc. Nephrol., 27*(7), 2148–2155.
43. Taylor, J. A., & Kuchel, G. A., (2006). Detrusor underactivity: Clinical features and pathogenesis of an underdiagnosed geriatric condition. *J. Am. Geriatr. Soc., 54*(12), 1920–1932.
44. Uetani, N., & Bouchard, M., (2009). Plumbing in the embryo: Developmental defects of the urinary tracts. *Clin. Genet., 75*(4), 307–317.
45. Van, K. P. E., Van, V. A. C., Heesakkers, J. P., Lycklama, Á N. A. A., Siegel, S., Jonas, U., Fowler, C. J., et al., (2007). Results of sacral neuromodulation therapy for urinary voiding dysfunction: Outcomes of a prospective, worldwide clinical study. *J. Urol., 178*(5), 2029–2034.
46. Weir, M. R., & Fink, J. C., (2005). Salt intake and progression of chronic kidney disease: An overlooked modifiable exposure? A commentary. *Am. J. Kidney Dis., 45*(1), 176–188.

Chapter 11

HUMAN DIGESTIVE SYSTEM

Contents

Unit Introduction

The human digestive system is responsible for carrying out the process of digestion. It consists of the digestive tract, which is a series of organs and structures that food and liquids pass through to be broken down and absorbed into the bloodstream. Additionally, the system includes organs that produce digestive juices and structures that aid in the elimination of waste.

Proper nutrition is essential for the body to function effectively. Certain nutrients serve as the building blocks for cellular components, while others regulate chemical reactions or provide energy through oxidation. However, many nutrients are initially in an unsuitable state for immediate use by the body. Digestion plays a crucial role in facilitating the necessary physical and chemical changes that these nutrients must undergo to become usable (Figure 11.1).

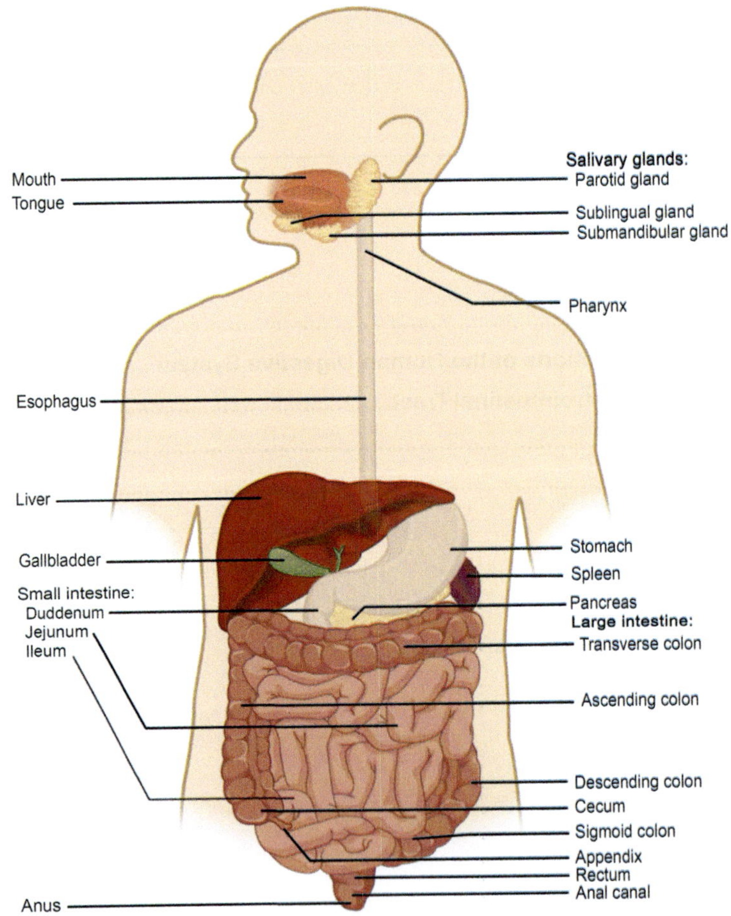

Figure 11.1. *Human digestive system.*

Source: https://courses.lumenlearning.com/suny-ap2/chapter/overview-of-the-digestive-system/.

Orientation and Directional Terms

Term	Definition	Illustration
Common bile duct	The common bile duct is a tube that carries bile from the liver and gallbladder to the small intestine. It's part of the biliary system and runs from the liver to the duodenum, the first part of the small intestine.	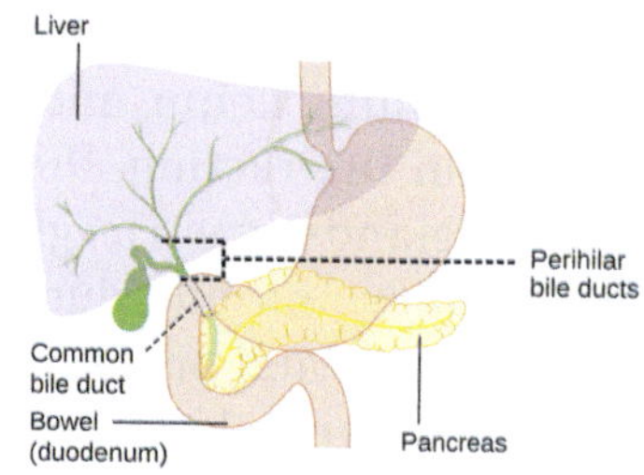
Defecation reflex	The defecation reflex is an involuntary reflex that occurs when the colon moves mass-like material into the rectum.	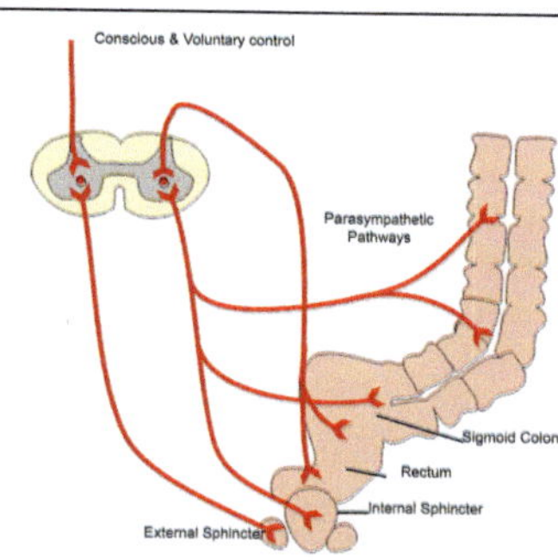
Duodenum	The duodenum is the first part of the small intestine. It is a C-shaped or horseshoe-shaped structure located in the upper abdomen, between the stomach and the jejunum.	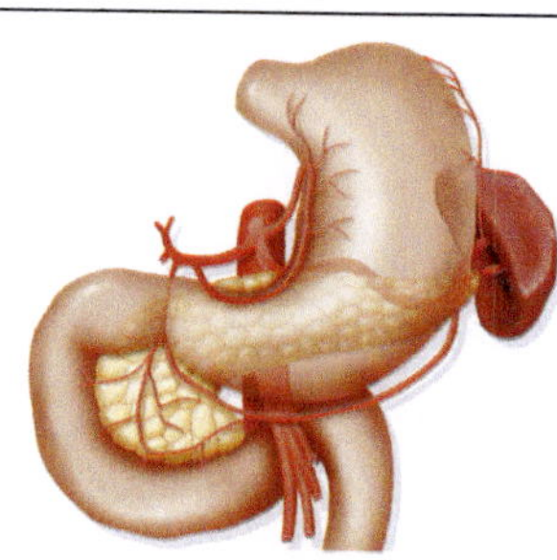
Ileocecal valve	The ileocecal valve (ICV) is a sphincter muscle in the small intestine that controls the flow of contents into the colon.	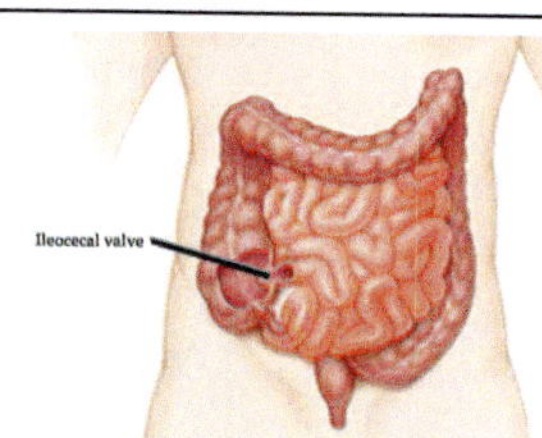
Periodontal membrane	The periodontal membrane, also known as the periodontal ligament, circumdental membrane, or periodontium, is a fleshy tissue that holds teeth in place and attaches them to adjacent teeth.	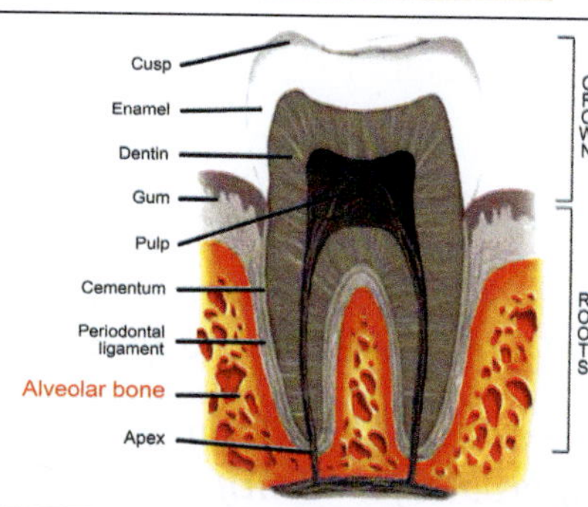

11.1. Structures and Functions of the Human Digestive System

Commencing at the lips, the gastrointestinal tract concludes at the anus. The oral cavity, also referred to as the mouth, comprises the tongue, which manipulates food and combines it with saliva; the pharynx, also known as the throat; the esophagus; the stomach; the small intestine, consisting of the jejunum, ileum, and duodenum; and the large intestine, composed of the sigmoid colon, culminating in the rectum, the ascending colon, the descending colon, and the cecum. The pancreas, salivary glands, gastric glands of the stomach lining, liver, and the liver's accessory organs, the gallbladder and bile ducts, are among the glands responsible for producing digestive secretions. These glands and organs all contribute to the ultimate elimination of indigestible waste as well as the physical and chemical breakdown of ingested food. This section presents a detailed account of their structures and functions (Figure 11.2).

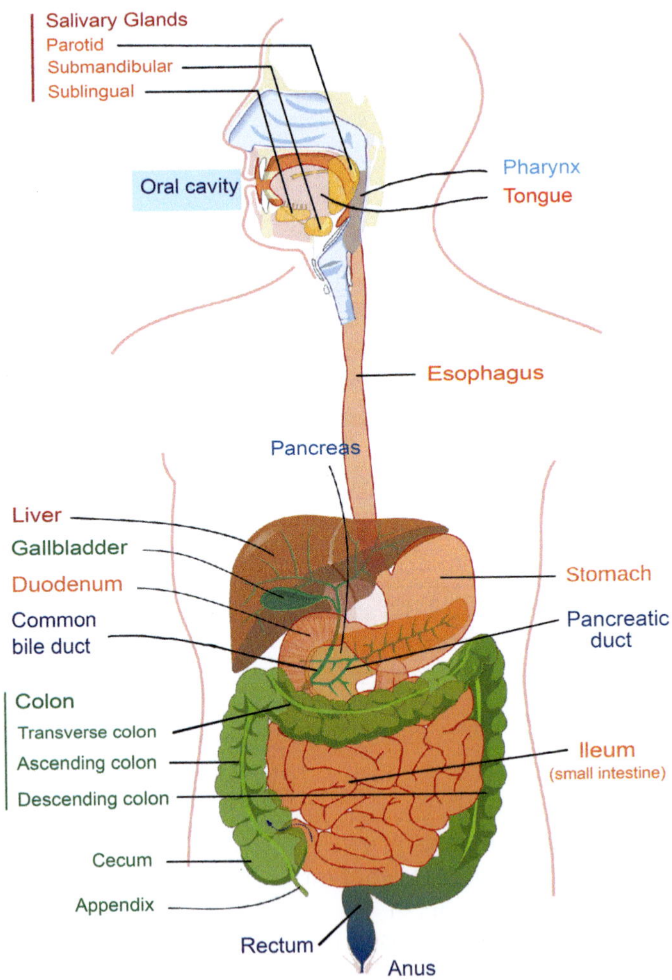

Figure 11.2. *The abdominal organs are supported and protected by the bones of the pelvis and ribcage and are covered by the greater omentum, a fold of peritoneum that consists mainly of fat.*

Source: Thomas, A. J. V., Muralidhar, A., Sathyarajasekaran, K., & Ilakiyaselvan, N., (2023). A deep-learning approach for identifying and classifying digestive diseases. Symmetry, 15(2), 379. https://doi.org/10.3390/sym15020379.

11.1.1. Mouth and Oral Structures

In reality, minimal food digestion takes place in the oral cavity. However, the oral cavity serves to prepare food for transit through the upper gastrointestinal tract and into the stomach and small intestine, where the primary digestive processes occur, via the process of mastication, or chewing. The initial mechanical process that food undergoes is mastication. The masseter, temporal, medial and lateral pterygoids, and buccinator muscles are the masticatory muscles that facilitate movement of the mandible during chewing. The force of the bite is not determined by the strength of the masticatory muscles, but rather by the sensitivity of the periodontal membrane that envelops and sustains the teeth (Figure 11.3).

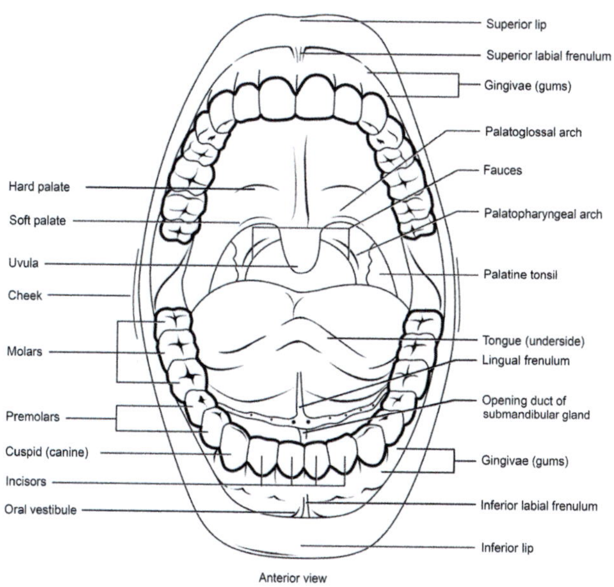

Figure 11.3. *Human mouth: Anterior view of the oral cavity.*

Source: https://courses.lumenlearning.com/suny-ap2/chapter/the-mouth-pharynx-and-esophagus/.

Sufficient digestion does not necessitate mastication. Nevertheless, through the process of fragmenting food into diminutive fragments and amalgamating it with saliva generated by the salivary glands, chewing does facilitate digestion. As chewing disperses saliva throughout the food aggregate, saliva lubricates and moistens desiccated food. A spherical aggregate of food, or bolus, is formed in part by the movement of the tongue against the cheeks and hard palate.

11.1.2. The Lips and Cheeks

The lips, which are two folds of flesh encircling the mouth, are made of mucous membrane, or mucosa, on the inside and skin on the outside. Mucus-secreting glands abound in the mucosa, and they work in tandem with saliva to provide sufficient lubrication for mastication and speech.

The sides of the mouth, or cheeks, share a similar structure and are continuous with the lips. The subcutaneous tissue of the cheek contains a unique fat pad that is referred to as the sucking pad. In infants, this pad is particularly large. The opening of the parotid duct, which originates from the parotid salivary gland, which is situated in front of the ear, is marked by a small elevation on the inner surface of each cheek, across from the second upper molar tooth. Four to five mucus-secreting glands, the openings of whose ducts face the final molar tooth, are located directly behind this gland.

11.1.3. The Roof of the Mouth

The hard and soft palates combine to form the concave roof of the mouth. The palatine portions of the maxillae, or upper jaws, and the horizontal sections of the two palatine bones combine to form the hard palate. A thick, somewhat pale mucous membrane that is continuous with the gums covers the hard palate. Firm fibrous tissue binds the membrane to the upper jaw and palate bones. The hard palate is in front of the soft palate, which is continuous with the mucous membrane covering the nasal cavity's floor posteriorly. The palatine aponeurosis, the glossopalatine and pharyngopalatine muscles, and a robust, thin, fibrous sheet make up the soft palate. The uvula is a tiny projectile that emerges freely from the back of the soft palate.

11.1.4. The Floor of the Mouth

Only when the tongue is raised is the floor of the mouth visible. The sublingual papilla, a small fold on either side of the prominent, elevated fold of mucous membrane known as the frenulum linguae that connects each lip to the gums, is where the submandibular salivary gland ducts open. The plica sublingualis, a ridge that extends outward and backward from each sublingual papilla, denotes the upper border of the sublingual salivary gland, which is located beneath the tongue, and is the surface where the majority of the gland's ducts open.

11.1.5. The Gums

The gums are made up of mucous membranes that are joined to the membrane encircling the jaw bones by dense fibrous tissue. Each tooth's base, or exposed portion, is surrounded by a collar-shaped formation of gum tissue. The gum tissues are rich in blood vessels, and the alveolar arteries, which supply the teeth and the spongy bone of the upper and lower jaws where the teeth are lodged, are also known as alveolar arteries because of their connection to the alveoli dentales, or tooth sockets.

11.1.6. The Teeth

The rigid, ivory structures discovered within the oral cavity are referred to as teeth. Teeth from various vertebrate species are commonly utilized for mastication, although they can also exhibit specialization. For instance, serpents possess exceedingly slender, pointed teeth that typically curve backwards; these teeth are employed for prey capture rather than chewing, as snakes ingest their food whole. In comparison to primates, including humans, the teeth of carnivorous mammals are keener; canines are lengthier, and premolars—which are better suited for shearing and cutting—lack flat grinding surfaces. Frequently, the more posterior molars are lost. However, canines are often entirely absent in herbivores such as cows and horses, which possess very large, flat premolars and molars adorned with intricate ridges and cusps. Flesh-consuming creatures like dogs, cats, and snakes are typically characterized by possessing sharp, pointed teeth that are ill-suited for chewing, whereas herbivores possess broad, flat teeth that are well-suited for chewing. Variations in teeth are a consequence of practical adaptations. Although few animals are capable of breaking down cellulose, herbivores must initially break down the cellulose cell walls enveloping the plant cells they consume in order for the contents of the cells to be exposed to the action of digestive enzymes. In contrast, the animal cells found in meat are directly susceptible to the action of digestive enzymes because they are not covered in indigestible material. Consequently, unlike herbivores, carnivores do not necessitate as much chewing. Given that they consume both plant and animal tissue, humans are omnivores, signifying that their teeth fall somewhere in between the extremes of specialization that carnivore and herbivore teeth achieve in terms of structure and function. A tooth consists of a crown and one or more roots. The crown is the visible part of the tooth above the gum line, while the root is the part that is not visible but anchors the tooth in the jawbone. Animals exhibit variations in the shapes of their crowns and roots. The teeth on one side of the jaw are mirror images of those on the other side. The upper teeth are different from the lower teeth and complement them. Humans typically have two sets of teeth throughout their lives. The first set, known as the milk, primary, or deciduous dentition, gradually develops between the ages of two and six months. The secondary set gradually replaces the primary teeth as the jaws grow and expand. Each quadrant of the mouth contains five permanent teeth and eight deciduous teeth, resulting in a total of 32 permanent teeth to replace the 20 deciduous teeth.

11.1.7. The Tongue

The tongue is a highly mobile muscular organ located on the floor of the mouth. It serves as an accessory organ for various oral motor functions such as chewing, swallowing, and speech. Working in conjunction with the cheeks, it can guide and hold food between the upper and lower teeth until the process of mastication is complete. Infants are able to suckle due to the tongue's ability to create negative pressure within the oral cavity. Taste buds, which are clusters of specialized epithelial cells on the tongue, play a crucial role as peripheral sense organs by transmitting stimuli from the oral cavity to the central nervous system. Additionally, the tongue's glands contribute to the production of saliva necessary for swallowing.

The tongue consists of a mass of fat and intricately striated (striped) muscles. The mucous membrane covering the tongue exhibits regional variations. Extrinsic muscles connect the tongue to the lower jaw, the hyoid bone (a U-shaped bone situated between the lower jaw and the larynx), the skull, the soft palate, and the throat. Mucous membrane folds anchor the tongue to the floor of the mouth and the epiglottis, a cartilaginous plate that covers the larynx.

11.1.8. Salivary Glands

When food enters the mouth, it is mixed with saliva produced by several glands. In addition to numerous minor glands, there are three main pairs of salivary glands: the parotid, submandibular, and sublingual glands. The parotid glands, the largest of the three pairs, are located on the side of the face below and in front of each ear. They are protected by sheaths that prevent excessive swelling during inflammation, such as in cases of mumps. The submandibular glands, which are round in shape, are located near the inner side of the lower jawbone in front of the sternomastoid muscle. The sublingual glands are positioned directly under the mucous membrane covering the floor of the mouth beneath the tongue (Figure 11.4).

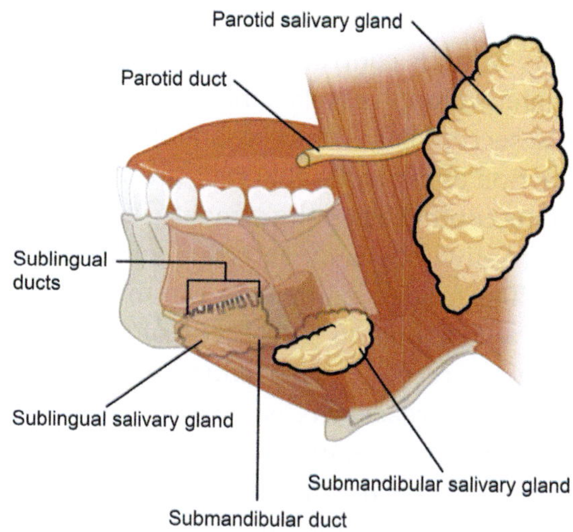

Figure 11.4. *Salivary glands. The three major pairs of salivary glands.*

Source: https://courses.lumenlearning.com/suny-ap2/chapter/the-mouth-pharynx-and-esophagus/.

The salivary glands, known as racemose glands, are so named because of the clustered arrangement of their secreting cells in rounded sacs called acini. These acini are connected to ducts that branch out freely. Within the acini are pyramidal secreting cells and flat, star-shaped myoepithelial cells that are believed to contract, similar to the cells in the breast that expel milk from the ducts.

The cells that secrete can either be mucous or serous in nature. The former secretes a watery fluid that contains the enzyme amylase, while the latter secretes mucin, the main component of mucus. The submandibular glands contain both mucous and serous secreting cells, with the serous cells outnumbering the mucous cells four to one. The parotid glands secrete cells of the serous type. The mucous cells that make up the acini of the sublingual glands are the main constituent.

The parasympathetic and sympathetic branches of the autonomic nervous system regulate the salivary glands. The parasympathetic nervous system controls acinar cell secretion and widens blood vessels. Constriction of blood vessels, secretion by acinar cells, and, most likely, contraction of myoepithelial cells are among the functions controlled by the sympathetic nervous system. Saliva normally secretes continuously, even when food is present in the mouth. One to one and a half to five liters of saliva are typically secreted in a 24-hour period. Saliva production increases in response to stimulation of the gums, tongue, or other parts of the oral cavity, as well as during chewing. Food is not necessary to stimulate salivation; shifting the jaws and tongue when the mouth is empty or even dry sand can elicit the same response. The unconditioned salivary reflex is the result of increased salivation following direct stimulation of the oral mucosa. Increased salivary flow may be triggered by a stimulus alone if a person discovers that a specific sight, sound, smell, or other stimulus is consistently linked to food. This reaction is referred to as the conditioned salivary reflex.

11.1.8.1. Saliva

Saliva functions as a lubricant and dissolves part of the food that has been chewed, making it easier for the food to pass through the subsequent sections of the digestive tract. Additionally, saliva contains the starch-digesting enzyme amylase (also known as ptyalin), which initiates the process of enzymatic hydrolysis by breaking down starch molecules into double sugars, maltose, and glucose. Starch is a polysaccharide composed of numerous sugar molecules linked in a continuous chain. Since many carnivores, including dogs and cats, lack amylase in their saliva, starch is not a common component in their diets. Saliva acts as the solvent for food ingredients, which is essential for substances to be in solution in order to stimulate the taste buds.

The composition of saliva varies, but its primary constituents are water, a variety of organic substances including salivary proteins, free amino acids, and the enzymes lysozyme and amylase, as well as inorganic ions that are similar to those typically found in blood plasma. Saliva has a slight acidity, but under normal circumstances, the bicarbonates and phosphates it contains act as buffers to maintain the pH, or hydrogen ion concentration, of saliva at a reasonably constant level.

Saliva's bicarbonate, chloride, potassium, and sodium concentrations are all directly correlated with the flow rate of these elements. Additionally, there is a direct correlation between blood carbon dioxide partial pressure and bicarbonate concentration. The concentration of chloride in the blood varies between 5 millimoles per liter at low flow rates and 70 millimoles per liter at high flow rates. Under comparable conditions, the sodium concentrations range from 5 millimoles per liter to 100 millimoles per liter. Saliva has a sharp, metallic taste when flow is brisk because the concentration of potassium in the blood is often higher than that in blood plasma, up to 20 millimoles per liter.

Saliva continuously flows through the mouth, keeping the teeth and oral cavity moist and relatively free of foreign objects, food particles, and sloughed epithelial cells. Saliva inhibits the growth of bacteria by eliminating materials that could be used as culture media. Due to the presence of the enzyme lysozyme, which can lyse, or dissolve, some bacteria, saliva serves a protective purpose. Saliva also acts as a vehicle for the body to expel a number of organic and inorganic materials, such as lead, potassium iodide, bromide, morphine, ethyl alcohol, mercury, and some antibiotics like streptomycin, penicillin, and chlortetracycline.

Saliva is not essential for life, but its absence causes a variety of problems. These include dry mucous membranes in the mouth, poor dental hygiene due to bacterial overgrowth, a significantly reduced sense of taste, and difficulty speaking.

11.1.9. Pharynx

The passageway connecting the mouth, nose, and esophagus to the larynx and esophagus is known as the throat or pharynx. The pharynx transports air to and from the trachea, or windpipe, during respiration and allows swallowed solids and liquids to pass into the esophagus, or gullet. Additionally, the Eustachian tube, which connects the pharynx to the middle ear cavity on both sides, equalizes the air pressure on the eardrum membrane, separating the middle ear cavity from the external ear canal. The pharynx resembles a flattened funnel in general shape. While it is fastened to the surrounding structures, it is sufficiently loose to allow the pharyngeal wall to slide against them during swallowing. The three pharyngeal constrictors, which form the main musculature of the side and rear pharyngeal walls and slightly overlap each other, are the principal muscles of the pharynx and are involved in the mechanics of swallowing (Figure 11.5).

The oropharynx, nasal pharynx, and laryngeal pharynx are the three primary divisions of the pharynx. The respiratory and digestive tracts share the oral pharynx, while the remaining two are airways. A palatine tonsil, so named because of its close proximity to the palate, is located on either side of the aperture that separates the mouth cavity from the oral pharynx. The glossopalatine arches are two vertical folds of mucous membrane that surround each palatine tonsil. The soft palate, seen above, divides the nasal pharynx from the oral pharynx. On the roof of the nasal pharynx is another pair of tonsils. The adenoids, or paranasal tonsils, are a component of the immune system. The pharyngeal tonsils obstruct the airway when they swell excessively, which happens frequently in childhood. The tongue root conceals the laryngeal pharynx and the lower portion of the oral pharynx.

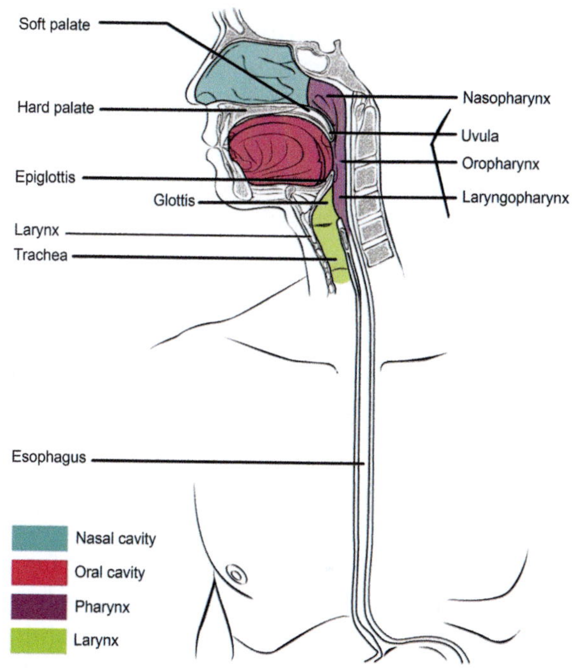

Figure 11.5. *Human pharynx. Sagittal section of the pharynx.*

Source: https://courses.lumenlearning.com/suny-ap2/chapter/the-mouth-pharynx-and-esophagus/.

The bolus is inserted into the pharynx during the first voluntary stage of deglutition, also known as swallowing. The tongue is retracted and depressed in the front, mastication stops, breathing is restricted, and the tongue is elevated and retracted in the back against the hard palate. The bolus is forced from the mouth into the pharynx by this action, which is caused by the powerful tongue muscles. The soft palate's elevation against the posterior pharyngeal wall prevents the bolus from entering the nasal pharynx. The larynx advances beneath the base of the tongue and rises as the bolus is forced into the pharynx. A quick peristaltic contraction, also known as a squeezing contraction, is initiated when the superior pharyngeal constrictor muscles contract. This contraction propels the bolus in front of the pharynx down the pharynx. The walls and structures of the lower pharynx are elevated to accommodate the approaching food mass. The bolus is directed to the pharynx by the epiglottis, a lid-like covering that protects the laryngeal opening. As the bolus approaches, the cricopharyngeal muscle, also known as the upper esophageal sphincter, which has been keeping the esophagus closed, relaxes and allows the bolus to pass through. The primary esophageal peristaltic contraction originates from the pharyngeal peristaltic contraction, which continues into the esophagus.

11.1.10. Esophagus

The esophagus, which transports food from the throat to the stomach, has a length of approximately 25 cm (10 inches) and a width that ranges from 1.5 to 2 cm (about 1 inch). The esophagus travels through the diaphragm and into the stomach, emerging from behind the heart and trachea and in front of the spinal column (Figure 11.6).

The esophagus is composed of four layers: the muscularis, tunica adventitia, submucosa, and mucosa. The mucosa consists of stratified squamous epithelium and contains numerous mucous glands. The submucosa is a thick layer of fibrous tissue that connects the muscularis and mucosa. Together, the mucosa and submucosa form long, longitudinal folds that give the esophageal opening a star-shaped cross section. The muscularis is comprised of two layers: an outer layer with longitudinal fibers and an inner layer with circular fibers. Both muscle groups wrap around the alimentary tract, but the outer muscle group has a slowly unwinding spiral that is almost longitudinal, while the inner muscle group has a tightly wound spiral that creates nearly circular windings. The tunica adventitia, the outer layer of the esophagus, is made up of loose fibrous tissue that connects the esophagus to nearby structures. Normally, the esophagus is empty except during swallowing, and the lumen, or channel, is effectively closed by the longitudinal folds of the mucosal and submucosal layers.

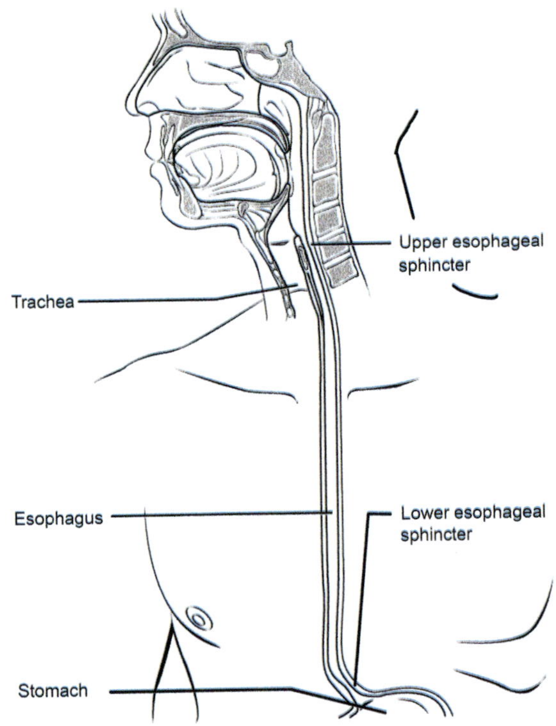

Figure 11.6. *Esophagus.*

Source: https://courses.lumenlearning.com/suny-ap2/chapter/the-mouth-pharynx-and-esophagus/.

The muscle that lines the upper third of the esophagus is striated (voluntary). The lower third is composed entirely of smooth muscle, while the middle third consists of a combination of striated and smooth (involuntary) muscle. Two circular muscles, known as sphincters, line the esophagus and act as drawstrings to close off passageways. Under normal circumstances, both sphincters remain closed, except during swallowing. The upper esophageal sphincter is located at the cricoid cartilage, which is a single ring-shaped cartilage forming the lower part of the larynx wall. This sphincter is called the cricopharyngeus muscle. The lower esophageal sphincter surrounds the portion of the esophagus that passes through the diaphragmatic hiatus, a hole in the diaphragm measuring 3 to 4 cm. The lower esophageal sphincter remains taut at all times, except during a descending contraction wave, allowing the release of gas (vomiting) or belching. Therefore, the lower esophageal sphincter plays a crucial role in preventing gastric reflux in the esophagus in response to changes in intragastric pressure or body position.

As previously mentioned, the pharynx serves as the origin of the primary esophageal peristaltic contractions, which propel food through the esophagus. A peristaltic wave that moves forward creates a pressure gradient and propels the bolus ahead of it, resulting in these contractions. The transit of material through the esophagus typically takes 10 seconds or less. When the bolus reaches the point where the esophagus meets the stomach, the lower esophageal sphincter relaxes, allowing the bolus to enter the stomach. However, in the middle or lower esophagus, bolus arrest may occur if the bolus is too large or if the peristaltic contraction is too weak. In such cases, local distension of the esophageal wall triggers secondary peristaltic contractions that initiate around the bolus and propel it into the stomach.

The passage of liquids through the esophagus after swallowing is partially influenced by the body's position and the force of gravity. When ingested horizontally or with the head-down, liquids follow a similar path as solids, moving ahead of the advancing peristaltic contraction. In animals with exceptionally long necks, such as giraffes, the esophageal peristaltic wave's high pressures and forceful contractions enable liquids to travel through the esophagus for considerable distances. However, when the body is upright, liquids enter the esophagus and descend gravitationally towards the lower end. They remain there for approximately 8 to 10 seconds until the lower esophageal sphincter opens and the peristaltic contraction occurs, emptying the liquids into the stomach.

11.1.11. Stomach

11.1.11.1. Anatomy

Food and liquids that have been swallowed are collected by the stomach, which then mixes and grinds them with gastric juice to make the food particles more soluble and smaller. The stomach's primary duties include initiating the breakdown of proteins and carbohydrates, converting food into chyme, and periodically releasing the chyme into the small intestine when the mixture's physical and chemical state allows it to progress to the next stage of digestion. The stomach is located directly below the diaphragm in the upper left section of the abdomen. The anterior abdominal wall, the liver, and a portion of the diaphragm are situated in front of the stomach. The colon, the left kidney, the left adrenal gland, the spleen, and the pancreas are positioned behind it. The left side of the stomach is convex, while the right side is essentially concave. The convex border is referred to as the greater curvature, and the concave border is known as the lesser curvature. When the stomach is empty, its mucosal lining folds repeatedly into long strips, or rugae, which tend to disappear when the stomach is enlarged (Figure 11.7).

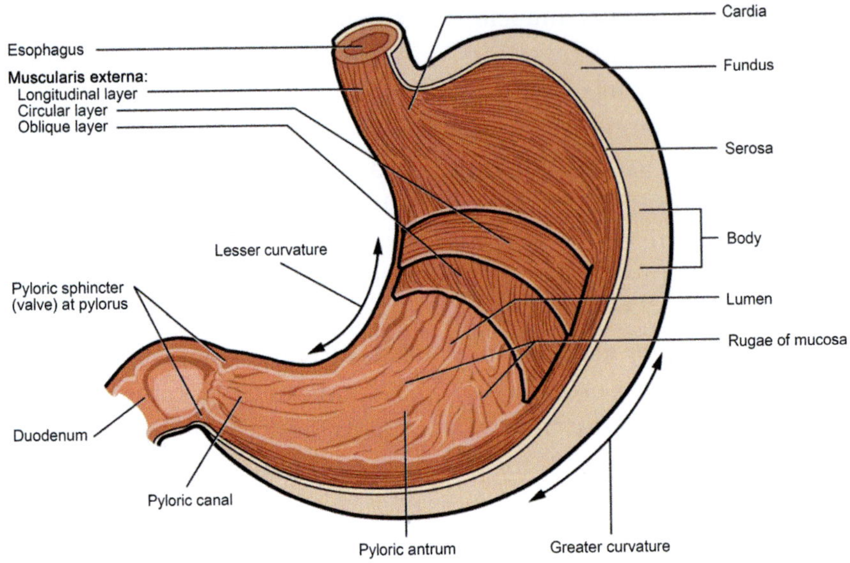

Figure 11.7. *Structures of the human stomach.*

Source: https://courses.lumenlearning.com/suny-ap2/chapter/the-stomach/

The stomach has three layers of muscle: an outer longitudinal layer, a middle circular layer, and an inner oblique layer. The inner lining consists of four layers: the serosa, the muscularis, the submucosa, and the mucosa. The mucosa is densely packed with gastric glands, which contain cells that produce digestive enzymes, hydrochloric acid, and mucus.

The cardia is the orifice through which the stomach and esophagus meet. The fundus is the uppermost portion of the stomach, situated above the esophageal entrance. The fundus often contains a gas bubble, especially after a meal, as it relaxes its muscular wall to accommodate the fluctuating volume of food that is ingested. The body, which makes up the majority of the stomach, is essentially used as a holding tank for liquids and food that have been swallowed. The bottom portion of the stomach, known as the antrum, resembles a funnel with its wide end connecting to the lower body and its narrow end to the pyloric canal, which empties into the duodenum, the upper division of the small intestine. The stomach's J-shaped shape is caused by the pyloric portion of the stomach, which consists of the antrum and the pyloric canal. This portion of the stomach tends to curve to the right, slightly upward, and backward. The stomach's exit into the duodenum is through the pylorus, which is the stomach's narrowest part. It has a diameter of about 2 cm, or nearly 1 inch, and thick smooth muscle loops encircle it.

There are three coats, or layers, to the muscles that make up the stomach wall. The esophageal longitudinal muscle coat and the external coat are continuous, known as the longitudinal muscle layer. The cardia separates longitudinal muscle fibers into two wide strips. The stronger one, located on the right, extends to encompass the stomach's adjacent anterior and posterior walls as well as its smaller curvature. The longitudinal fibers on the left originate from the esophagus and extend across the fundus' dome to accommodate the greater curvature. They then join the longitudinal fibers that descend over the lesser curvature at the pylorus. The small intestine's longitudinal muscle is formed by the longitudinal layer continuing into the duodenum.

The stomach is entirely covered by the middle, or circular, muscular layer, which is the strongest of the three. The lower part of the stomach, especially the area over the antrum and pylorus, is where the circular fibers of this coat are most developed. The pyloric sphincter is formed at the pyloric end of the stomach by a significant thickening of the circular muscle layer. Connective tissue divides this muscular ring from the duodenum's circular muscle by a small amount.

The oblique muscular layer, which is the innermost layer of smooth muscle, is weakest as it approaches the pylorus and strongest in the fundus region. Without exerting additional pressure on the stomach, it is capable of expanding to accommodate more than one liter (approximately one quart) of food or liquids. When hydrochloric acid comes into contact with the mucosa of the antrum, a neural reflex is partially responsible for the receptive relaxation of the upper part of the stomach to accommodate a meal. This reflex may be triggered by the release of the hormone known as vasoactive intestinal peptide. The dilation of the stomach's body caused by food initiates a neurological reflex that stimulates muscular contractions in the antrum.

11.1.11.2. Blood and Nerve Supply

The stomach receives arterial blood through various branches of the celiac trunk. The celiac trunk, a short and wide vessel, is a major conduit that carries arterial blood from the heart to the systemic circulation. Venous blood from the stomach is returned to the venous system through the portal vein, which then transports it to the liver.

Both the parasympathetic and sympathetic branches of the autonomic nervous system supply the stomach with nerve fibers. The parasympathetic nerve fibers are carried by the vagus nerve, also known as the tenth cranial nerve. The vagus nerve passes through the diaphragm's opening alongside the esophagus. The anterior portion of the stomach is supplied by the left vagus nerve, while the posterior portion is covered by branches of the right vagus nerve. Sympathetic branches of the celiac, or solar, plexus, a network of nerves, follow the arteries of the stomach into its muscular wall.

11.1.11.3. Stomach Contractions

There are three different kinds of stomach motor activity that have been noted. The first is a small wave of stomach wall contraction that initiates in the upper portion of the organ and gradually descends over it towards the pyloric sphincter. This type of contraction causes a slight indentation in the stomach wall. Retrograde waves frequently sweep the pyloric sphincter, the antrum, and the junction of the antrum and the stomach body, resulting in back-and-forth movement, mixing, and crushing of the stomach contents. Although it exhibits peristaltic characteristics, the second type of motor activity is also a contracting wave. The contraction begins in the upper region of the stomach and gradually moves down towards the pyloric sphincter. This type of gastric contraction deeply indents the stomach wall, completely blocking the stomach lumen or cavity as the peristaltic wave approaches the antrum, compartmentalizing the stomach. The material ahead of the contracting wave is then propelled through the pyloric sphincter and into the duodenum as it passes over the antrum. The purpose of this type of contraction is to pump the contents of the stomach antrum past the pyloric sphincter. When recorded from the gastric antrum, the stomach's peristaltic contractions and mixing occur at a steady rate of three contractions per minute. At two-hour intervals following meals, a wave of peristalsis sweeps along the lower half of the stomach and throughout the entire intestine to the proximal colon. Eating can inhibit these peristaltic waves, and the hormone motilin can also induce them. The third type of gastric motor activity can be accurately characterized as a tonic, or prolonged, contraction of all stomach muscles. During the tonic contraction, the stomach lumen shrinks as the entire gastric wall contracts simultaneously. This activity explains the stomach's ability to adapt to different volumes of gastric content. While mixing contractions and peristaltic contractions typically occur alongside the tonic contraction, the tonic contraction is independent of the other two types of contractions. During food digestion, smaller particles pass through the pyloric sphincter, which briefly opens as a peristaltic wave passes through the antrum towards it. This allows the duodenum to "sample" the contents of the stomach.

11.1.11.4. Gastric Mucosa

The gastric mucosa is a mucous membrane that lines the inside of the stomach. Tall columnar epithelial cells secrete a thick layer of mucus that covers the mucosa at all times. The glycoprotein known as gastric mucus has two functions: it lubricates food particles to facilitate their movement through the stomach and forms a protective layer over the lining epithelium of the stomach cavity. The surface layer of the stomach secretes bicarbonate from the underlying mucosa, aiding in the formation of this protective layer that acts as a defense mechanism against the stomach's own protein-lyzing enzymes. The acidity, or hydrogen ion concentration, of the mucous layer is measured at pH7 (neutral) near the epithelium and increases to pH2 (acidic) at the luminal level. When the gastric mucus is extracted from the surface epithelium, tiny pits called foveolae gastricae can be observed under a magnifying glass. The surface epithelium contains between 90 and 100 gastric pits per square millimeter (58,000 to 65,000 per square inch). Each gastric pit receives secretions from three to seven distinct gastric glands. The muscularis mucosae, a thin layer of smooth muscle, is located beneath the gastric mucosa. The submucosa, a loose layer of connective tissue, connects the gastric mucosa to the muscles in the stomach walls.

There are six distinct cell types found in the gastric mucosa. The gastric glands contain five common cell types in addition to the tall columnar surface epithelial cells previously mentioned.

1. Mucoid cells secrete gastric mucus and are present in all types of gastric glands. Mucoid cells are the predominant cell type found in the gastric glands in the cardiac and pyloric areas of the stomach. The necks of the glands in the body and fundic parts of the stomach are lined with mucoid cells.
2. Zymogenic, or chief, cells are mainly located in gastric glands in the body and fundic portions of the stomach. These cells secrete pepsinogen, which is converted into the proteolytic enzyme pepsin. There are two varieties of pepsinogen, known as pepsinogen I and pepsinogen II. Both are produced in the mucous and zymogenic cells in the glands of the body of the stomach, but the mucous glands located elsewhere in the stomach produce only pepsinogen II. Stimuli that induce gastric acid secretion, particularly vagal nerve stimulation, also promote the secretion of the pepsinogens.
3. Gastrin cells, also known as G cells, are distributed throughout the antrum. These endocrine cells secrete the acid-stimulating hormone gastrin in response to decreased acidity of the gastric contents when food enters the stomach and gastric distention. Gastrin then enters the bloodstream and is transported to the mucosa of the body of the stomach, where it binds to receptor sites on the outer membrane

of the parietal cells (described below). The formation of the gastrin-receptor complex triggers an energy-consuming reaction mediated by the presence of the enzyme ATPase, bound to the membrane, which leads to the production and secretion of hydrogen ions in the parietal cells.

4. Parietal, or oxyntic, cells, which are located in the glands of the body and fundic portions of the stomach, secrete hydrogen ions that combine with chloride ions to form hydrochloric acid (HCl). The acid that is produced drains into the lumen of the gland and then passes through to the stomach. This process occurs only when one or more types of receptors on the outer membrane of the parietal cell are bound to histamine, gastrin, or acetylcholine. Prostaglandins, hormonelike substances that are present in virtually all tissues and body fluids, inhibit the secretion of hydrochloric acid. The drugs omeprazole (Losec or Prilosec) and lansoprazole (Prevacid) also inhibit acid secretion by the parietal cells and are used as treatments for peptic ulcer. Parietal cells produce most of the water found in gastric juice; they also produce glycoproteins called intrinsic factor, which are essential to the maturation of red blood cells, vitamin B12 absorption, and the health of certain cells in the central and peripheral nervous systems.
5. Endocrine cells called enterochromaffin-like cells, due to their staining characteristics, are scattered throughout the body of the stomach. These cells secrete several substances, including the hormone serotonin.

11.1.11.5. Gastric Secretion

Every day, the gastric mucosa secretes between 1 and 2 liters of gastric juice. This gastric juice serves to prepare food for further digestion in the small intestine. It accomplishes this by solubilizing food particles, initiating the breakdown process (particularly for proteins), and transforming the stomach contents into a semi-liquid mass called chyme. Gastric juice is composed of water, hydrogen chloride, electrolytes (such as sodium, potassium, calcium, phosphate, sulfate, and bicarbonate), and organic materials (including mucus, pepsins, and protein). The composition of gastric juice can vary. Due to its high concentration of hydrochloric acid, this juice has a high level of acidity and is rich in enzymes. As previously mentioned, the membrane on the surface of the epithelial cells lining the stomach lumen protects the stomach walls from the digestive juices. This membrane contains lipoproteins that are resistant to acid attack. Certain mammals, such as calves, possess the enzyme renin, which causes milk proteins to clump together, removing them from solution and increasing their susceptibility to the action of a proteolytic enzyme.

Gastric secretion can be divided into three phases (cephalic, gastric, and intestinal), each of which stimulates the gastric mucosa to release gastric juice through specific mechanisms. These secretion phases are interconnected, demonstrating the relationship between neural and humoral pathways.

Taste, smell, sight, and sound are the stimuli that cause the cephalic phase of gastric secretion to occur. This stage of gastric secretion is reflex mediated through the vagus nerve (10th cranial). When vagal stimulation occurs, either directly through electrical impulses or indirectly through stimuli received through the senses, gastric juice is secreted. This mechanism of stomach secretion was first demonstrated by Russian physiologist Ivan Petrovich Pavlov in a now-famous canine experiment.

During the gastric phase, the vagus nerve and gastrin play important roles in regulating stomach acidity after a meal. Proteins help buffer the acidity of gastric contents to maintain a pH of around 3 for about 90 minutes. Acid is continuously secreted during this phase in response to distension and the release of peptides and amino acids from protein digestion. The presence of free amino acids and peptides stimulates the release of gastrin into the bloodstream. Mechanical, chemical, and hormonal factors all contribute to the gastric secretory response to eating. This phase ends once the food has fully emptied from the stomach.

Due to the intricate stimulatory and inhibitory processes involved, the intestinal phase is not completely understood. Chyme inhibits acid secretion while simultaneously promoting gastric acid secretion through the circulation of amino acids and small peptides. One significant factor preventing the release of gastrin is the secretion of gastric acid. Gastrin is not released if the antral contents' pH drops below 2.5. Glucagon and secretin are two hormones that are released from the small intestine by byproducts of digestion, particularly fat, and they also inhibit the secretion of acid.

11.1.11.6. Absorption and Emptying

Although the stomach only absorbs a few digestion products, it can absorb various other substances such as glucose, amino acids, and some fat-soluble substances. The pH level of the stomach determines the absorption rate of different substances. For example, at a low pH, acidic environment, aspirin is absorbed quickly, while at a higher pH, more basic environment, absorption is slower. Water can easily move from the stomach contents into the blood through the gastric mucosa. However, the overall absorption of water from the stomach is limited because water can move just as easily from the blood back into the stomach. The absorption of water and alcohol can be hindered by the presence of food, especially fats, which can delay gastric emptying. Most water is absorbed in the small intestine regardless of the situation.

The physical and chemical makeup of the meal affects how quickly the stomach empties. Proteins empty faster than fats, fluids empty faster than solids, and carbohydrates empty faster than proteins. The duodenal bulb and the second part of the duodenum relax, enabling the stomach to empty when food particles are small enough and almost soluble, and when receptors in the duodenal bulb—the area of attachment between the duodenum and the stomach—have a fluidity and a concentration of hydrogen ions that meet certain criteria. The pressure in the duodenal bulb increases more than the pressure in the antrum during a duodenal contraction. By closing, the pylorus stops food from refluxing into the stomach. While the sympathetic division of the autonomic nervous system may also be involved, the vagus nerve plays a major role in controlling emptying. The function of a number of the digestive tract's peptide hormones in physiological conditions is unknown, although they do affect intragastric pressure and stomach movements.

11.1.12. Small Intestine

The main component of the digestive system is the small intestine. The small intestine's main functions include the production of enzymes and other components necessary for digestion, the mixing and transportation of intraluminal materials, and the absorption of nutrients. The small intestine is where most of the processes occur that break down proteins, fats, and carbohydrates into simpler organic compounds.

11.1.12.1. Anatomy

In terms of anatomy, the small intestine is the longest segment of the digestive tract, measuring 670 to 760 cm (22 to 25 feet) in length and 3 to 4 cm (approximately 2 inches) in diameter. It begins at the pylorus, the junction between the stomach and colon, and ends at the ileocecal valve, the junction between the colon and stomach. The small intestine consists of three main functional segments: the duodenum, jejunum, and ileum.

The duodenum forms a C-shaped curve around the head of the pancreas and is approximately 23 to 28 cm (9 to 11 inches) long. It is located retroperitoneally, meaning it is situated behind the peritoneum, the membrane that lines the abdominal wall, unlike the rest of the small intestine. The duodenal bulb, which is the first segment of the small intestine, is the widest section. It is positioned horizontally and partially lies behind the wide end of the gallbladder. From the pylorus, it travels to the right and back. Pancreatic juice and bile enter this part of the duodenum through the duodenal papilla (papilla of Vater), which descends vertically in front of the hilum of the right kidney (the point of entry or exit for blood vessels, nerves, and ureters). The fourth section of the duodenum ascends to the left side of the second lumbar vertebra (at the level of the small of the back), then sharply bends downward and forward to connect with the jejunum, the second part of the small intestine. The third section of the duodenum runs horizontally to the left in front of the aorta and the inferior vena cava (the principal channel for the return of venous blood from the lower part of the body and the legs to the heart). This segment of the small intestine is supported by the ligament of Treitz, forming an acute angle known as the duodenojejunal flexure. The jejunum constitutes approximately 40% of the small intestine and, similar to the ileum, is characterized by numerous convolutions. It is connected to the posterior abdominal wall by a membrane known as the mesentery. The remaining 60% of the small intestine is referred to as the ileum, with no distinct boundary between the jejunum and the ileum. Generally, the jejunum is situated in the upper left part of the abdomen below the 10th rib, while the ileum is located in the lower right part. The ileum connects to the large intestine at its terminal end.

The muscular coats of the small intestine are consistently arranged along its entire length. The outer longitudinal layer is thinner compared to the inner circular layer. The peritoneum lines the outermost layer of the small intestine.

11.1.12.2. Blood and Nerve Supply

The small intestine is supplied with blood by the superior mesenteric artery, a branch of the abdominal aorta, and the superior pancreaticduodenal artery, a branch of the hepatic artery. These vessels travel between layers of the mesentery, the membrane connecting the intestines to the abdominal cavity wall. They give off large branches that form connecting arches, from which smaller branches enter the wall of the small bowel. Blood from the intestine is returned via the superior mesenteric vein, which along with the splenic vein, forms the portal vein that drains into the liver.

Both parasympathetic and sympathetic innervation exist in the small intestine. One source of parasympathetic innervation is the vagus nerve. The sympathetic nervous system is innervated by branches of the superior mesenteric plexus, a nerve network situated beneath the solar plexus that follows blood vessels into the small intestine and ultimately ends in the Meissner plexus in the submucosa and the Auerbach plexus between the circular and longitudinal muscle coats. These two plexuses are connected by a profusion of adrenergic (sympathetic) and cholinergic (parasympathetic) fibrils.

11.1.12.3. Contractions and Motility

Electrical impulses initiate when calcium ions enter the muscle cell, regulating the contractions of the circular and longitudinal muscles. The duodenal pacemaker sends electrical impulses down the small intestine at a rate of 11 cycles per minute in the duodenum and 8 cycles per minute in the ileum. These electrical alterations are propagated in the longitudinal muscle layer of the small intestine wall. Spike-like electrical charges may occur simultaneously with the slow-wave electrical activity. When the circular muscle layer of the intestinal wall contracts to create a segmenting contraction, it produces this specific electrical activity. The myofibrils, which are the contracting elements of the muscle tissues, contract due to the depolarization of the muscle cell membranes, resulting in an excess of positive charges inside the cell. The pace at which the muscle cell membrane depolarizes determines the speed of these contractions. Subsequently, the contraction of the two spiral muscle layers leads to the motor activity that facilitates the mixing and transportation of food through the small intestine.

Transporting and mixing intraluminal contents are the main functions of the small intestine's movements. One feature of small intestine motility is the smooth muscle that makes up the intestinal wall's intrinsic capacity for spontaneous and periodic contraction. There is no extrinsic nerve supply to the small intestine causing this phenomenon. Other messenger substances and receptors that can control smooth muscle activity are found in the myenteric plexus, which is a network of nerve fibers in the intestinal wall. These substances and receptors include somatostatin, serotonin (5-hydroxytryptamine), and enkephalins. There are at least seven of these substances in and around the smooth muscle, and their specific functions are not entirely clear. There are pressure gradients between adjacent segments of the organ caused by the small intestine's contractions. Transport within the small intestine is primarily carried out by the pressure gradients. Peristaltic contractions and segmenting contractions are the two recognized forms of motor activity.

The segmenting contraction, a localized circumferential contraction primarily of the intestinal wall's circular muscle, is the main motor action of the small intestine. The intestinal chyme is mixed, separated, and agitated by segmenting contractions. Less than 1 to 2 cm (about 1 inch) of the intestinal wall is involved in this brief contraction, which constricts the lumen and tends to divide its contents. The number of segmenting contractions gradually decreases as the chyme passes from the duodenum to the ileum. This has been referred to as the small intestine motility "gradient." Segmenting contractions can occur in a regular or rhythmic pattern and at a maximum rate for that specific small intestine site, despite the fact that they typically occur in an irregular manner (rhythmic segmentation). Only a small portion of the small intestine may experience rhythmic segmentation, or the segmentation may occur gradually, with each segmenting contraction happening slightly below the one before it (progressive segmentation).

A peristaltic contraction is a moving ring or wave of contraction that travels through a section of the gastrointestinal tract. It typically occurs over a short distance, around 6 cm, and moves at a speed of 1 to 2 cm per minute. This type of movement in the small intestine helps to push the contents of the intestine downward, moving one segment at a time.

A peristaltic contraction known as the "peristaltic rush" may occur over a significant portion of the small intestine when there is an inflammatory condition of the small bowel or when irritating substances are present in the intraluminal contents. Peristaltic rushes are often linked to diarrhea caused by common infections. The majority of cathartics cause diarrhea by irritating the intestinal mucosa or by increasing the contents, especially when it comes to fluids.

11.1.12.4. Absorption

The small intestine is estimated to have a total absorptive surface area of 4,500 square meters (5,400 square yards), despite only measuring 3 to 4 cm in diameter and 7 meters in length. The mucosa's distinct structure, which is arranged in concentric folds that resemble transverse ridges, provides an enormous absorptive surface. These folds, called plicae circulares, measure roughly 3 mm (0.01 inch) thick and 5 to 6 cm (2 inches) in length. The small intestine is covered in plicae circulares, with the exception of the bulb, or first part, of the duodenum, which is often smooth and flat with a few longitudinal folds. The plicae circulares, also known as valves of Kerckring, are found in the upper and lower sections of the jejunum and duodenum, respectively. As they get smaller, they eventually vanish in the lower ileum. The intestinal wall is normally circumscribed by the folds between half and two-thirds of the way; on rare occasions, a single fold may spiral the wall for three or four full turns. The number of plicae circulares in the small intestine is thought to be 800, and they multiply the outer surface area of the lining of the small intestine by five to eight times.

Villi are microscopic projections that are another characteristic of the mucosa, significantly increasing its surface area. The height of the villi typically ranges from 0.5 to 1 mm, with diameters ranging from about one-third to one-eighth of their height. The tall columnar cells that cover the villi, resembling empty goblets after releasing their contents, are referred to as goblet cells. Goblet cells, dispersed among the surface epithelial cells that cover the villi, produce mucin, the main component of mucus.

Liebkühn's glands, also known as intestinal glands, are depressions located at the base of the mucosal villi. The cells lining these glands extend over the surface of the villi and upward. Alpha granules, also known as eosinophilic granules, are found inside the epithelial cells known as Paneth cells, located at the base of the glands. They are named this way because they absorb the rose-colored stain eosin. Despite the possibility that they contain immunoglobulins and the bactericidal enzyme lysozyme, their exact purpose remains unknown.

The goblet cells indicated above, endocrine cells—which are explained below—and undifferentiated cells—which possess the capacity to change in order to replace losses of any cell type—are the other three cell types found in the Lieberkühn's glands. The undifferentiated cells in these glands are primarily responsible for secretion and cell renewal. The average lifespan of undifferentiated cells is 72 hours, after which they run out of energy and die.

Different levels of the small intestine have differing villi in terms of appearance and shape. The villi in the duodenum are large, densely packed, and often shaped like leaves. The diameter of each individual villus in the jejunum is between 110 and 135 μm, and its height ranges from 350 to 600 μm (one inch contains approximately 25,000 μm). The interior of each individual villus is composed of smooth muscle fibers, a central lattice, or channel for lymph, a rich network of blood vessels, and a variety of dispersed cells. The central lacteal is surrounded by smooth muscle cells, which perform the pumping action necessary to initiate the lymph flow out of the villus. At the tip of the villus, a tiny central arteriole, or minute artery, branches off to create a capillary network. The capillaries then empty into a collecting venule that extends to the base of the villus. The rough, specialized surface of the epithelial cells is a remarkable characteristic of the mucosal villi. In comparison to the plasma membrane on the epithelial cells at the side and base of the villus, this plasma membrane, also known as the brush border, is thicker and richer in proteins and lipids. Water and other solutes are transported through solvent drag and active transport via pores in the surface epithelium of the mucosa. In other words, solutes are transported by a flowing stream of water, which increases the solute concentration on the side of the membrane where the water originally originated. The different pore sizes in the ileum and jejunum account for the varying rates of water absorption in these two locations. The term "tight junction" refers to the contact zone that connects the enterocytes near their apex. It is believed that these junctions have closed pores at rest and dilate when absorption is required. The "fuzzy coat," a layer of glycoprotein containing partially digested nutrients, is fused to the brush border. It consists of individual microvilli that are approximately 0-1 μm in diameter and 1 μm in height. Each epithelial cell can have up to 1,000 microvilli. Due to the microvilli increasing the absorbing surface by about 25 times, they play a crucial role in the digestion and absorption of intestinal contents. The enzymes disaccharidase and peptidase, which hydrolyze polypeptides to monosaccharides and dipeptides to amino acids, respectively, are also secreted by them. Different levels of molecular receptors for specific substances are present on the surfaces of microvilli in the small intestine. This could explain the selective absorption of certain substances at specific locations, such as vitamin B12 that is bound to intrinsic factor in the terminal ileum. The selective absorption of calcium and iron in the duodenum and upper jejunum may also be explained by these receptors. Additionally, the microvillus membrane contains transport proteins that facilitate the passage of amino acids, D-glucose, and sodium ions.

Myosin is located in the brush border, while actin is found in the core of the microvillus. Since these proteins are essential for contractility, it is likely that the motor activity of the microvilli initiates the stirring and mixing processes that occur in the lumen of the small intestine.

Similar to the mucosa of the stomach, the muscularis and submucosa are located beneath the mucosa of the small intestine. The submucosa is composed of loose connective tissue and is densely packed with lymphatic and blood vessels. Brunner's glands consist of tubules that twist and branch multiple times, as well as acini, which are round sacs found in the submucosa of the duodenum. These glands secrete into the base of Lieberkühn's glands in the duodenum. While their exact function is unknown, they secrete a clear liquid that is mixed with bicarbonate, mucus, and a weak proteolytic enzyme.

Solitary nodules of lymphatic tissue are present in the submucosa of the jejunum. Peyer patches are collections of nodules in the ileum that contain more lymphatic tissue.

11.1.12.5. Secretions

The small intestine receives digestive secretions from various sources. Secretions into the small intestine are regulated by hormones and nerves, including the vagus nerve. Local mechanical or chemical stimulation of the intestinal mucous membrane is the most effective stimulus for secretion. Food particles and chyme constantly provide these stimuli in the intestine. Gastric secretions from the stomach are present in the chyme that is emptied into the duodenum and continue to be digested temporarily in the small intestine. The pancreas, a large gland that produces hormones and digestive enzymes, is one of the main sources of digestive secretions.

The pancreas empties its secretions into the duodenum through the major pancreatic duct (duct of Wirsung) in the duodenal papilla (papilla of Vater) and the accessory pancreatic duct located a few centimeters away. Pancreatic juice contains enzymes that break down carbohydrates, lipids, and proteins.

Liver secretions travel through the gallbladder and the duodenal papilla to reach the duodenum via the common bile duct.

Different sections of the intestine have slightly different sucus entericus compositions, which are mixtures of substances secreted into the small intestine. Even in the presence of stimulation, very little fluid is secreted, with the exception of the duodenum. The secretion has a higher mucus content in the duodenum, for instance, the location of the Brunner's glands. The small intestine secretes a thin, colorless or slightly straw-colored fluid that contains organic material, water, inorganic salts, and mucus particles. Other bodily fluids frequently contain inorganic salts, with a higher bicarbonate concentration than blood. Cell debris and enzymes, such as a pepsin-like protease (found only in the duodenum), an enzyme called lipase, an amylase, two or more peptidases, sucrase, maltase, enterokinase, alkaline phosphatase, nucleophosphatases, and nucleocytases, make up the organic matter aside from mucus.

11.1.13. Large Intestine

The fluids emptied into it from the small intestine are stored in the large intestine, also known as the colon. At 150 cm (5 feet), it is less than one-quarter the length of the small intestine, but it has a much larger diameter than the small intestine (approximately 2.5 cm, or 1 inch, as opposed to 6 cm, or 3 inches, in the large intestine). The colon's main purposes are to absorb water, store feces until they can be expelled by defecation, and maintain the blood's osmolality, or solute level, by excreting and absorbing electrolytes—substances like sodium and chloride that take on an electrical charge in solution. Additionally, the large intestine secretes mucus, which facilitates the passage of intestinal contents through the bowel and helps to lubricate them. About 1.5 to 2 liters (or roughly 2 quarts) of chyme flow through the ileocecal valve, which divides the small and large intestines, each day. By absorption in the colon, the chyme is reduced to about 150 ml (5 fluid ounces). The remaining indigestible material, dead bacteria, sloughed-off mucosal cells, and food remnants that the bacteria were unable to break down make up the feces (Figure 11.8).

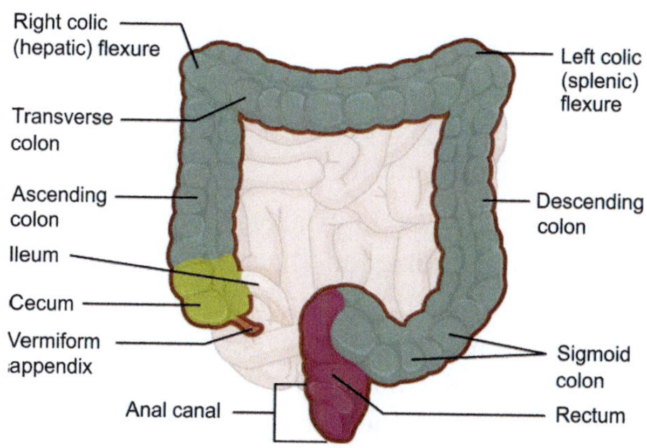

Figure 11.8. *Structures of the human large intestine, rectum, and anus.*

Source: https://courses.lumenlearning.com/suny-ap2/chapter/the-small-and-large-intestines/.

The mucosa of the large intestine is punctuated with numerous crypts that absorb water and are lined with mucus-secreting goblet cells. At the lower end of the rectum, the circular and longitudinal muscle layers terminate in the internal and external anal sphincters.

Additionally, the colon houses a significant amount of bacteria that produce niacin, thiamin, and vitamin K, which are vital for various metabolic processes and the proper functioning of the central nervous system.

11.1.13.1. Anatomy

The large intestine is composed of five main parts: the cecum, ascending colon, transverse colon, descending colon, and sigmoid colon. The cecum, located in the right iliac fossa, serves as the first part of the large intestine. It is connected to the ileum, the terminal portion of the small intestine, by the ileocecal valve. The circular muscle fibers of the ileum and cecum combine to form the circular sphincter muscle of the ileocecal valve.

The ascending colon extends from the cecum, at the level of the ileocecal valve, to the hepatic flexure. The hepatic flexure is a bend in the colon situated behind and beneath the right lobe of the liver, in contact with the right kidney and the posterior abdominal wall. The ascending colon is surrounded by the peritoneum, except for its posterior surface.

The location of the transverse colon varies, primarily depending on the distention of the stomach. However, it is typically found in the subcostal plane or at the level of the tenth rib. The transverse colon ascends to the splenic flexure, a bend on the left side of the abdomen that may cause indentation of the spleen. A peritoneal fold connects the transverse colon to the diaphragm, opposite the 11th rib.

The descending colon travels to the iliac crest, which is the upper border of the hipbone, via the left side of the posterior abdominal wall, the left kidney, and downwards. The peritoneum is more likely to encircle the descending colon than the ascending colon.

It is customary to separate the iliac and pelvic portions of the sigmoid colon. The iliac colon extends from the inner border of the psoas muscle, located in the left iliac fossa, to the crest of the ilium, or upper border of the hipbone. The peritoneum typically covers the iliac colon, just like it does the descending colon. The pelvic colon is situated in the true pelvis, which is the lower portion of the pelvis. It forms one or two loops, bending back and sharply turning downward at the midline to become the rectum, and reaching across to the right side of the pelvis.

There are clear distinctions between the layers that comprise the wall of the colon and the small intestine, but there are also some similarities. The colon's external aspect is distinct from the small intestine's due to characteristics referred to as the haustra, appendices epiploicae, and taeniae. The taeniae are three lengthy, uniformly spaced longitudinal muscle bands that measure one centimeter in width around the colon's circumference. There is a thin layer of longitudinal muscle fibers in between the thick bands of taeniae. Due to the fact that the taeniae are marginally shorter than the large intestine, the intestinal wall contracts, creating what are known as haustra, or circular furrows, that vary in depth. Beneath the covering membrane are collections of fatty tissue known as the appendices epiploicae. They typically form two rows on the transverse colon, but one row on the ascending and descending colon.

The inner surface of the colon lacks the plicae circulares and villi found in the small intestine. Instead, it is lined with crypts that contain mucous glands and goblet cells. While there are numerous isolated lymphatic nodules, Peyer patches are absent. The colonic mucosa is characterized by deep tubular pits that become deeper towards the rectum.

Contraction of the inner layer of the large intestine's muscle tightly coils around the colon, compartmentalizing the lumen and its contents. In contrast, the outer layer follows a loose, undulating course. When this muscle contracts, the contents of the colon move both forward and backward. These muscle actions are influenced by the contents, particularly the amount of undigested fiber.

11.1.13.2. Blood and Nerve Supply

The hypogastric branch of the internal iliac artery, which supplies blood to the pelvic walls and viscera, the genital organs, the buttocks, and the inside of the thighs, along with the superior and inferior mesenteric arteries, both of which are branches of the abdominal aorta, provide the arterial blood supply to the large intestine. These vessels form a continuous row of arches that lead into the large intestine. Similar to the venous arches formed by arteries, venous blood is drained from the colon through branches, which eventually empty into the inferior and superior mesenteric veins, ultimately forming the portal vein by joining the splenic vein. The innervation of the large intestine is similar to that of the small intestine.

11.1.13.3. Contractions and Motility

Contraction and motility of the large intestine are facilitated by local contractions and retrograde propulsions, ensuring good contact with the mucosa and mixing of the contents. Colonic motility is promoted by factors such as mastication, fat, unabsorbed bile salts, bile acids, and the peptide hormones gastrotine and cholecystokinin. On the other hand, motility is inhibited by hormones like secretin, glucagon, and vasoactive intestinal peptide. Compared to the small intestine, the muscles of the colon exhibit more intricate electrical activity. The rectum and the lower (distal) half of the colon differ from the basic rhythmic movements of the colon. Slow-wave activity generates 11 cycles per minute, causing contractions to move from the ascending colon to the descending colon, while the sigmoid colon and rectum exhibit six cycles per minute of slow-wave activity. Local contractions of the colon move at a rate of 4 cm (1.66 inches) per second in a distal direction. Retrograde movements, on the other hand, predominantly occur in the proximal (upper) colon.

11.1.14. Rectum and Anus

The midsacrum, the triangular bone located between the two hipbones and near the base of the spine, is where the rectum begins. The rectum is a continuation of the sigmoid colon and it ends in a widened section called the rectal ampulla. In males, the rectal ampulla is in contact with the posterior vaginal wall, while in females, it is in contact with the rear surface of the prostate. The rectal ampulla is situated posteriorly, in front of the coccyx, which is a small bone at the base of the spine.

The rectum is covered by peritoneum only on its sides and front. The peritoneum, which is a fold of tissue that connects the colon to the back wall of the abdomen and pelvis (known as the mesocolon), disappears at the end of the pelvic colon. As the rectum descends, it gradually loses the peritoneal covering on its sides until only the front remains covered. The anterior peritoneal covering is also folded back onto the vagina, prostate, and bladder, approximately 7.5 cm (3 inches) from the anus.

Colic taeniae spread out to form a broad external longitudinal muscle coat near the end of the sigmoid colon and the start of the rectum. Muscle fibers of the circular and longitudinal coats often intermingle at the bottom of the rectum. The thick, rounded internal anal sphincter muscle marks the termination of the internal circular muscle coat. The smooth muscle fibers of the rectum merge with the striated muscle fibers of the levator ani, also known as the pelvic diaphragm, a broad muscle that comprises the pelvic floor. The second sphincter, known as the external anal sphincter, consists of striated muscle and is composed of the subcutaneous, superficial, and deep external sphincters. The external sphincters are innervated by the pudendal nerves and are under somatic (voluntary) control, while the internal sphincters are composed of smooth muscle and are innervated by the autonomic nervous system.

Similar to the mucosal lining of the sigmoid colon, the rectum's mucosa becomes thicker and more vascularized, particularly in the lower rectum. Arterial blood supply to the rectum and anus is provided by the right and left internal iliac arteries, as well as branches from the inferior mesenteric artery. The internal and external hemorrhoidal veins form an extensive network of veins that drain blood from the anal canal and rectum.

The rectal ampulla contains two or three sizable, crescent-shaped folds that are referred to as rectal valves. The circular muscle and submucosa invaginate, or infold, to form these valves. A few centimeters above the pectinate line—the point where the squamous mucous membrane of the lower rectum and the skin lining the lower portion of the anal canal meet—the columnar epithelium of the rectal mucosa, innervated by the autonomic nervous system, changes to the stratified squamous (scalelike) type, innervated by the peripheral nerves.

A mass peristaltic movement moves the accumulated feces from the colon's descending and sigmoid sectors once or twice every 24 hours. The urge to defecate arises when the rectum, which is normally empty, becomes filled with gas, liquid, or solid to the point where the intraluminal pressure rises to a particular level.

At the point where the rectum and the anal canal converge, the musculus puborectalis creates a sling and is always taut. As a result, the lower rectum becomes angular, which prevents the lumens of the rectum and the anal canal from being continuous—a condition necessary for continence. When the distal and pelvic colon's longitudinal muscles contract and the sling of muscle relaxes, continuity between the lumina of the two sectors is restored. The distal colon shortens as a result, elevating the pelvic colon and eliminating the angle it normally forms with the rectum. The passage's straightening and shortening makes evacuation easier.

The voluntary effort required to precede the act of defecation likely results in stimuli that amplify the visceral reflexes, though these primarily stem from the distension of the rectum. Defecation reflex control centers are located in the ganglionic plexus of the colon, two areas of the spinal cord, and the brain's hypothalamus. These reflexes cause the internal anal sphincter to relax.

11.1.15. Liver

The liver is the largest and most complexly functioning gland in the body. The liver's primary roles include participating in the metabolism of fat, protein, and carbohydrates; synthesizing bile acids and cholesterol; initiating the formation of bile; conducting bilirubin transport; metabolizing and transporting specific drugs; and regulating the movement and storage of carbohydrates (Figure 11.9).

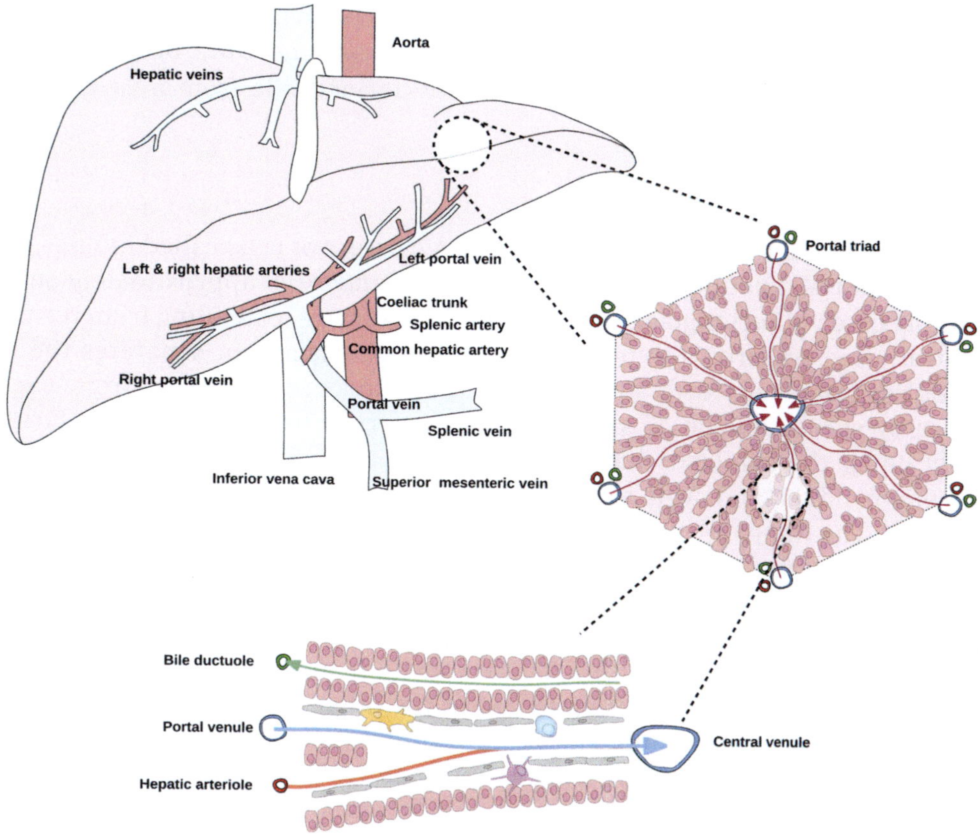

Figure 11.9. *Human liver.*

Source: By Gwilz – Own work, CC BY-SA 4.0, https://commons.wikimedia.org/w/index.php?curid=99416651.

11.1.15.1. Gross Anatomy

Located under the lower right rib cage, the liver occupies a significant portion of the upper right abdomen, extending slightly into the upper left quadrant. Typically weighing between 1.2 and 1.6 kg (2.6 to 3.5 pounds), the liver tends to be larger in men than in women. Its measurements can vary, with a horizontal range of 20 to 22 cm, a vertical extension of 15 to 18 cm, and a thickness ranging from 10 to 13 cm. Divided into a larger right lobe and a smaller left lobe, the liver is connected to the diaphragm by the falciform ligament on its anterior side and by the teres ligament on its inferior side. The organ is enveloped by a protective tissue capsule, part of which connects to the parietal peritoneum lining the walls of the abdomen and diaphragm.

The liver receives blood from two sources: the hepatic artery, which carries fully oxygenated blood from the celiac axis, and the portal vein, which receives partially oxygenated blood from various organs including the spleen, pancreas, and gastrointestinal tract. These blood vessels enter the liver through the portal hepatis on its inferior surface, anatomically separating the quadrate and caudate lobes. The portal vein is formed by the convergence of the splenic vein and the superior mesenteric vein. At the porta hepatis, the portal vein divides into two major branches, each supplying blood to one of the main lobes of the liver. The porta hepatis is also the exit point for the hepatic ducts. These ducts represent the final stage in a network of smaller bile ductules distributed throughout the liver, which transport newly formed bile from liver cells to the small intestine through the biliary tract.

11.1.15.2. Microscopic Anatomy

The liver's microscopic structure, composed of uniform clusters of cells called lobules, is where the liver performs its essential functions. Each lobule, with a diameter of approximately one millimeter, consists of multiple cords of rectangular liver cells, or hepatocytes, extending from terminal hepatic venules, or central veins, towards a thin layer of connective tissue that separates the lobule from neighboring lobules. Liver cell cords are one cell thick and are separated from each other on multiple surfaces by spaces known as sinusoids, also referred to as hepatic capillaries. The thin endothelial cells lining the sinusoids have apertures through which the hepatocytes' finger-like projections, or microvilli, extend. This allows the hepatocytes to directly access the bloodstream within the sinusoids. The Kuppfer cell, the other major cell of the liver, attaches itself to the sinusoid wall and extends into its lumen. It functions as a phagocyte, engulfing and killing other cells or foreign objects. Tiny gaps, known as Disse spaces, exist between the sinusoidal endothelium and the hepatocyte, most likely for lymphatic transport. Hepatocytes are connected to each other on adjacent surfaces by dense, tight junctions. These junctions are punctured by tiny passageways called canaliculi, which serve as the terminal ends of the biliary system and collect bile from the hepatocyte. The hepatic duct, eventually emerging from the porta hepatis, is formed when these canaliculi unite with additional canaliculi to form progressively larger bile ducts (Figure 11.10).

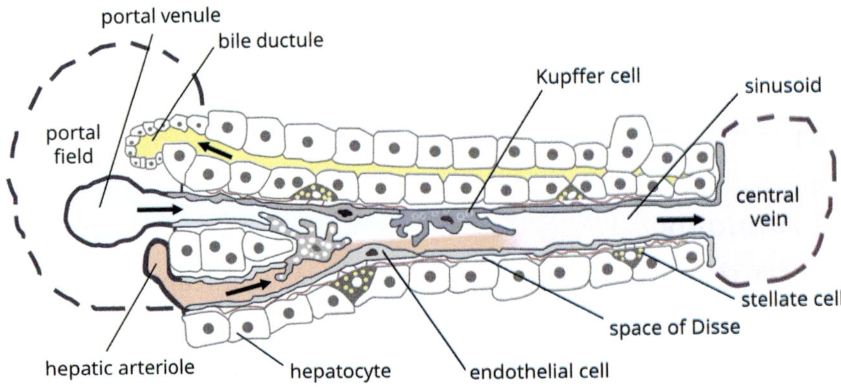

Figure 11.10. *Microscopic structure of the human liver.*

Source: By Originally by Frevert, U., Engelmann, S., Zougbédé, S., Stange, J., Ng, B., et al. Converted to SVG by Viacheslav Vtyurin who was hired to do so by User:Eug. – Based on the research article "Intravital Observation of Plasmodium berghei Sporozoite Infection of the Liver," PLoS Biology, doi:10.1371/journal.pbio.0030192.g011, CC BY 2.5, https://commons.wikimedia.org/w/index.php?curid=14388642.

Liver cells, or hepatocytes, have direct access to the liver's blood supply through small capillaries called sinusoids. Hepatocytes carry out many metabolic functions, including the production of bile. Kupffer cells line the liver's vascular system; they play a role in blood formation and the destruction of cellular debris. Hepatocytes constitute approximately 80% of the liver's volume. The cytoplasm of these cells, located around the nucleus, contains numerous mitochondria that provide the necessary energy for the liver cell's various metabolic and synthetic processes. The cytoplasm also contains the endoplasmic reticulum, a network of elongated tubules that house numerous enzymes essential for liver function. Some of the endoplasmic reticulum's membranes have a granular or rough appearance due to the presence of ribosomes. These ribosomes are responsible for synthesizing specific polypeptide (protein) chains by removing the amino group (deamination) and converting it into glucose through gluconeogenesis. Gluconeogenesis produces ammonia, which hepatocytes convert to urea using the urea cycle. The liver's vital processes, such as drug and hormone metabolism, as well as cholesterol synthesis, are carried out by cytochromes. Cytochromes are combinations of heme from hemoglobin and various proteins, along with specific enzymes found in the nonribosomal, or smooth, endoplasmic reticulum. Furthermore, hepatocytes conjugate with fat-soluble metabolic and foreign substances, including the carbohydrate components of bilirubin, resulting in their solubility in water. The byproduct of hemoglobin metabolism, bilirubin, is created in lymphatic and bone marrow tissue before being bound to plasma albumin and transported to the liver. It is secreted at the hepatocytic sinusoidal membrane and then transported to the smooth endoplasmic reticulum, where it combines with glucuronic acid molecules to become water-soluble and is excreted in bile. The Golgi apparatus, located between the endoplasmic reticulum and the canaliculus, serves as a transfer point for newly synthesized proteins and other products before they are sent to other parts of the cell or expelled from the cell. Lysosomes, an essential part of the cytoplasm, store pigments like iron and copper and aid in the breakdown of substances like glycogen or foreign particles. The nucleus of the hepatocyte controls cell reproduction and transfers genetic information in the form of messenger ribonucleic acid (mRNA) from deoxyribonucleic acid (DNA) to organelles in the cytoplasm.

11.1.16. Biliary Tract

11.1.16.1. Anatomy

The right and left hepatic ducts, two sizable ducts that split two lobes on the right side of the liver, emerge at the porta hepatis, marking the beginning of the biliary tract. These 1 to 2 cm (roughly half an inch) ducts come together just below the porta hepatis to form the hepatic duct. This duct then travels another 2 to 3 cm before joining the cystic duct, which originates from the gallbladder. The resulting common bile duct descends through the pancreatic head. The hepatopancreatic ampulla (ampulla of Vater), which is located in the wall of the inner curve of the descending duodenum, is where it is typically joined by the main pancreatic duct (duct of Wirsung). It ends in the lumen of the duodenum at a 2- to 3-cm elevation known as the duodenal papilla (papilla of Vater) (Figure 11.11).

The average length of the common bile duct is approximately 10 cm. Bile flow into the intestine is regulated by the hepatopancreatic sphincter, also known as the sphincter of Oddi. The cystic duct, ranging from 2 to 3 cm in length, ends in the gallbladder which can hold about 50 ml of fluid. The cystic duct is lined with a spiral mucosal elevation called the valve of Heister. The gallbladder is usually situated partially beneath the right lobe of the liver.

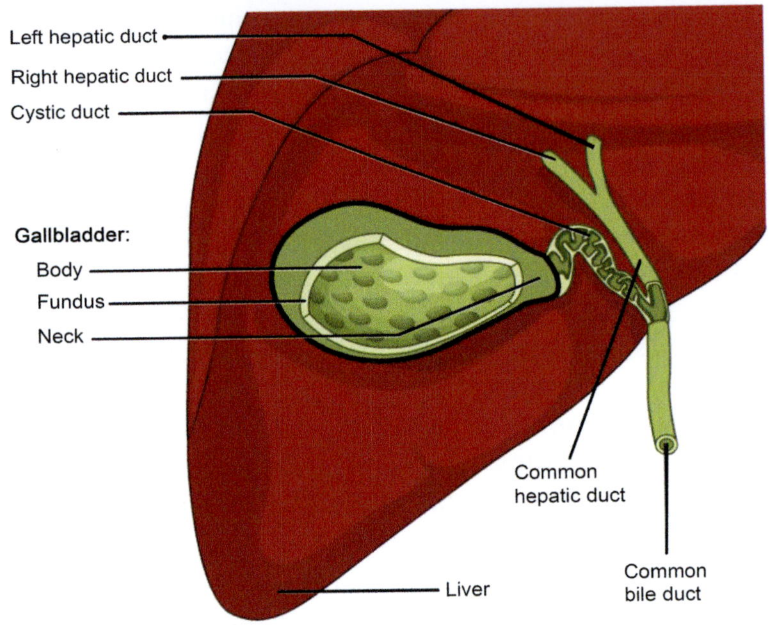

Figure 11.11. *The gallbladder and bile ducts in situ.*

Source: https://courses.lumenlearning.com/suny-ap2/chapter/accessory-organs-in-digestion-the-liver-pancreas-and-gallbladder/.

11.1.17. Bile

Bile's principal role in digestion is to facilitate fat breakdown and dispersion in the lumen of the small intestine. The formation of bile first occurs in the hepatocyte, or liver cell, and the secretion rate of bile acids into the bile canaliculi, or bile channels, largely governs this process. However, there are other factors that influence bile flow in addition to the secretion of bile acids. Specifically, it appears to depend on the secretion of sodium by the hepatocyte and is also partially regulated by intestinal hormones such as secretin, cholecystokinin (CCK), and gastrin.

Almost the entire bile acid pool, which amounts to approximately 3 grams (0.01 ounce) at any given time, is stored in the gallbladder as a reserve. Hepatic bile undergoes concentration during its passage through the biliary tract, reducing its initial volume to as little as one-tenth. This concentration is achieved through the selective reabsorption of bicarbonate, chloride, and water. Since the gallbladder is primarily responsible for this concentration process, the bile that is expelled from this organ is considerably thicker and darker than the bile that is expelled from the liver, due to the higher concentration of pigments.

When the duodenum becomes distended, particularly after consuming a meal containing fat, the hormone CCK is secreted. This hormone triggers the contraction of the muscular layer of the gallbladder.

In addition to inorganic ions such as sodium, potassium, calcium, magnesium, chloride, and bicarbonate, bile also includes protein and bilirubin. The latter gives bile its dark amber color in concentrate and golden color in diluted solutions. Bile is highest in cholesterol, phospholipids (mainly phosphatidyl choline or lecithin), and bile acids, which are produced from hepatocyte cholesterol. Four-ringed sterols like cholesterol are produced by the liver and intestinal lining or absorbed from food. Normally insoluble in aqueous secretions, cholesterol is transported in bile as colloidal solutions consisting of mixed aggregates of complexes with lecithin and bile acids. Cholesterol crystallizes when there is insufficient lecithin and bile acid present. The liver produces chenodeoxycholic acid and cholic acid, two forms of primary bile acid, from cholesterol. Bacterial action in the lower intestine dehydroxylates (removes one of the hydroxyl groups from) cholic acid, resulting in deoxycholic acid. As a result of being absorbed from the intestine and returned to the liver, this secondary bile acid is visible in bile. In the intestine, chenodeoxycholic acid is likewise dehydroxylated to form lithocholic acid, a trace amount of which is reabsorbed and manifests as normal bile.

11.1.18. Pancreas

The pancreas is an elongated, slender gland that resides posterior to the spleen and stomach, spanning horizontally across the upper abdomen. The inferior vena cava, the abdominal aorta, and the vertebral column come into contact with the central portion of the pancreas (Figure 11.12).

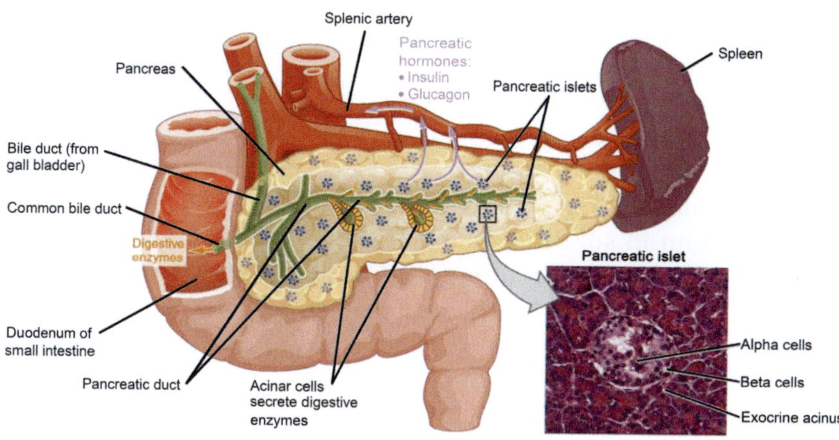

Figure 11.12. *Structures of the human pancreas.*

Source: https://courses.lumenlearning.com/suny-ap2/chapter/the-endocrine-pancreas/.

Acinar cells produce digestive enzymes, which are secreted into tiny ducts that feed into the pancreatic duct. Islets of Langerhans are clusters of cells that secrete hormones such as insulin and glucagon directly into a capillary network, which also joins the pancreatic duct.

An endocrine (ductless) and exocrine (ductal) gland, the pancreas serves both functions. The endocrine tissue, located in the islets of Langerhans, produces at least two crucial hormones (glucagon and insulin) that regulate carbohydrate metabolism. On the other hand, the exocrine tissue, also known as acinar tissue, produces significant digestive enzyme precursors that are transported to the small intestine. The pancreas also produces two additional hormones, somatostatin and vasoactive intestinal polypeptide, which play critical roles in regulating intestinal secretion and motility.

Each acinar cell has a truncated pyramid shape and is arranged around a central ductal lumen. These central ducts empty into larger intercalated and collecting ducts, which eventually connect to the pancreatic duct (duct of Wirsung). The pancreatic duct then enters the hepatopancreatic ampulla (ampulla of Vater) of the duodenum, where it is often joined by the common bile duct in approximately 80% of cases. Occasionally, the junction with the common bile duct is proximal to the ampulla, and in a few instances, the pancreatic duct and common bile duct connect to the duodenum separately.

11.1.18.1. Acinar Cells

Over 95% of the cellular population of the exocrine pancreas is composed of acinar cells. Within the intestine, these cells generate a variety of digestive proteins, or enzymes, primarily involved in the breakdown of dietary proteins (lipases), fats (lipases), and carbohydrates (amylases). Additional protein secretions include a trypsin inhibitor, a "stone protein" that maintains calcium in solution, as well as various serum proteins such as albumin and immunoglobulins.

The majority of enzymatic proteins in the acinar cells are synthesized on ribosomes from amino acids that are transported to the pancreas via the bloodstream. The Golgi apparatus then modifies enzyme precursors, which are subsequently concentrated into membrane-wrapped zymogen granules that are stored in the cytoplasm prior to secretion. The release of enzymatic secretions is mediated by stimulants such as cholecystokinin (CCK), which is released in response to the presence of dietary fat, amino acids, hydrochloric acid, and acetylcholine. Acetylcholine is produced in response to the sensory aspects of feeding, as well as the physical effects of chewing and swallowing. Secretin, on the other hand, is a hormone released from the duodenum upon the introduction of gastric acid.

The zymogen granules migrate to the apex of the acinar cell and are extruded into the central ductal lumen upon binding of specific receptor sites on the acinar membrane with CCK or acetylcholine. Acinar cells and small ductal cells produce more bicarbonate, sodium, water, and enzymes when acinar receptors are bound by vasoactive intestinal polypeptide or secretin. As a result, the actively secreting pancreas secretes bicarbonate in place of chloride and sodium in place of hydrogen, leading to an increase in the acidity of the blood. Bicarbonate and enzymes are produced by the acinar cells when bound by CCK.

When CCK and acetylcholine are lacking, as in the case of fasting individuals or patients receiving intravenous nutrition, the acinar cells produce significantly less zymogen. After the pituitary gland is removed, pancreatic atrophy also occurs, most likely as a result of the lack of growth hormone. Therefore, pancreatotrophic, or pancreas-feeding, hormones include growth hormone, acetylcholine, and CCK. It appears that the pancreas secretes an unidentified hormone that provides nutrition, or trophic support, to the liver.

11.1.18.2. Islet Cells

Alpha (or A), beta (or B), and delta (or D) are the names of the three different types of islet cells that make up approximately 2% of the pancreatic mass. About 20–35% of islet cells are alpha, 75–75% are beta, and 5% are delta. Beta cell granules contain insulin, which has the opposite effects of glucagon and causes the liver to break down glycogen and raise blood glucose levels. Alpha cell granules only contain glucagon. Somatostatin, which is present in delta cell granules, inhibits the release of insulin and glucagon.

11.2. Features of the Gastrointestinal Tract

11.2.1. General Features of Digestion and Absorption

Digestive products are absorbed through four different pathways: endocytosis, passive diffusion, facilitated diffusion, and active transport. Active transport occurs when a material is moved through the absorbing cell's membrane in opposition to an electrical or chemical gradient. This process is carrier-mediated, meaning that the substance is momentarily bound to another substance, transported through the cell membrane, and then released. Energy is required for active transport, and it can be inhibited by other substances through competitive inhibition, where molecules with similar structures compete for the carrier's binding site.

Passive diffusion, on the other hand, does not require energy or a carrier. Assisted diffusion, also known as facilitated diffusion, does not require energy either, but it involves a protein molecule called a carrier that is located outside the cell membrane. The carrier binds to the material to be transported and facilitates its movement into the cell. There may be a competitive barrier for the carrier.

When the substance to be absorbed crosses the cell membrane and is taken into the interior of the cell, this process is known as endocytosis.

The duodenum, despite being the shortest part of the small intestine, plays a crucial role in the process of food absorption. The jejunum, located in the middle section, is where food absorption occurs most frequently. In addition to gastric acid-saturated chyme, the duodenum receives secretions from the pancreas and liver. In the duodenum, the intestinal contents are adjusted to be isotonic with blood plasma, ensuring that the pressures and volumes of the intestinal contents are equal to those of blood plasma. This equilibrium prevents water loss or gain for the cells on either side of the barrier.

The stomach secretes acid, which is then neutralized by the pancreas' bicarbonate. This process brings the intestinal contents to the ideal pH, allowing the digestive enzymes to function efficiently on their substrates. Several key gastrointestinal hormones regulate pancreatic secretion, gastric emptying, gallbladder contraction, and stomach secretion. These hormones, along with neural impulses from the autonomic nervous system, provide the autoregulatory mechanisms for regular digestive processes.

The small intestine efficiently absorbs most salts, minerals, and water. Sodium absorption is an active process that requires metabolic energy from epithelial cells in the mucosa. This process transports sodium from the intestinal lumen across the mucosa against concentration and electrochemical gradients. Sodium ions are more easily absorbed from the jejunum compared to other parts of the small intestine. Chloride is also absorbed in the small intestine, likely due to the absorption of sodium.

Approximately 5% of sodium is absorbed at the same rate as potassium. Potassium is believed to diffuse through the intestinal mucosa either passively or with the assistance of water absorption. It appears that the absorption of electrolytes, substances that dissociate into ions in a solution, occurs prior to water absorption. While this process primarily occurs in the jejunum, water is absorbed throughout the entire small intestine. Water can freely flow through the intestinal mucosa in both directions, but it tends to flow towards the hypertonic solution, which is the solution with a net flow of water, and away from the hypotonic solution. Consequently, if the contents of the lumen are hypotonic, water quickly flows from the lumen to the blood. Conversely, if the contents are hypertonic, water enters the intestinal lumen from the blood at a faster rate. This two-way water flow helps maintain the intestinal contents in an isotonic state.

11.2.2. Digestion and Absorption of Specific Nutrients

11.2.2.1. Carbohydrates

Carbohydrates are broken down into monosaccharides such as glucose, fructose, and galactose, or disaccharides such as sucrose, lactose, maltose, and dextrin. These simpler molecules are obtained by breaking down complex carbohydrates known as polysaccharides. The main polysaccharide in the diet is amylose, which constitutes 20% of carbohydrate intake. Amylose consists of a linear chain of glucose molecules linked together, while the majority of starch is amylopectin, which contains branched chains linked at intervals along the main chain.

Salivary amylase partially breaks down starch, while pancreatic amylase rapidly breaks down starch in the duodenum. However, the effect of this enzyme on the branched chains of amylopectin and the linkages within cellulose molecules is negligible. This explains why humans are unable to digest cellulose. Pancreatic juice contains various types of amylase, which hydrolyze complex carbohydrates into disaccharides and trisaccharides, as well as amylopectins into dextrins. The disaccharidase enzymes lactase, maltase, sucrase, and trehalase are located in the brush border (composed of ultrafine microvilli) and the surface membrane of the epithelial enterocytes. They hydrolyze maltose and dextrins to produce the monosaccharides glucose, galactose, and fructose. The liver cell combines glucose with phosphate to form glycogen, a complex polysaccharide that is either stored in the hepatocyte for metabolic use or transported to peripheral tissues as one of the two monosaccharide components of table sugar (sucrose) and milk sugar (lactose). For these conversions and the translation of other dietary monosaccharides (fructose from sucrose and galactose from lactose) into glucose, the hepatocyte possesses specific enzyme systems. By the process of gluconeogenesis, the hepatocyte, or liver cell, is also capable of converting some amino acids and the byproducts of glucose metabolism, such as lactate and pyruvate, into glucose.

While glucose and galactose are transported by an energy-consuming process that likely involves binding to a particular protein carrier with sodium ions attached, fructose appears to be absorbed by simple diffusion. The sugar is released inside the enterocyte, sodium is pumped out, and the sugars then diffuse into the circulation along a concentration gradient.

11.2.2.2. Proteins

In order to digest protein, the complex molecule must first be broken down into peptides, each of which has a number of amino acids, and then into individual amino acids. The pepsins are digestive enzymes that the stomach secretes when it senses acidity. This process is known as proteolysis. About 10% to 15% of the digestion of proteins is done by the pepsins. Their peak activity occurs during the first hour of digestion, and their capacity to digest protein is limited by the need for an acidic pH range of 1 to 3. Since trypsins, which are proteolytic enzymes secreted by the pancreas, are far more potent than pepsins, the duodenum and upper jejunum are where most protein digestion takes place. Therefore, protein digestion is typically not hampered even after the stomach is completely removed.

Protease precursors that are inactive in pancreatic secretion can become active by interacting with enterokinase, an enzyme secreted from the microvillous part of the enterocytes in the duodenal and jejunal mucosa. Enterokinase, which is released from duodenal lining cells by the action of bile acids and CCK, activates trypsinogen in the intestine. The cleavage of six terminal amino acid residues from trypsinogen causes trypsin to activate. Free trypsin acts as an activator for the other proteases. These proteases ultimately reduce dietary proteins to single amino acids and small polypeptide chains of two to six amino acids. Chymotrypsin, elastase, and other pancreatic proteases are all activated by trypsin. Known as endopeptidases, trypsin, chymotrypsin, and elastase are in charge of the first hydrolysis that breaks down protein chains into peptides. The subsequent process involves the hydrolysis of these peptides into smaller molecules and ultimately individual amino acids, which is catalyzed by the pancreatic enzyme carboxypeptidases.

Peptidase activity initiates in the mucus and brush border, located outside the enterocytes, and continues within the cell. It appears that various peptidases are involved in the different stages of protein breakdown into amino acids. Similarly, distinct transport mechanisms are involved in the movement of different peptides. A carrier protein participates in an energy-demanding process that transfers dipeptides—peptides that hydrolyze to release two amino acids—and tripeptides—peptides that hydrolyze to release three amino acids—from the surface brush border into the cell. Consequently, small peptides containing only a few amino acids are directly absorbed. The enterocyte is where the majority of peptide breakdown into amino acids occurs. It is interesting to note that small peptides are absorbed more rapidly than amino acids. In fact, the specific mechanism governing amino acid absorption remains largely unknown. It is well established that while some amino acids share a single transport system, others have unique ones. The classification of amino acids by a group can be based on their optical rotatory properties, specifically their ability to rotate polarized light in terms of reactivity, acidity (pH), and whether they rotate to the left (levorotatory) or to the right (dextrorotatory). Levorotatory amino acids are absorbed much more quickly compared to dextrorotatory amino acids. Levorotatory amino acids are actually absorbed practically as fast as they are liberated from proteins or peptides. The active transport of neutral amino acids depends on specific structural arrangements; if these arrangements are disrupted, active transport will not occur. The rate of transportation of basic amino acids, which are acidic (pH greater than 7), is only 5–10% of that of neutral levorotatory amino acids.

11.2.2.3. Fats

Triglycerides are the primary form of stored fat in diets. For fat to be transported from the intestinal lumen to the absorptive cells, it must be soluble in water. Numerous elements, including the triglycerides' long fatty acid chains, are crucial in determining this solubility. Triglycerides are insoluble in water and consist of three long chains of fatty acids (LCFA) linked to a glycerol framework. The remaining fats are medium-chain triglycerides (MCT), which the small intestine's mucosa can absorb whole. Phospholipase, esterase, colipase, and lipase are among the lipases that break down MCTs into free monoglycerides and medium-chain fatty acids (MCFA), which are more water-soluble than LCFAs and flow through cells swiftly before entering the portal circulation and ultimately reaching the liver. Before fat can be digested to its best potential, lipases need bile acids to form micellar solutions in the intestinal lumen.

The pancreatic enzyme lipase targets the long-chain fatty acids that are linked to triglycerides. One of the three fatty acid chains remains attached to the glycerol after the other two break off (forming a monoglyceride). Pancreatic lipase, however, is not active when there is an excess of bile salt present. There may be lipase in gastric juice, but it cannot break down MCFAs and LCFAs because there isn't much small-chain fatty acid in food. As a result, the stomach does not digest much. Lipase, an additional pancreatic enzyme, binds to the bile salts, freeing lipase to attack the triglycerides. These splitting processes produce monoglycerides, which unite to form a complex known as a micelle. Water solubility of fat components is made possible by the micelle. The micelle is formed with bile salts arranged around the outside with hydrophobic ends facing inside and hydrophobic fatty acids, monoglycerides, phospholipids, and cholesterol, as well as the fat-soluble vitamins A, D, E, and K, in the center. This is because bile salts have a hydrophobic, or water-repelling, and a hydrophilic, or water-attracting, region.

The "unstirred" layer is a layer of fluid that covers the surface cells of the small intestine mucosa. The micelles must pass through this layer to reach the cell membranes. The rate of diffusion through the undisturbed layer is determined by the gradient in concentrations of the different components of the transport system from the intestinal lumen to the cell membrane, as well as the thickness of the layer. Below the unstirred layer lies the "fuzzy coat," a glycoprotein layer primarily composed of mucus. The brush border on the surface of the cell membrane is visible beneath the fuzzy coat. Due to their solubility in lipids, fatty acids and monoglycerides can easily permeate the two lipid layers. After passing the brush border and fuzzy coat, the micelle enters the cells of the intestinal lining tissues. A carrier protein absorbs the fatty acids and monoglycerides and transports them to the endoplasmic reticulum, a tubular structure filled with enzymes located inside the cell, while the micelle breaks down and the bile salts return to the lumen. At this stage, an enzyme called acyltransferase acts as a catalyst to regenerate the triglyceride.

Triglycerides travel to the Golgi apparatus membrane, which is another tubular structure, where they are encapsulated into vesicles known as chylomicrons. These vesicles have a spherical shape with a phospholipid-and/or apoprotein-coated exterior and a completely triglyceride interior, with the exception of a trace amount of cholesterol. The chylomicrons then move towards the cell membrane, traverse it, and are drawn towards the lacteals, which are the fine branches of the lymphatic system. From there, the chylomicrons proceed to the thoracic duct. The entire absorption process, from the creation of micelles to the exit of the cells and entry into the lacteals, takes approximately 10 to 15 minutes.

Pancreatic lipase converts medium-chain triglycerides into medium-chain fatty acids. These water-soluble fatty acids easily dissolve into the micelles. Eventually, they traverse the enterocyte's membrane, enter the capillary branches of the portal vein, and ultimately reach the liver.

When hepatic glucose and glycogen stores are depleted or unavailable for metabolic use (as in diabetic ketoacidosis), the liver metabolizes fat by converting stored fatty acids to their energy-releasing form, acetyl coenzyme A (acetyl CoA). When carbohydrates, protein, or fat exceed the liver's glycogen needs or the tissues' glucose needs, the liver also contributes to the synthesis of storage fats, or triglycerides. Additionally, the liver synthesizes lipoproteins, which are proteins that transport lipids in the blood, such as fats, cholesterol, and phospholipids, which are components of cell membranes.

11.2.2.4. Fat-Soluble Vitamins

Fat-soluble vitamins enter the lymphatic system with chylomicrons. Before entering the chylomicron, vitamin A, initially present as the precursor beta-carotene, is converted to retinol, which is then combined with fatty acids. Vitamins D and D3 passively diffuse into the chylomicron. In cases of biliary tract obstruction leading to jaundice, the intestine loses its supply of bile salts, compromising vitamin K absorption and increasing the risk of bleeding. Eggs contain a mixture of tocopherols, a form of vitamin E produced by plants like wheat, soybeans, and corn (maize). Along with other lipids in the micelle, it is transported through the enterocyte and finally stored in the liver.

11.2.2.5. Calcium

Calcium is necessary for the synthesis of bone, as it is a component of the material that holds neighboring cell walls together. Additionally, it is essential for the excitability of muscle and nerve cells, enabling them to respond to stimuli. The primary sources of calcium include dairy products and milk, where it is bound to proteins, as well as vegetables, where it is bound to oxalates (the salt of oxalic acid) and phytates (phytotic acid).

The conditions in the lumen of the small intestine have a significant impact on calcium absorption. The duodenum absorbs the majority of the calcium, which is converted to a salt by the stomach's acid secretion. The ileum precipitates any unabsorbed calcium, which is then expelled in the stools. High levels of magnesium, oxalates, and excess fatty acids can obstruct the absorption of calcium. However, lactose, the sugar found in milk, aids in the body's absorption of calcium.

An energy-intensive process traverses the brush border of the enterocyte cell membrane to assimilate calcium. This process relies on vitamin D, and inadequate amounts result in the cessation of active calcium transport. Growth hormone from the pituitary gland and parathyroid hormone (parathormone) also impact the absorption of calcium. One-third of the 1,200 mg of calcium in an average diet is absorbed. Around 99% of the calcium in the blood is reabsorbed by the kidneys during blood flow. Consequently, excessive calcium losses occur in both malabsorption states and kidney failure. In the event of a calcium deficiency, the skeletal structure becomes weakened and more pliable as calcium is reabsorbed from the bone.

11.2.2.6. Magnesium

About two-thirds of the 300 mg of magnesium found in an average diet is absorbed. The kidneys eliminate half of the absorbed magnesium, and they have the ability to control the amount between 1 and 150 millimoles per day. Both the thyroid hormone calcitonin and the parathyroid hormone parathormone have an impact on this regulation. The transmission of neuromuscular signals depends on magnesium. Additionally, it plays a significant role as a cofactor in the synthesis of nucleic acid and the enzymatic processes that create the bone matrix. Overuse of diuretics, chronic renal failure, chronic alcoholism, uncontrolled diabetes mellitus, and intestinal malabsorption can all lead to magnesium deficiency.

There is an inverse relationship between magnesium and calcium. As a result, food that is low in magnesium absorbs more calcium from it. Calcium is released from bone when there is a low magnesium level in the blood. Supplemental magnesium is part of the treatment for malabsorption-related hypocalcemia.

11.2.2.7. Hematinics

Hematinics are substances necessary for the correct synthesis of blood components. Hematinics include iron, vitamin B12, and folic acid. Additionally, vitamin D may contribute to preserving hemoglobin and promoting the production of new blood cells by supporting bone health, which serves as the reservoir for new blood cells.

11.2.2.8. Folic Acid

Folic acid, also known as pteroylglutamic acid, is essential for cell division and nucleic acid synthesis. Folic acid deficiency impairs the maturation of red blood cells (erythrocytes). Folic acid is produced by plants and bacteria, and it is hydrolyzed to folic acid by the digestive system. Milk and fruit are the primary food sources of folic acid, providing an average of 500 micrograms per day. The liver stores folic acid.

A prerequisite for absorption, the hydrolysis of the folates occurs on the brush borders of the jejunal enterocytes and is completed in the lysosomes, which are cellular structures that are part of the intracellular digestive system and contain a variety of hydrolytic enzymes. Anemia arises when the hydrolysis of folates is disrupted. Certain medications, particularly phenytoin, which is used to treat epilepsy, and the long-term use of sulfonamides, which are used to suppress disease, can impede this process. In the enterohepatic circulation of the liver, pteroylglutamic acid receives a methyl group addition that is eliminated in the bile. Approximately 100 micrograms are used daily. The absorption process remains unclear.

11.2.2.9. Vitamin B_{12}

Because it contains cobalt, vitamin B12, also known as cobalamin, is necessary for the development of red blood cells. It is a coenzyme that supports the enzymes involved in the transfer of folate into the interior of cells. Vitamin B12 is produced through bacterial metabolism. Despite the fact that bacteria in the colon also produce it, vitamin B12 is not absorbed there. In food, vitamin B12 is present in bound forms, which are released in the stomach and small intestine through proteolytic activity. The glycoprotein called intrinsic factor (IF), produced by the parietal cells that also produce hydrochloric acid, binds to vitamin B12. The transport of vitamin B12 requires intrinsic factor, and the B12 protein complex, known as transcobalamin II, is necessary for its movement from the intestine to the rest of the body. Once the IF is attached, the bound vitamin cannot be further broken down by proteases. Only the distal 100 cm of the ileum, particularly the final 20 cm, is absorbed. In this region, the complex attaches to receptors in the brush border of the enterocytes. The process of vitamin B12 going from its presence in food to its appearance in the peripheral blood through the hepatic veins and enterohepatic circulation is a slow one, taking three hours. A daily intake of one microgram of vitamin B12 is required. The liver is the primary storage site for vitamin B12.

11.2.2.10. Iron

Iron is required for the production of hemoglobin, the molecule in red blood cells that carries oxygen. Additionally, it plays a significant role in intracellular metabolism as a cofactor. The primary sources of iron in the diet are seeds, nuts, meat, and eggs. Humans are unable to excrete excess iron that has been absorbed beyond the daily requirement of 1 mg; the average daily diet contains about 20 mg of iron. Both vitamin C and stomach acid inhibit the formation of insoluble iron complexes. Low molecular weight iron complexes are stabilized by certain amino acids found in dietary protein. Iron absorption is hindered by certain food additives, vegetable-derived phosphates and phytates, and the inhibition of acid secretion. In the duodenum, iron is predominantly absorbed through energy-dependent metabolic activity. When enterocytes on the surface of the intestine die and are expelled, the majority of the iron remains trapped within them. The body's ability to store iron seems to influence the amount of iron lost; however, this can be overcome by taking extremely high oral doses of iron. Alcohol accelerates absorption in the duodenum and stomach. By binding to transferrin, a plasma protein that carries iron, the iron within enterocytes is transported. It then enters the portal circulation and the liver after leaving the intestine. The rate of absorption increases from less than 1 mg per day to 1.5 mg or more when iron loss is increased, as in the case of bleeding disorders and heavy menstruation.

11.2.2.11. Vitamin D

In essence, vitamin D is a hormone that originates from two sources. Firstly, a sterol compound known as dehydrocholesterol in the liver is converted into vitamin D3 through photosynthesis, facilitated by UV radiation from the Sun. This supplies all the necessary vitamin D3 for humans. In the absence of sunlight exposure, dietary supplements are required. The primary sources of vitamin D include eggs, liver, fortified bread, and milk. Insufficient intake of vitamin D and lack of sunlight exposure can lead to vitamin D deficiency. Infections or resections of the small intestine may also contribute to malabsorption, potentially resulting in conditions such as rickets and osteomalacia, characterized by bone softening.

Vitamin D is incorporated into micelles in the jejunum along with fatty acids and bile salts. Subsequently, as provitamin D1, vitamin D is absorbed in the ileum and enters the bloodstream through the portal vein. It then travels to the liver via a specific blood protein called alpha-1-globulin, where it undergoes hydroxylation to become cholecalciferol, the initial step in its chemical transformation into the active hormone. The derivatives are transported by the liver to various tissues, including the skin, bone, and parathyroid glands. Vitamin D influences the permeability of calcium in the intestine through the brush borders of enterocytes. The body's ability to produce hemoglobin can be influenced by vitamin D levels. For instance, anemia can occur in people with low vitamin D levels, but vitamin D supplements can raise hemoglobin levels in these individuals. It is unclear how vitamin D affects hemoglobin production, but studies have indicated that it might protect the oxygen-carrying molecule by acting as an anti-inflammatory agent. Additionally, in the presence of erythropoietin, a hormone primarily produced in the kidneys that affects the rate of red cell production, vitamin D has also been shown to enhance the production of red blood cells.

11.2.2.12. Intestinal Gas

The gurgling noises, known as borborygmi, are caused by the passage of gas through the intestines. The gastrointestinal tract typically contains 200 milliliters of gas while at rest. There are variations in its composition: nitrogen makes up 20–90% of it, oxygen makes up 10%, hydrogen makes up 50%, methane makes up 10%, and carbon dioxide makes up 10–30%. Particularly during eating and talking, the majority of the air that people swallow is either absorbed in the stomach or regurgitated (such as when they belch). Frequent swallowing of air due to anxiety or fast eating can result in belching or increased flatus in the colon. The breakdown of dietary triglycerides to fatty acids in the jejunum produces some of the carbon dioxide that is generated in the small intestine, although some of it is caused by the interaction of hydrogen ions of gastric acid with bicarbonate. Rectal flatus with elevated carbon dioxide levels indicates colonic bacterial activity. Methane is not produced by any cell and is only generated in the colon by bacteria acting on fermentable food remnants; however, since not everyone is able to produce methane, this process appears to be influenced by genetics. When the diet contains an excess of vegetable saccharides, the amount of hydrogen produced by colon bacteria is noticeably increased.

This is especially apparent, for example, after consuming beans. In malabsorption states, gas is more frequently to blame for the buoyancy of stools than excessive residual fat.

The direction of gas movement is determined by the gradient between the partial pressures of specific gases in the intestinal lumen and the partial pressures of gases in the circulating blood (or the pressure exerted by each gas in a mixture of gases). Consequently, oxygen diffuses from the blood into the intestine because the colon typically exhibits low pressure. Due to the gradient created by the carbon dioxide, methane, and hydrogen generated by the metabolic processes of commensal bacteria, nitrogen from the blood diffuses into the intestine. This occurs because nitrogen in the colon reduces partial pressure, thereby promoting the entry of nitrogen from the blood into the intestine. In cases where lactase, the enzyme responsible for breaking down lactose (milk sugar), is absent from the group of disaccharidases in the small intestine, lactose enters the colon undigested. Unhydrolyzed lactose in an individual deficient in lactase enters the colon, where the quantity of lactose typically found in a glass of milk can release the equivalent of two to four cups (500–1,000 ml) of gas (hydrogen) through bacterial fermentation. Around 50% of the gas is expelled as flatus, while the remaining 15% dissolves back into the blood. The hydrogen produced in the colon is partially absorbed, travels to the lungs through the bloodstream, and diffuses into the respiratory passages, where it is readily detectable. The duration required for hydrogen to emerge in the breath following the consumption of a standard glucose or lactose load serves as a marker for the presence of bacterial colonization in the upper gastrointestinal tract. Within 30 minutes of ingesting the sugar load, the presence of hydrogen indicates a significant small intestine colonization.

11.2.3. Hormones of the Gastrointestinal Tract

11.2.3.1. Production and Secretion of Peptides

Signals received at the cell membranes of specialized cells in the digestive system, which are involved in motor and secretory functions, control their activity. Amino or peptide "messenger" molecules deliver these signals to the target cell from either endocrine or nerve cells. These substances either diffuse into the surrounding tissue spaces when secreted, affecting nearby target cells, or they are absorbed by the circulating blood and reach distant target cells. The messengers in both cases are hormones; however, the term "paracrine" refers to messengers that act locally, while "endocrine" refers to messengers that act distantly.

A peptide is an amino acid chain made up of several amino acids. Each peptide has its own unique ordered sequence of amino acids. The peptide's biological activity, such as the capacity to stimulate target cells, may only reside in a small portion of the chain, for instance, a four- or five-amino-acid sequence. In other cases, the entire chain needs to be intact to achieve this effect. For example, delta (D) cells, which are responsible for producing the hormone somatostatin, are found throughout the entire gastrointestinal tract. Somatostatin inhibits the production of acid in the stomach, intestinal motility, and pancreatic release of digestive enzymes. It is locally diffused from D cells in the vicinity of the target tissue to produce these effects. On the other hand, the hormone known as gastrin (G) is secreted into the bloodstream by the granular gastrin (G) cells found in the mucosa of the gastric antrum, the lower portion of the stomach.

Another example of a portion of the molecule's biological potential is the hormone gastrin. These fractions can initiate intracellular processes that lead to the synthesis of acid because their molecular structure corresponds to the receptor site on the target cell's membrane. The G cells in the duodenum and jejunum of the small intestine primarily produce a messenger peptide with 34 amino acids, whereas the G cells in the antrum of the stomach primarily produce a messenger peptide with 17 amino acids in sequence. The shorter peptide is more potent. The chain can only be broken down into four amino acids (the tetrapeptide), but even then, the cleaved amino acid chain still exhibits biological activity, albeit with less potency than the larger gastrin molecules, as long as the fragment is located at the amino terminal of the entire molecule and the sequence remains unchanged.

It has been discovered that some messenger peptides are produced in neural elements of the gastrointestinal tract rather than in endocrine cells and are released during nerve electrical discharge. Vasoactive intestinal peptide (VIP), for instance, is widely distributed in the gut's nervous system, including the submucosal and myenteric nerve plexuses. VIP is released from nerve terminals in the brain. VIP occasionally coexists with the autonomic parasympathetic nervous system's messenger molecule, acetylcholine. The release of VIP affects the long peristaltic movements in the intestine, the receptive relaxation of the pyloric and esophageal sphincters, and the secretion of electrolytes from the small intestine mucosa.

Within the gastrointestinal tract, 18 distinct endocrine cells have been identified. However, it is likely that some of these, along with their unique peptides, are evolutionary remnants that served a different purpose during earlier stages of human development, while others might represent distinct phases of the same endocrine cell's maturation.

Agonists are peptides that attach to receptors on target cells and cause the cell to respond. Antagonists are those that bind to the receptor but do not initiate any internal processes. The basis for using histamine (H2) receptor blockers to treat peptic ulcer disease lies in the ability of their antagonists to occupy receptors and thereby prevent access to an agonist. Antagonists, one of the main causes of peptic ulcers, prevent histamine from initiating the synthesis of hydrochloric acid by binding to the receptors on the parietal cells.

Comparable occurrences either increase or decrease the synthesis of messenger peptides in the endocrine or neural cells that produce them. For example, when a meal is consumed, gastrin granules are released from the G cells. The buffering effect of the food keeps the concentration of hydrogen ions (acidity) low, but the release of gastrin continues. As digestion progresses and the stomach begins to empty, the food's neutralizing effect decreases, causing the acidity to rise. The release of gastrin stops when the stomach contents in contact with the antrum's mucosa reach a specific acidity level (pH of 2.5 or less). If this mechanism malfunctions, the stomach secretes acid inappropriately when it is empty, which can lead to peptic ulcers in the duodenum. Certain endocrine cells have microvilli on their surface that extend into the lumen of the gland or the main channel of the stomach or intestine. These cells likely have the ability to continuously "sample" the contents of the lumen in their surrounding area.

Excessive peptide hormone production and secretion cause the target cell population to grow, potentially resulting in larger individual cells. This phenomenon is known as trophism and can be compared to work hypertrophy, which is the enlargement of skeletal muscle in response to appropriate exercise. Trophism of this nature is observed in certain disease states involving hormones in the gastrointestinal tract.

In cases where a tumor of G cells (gastrinoma) in the pancreas secretes gastrin, there is no mechanism to halt its secretion into the blood. As a result, the process continues unabated, leading to excessive acid production and a significant increase in the number of parietal cells in the stomach. This, in turn, leads to intractable and complex peptic ulceration, overwhelming the mucosa of the upper gastrointestinal tract against autodigestion.

11.2.4. Individual Hormones

11.2.4.1. Insulin

The pancreatic beta (B) cells secrete insulin in response to a decrease in glucagon levels and an increase in plasma glucose concentration. Insulin promotes the uptake of glucose, a type of carbohydrate, into the stores found in adipose (fatty) and muscle tissue. The medication insulin is used to treat diabetes mellitus.

11.2.4.2. Glucagon

When the concentration of plasma glucose falls, pancreatic alpha (A) cells release glucagon, which has the opposite effects of insulin. Glucagon promotes the liver's process of converting glycogen to new glucose (gluconeogenesis). Additionally, it lessens the secretion of pancreatic and stomach secretions. Conditions that cause a decrease in blood sugar levels are treated with glucagon.

11.2.5. Somatostatin

Somatostatin, a peptide released by the delta (D) cells, is triggered by food, especially when fat enters the duodenum. It acts as an inhibitory modulator of the release of gut hormones such as insulin, gastrin, and others, as well as the secretion of pepsin and acid. It inhibits the motility of the intestines and gallbladder and prevents the pancreas from secreting lipase.

11.2.5.1. Serotonin

Serotonin, also known as 5-hydroxytryptamine, is an amine that is produced in enterochromaffin cells (EC) and other related cells known as enterochromaffin-like cells (ECL) from the amino acid 5-hydroxytryptophan. These cells also secrete kinins and histamine, which serve as important messengers in blood vessels and glandular secretions. Serotonin exhibits paracrine effects. The gastrointestinal tract harbors a significant number of EC and ECL cells.

11.2.5.2. Cholecystokinin

Cholecystokinin, a peptide released by the I cells in response to the emptying of stomach contents into the duodenum, induces gallbladder contraction, sphincter relaxation to close the bile duct, and increased enzyme production by the pancreas. Cholecystokinin is utilized in pancreatic function tests and radiological gallbladder examinations due to its ability to enhance intestinal peristalsis.

11.2.6. Gastric Inhibitory Peptide

Gastric inhibitory peptide is secreted by the K cells. In response to elevated blood sugar, it increases the production of insulin and prevents the small intestine from absorbing water and electrolytes. Individuals with duodenal ulcers, chronic pancreatic inflammation, and obesity-related diabetes tend to have higher cell counts.

11.2.6.1. Intestinal Glucagon

Intestinal glucagon, also known as enteroglucagon, is secreted by the L cells in response to the presence of triglycerides and carbohydrates in the small intestine. It exerts a potent trophic effect on mucosal structures and regulates intestinal motility.

11.2.7. Motilin

A high blood level of motilin promotes the

contraction of the fundus and antrum, which accelerates the emptying of the stomach. It increases the squeeze pressure of the lower esophageal sphincter and contracts the gallbladder. Motilin is secreted between meals.

11.2.8. Neurotensin

Neurotensin is a substance released by the N cells of the ileum in response to fat in the small intestine. It relaxes the lower esophageal sphincter, regulates motility, and prevents the vagus nerve from stimulating the secretion of acid and pepsin.

11.2.8.1. Pancreatic Polypeptide

Pancreatic polypeptide is secreted by special endocrine cells, or "PP" cells, in reaction to protein meals. Its role is closely linked to cholinergic and vagal activity. Diabetes usually results in an increase in pancreatic polypeptide levels.

11.2.8.2. Secretin

Secretin, which is secreted by the S cells in the duodenum in response to meals and the presence of acid in the duodenum, stimulates the pancreas to produce more bicarbonate.

11.2.8.3. Vasoactive Intestinal Peptide

Vasoactive intestinal peptide (VIP) is locally produced in the gastrointestinal tract by endocrine cells and nerve endings. It plays a role in inhibiting the release of gastrin and acid secretion, stimulating bicarbonate secretion from the pancreas, and promoting the secretion of water and electrolytes by the intestines. Additionally, it relaxes sphincters and slows down intestinal transit time. Other peptide messengers found in the brain and gastrointestinal tract include substance P, endorphins, enkephalins, and bombesin.

11.2.8.4. Substance P

Substance P, which is abundant in the myenteric plexus and vagus nerves, increases the production of saliva, smooth muscle cell contraction, and inflammatory responses in tissues. However, it is unclear if substance P serves any significant purpose beyond being an evolutionary remnant.

11.2.8.5. Endorphins and Enkephalins

The myenteric plexus and the vagus nerves contain the molecules endorphins and enkephalins, each consisting of five amino acids. These molecules bind to the same receptors as opiate substances derived from opium, such as morphine, and can be counteracted by the opiate antagonist naloxone. While enkephalins may have a paracrine role in regulating smooth muscle activity in the gastrointestinal tract, and endorphins may be involved in regulating the release of other peptides from endocrine cells in the digestive system, there is no evidence to support the idea that endorphins and enkephalins function as circulating hormones.

11.2.9. Bombesin

Bombesin, a peptide found in the intrinsic nerves of the gastrointestinal tract, stimulates the release of gastrin and pancreatic enzymes, as well as the contraction of the gallbladder. However, these actions may be overshadowed by the hormone cholecystokinin, which has similar effects and is secreted by the intestinal mucosa. The physiological significance of bombesin remains uncertain, as it is unclear whether it plays a role in the body or if it is a remnant of evolutionary traits.

11.2.10. Prostaglandins

Prostaglandins are hormone-like molecules that play a role in the contraction and relaxation of the smooth muscle in the gastrointestinal tract. By promoting the secretion of mucus and bicarbonate by the mucosa, prostaglandins can also protect the gastrointestinal tract from damage caused by various insults, including boiling water, alcohol, aspirin, bile acids, and stress. This process then stimulates the migration of cells to the surface to replace and repair the mucosal lining.

11.2.11. The Gastrointestinal Tract as an Organ of Immunity

The gastrointestinal tract serves as an organ of immunity. Ingested toxins and chemicals, such as medications and food additives, viruses, bacteria, parasites, and foreign plant proteins, can constantly pose harm to the body. The interface between the sterile interior of the body and the external environment is composed of the skin, respiratory system, and digestive system, all of which are exposed to these insults.

The body's defense is heavily reliant on the lymphatic system and lymphocytes. Lymphoid tissue, which is divided into three sectors, occupies a significant portion of the digestive tract. The first sector includes the appendix, pharyngeal tonsils, and Peyer's patches, which are large nodular aggregates dispersed throughout the small intestine. The second sector consists of lymphocytes and plasma cells that make up the basement membrane, or lamina propria, of the small intestine. This region of loose connective tissue extends into the villi and lies above the supporting tissue of the mucosal lining. The third sector is comprised of lymphocytes located in the spaces between the epithelial cells of the mucosa. The defense mechanism of the gastrointestinal tract is based on the interaction between these lymphatic system cells and potentially harmful substances.

Lymphocytes are categorized into two types: type B and type T, depending on their point of origin in the body. Type B lymphocytes originate in the bone marrow while Type T lymphocytes originate in the thymus gland situated in the chest. Both of these types are transported to the peripheral lymphoid structures like the spleen, Peyer patches, intestinal mesentery lymph nodes, peripheral lymph glands, and the spaces between the mucosal epithelial cells.

Initially, lymphocytes are immature. When T lymphocytes (T cells) recognize foreign substances, they undergo a maturation process where they divide and transform into various subclasses. The first subclass is known as "helper" T cells, which mediate immune function. The second subclass is "suppressor" T cells that regulate and manage immune responses. The third and final subclass is "killer" T cells or cytotoxic T cells that have the power to destroy other cells. Killer T cells are the most abundant type of lymphocytes found in the spaces between the mucosal epithelial cells.

When a foreign substance, called antigen, enters the body, it activates a type of white blood cell called B cell. B cells mature and transform into plasma cells, which produce immunoglobulin (Ig) – also known as antibodies. There are five types of immunoglobulin: IgA, IgM, IgG, IgD, and IgE. B cells and plasma cells are primarily located in the spaces of the basement membrane. To transport antigenic material, specialized cells called M cells cover epithelial cells of the mucosa and transport the material into vesicles. These vesicles are then moved through the cell and surrounding spaces to activate the immune response.

Lymphocytes from Peyer's patches travel through lymph vessels to reach the mesentery nodes. From there, they enter the thoracic duct, which is a channel that collects lymphatic branches from the abdomen and connects the left internal jugular and left subclavian veins. The thoracic duct then carries these lymphocytes through the thorax and empties them into the vein system. The lymphocytes are then distributed to other organs and returned to the colon. These migrated lymphocytes fill gaps between epithelial cells and populate the basement membrane.

IgA, IgM, IgE and IgG are immunoglobulin classes produced by various cells in different organs. IgA is produced by the majority of plasma cells in the basement membrane and mesenteric nodes. Plasma cells in the spleen and peripheral lymph nodes produce IgG. IgM and IgE are produced to a lesser extent. The IgA produced by plasma cells is secreted into the intestinal lumen, where it is known as "secretory IgA." This IgA differs molecularly from IgA found in blood circulation. The mucosa's epithelial cells secrete a glycoprotein along with the substance. When this material binds to the IgA molecule, it prevents protein-splitting enzymes from breaking it down. This IgA complex can attach itself to bacteria and viruses, preventing their growth and reducing their ability to infiltrate tissue. It can also neutralize poisonous substances.

IgE is produced by B cells and covers mast cells. These cells are specialized to respond to allergic reactions that are caused by parasites and worms. Already-matured immunoglobulin, which is abundant in colostrum (the first secretion secreted by nursing breasts), protects newborns. Over time, the immune system's lymphocytes and other cells adapt to deal with the increasing variety of insults that an infant's gastrointestinal tract is subjected to. The body also grows tolerant to potentially harmful substances in this way. However, if tissue invasion occurs despite these defense mechanisms, a systemic immune response is triggered. Fever and a sharp rise in white blood cell counts are two characteristics of this reaction that point to an illness.

A Closer Look

Gallbladder

The gallbladder is a muscular sac that stores and concentrates bile, a fluid produced by the liver and essential for digestion. It is located beneath the liver and has a capacity of about 50 ml (1.7 fluid ounces). The inner surface of the gallbladder wall is lined with mucous-membrane tissue akin to that of the small intestine. The cells of the mucous membrane have microscopic projections called microvilli, which increase the area of fluid absorption. The bile stored in the gallbladder is about 5 times more concentrated than when it was produced in the liver because of the absorption of water and inorganic salts from the bile by the cells of the mucous membrane.

The vagus nerve of the parasympathetic system and the hormone cholecystokinin stimulate the contraction of the gallbladder's muscle wall. This contraction results in the discharge of bile via the bile duct into the duodenum of the small intestine. The bile duct is composed of three branches, which form the shape of the letter Y. The common bile duct is the lower segment and terminates in the duodenal wall of the small intestine. The sphincter of Oddi, located at the end of the common duct, regulates the flow of bile into the duodenum. The hepatic duct, which leads to the liver, is the upper right branch. The cystic duct, which passes to the gallbladder, is the upper left branch.

Bile flows from the two lobes of the liver into the hepatic and common bile ducts. If there is food present in the small intestine, the bile will continue directly into the duodenum. If not, the sphincter of Oddi will close, and bile flowing down the common duct will accumulate and be forced back up the tube until it reaches the open cystic duct. The bile then flows into the gallbladder, where it is stored and concentrated until needed. When food enters the duodenum, the common duct's sphincter opens, the gallbladder contracts, and bile enters the duodenum to aid in the digestion of fats.

The gallbladder can be subject to many disorders, primarily the formation of solid deposits called gallstones. Despite its activity, it can be surgically removed without serious effect.

Summary

- The digestive system in humans, which the body employs to carry out the process of digestion. The digestive tract, or the collection of organs and structures that food and liquids traverse in order to be transformed into forms that can be assimilated into the bloodstream, constitutes the majority of the human digestive system
- The lips, which are two folds of flesh encircling the mouth, are composed of mucous membrane, or mucosa, on the inside and skin on the outside.
- The hard and soft palates combine to constitute the concave roof of the mouth. The palatine portions of the maxillae, or upper jaws, and the horizontal sections of the two palatine bones combine to form the hard palate.
- The salivary glands are named racemose glands due to their clustered arrangement of secreting cells in sacs called acini.
- The passageway connecting the oral cavity, nasal cavity, and esophagus to the larynx and esophagus is commonly referred to as the throat or pharynx. The pharynx facilitates the movement of air to and from the trachea, or windpipe, during respiration and allows ingested solids and liquids to pass into the esophagus, or gullet.
- The esophagus, which conveys food from the pharynx to the stomach, has a length of approximately 25 cm (10 inches) and a width that ranges from 1.5 to 2 cm (about 1 inch).
- The cardia serves as the opening where the stomach and esophagus meet. The fundus represents the uppermost portion of the stomach, situated above the entrance of the esophagus.
- The gastric mucosa is a mucous membrane that coats the interior of the stomach. Tall columnar epithelial cells secrete a dense layer of mucus that envelops the mucosa consistently.
- Gastric secretion can be classified into three phases (cephalic, gastric, and intestinal) that depend on distinct mechanisms to stimulate the gastric mucosa for the purpose of releasing gastric juice.
- The small intestine has three primary functions, which are producing enzymes and other essential components for digestion, mixing, and transporting intraluminal materials, and absorbing nutrients. On the other hand, the large intestine consists of five main parts, which are the cecum, ascending colon, transverse colon, descending colon, and sigmoid colon.

References

1. Bhatia, A., Shatanof, R. A., & Bordoni, B., (2023). *StatPearls* [Internet]. StatPearls Publishing; Treasure Island (FL). Embryology, Gastrointestinal.
2. Chojnowska, S., Baran, T., Wilińska, I., Sienicka, P., Cabaj-Wiater, I., & Knaś, M., (2018). Human saliva as a diagnostic material. *Adv. Med. Sci., 63*(1), 185–191.
3. Ellingsgaard, H., Hauselmann, I., Schuler, B., Habib, A. M., Baggio, L. L., Meier, D. T., Eppler, E., et al., (2011). Interleukin-6 enhances insulin secretion by increasing glucagon-like peptide-1 secretion from L cells and alpha cells. *Nat. Med., 17*(11), 1481–1489.

4. Farooqi, N., & Tuma, F., (2023). *StatPearls* [Internet]. StatPearls Publishing; Treasure Island (FL). Intestinal Fistula.

5. Fieker, A., Philpott, J., & Armand, M., (2011). Enzyme replacement therapy for pancreatic insufficiency: Present and future. *Clin. Exp. Gastroenterol., 4*, 55–73.

6. Fish, E. M., & Burns, B., (2022). *StatPearls* [Internet]. StatPearls Publishing; Treasure Island (FL). Physiology, Small Bowel.

7. Flemström, G., & Isenberg, J. I., (2001). Gastroduodenal mucosal alkaline secretion and mucosal protection. *News Physiol. Sci., 16*, 23–28.

8. Kalra, A., Wehrle, C. J., & Tuma, F., (2023). *StatPearls* [Internet]. StatPearls Publishing; Treasure Island (FL). Anatomy, Abdomen and Pelvis, Peritoneum.

9. Krause, W. J., (2000). Brunner's glands: A structural, histochemical, and pathological profile. *Prog. Histochem. Cytochem., 35*(4), 259–367.

10. Law, N. M., Bharucha, A. E., & Zinsmeister, A. R., (2002). Rectal and colonic distension elicit viscerovisceral reflexes in humans. *Am. J. Physiol. Gastrointest. Liver Physiol., 283*(2), G384–389.

11. Mohamed, M., Thio, J., Thomas, R. S., & Phillips, J., (2020). Pernicious anaemia. *BMJ., 369*, m1319.

12. Nicosia, M. A., Brasseur, J. G., Liu, J. B., & Miller, L. S., (2001). Local longitudinal muscle shortening of the human esophagus from high-frequency ultrasonography. *Am. J. Physiol. Gastrointest Liver Physiol., 281*(4), G1022–1033.

13. Portincasa, P., Di Ciaula, A., Wang, H. H., Palasciano, G., Van, E. K. J., Moschetta, A., & Wang, D. Q., (2008). Coordinate regulation of gallbladder motor function in the gut-liver axis. *Hepatology, 47*(6), 2112–2126.

14. Qin, J., & Pei, X., (2018). Isolation of human gastric epithelial cells from gastric surgical tissue and gastric biopsies for primary culture. *Methods Mol Biol., 1817*, 115–121.

15. Shaydakov, M. E., & Tuma, F., (2023). *StatPearls* [Internet]. StatPearls Publishing; Treasure Island (FL). Operative Risk.

16. Srikumar, K., & Premalatha, R., (2003). Effect of gastrointestinal proteases on purified human intrinsic factor-vitamin B12 (IF-B12) complex. *Indian J. Biochem. Biophys., 40*(2), 139–142.

17. Vegesna, A. K., Chuang, K. Y., Besetty, R., Phillips, S. J., Braverman, A. S., Barbe, M. F., Ruggieri, M. R., & Miller, L. S., (2012). Circular smooth muscle contributes to esophageal shortening during peristalsis. *World J. Gastroenterol., 18*(32), 4317–4322.

INDEX

I

J

K

L

Printed and bound by CPI Group (UK) Ltd, Croydon, CR0 4YY
18/09/2026
14965061-0007